EVERYBODY'S  **DS . . .**

ORGANIC, NATURAL,
UNPROCESSED . . . WHICH IS BEST?

At last, there is a handy, one-stop source for answers to all of your questions about eating well for optimal health—for you and the environment. Wholefoods are the defenders of good health, from antioxidant-rich to immunity-boosting choices. And let's not forget about great taste! Treats such as red wine, blueberries, pomegranate juice, and dark chocolate are some of the most wholesome choices you can make.

Let the bestselling nutrition experts guide you through today's world of food choices with complete nutrition breakdowns of wholesome brands and generic foods. A wealth of great advice delivered in an accessible and easy-to-use format.

Pick up

THE HEALTHY WHOLEFOODS COUNTER

and find out what to buy and eat
when good health is the order of the day!

Books by Annette B. Natow and Jo-Ann Heslin

The Calorie Counter
(*Fourth Edition*)

The Cholesterol Counter
(*Seventh Edition*)

The Complete Food Counter
(*Second Edition*)

The Diabetes Carbohydrate and Calorie Counter
(*Third Edition*)

Eating Out Food Counter

The Fat Counter
(*Sixth Edition*)

The Healthy Heart Food Counter

The Healthy Wholefoods Counter

The Most Complete Food Counter
(*Second Edition*)

The Protein Counter
(*Second Edition*)

The Ultimate Carbohydrate Counter

The Vitamin and Mineral Food Counter

Published by POCKET BOOKS

THE
HEALTHY WHOLEFOODS COUNTER

Annette B. Natow, Ph.D.

Jo-Ann Heslin, M.A., R.D.

With the Assistance of Karen J. Nolan, Ph.D.

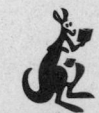

POCKET BOOKS

New York   London   Toronto   Sydney

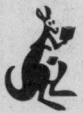
Pocket Books
A Division of Simon & Schuster, Inc.
1230 Avenue of the Americas
New York, NY 10020

Copyright © 2008 by Annette B. Natow and Jo-Ann Heslin

All rights reserved, including the right to reproduce this book or portions thereof in any form whatsoever. For information address Pocket Books Subsidiary Rights Department, 1230 Avenue of the Americas, New York, NY 10020

First Pocket Books paperback edition January 2008

POCKET and colophon are registered trademarks of Simon & Schuster, Inc.

For information about special discounts for bulk purchases, please contact Simon & Schuster Special Sales at 1-800-456-6798 or business@simonandschuster.com.

Cover design by Heather Kern

Manufactured in the United States of America

10   9   8   7   6   5   4   3   2   1

ISBN-13: 978-1-4165-5253-6
ISBN-10:   1-4165-5253-7

*To our families, who support us
through every project:*

**Harry, Allen, Irene, Sarah, Meryl, Marty, Laura,
George, Emily, Steven, Rebecca, Joseph, Kristen,
Brian, Karen, and John**

ACKNOWLEDGMENTS

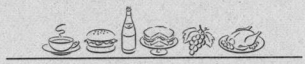

For graciously sharing her knowledge: Karen J. Nolan, Ph.D.

For all her continuous support and help, our agent, Nancy Trichter.

For her suggestions and editing skills, Sara Clemence.

Without the tireless cooperation of Stephen Llano and the production department at Pocket Books, *The Healthy Wholefoods Counter* would never have been completed.

A special thank-you to our "volunteer" readers for their suggestions and criticisms: Jonesie Clemence, Betty Goldblatt, and Jean Schwarsin. You were all good sports and had great ideas. We appreciate the time and effort you put into this project.

A very special thank-you to our editor, Micki Nuding.

"The earth's greatest bank of energy is the sun; its currency is light and heat. These man cannot 'cash in' directly. They have to go through a great clearing house, the plant world, before they become available for the human economy."

Mary Swartz Rose, Ph.D.
Feeding the Family
The Macmillan Company, 1919

CONTENTS

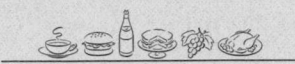

INTRODUCTION

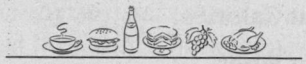

What's good for the earth is good for you.

America's food supply is "greening." Organic, natural, sustainable, free range, vegetarian, whole grain, antibiotic-free, eco-friendly—which are the best to buy?

You want answers about planet-friendly, healthy eating options. *The Healthy Wholefoods Counter* has the answers you need in an easy-to-read question-and-answer format.

Our goal is not to persuade you but to inform you. You may already have strong opinions about organic versus conventionally grown fruits and vegetables. Or you may be wondering which is best. You may not eat meat, or you may only buy grassfed beef. You may feel unprocessed foods are better. Or you may see fortified and functional foods as an important part of your healthy diet. There are many ways to eat well, and what's best for one person isn't always best for another.

Today, we expect food producers to give us some assurance about the backstory of the foods we buy. We want to know that the world's resources aren't being depleted so that we can eat. We want to know that food brings to our table the qualities of the land from which it is grown. We want to know where our food comes from.

Was the broccoli grown on a huge industrialized farm or a smaller sustainable farm? Was the milk produced on a highly mechanized farm, where cows are pumped with growth hormones to produce more milk, or on an organic farm? We want to know we can trust the farm or company to be good stewards of the earth. And last, but probably most important, we want assurances that our food is good for us and will help protect our health and prevent disease.

Because almost half of all food purchases are made in supermarkets, we've laid out *The Healthy Wholefoods Counter* like the supermarket aisles. As we go up and down the aisles we'll explore and explain all the different food choices available, and, we hope, clarify some of your concerns and answer most of your questions. So—let's get started.

Bottom line: Focus on wholefoods—tasty, healthy, and planet-friendly.

We can't separate ourselves from the earth that feeds us.

HOW DOES YOUR GARDEN GROW?

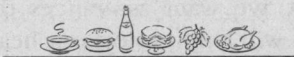

The last 100 years has seen a revolution in every aspect of our food environment.

Some things to consider when it comes to wholefoods:

- Every year the U.S. population grows by 3 million, and 3 million acres of farmland are lost to development.
- Looking at food from an ecological perspective makes us think of everything that happens from the soil to our table.
- Using fewer chemicals, pesticides, fertilizers, antibiotics, and growth stimulators should mean healthier soil, air, animals, and ultimately us.
- Your health isn't just about your body; what's good for the earth is good for you, too.

As we've moved away from traditional and organic farming methods toward highly mechanized, monoculture-based agriculture, has the improvement in seed stock improved the quality of our food? Has modern agriculture, with its focus on yield, fulfilled its promise to enrich our food supply? Are our soil and water resources burdened by the use of chemical fertilizers and pesticides?

Interestingly, few studies examine these problems. Health professionals seem more concerned with public health issues, such as the growing rate of obesity and the poor quality of people's diet, than with the nutrient content of individual foods. You, on the other hand, are probably very interested in those issues.

More Americans are regularly shopping at farmer's markets. Organic foods are readily available in every local supermarket, and the demand for these products grows at the rate of 20% yearly. Smaller, natural, healthier brands are finding their way onto supermarket shelves. And the concept of *food miles* is becoming widely understood, as more people want to protect the environment by buying food that isn't transported thousands of miles.

Is it true that our fruits and vegetables have fewer nutrients today?

There is limited research in this area, but evidence does show that the nutrient content of some foods has decreased modestly over the last century. The amounts lost are tiny, but the trend is definitely down. Plants selectively bred to grow faster and larger may not be able to gather nutrients from the soil as quickly before harvest. This has been referred to as the *dilution effect*—bigger but not necessarily better.

What does the term "organic" truly mean?

In 2002, the United States Department of Agriculture (USDA) finally standardized organic foods labels and for the first time, no matter what state you live in, organic standards are the same. Foods must be certified organic to use the USDA seal, but the use of the seal is voluntary.

The USDA organic standards ensure that certified fruits, vegetables, and grains have been grown without fungicides, pesticides, insecticides, chemical fertilizers, and herbicides. And it guarantees that the foods have not been irradiated, genetically modified, or treated with human or industrial waste.

The organic label does not mean the food is safer or healthier. The nutrient content of organic foods is virtually the same as that of nonorganic foods. *Organic* simply refers to the method of growing crops or raising animals. Farmers committed to the process feel that they are protecting the environment and treating animals in a more humane manner. Some argue that the higher price of organic foods is the true cost of farming without government subsidies.

Certified organic meat and poultry are fed organic grain, without hormones or antibiotics, and the animals have spent time outdoors, though the amount of time is not specified. For more information on organically raised meat, fish, and poultry, see pages 55, 68, and 78.

The most complicated thing about the labeling standards is that they provide for 4 levels of organic certification.

- **100% organic:** Products labeled 100% organic must contain only organic ingredients. The USDA organic seal can be used on the label.
- **Organic:** These products must have at least 95% organic ingredients. The USDA seal is allowed to be displayed on the front panel of the package.
- **Made with organic ingredients:** These foods must have at least 70% organic ingredients. The

label may read "Made with organic ingredients," but the USDA seal may not be used.

- **Products with less than 70% organic ingredients:** The USDA seal may not be used and the products cannot make any statement about organic on the front of the package; organic ingredients can only be identified in the ingredients listing.

SHOPPING TIP—

Look for the USDA organic seal on foods you buy.

Is there a difference between certified organic and organic?

For the most part, the terms are the same. *Certified organic* means a certifying agent, such as the USDA, has inspected or overseen the production. Small organic farms often decide to forgo the cost of certification, and therefore they can't use the USDA organic seal.

SHOPPING TIP—

PLU (Product Look Up)

These codes are those annoying little stickers you need to peel off fresh fruit and vegetables. The PLU codes for organic foods all start with a 9.

Are organic foods healthier?

There is some evidence that organic produce may have more antioxidants than conventionally grown plants. But the difference isn't enormous. Because organics can't be treated to delay ripening, they may be somewhat fresher than typical products because of their shorter shelf life. But they will also spoil more quickly. Most shoppers buy organic foods to avoid the pesticides and chemicals found in conventional foods.

For more information on pesticide residues on fruits and vegetables, go to pages 15 to 30.

Should I try to eat mostly organic foods?

A simple question, but the answer has gotten complicated. At least 40% of all U.S. shoppers have bought organic food, and mainstream consumers are looking for and buying more and more such products weekly. The organic market has become so successful that its very success may jeopardize its ideals. Why? There simply isn't enough organic food to meet the demand. If we could produce enough organic food in the U.S. to meet demand, we would recommend using mostly organic.

What was once the domain of small local farmers has become the latest marketing focus of corporate food giants. Of the 9 million-plus dairy cows in this country, fewer than 150,000 are organic. Where is all the organic milk, plus the organic butter, cheese, and yogurt, going to come from to line our supermarket shelves? The answer is global. Organic powdered milk is being shipped from New Zealand and elsewhere. Organic produce is being grown in China, Sierra Leone, and Brazil.

You might be thinking, Who cares where the organic foods come from, as long as they are organic? And you might be right. But do foreign governments interpret and impose the same standards? Is shipping organic fruit thousands of miles truly eco-friendly? Can giant corporate organic farms support environmental practices, humane animal husbandry, and exist side by side with smaller farms? Or will future organic farming become just another segment of industrial agribusiness? The explosion of the organic foods market is in its infancy; only time will tell if it can withstand these growing pains.

YOU SHOULD KNOW—

One hundred and thirty countries ship food to the U.S., with Canada, Mexico, and China leading the way. In 2007, the Food and Drug Administration (FDA) inspected only 1% of incoming international food shipments due to severe understaffing. With increasing globalization of our food supply, this needs to change.

Should we be supporting sustainable agriculture to promote healthier plants and a healthier world?

Most of the food consumed in the U.S. travels an average of 1,500 miles to reach your table. Pears in winter can come from Argentina, melons from Mexico, and kiwis from Australia. The concept of *food miles* is gaining more and more attention. In addition to the cost of growing methods that may use up large amounts of water, pesticides, and fertilizers, you must include the cost of fuel and extra packaging that enable fresh fruits and vegetables to make the long journey to you.

Sustainable agricultural growing methods, on the other hand, are committed to using only those resources that the earth can replenish and producing pollutants at a rate that effectively can be removed from the environment. The goal is no net depletion of the world's resources or accumulation of waste.

Practically speaking, this means buying fruits and vegetables grown locally. In an urban area, which can be defined as anywhere within a 5- or 6-hour drive from the city, this means eliminating the need for long-distance transportation from field to table. You'll need to eat foods seasonally produced—no watermelon in the winter if you live in the Northeast. Farmers markets are great resources for local produce, and they are springing up everywhere. Supporting sustainable agriculture is a way to vote with your buying power, to let supermarkets and restaurants know it's important to take care of the earth.

TO LEARN MORE—

About sustainable agriculture, go to

www.sustainabletable.org

and

www.localharvest.org

and

www.biodynamics.com

How can I tell if my fruits and vegetables are grown locally?

Most of the time, you can't. If you are shopping in a farmers market, you can confidently assume the farmer didn't drive 3 days to bring you watermelons. If, however, you live in Maine, you can be sure your watermelon in December wasn't grown down the road. To eat locally, eat foods that are in season.

Most of the fresh produce in the U.S. is trucked to your

store. Very light perishable items, like herbs, may be shipped air freight, but little else is.

In a large supermarket chain, the trip for a head of broccoli from the field to your table could take a week to 10 days, and goes something like this—field, local warehouse, regional distribution center, refrigerated truck, supermarket chain distribution center, a second truck, local supermarket's backroom storage area, the produce counter, and finally your dinner table. The broccoli you're eating could be a seasoned traveler!

What is an ecological footprint?

It's the imprint humanity makes on the earth. Today, humanity's ecological footprint is over 23% larger than what the planet can regenerate. We are living off nature's credit card, taking more than we give back. It takes 1 year and 2 months for the earth to produce what we use in a single year. By measuring the ecological footprint of an individual, city, nation, or all of humanity, we can manage resources—soil, water, air, and nonrenewable resources—more responsibly. The goal is sustainability: Our demand on nature should be in balance with the resources it can provide. The Global Footprint Network wants decision makers throughout the world, from individuals to nations, to use the footprint as a tool to manage the planet's resources more responsibly and to appreciate their limits.

TO LEARN MORE—

About the Global Footprint Network, go to www.footprintnetwork.org.

To evaluate your individual ecological footprint, take the Ecological Footprint Quiz: www.ecofoot.org.

Doesn't fresh produce need to show the country of origin on its label?

It's COOL. In 2002, Congress passed a law requiring Country Of Origin Labeling—COOL. It will take until the end of 2008 to fully implement the law, making all fresh fruits, vegetables, meat, and fish officially COOL. This law is a great labeling tool for consumers, because once you know where the food comes from, you can make judgments about its freshness and decide whether you want to buy products that have logged that many food miles.

What is a locavore?

Begun in San Francisco, locavores are people who have agreed to eat nothing—or almost nothing—but food produced within 100 miles of their home. They are hoping to encourage all of us to eat locally and preserve farmland around major cities, embracing locally grown foods as an eco-healthy choice. People are encouraged to try the 100-mile diet for a month in the hope that it inspires them to eat seasonally.

I've heard about a group called Slow Food. What is it?

The Slow Food movement was founded in 1986 by Carlo Petrini, a well-known food writer and activist, in response to the planning of a quick-service restaurant in Piazza di Spagna in Rome. In 20 years, the movement has grown to 850 groups worldwide with over 80,000 members. Its philosophy is eco-gastronomy—a desire to have people rediscover the joys of eating while at the same time understanding where their food comes from, who makes it, and how it is made.

The group supports sustainable agriculture and biodiversity, seasonal eating, and local, artisanal food producers. The Slow Food movement has cataloged forgotten or marginalized animal breeds and plants to protect them from disappearing from our food supply. They have also supported small producers of traditional foods to keep their production methods alive. And they have created networks of small farmers, producers, and distributors to help them promote their products.

TO LEARN MORE—

About Slow Food, go to www.slowfood.com.

What is biodynamic farming?

Biodynamic farming is the oldest nonchemical agriculture movement in the world. It predates organic farming, and the ecological concern is more vigilant. Biodynamic farmers adopt overall farming methods that preserve water, energy, and land resources, while allowing natural livestock behaviors. The Biodynamic Farming and Gardening Association (BDA), a nonprofit organization open to the public, was formed in the U.S. in 1938 to promote and support biodynamic agricultural methods. Demeter, an international ecological association, certifies biodynamic farms and allows foods from these farms to use the Demeter brand.

TO LEARN MORE—

About the Biodynamic Farming and Gardening Association, go to www.biodynamics.com, *and about Demeter-International, go to* www.demeter.net

---

Are genetically engineered foods safe?

We simply don't know. There are a lot of strong opinions but not enough hard science to definitively say whether genetically engineered (GE) foods are safe or unsafe. And the safety issue is twofold: safe for humans and safe for the environment.

Here's what we do know. *Genetic engineering* is a process by which a gene is manipulated to achieve a desired characteristic. A tomato can be engineered to produce its own pesticide or corn can be altered to resist an herbicide. This may sound good to a farmer, but many Americans are suspicious.

Biotechnology has become the fastest-adopted crop technology in recent history. If you live in the U.S., you have eaten genetically engineered food. A large percentage of the corn and soybeans grown here are from genetically engineered plants. It's estimated that 70% of all foods in the supermarket have at least one genetically engineered ingredient. A great deal of the cheese we eat today is produced using genetically modified organisms. In the past, the enzyme used to "start" cheese came from an animal source. With the newer process, more cheese varieties can be considered Kosher or acceptable to those who don't eat meat.

Currently, most genetically engineered crops are altered to protect plants against natural enemies like fungi and pests. In the future, the same process could be used to nutritionally enhance foods. An experimental tomato high in folic acid has been developed, but remains in the research pipeline, not on the market. What concerns most shoppers is that there is no way to tell if the foods they are buying are genetically modified, because GE foods do not have to be labeled.

There have been a lot of negative headlines about GE foods. The anti-GE lobby strongly believes we can't predict the long-term effect on human health when we tinker with plant and animal genes. The process of genetic engineering has not been shown to be inherently dangerous, but there is always the possibility of unintended changes in the composition of foods.

We need much more scientific evidence that these crops are safe for the environment, safe for neighboring non-GE plants, and safe for humans. The future of genetically engineered agriculture will depend on how shoppers respond to these products, and no one is sure what to expect. In the meantime, you should know that genetically engineered foods are not allowed in organic food production.

YOU SHOULD KNOW—

Genetically Engineered Foods
Currently on the Market

Soy and soy products	*Cantaloupe*
Corn and corn products	*Sugar beets (sugar)*
Canola oil	*Radicchio*
Alfalfa	*Flax*
Tomatoes	*Papaya*
Potatoes	*Squash*
Rice	*Wheat*

THE ULTIMATE SUPERFOODS—FRUITS AND VEGETABLES

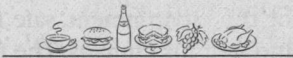

Keep it simple—eat more fruits and vegetables.
Aim for 5 or more servings a day.

Even the most humble fruit or vegetable is a complex collection of healthy, wholesome compounds that function in a dynamic and interdependent way. You don't need to understand all the science behind each compound or interaction to reap the health benefits. Your current fruit and vegetable intake can protect you against health problems in the future.

Fruits and vegetables are loaded with vitamins and minerals and are good sources of fiber. Even more important than that, they are an excellent source of *phytochemicals*. These are compounds that protect plants from bacteria, fungi, damaging free radicals, and high levels of ultraviolet light. When you eat fruits and vegetables, the phytochemicals wind up in your tissues and protect you as well.

Here are just a few of the health benefits you gain when you eat fruits and vegetables daily. They . . .

- help protect you from heart disease, high blood pressure, and stroke
- reduce your risk for cancer
- protect your eyes against cataracts and macular degeneration
- protect your lungs against pulmonary disease
- help to keep your weight down
- support bone health and prevent osteoporosis
- help to prevent birth defects
- reduce a man's risk of an enlarged prostate
- keep your brain younger and protect against dementia
- reduce skin wrinkling

Plants contain *thousands* of phytochemical compounds that can protect you from disease. Here are just a few.

PHYTOCHEMICALS IN FOODS

Phytochemicals	Foods	Health Benefits
Beta-carotene	Apricots, mango, papaya, carrots, sweet potato, spinach, pumpkin, orange, peppers	Neutralizes free radicals Prevents cell damage
Lutein Zeaxanthin	Kale, collards, spinach, corn, field greens	Anticancer Prevents cell damage Maintains healthy vision
Lycopene	Tomato, red peppers, pink grapefruit, guava, watermelon, pomegranate	Anticancer Maintains prostate health

Phytochemicals	Foods	Health Benefits
Anthocyanidins Ellagic acid	All berries, cherries, red grapes	Prevents cell damage Maintains healthy brain function Anticancer Reduces cholesterol
Catechins Epicatechins Procyanidins	Apple, grapes	Maintains a healthy heart
Flavanones	Orange, grapefruit	Prevents cell damage Strengthens immune system
Flavonols	Apple, onion, broccoli	Prevents cell damage Strengthens immune system
Proantho-cyanidins	Cranberries, apple, strawberries, grapes	Maintains healthy urinary tract Maintains a healthy heart
Sulforaphane	Cauliflower, broccoli, broccoli sprouts, cabbage, kale, horseradish	Strengthens immune system
Caffeic acid Ferulic acid	Apple, pear, orange	Prevents cell damage Maintains healthy vision Maintains a healthy heart

(continued)

Phytochemicals	Foods	Health Benefits
Diallyl sulfide *Allyl methyl* *trisulfide*	Garlic, onion, leeks, scallions, chives	Strengthens immune system Maintains a healthy heart Anticancer
Dithiolthiones	Broccoli, bok choy, collards, cabbage	Strengthens immune system
Capsaicin	Chili peppers	Interferes with cancer development Helps prevent blood clots
Isoflavonoids *Phytic acid* *Saponins* *Phytosterols*	All varieties of beans	Anticancer Maintains a healthy heart Reduces cholesterol
Diadzein *Genistein* *Lignans* *Saponins*	Soybeans	Anticancer
Resveratrol	Red grapes, grape juice	Prevents cell damage Curbs tumor growth Reduces cholesterol
Quercetin *Luteolin* *Phthalides*	Celery, lettuce, cranberries	Anticancer Lowers blood pressure

Why are the antioxidants in fruits and vegetables so important?

Antioxidants are needed to protect the health of cells. Using oxygen in the body is critical to life, but in the process, damaging compounds called *free radicals* are formed. It's believed that free radicals promote cancer, heart disease, dementia, cataracts, and macular degeneration, and they may contribute to aging. Natural plant compounds like phytochemicals, vitamins, and minerals act as antioxidants, seeking out and deactivating free radicals. This stops the damage that could be caused by free radicals and protects you from diseases.

One test, the Oxygen Radical Absorbance Capacity (ORAC) analysis, measures the antioxidant capacity of foods. The more free radicals a food can absorb and deactivate, the higher the ORAC score. Researchers suggest we consume 3,000 to 5,000 ORAC units a day, but most of us average only 1,200 because we eat so few fruits and vegetables. An average serving has 600 to 800 ORAC units, and many have much more. If we eat the recommended 5 servings of fruits and vegetables a day, we'll easily meet the ORAC recommendation.

ORAC UNITS IN A SERVING

Fruit	ORAC Units	Vegetable	ORAC Units
Blueberries, 1 cup	5,486	Kale, cooked, 1 cup	2,301
Pomegranate, 1	5,098	Spinach, cooked, 1 cup	2,268
Goji berries, 1 ounce	5,054	Broccoli, cooked, 1 cup	1,342
Blackberries, 1 cup	4,654	Brussels sprouts, cooked, 5	980
Strawberries, 8	3,520	Sweet red peppers, raw, 1 medium	862
Prunes, 6	3,297	Spinach, raw, 3 cups	756
Dried cherries, ¼ cup	3,060	Onion, raw, 1 medium	595
Raspberries, 1 cup	2,789	Corn, canned, 1 cup	420
Orange juice, 8 ounces	2,500	Eggplant, cooked, 1 cup	390
Orange, 1 medium	1,125	Sweet potato, baked, 1 medium	336
Raisins, ¼ cup	1,026	Cauliflower, cooked, 1 cup	136
Plums, 1	949		
Tangerine, 1	900		
Cherries, 20	893		
Red grapes, 20	739		
Kiwi, 1	542		
Pink grapefruit, 1 medium	180		
Cantaloupe, ½	157		

At this point, you might be feeling a little overwhelmed by the list of phytochemicals and ORAC values. But we can make it very simple: Eat a rainbow every day.

You don't need to worry about which specific fruit or vegetable contains which phytochemical or antioxidant, or what its ORAC score is. By eating a wide variety of colored plants you will eat a wide array of phytochemicals, antioxidants, vitamins, minerals, and fiber.

EAT A RAINBOW EVERY DAY

Green	Deep Yellow or Orange	Red
Avocado	Apricot	Cherries
Green apple	Cantaloupe	Cranberries
Green grapes	Grapefruit	Pomegranate
Honeydew	Mango	Pink or red grapefruit
Kiwis	Papaya	Red grapes
Green pears	Peach	Strawberries
Asparagus	Pineapple	Watermelon
Broccoli	Carrots	Beets
Green Beans	Yellow pepper	Red onion
Green Cabbage	Sweet corn	Red peppers
Leafy Greens	Sweet potato	Red potatoes
Green peppers	Winter squash	Rhubarb
Zucchini		Tomato

Purple and Blue	Tan and Brown	White
Blackberries	Brown pear	White peach
Blueberries	Dates	Cauliflower
Dried plums	Figs	Jicama
Plums	Raisins	Parsnips
Eggplant	Mushrooms	Turnips
Purple potatoes		Potatoes

YOU SHOULD KNOW—

These foods may be fun to eat, but you can't count them toward your daily fruit and vegetable intake because of their high fat, sugar, or sodium content:

Deep-fried, battered vegetables

Candy- or chocolate-coated dried fruits

Heavily sugared or salted food—dill pickles, olives, or candied fruits

Fruit leathers or fruit roll-ups

Fruit or vegetable drinks with a small percentage of real juice

---

Can you give me some suggestions on how to eat 5 or more servings of fruits and vegetables a day?

At first that may seem like a lot, but one serving is smaller than you may realize. Eating a cup of cooked broccoli or green beans for dinner counts as 2 servings. We often eat large fruits, which could easily add up to 1½ to 2 servings. Most of us drink more than one serving of juice, which is only ¾ cup or 6 ounces. And a leafy salad at lunch or dinner could easily satisfy 3 to 4 servings. It's actually much easier than you think to eat 5 or more servings of fruits and vegetables each day.

One serving equals:

- 1 cup leafy greens (spinach, kale, field greens, romaine, lettuce)
- ½ cup raw or cooked cut-up fruits or vegetables
- ½ cup cooked dried beans or peas
- 1 medium whole fruit (apple, banana, orange)
- ¼ cup dried fruits (raisins, cranberries, apricots, cherries, mixed berries)
- ½ cup freeze-dried fruits or vegetables (corn, peas, blueberries)
- ¾ cup 100% fruit or vegetable juice

TAKE-OUT TIP—

Order More Fruits and Vegetables

We take out or eat out one third of all the food we eat, but we rarely order fruits or vegetables.

What do I do if I just hate vegetables?

If you are a dedicated vegetable hater and have vowed to eat nothing green, fruits make a great alternative, offering many of the same nutrition benefits. Don't like green beans? Consider sliced peaches or a dish of blueberries.

Every fruit provides a wide array of vitamins, minerals, and disease-protecting phytochemicals that add up with multiple servings. Don't count out those fruits, like apples, that seem to be low in important nutrients, because the fiber found in apples is similar to the "heart healthy" fiber found in oatmeal. Remember the old saying, "An apple a day keeps the doctor away."

YOU SHOULD KNOW—

An Apple Peel a Day May Keep Cancer at Bay.

Cornell researchers have identified a dozen compounds—triterpenoids—in apple peels that either inhibit or kill cancer cells.

The following table will help you compare fruits. All values are given for a 1 cup serving so you can easily compare one against the other. The values are for fruits with edible skins that have been cut up but not peeled, such as grapes, peaches, plums, and cherries. When the peel is not eaten, such as with watermelon, cantaloupe, or pineapple, the values reflect a 1 cup serving of cut-up, peeled fruit. When you peel fruit you lower the fiber content, so eat it unpeeled whenever possible.

Fruit	Rich in*	Calories/Cup
Apple	Fiber	57
Apricots	Fiber, vitamins A & C, potassium	79
Banana	Fiber, vitamin C, potassium	134
Blackberries	Fiber, vitamin C, potassium	62
Blueberries	Fiber, potassium	83
Cantaloupe	Vitamins A & C, potassium	60
		(continued)

Fruit	Rich in*	Calories/Cup
Cherries	Fiber, vitamin C, potassium	74
Grapes	Vitamin C, potassium	110
Guava	Fiber, vitamins A, C & folic acid, potassium	112
Honeydew	Vitamin C, potassium	61
Kiwis	Fiber, vitamins C & folic acid, potassium	108
Mango	Fiber, vitamins A & C, potassium	107
Nectarine	Fiber, vitamin C, potassium	61
Orange	Fiber, vitamins C & folic acid, potassium	85
Papaya	Fiber, vitamins A, C & folic acid, potassium	55
Peach	Fiber, vitamins A & C, potassium	66
Pear	Fiber, vitamin C, potassium	96
Pineapple	Fiber, vitamin C, potassium	74
Plums	Fiber, vitamins A, C & folic acid, potassium	76
Raspberries	Fiber, vitamin C, potassium	64
Strawberries	Fiber, vitamin C, potassium	49
Tangerine	Fiber, vitamins A & C, potassium	103
Watermelon	Vitamins A & C, potassium	46

* A rich source = 2 or more grams of fiber; or 10% or more of the daily requirement for vitamins A, C, or folic acid; or 10% or more of the daily requirement for potassium in a 1-cup serving.

SHOPPING TIP—

Like the convenience of prepackaged, cut-up fruit? A recent research study shows it retained its nutritional quality just as well as fresh fruit. Less work, and equally good for you.

Are newer, exotic fruits better for me than the usual ones?

Goji berries, acai berries, pomegranates, and mangosteens, among others, are getting a lot of press lately. There is nothing wrong with expanding your fruit intake by eating some of these, but many of our homegrown varieties—

blueberries and tart cherries—are just as nutritious, if not more so. And the homegrown fruits don't have to travel thousands of miles to your kitchen, which helps preserve the earth's valuable resources.

Is it wise to buy only organic fruits and vegetables?

Nutritionally, organic and conventionally grown fruits and vegetables are remarkably similar. Most people choose organic produce to reduce the pesticide and chemical residues. Organic produce is grown without synthetic chemicals, including fertilizers, herbicides, pesticides, and fungicides. In conventional farming, the chemicals used may leave a residue on fruits and vegetables. Little is known about the long-term effects of these low-level residues on our health. Some feel it is of little consequence; others are concerned.

Recognize that small amounts of pesticide residues are unavoidable, even on organic crops. Wind and water can spread pesticides and some residue remains in the soil for years after land is certified organic. Some produce is more likely to have pesticide residue because of its structure. And in some cases, like bananas, you eliminate the residue by simply peeling the fruit before eating.

The Environmental Working Group, a nonprofit consumer activist organization, evaluated government data on fruits and vegetables to assess their pesticide residue. They believe you can reduce your pesticide intake by up to 90% by simply buying organic for those varieties of produce with the highest residue. Much conventionally grown produce is actually low in residue. The following chart will help you spend your organic dollars wisely. For more information on organic foods, see pages 4 to 8.

PESTICIDE RESIDUE IN PRODUCE

Lowest Pesticide Levels	Highest Pesticide Levels
Onions	Peaches
Avocado	Apples
Sweet Corn (frozen)	Sweet bell peppers
Pineapples	Celery
Mango	Nectarines
Asparagus	Strawberries
Sweet peas (frozen)	Cherries
Kiwis	Pears
Bananas	Grapes (imported)
Cabbage	Spinach
Broccoli	Lettuce
Papaya	Potatoes
Blueberries	Carrots
Cauliflower	Green beans
Winter squash	Hot peppers
Watermelons	Cucumbers
Sweet potatoes	
Tomatoes	
Honeydew melons	
Cantaloupe	
Mushrooms	
Tangerines	

Source: www.foodnews.org

Which are best—fresh, frozen, or canned vegetables?

When we talk about vegetables being "fresh," there's garden fresh and then there's market fresh. For example, green beans picked from the garden are the freshest, richest in vitamins and taste. Green beans at the store are market fresh, shipped in from anywhere from a neighboring county to a neighboring country. Days or weeks can go by from the time the green beans leave the fields and land in your shopping cart. Vitamins break down over time. Some vitamin C and folic acid will be lost, but there is no way to judge how much loss has occurred. Appearance can be an indicator—for example, wilted or mushy green beans have probably been stored poorly and for too long. Green, crisp, firm green beans are definitely younger, fresher, and more vitamin rich.

Would frozen be a better choice? When green beans are not in season locally, yes. Frozen produce is closest to fresh in vitamin content, because it is processed and frozen very quickly after picking. The key to maintaining quality is handling. Vegetables should be frozen but loose in the bag. If the vegetables are frozen in a block, it usually means they have been partially thawed and refrozen one or more times, destroying some of their taste and overall quality.

Canned vegetables are almost always mushier in texture than fresh or frozen. Because they are preserved in water and salt, the sodium content is higher, and some of the vitamins will dissolve into the canning liquid. But given the choice to eat canned vegetables or no vegetables, canned is a good choice. Most of us normally eat a combination of all three—fresh, frozen, and canned.

What's the best way to cook vegetables to maintain their nutritional value?

It's been estimated that 50% of vitamins are lost in cooking. There are things you can do to lessen the loss.

Microwaving is the kindest to vitamins—short cooking time, moderate heat, and little water. Steaming is a close second. Stir-frying is also gentle on vitamins because it cuts down on water and the vegetables cook more quickly. The downside is that you need to add some fat to your normally fat-free vegetable. Boiling is the most destructive.

You can recycle some of the lost vitamins by using the vegetable water in soups, sauces, and other recipes.

For maximum nutrition and taste, use fresh vegetables within 3 days of purchase, keep frozen vegetables frozen, and cook all vegetables quickly, using as little water as possible and keeping the lid on for faster cooking. There is no such thing as a bad vegetable, because all provide some vitamins, even when handled and cooked poorly, and nothing you can do in storage or cooking destroys minerals.

When grapes or berries have a cloudy film, does that mean they are old or have a chemical residue?

Quite the contrary: The "bloom"—the waxy, silvery white substance on the surface of grapes, blueberries, and plums—is natural. It acts as a barrier against insects and bacteria and helps seal in the fruit's moisture. The bloom is actually a sign of freshness that fades with time and handling.

Are waxed fruits and vegetables safe to eat?

Food waxes are merely a nuisance, not a health problem. Food-grade waxes are made from vegetables, beeswax, or carnauba, which are the leaves of palm trees. Food-grade shellac can also be used. Waxes are fats your body does not absorb, so they just slide through your digestive tract and are excreted. Animal experiments have shown no risk from food wax when eaten in amounts up to 10% of the animal's diet. We eat far less over a lifetime. One gallon of wax can cover 12,000 pounds of fruit. Avocados, cantaloupes, pumpkins, clementines, oranges, grapefruits, apples, cucumbers, and peppers may all be waxed to preserve moisture, prevent bruising, protect against mold, and extend shelf life. You can't wash it off, so if you are concerned about eating wax, only buy unwaxed, or peel waxed produce before eating.

Wouldn't it be easier to just take a vitamin and mineral supplement?

Most healthy-eating messages focus on foods, not supplements—and for very good reason. Supplements of any nutrient should be considered just that—additions to healthy eating, not substitutes for healthy foods.

Nutrients work together in foods, much as instruments in an orchestra blend to produce a sound that one instrument cannot make by itself. The music that results from the individual instruments is a balance of tones and harmonies. The ultimate value of eating wholefoods is similar: a blend of many compounds working together. When we isolate a compound, or supplement one nutrient in large amounts, the overall harmony or working relationships change—and the change may not always be good.

We know that beta-carotene in foods offers protection from cancer. But in a well-designed study, when smokers were supplemented with beta-carotene, their risk of lung cancer actually went up. Did the extra beta-carotene tip the scales in favor of tumor promotion? Did the beta-carotene have to be naturally occurring in plants, working with other compounds, to offer protection? Or maybe it isn't the beta-carotene that's protective against lung cancer, but some other substance we have yet to discover that is also found in foods high in beta-carotene. We simply don't know.

If we depend on supplements instead of food, we short-change ourselves of health-promoting substances that are more effectively packaged in food than in a pill or bottle.

The message stays the same: **focus on tasty, healthy, planet-friendly wholefoods.**

To demonstrate even further how much we still have to learn about wholefoods, a recent study showed that flavonoids, a family of phytochemicals, are very weak antioxidants in the human body. Nonetheless, they offer strong protection against cancer and heart disease. How can that be?

In a test tube, flavonoids are very strong antioxidants. But the human body perceives them as foreign compounds and quickly excretes them in the urine and bile. Yet, in the process of getting rid of flavonoids, the body makes enzymes that also help to get rid of mutagens and carcinogens, protecting you against cancer. Flavonoids also activate a compound called nitric oxide, which protects your blood vessels against inflammation and lowers your blood pressure, both of which protect you against heart disease. So the flavonoids themselves do very little, but they set into motion reactions that promote health. This may sound complicated, but the take-home message is simple: Eat more fruits and vegetables and you'll be healthier.

YOU SHOULD KNOW—

As globalization threatens indigenous societies, it is impacting children's health. Parents who know more about plants—how to use and eat them—have healthier children. As modern society intrudes, this knowledge base is being lost.

BEANS—
THE FORGOTTEN
VEGETABLE

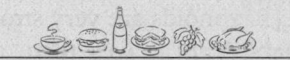

Beans are a humble vegetable, most often considered a poor man's meat or a vegetarian staple. For most of us, beans are only an occasional food—a side order of beans and rice, chickpeas scattered on a salad, or a bowl of split-pea soup on a cold day. Many people are surprised that beans are actually a vegetable, because they seem to straddle more than one food group—vegetable, protein, and carbohydrate.

That combination is exactly why beans qualify as a nutrition superstar. They are high in protein, like meat, fish, poultry, and eggs, while being packed with vitamins, minerals, and phytochemicals like their vegetable cousins. Add to that their being rich in complex carbohydrates and fiber, low in fat and sodium, and cholesterol-free.

WHAT ONE CUP OF BEANS PROVIDES

Nutrient	% Daily Requirement*
Calories	12
Carbohydrates	13
Fiber	53
Protein	33
Fat	4
Cholesterol	0
Folic Acid	69
Potassium	18
Calcium	8
Iron	28
Sodium	Less than 1

* Based on 2,000 calories per day and averaged from 13 bean varieties

---

It's All in the Shape

Beans belong to a family of plants called legumes. Legumes are all similar in nutritional value, but different in shape:

Beans: oval or kidney shaped
Peas: round
Lentils: flat, disklike

Which are the best beans to eat?

Like vegetables, all beans are good for you, so eating a wide variety is the smartest thing to do. As you can see from the table above, all beans are high in fiber, protein, iron, and folic acid, and provide a healthy amount of many other nutrients. In addition, all are excellent sources of phytochemicals.

Red beans are also called Mexican beans. They have more antioxidants than blueberries and are the top source of iron.

Kidney beans can be large or small, dark red or pink. They rank at the top of the antioxidant list and are the best source of fiber.

Blackeyed peas, also called cowpeas or field peas, are an excellent source of folic acid, with 1 cup providing 90% of your day's supply.

Black beans are also called turtle beans or bayo beans. They are another antioxidant superstar and an excellent source of minerals.

White beans are also called navy or great northern beans. They are an excellent source of minerals and fiber.

Lima beans can be baby or regular size and are also called butter beans. They are the top source of potassium among beans, as well as being an excellent source of phytochemicals.

Pinto beans are also called calico beans. They are an excellent source of minerals and contain as much antioxidant power as blueberries.

Cranberry beans are also called Roman beans. They provide almost a day's supply of folic acid and close to 10% of calcium in 1 cup.

Soybeans are the protein powerhouse, providing 60% of your daily need in 1 cup.

Counting Beans

1 (15-ounce) can beans = 1½ cups cooked beans
1 pound dry beans = 2 cups uncooked beans
1 pound dry beans = 6 cups cooked beans

Aren't canned beans very high in sodium?

Compared to cooked dry beans, which have hardly any, yes. But canned beans are a great alternative to dry when you have little time to cook. And if you drain and rinse canned beans before you eat them or add them to a recipe, you can reduce the sodium content by at least 40%.

Also, look for frozen cooked dry beans. They are becoming more and more available and are as low in sodium as the dry variety.

YOU SHOULD CONSIDER—

Meatless Monday

This is a national health campaign that encourages Americans to go meatless one day a week to reduce their consumption of saturated fat and to prevent heart disease, stroke, diabetes, and cancer.

www.meatlessmonday.com

The Most Versatile Bean—Soy

Soybeans, edamame, and all things made of soy were the darlings of the food industry not too long ago, touted as the cure-all for heart disease, breast cancer, hot flashes, and osteoporosis. As with many areas of evolving research, the promise did not measure up to the hype. Does that mean we should stop eating soybeans and soyfoods? Not at all. Soybeans and many of the foods made from soy are excellent foods—just not the health miracle once promised.

How are soybeans different from other beans?

Soybeans are unique among all plant foods because of their protein content and quality, equal to that found in milk, meat, or eggs. The soybean is 40% protein, 20% oil, 35% carbohydrate, and 5% minerals and other active compounds. Most important among these are isoflavones, powerful estrogen-like phytochemicals that have been linked to reducing the risk for breast cancer and relieving symptoms of menopause.

If soybeans and soyfoods are so nutritious, why don't they offer more disease protection?

Soybeans offer a great example of the wholefood principle, plus the importance of eating well throughout life. The early promising data about the ability of soy to protect against heart disease and cancer were drawn from studies of traditional Asian diets that were rich in soy, but were also rich in vegetables, low in fat, and used smaller portions. In addition, the people studied ate this way throughout their lives.

In contrast, American diets are far more energy dense, contain more food, more fat, and more sugar. When soy was added to this eating pattern the disease protection potential was much smaller.

The Asian diets also contained more soybeans, tofu, tempeh, miso, soybean oil, and soy sauce. The American diets contained "second generation" soy-based products, foods made from soy flour, soy protein, or soy protein isolate, like veggie burgers, meat substitutes, and soy cereals. Depending on the processing, the amount of isoflavones can vary dramatically. In a free-living population, it is hard to get an accurate value on the amount of isoflavones eaten from soyfoods, making it almost impossible to measure the health benefits.

SOY MANY CHOICES

Soyfood	Description	Isoflavone Level
Edamame	Young green soybeans sold frozen in the pod or shelled	High
Soybeans	Black, yellow, or brown, sold dried, frozen, or canned	High
Soynuts	Roasted soybeans available plain, salted, or flavored	High
Tempeh	Dense bean cake made from fermented soybeans with a chewy texture	High
Soymilk	Milk substitute, available lowfat, flavored, and fortified with calcium and vitamin D	Moderate to high*
Soy yogurt	Yogurt substitute made from cultured soymilk; available lowfat and flavored	Moderate to high*
Tofu	Soymilk coagulated to form a curd, available firm, medium, or soft	Moderate to high*
Soy flour	Made from ground roasted soybeans	Moderate
Soy cereal	Available in various shapes and flavors, can be sweetened	Moderate to low*
Soynut butter	Similar to peanut butter	Moderate to low*

Soyfood	Description	Isoflavone Level
Frozen soy desserts	Similar to ice cream	Low*
Meat substitutes	Made from soy protein	Low*

*Varies by brand and degree of processing

Does soy offer protection against heart disease?

Yes. Soy can help to reduce bad LDL cholesterol, because it contains natural plant sterols, and it helps reduce inflammation, which can lead to plaque buildup in the arteries. Research showed the protection was more likely when whole soyfoods, like soynuts, were eaten regularly rather than processed soyfoods or soy supplements. Eating any type of soyfood will reduce the amount of saturated fat and cholesterol in your diet if you eat them instead of meat, milk, or cheese.

Does soy protect against or cause breast cancer?

Some groups of women who eat a lot of soy have a lower risk of breast cancer. But these women have eaten soyfoods since they were teenagers, and also have eaten a vegetable-based Asian diet. So we are not sure if it was the soy or the diet or the two combined. Starting to eat soyfoods as an adult in the hope of protecting again breast cancer may not work.

There is also concern that increased consumption of the estrogen-like isoflavones found in soy could promote the growth of precancerous or malignant cells. This could be especially important for women who are at high risk for developing breast cancer, or those who have estrogen-sensitive breast cancer. But another long-term study has found no effect from isoflavones on cancer risk.

The American Cancer Society suggests moderation. It recommends that breast cancer survivors eat moderate amounts of soyfoods and not use isoflavone supplements. For everyone else, using some soyfoods is fine; overdoing it in the hope of some perceived health benefit is probably not wise until we learn more.

> **YOU SHOULD KNOW—**
>
> *A moderate amount of soy is 1 serving of a soyfood, 1 cup of soymilk, a few ounces of tofu, or a handful of soynuts daily.*

What the evidence says about soy and the reduction of

- **hot flashes:** Modestly reduces number of episodes; effect varies among women.
- **vaginal dryness:** There is no effect.
- **dementia:** Results to date are not promising, and some studies show a slight increase with high consumption.
- **normal aging:** Could have promise but much more research is needed.
- **osteoporosis:** The effects are modest and more beneficial to the spine than the hip.
- **prostate cancer:** May protect against the progress of dormant cancer, with the most protection seen in men over 60, but offers no benefit against advanced cancer.

THE SHELL GAME—
NUTS AND SEEDS

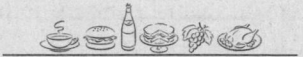

A handful, not a canful.

In the last few years, nuts and seeds have gone from forbidden foods to healthy choices. They were once considered too high in fat to eat regularly, but we now know that a small serving of nuts daily is a healthy eating habit because they are rich in "good" fats. Nuts are unique in their nutrition chemistry, made up of unsaturated fats, protein, fiber, vitamins, minerals, and powerful antioxidants.

YOU SHOULD KNOW—

Nuts and seeds are all the embryo of a new plant. Tree nuts, like almonds and walnuts, are seeds wrapped in a hard shell. Groundnuts are seeds that grow underground, like peanuts.

Which is the most nutritious nut or seed?

Like vegetables, all nuts and seeds are good for you, so eating a wide variety is the smartest thing to do.

Almonds are a top source of alpha-tocopherol, a form

of vitamin E that is believed to be heart healthy. Eating them regularly may slow the effects of aging and boost the immune system.

Brazil nuts are an excellent source of the mineral selenium. Just 1 nut provides 160% of your daily need. Selenium is needed for proper thyroid and immune function, and helps protect you against cancers of the prostate, liver, and lungs.

Cashews are an excellent source of zinc, needed for healthy vision and a healthy immune system. Cashews also contain cholesterol-lowering phytosterols.

Coconuts come from tropical palm trees. Higher in saturated fat, coconuts cannot claim the health benefits of other nuts and should be eaten in moderation.

Flaxseeds can be brown or yellow in color and can add crunch to foods, but they must be ground to release their health-promoting properties. Rich in omega-3 fats, lignans, phytoestrogens, and fiber, flax is protective against heart disease, diabetes, autoimmune diseases and inflammatory disorders. One tablespoon of flaxseeds has as much fiber as ½ cup of oat bran.

Hazelnuts are also called filberts. These two nuts are so similar that experts can't tell them apart, but they do grow on different but related trees. Hazelnuts are very high in heart-healthy monounsaturated fats.

Hempseeds have a lower fat content than other nuts or seeds, and a higher fiber content than any grain. They can be ground into flour. Hemp is rich in antioxidants and in anticancer, heart-healthy phytosterols.

Macadamia nuts are the highest in total fat and calories, but rich in monounsaturated fats and an excellent source of a B vitamin, thiamin.

Peanuts are technically beans, but nutritionally they parallel nuts. Peanuts have more protein than other nuts and they are rich in the phytochemical resveratrol, found in red grapes and red wine, and in saponins, which have anticancer properties.

Pecans are the highest-ranking nut on the ORAC scale (see pages 19 to 20), which makes them very rich in antioxidants. Pecans are also rich in cholesterol-lowering phytosterols and in gamma-tocopherol, which inhibits cancer cell division.

Pine nuts are also called pignolis, pignolias, piñons, and Indian nuts. They are tiny, torpedo-shaped kernels harvested from pine trees. Pine nuts are rich in manganese, are a good source of copper, magnesium, and zinc, and are an excellent source of cholesterol-lowering phytochemicals.

Pistachios are rich in fiber. They are a top source of potassium, which keeps blood pressure normal, and they have the highest amount of cholesterol-lowering phytosterols.

Pumpkin seeds can be dried or roasted. They are lower in fat and higher in protein than most seeds, and are rich in potassium, iron, and zinc.

Sesame seeds are rich in potassium, calcium, magnesium, phosphorus, iron, and zinc. They are ground to a paste to make tahini.

Sunflower seeds are rich in protein, polyunsaturated fats, fiber, magnesium, and copper. They are widely used for oil and to make margarine.

Walnuts are rich in heart-healthy alpha-linolenic acid, the same type of omega-3 fat found in fish. Walnuts also contain cholesterol-lowering phytosterols, and are rich in gamma-tocopherol, which inhibits cancer cell division.

YOU SHOULD KNOW—

Oils pressed from nuts and seeds do not contain all the health-promoting compounds found in the wholefood.

ONE SERVING EQUALS

Nuts	Serving Size	Calories
Almonds	1 ounce (24 nuts)	167
Almond butter	2 tablespoons	202
Brazil nuts	1 ounce (8 nuts)	186
Cashews	1 ounce (18 nuts)	160
Cashew butter	2 tablespoons	188
Hazelnuts	1 ounce (20 nuts)	188
Macadamia nuts	1 ounce (11 nuts)	200
Macadamia butter	2 tablespoons	230
Peanuts	1 ounce (30 nuts)	170
Peanut butter	2 tablespoons	188
Pecan halves	1 ounce (15 halves)	187
Pine nuts	1 ounce (160 nuts)	161
Pistachios	1 ounce (47 nuts)	190
Walnut halves	1 ounce (14 halves)	190

Seeds	Serving Size	Calories
Flaxseeds	2 tablespoons	70
Hemp seeds	2 tablespoons	160
Pumpkin seeds, hulled	2 tablespoons	148
Sesame seeds	1 tablespoon	48
Sesame butter	2 tablespoons	190
Sunflower seeds, hulled	2 tablespoons	103
Sunflower butter	2 tablespoons	186

Staying Fresh

Nuts in the shell will keep for a year. Shelled nuts will stay fresh for 6 months in the refrigerator and up to a year in the freezer.

A Handful of Nutty Suggestions

- To enhance flavor, roast nuts for 5 to 10 minutes at 350°F.
- Eat unsalted, dry-roasted nuts instead of oil-roasted, sugared, salted, or chocolate-covered nuts.
- Swap saturated fats like cheese or butter for polyunsaturated fats like nuts and nut butters.
- Pair up nutrition powerhouses: apple + peanut butter, oatmeal + sunflower seeds, steamed spinach + slivered almonds, dried fruits + nuts.
- Roasting nuts does not create trans fat.

WHOLE-GRAIN EVERYTHING

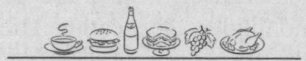

Keep it simple—eat mostly whole grains.
Aim for at least 3 servings a day.

Some things to consider when it comes to whole grains:

- Whole grain foods are nutrient and fiber rich; they help protect your health and maintain your weight.
- Do you need whole grain foods that are highly fortified or packed with extra protein? Probably not, because whole grains are valuable just the way nature designed them.
- Whole grains don't need to be sweetened to be tasty, but a little sweetness won't detract from their value.

Why are whole grains so healthy?

Eating whole grains every day reduces your risk for diabetes, cancer, high blood pressure, and high cholesterol, and will keep you slimmer. Making this one simple change in your diet can reap some pretty big results—and this is one of the easiest food switches you can make! It's hard to get people to eat more fruits and vegetables. Others refuse to give up their favorite fatty foods or desserts. But switching from white bread to whole wheat bread isn't that big a step, and it will yield impressive health benefits.

Those who eat whole grains regularly weigh less than those who don't, because whole grains provide a feeling of satisfaction and fullness after eating. The fiber in whole grains reduces the absorption of dietary cholesterol, and the naturally occurring plant sterols lower bad LDL cholesterol. If that isn't enough, whole grains are rich in antioxidants and phytochemicals that act like bodyguards, protecting cells from damaging free radicals that can trigger disease and signs of aging. When grains are refined, many of these natural health-promoting agents are removed, including fiber, vitamin, minerals, phytosterols, and antioxidants.

YOU SHOULD KNOW—

We're Falling Short

Only 8% of U.S. adults eat 3 or more servings of whole grains a day and 42% eat none. Aim for 3 a day.

I'm confused: What is the difference between whole grain and fiber?

Fiber makes up the outer covering of the whole grain. A kernel is the entire grain seed, and it's made up of 3 parts: bran, germ, and endosperm. Bran, the outer protective layer, is made up mostly of fiber. The germ is the embryo of the kernel, which can sprout into a new plant. The endosperm is the largest part of the kernel, made up of protein and carbohydrate. It provides food for the germ to grow.

All parts of the whole grain kernel offer valuable nutrients. The bran provides fiber and minerals. The endosperm gives you protein and carbohydrate. The germ gives you vitamins, minerals, and healthy fats. Eating the entire grain gives you the full benefit of all three. Whole wheat bread is made from flour from the entire wheat kernel. White bread is made from flour from just the endosperm.

I'm trying to limit carbs. How can I eat enough whole grains?

Eating 3 whole grain servings daily will easily fit into a low-carb plan. Most of us will eat more. As we discuss beginning on page 124, people choose to eat varying amounts of carbohydrates or grain foods daily. We all need some, and our choices should be whole grain whenever possible.

Keep the recommended serving sizes in mind when you're counting up the number of daily servings. If you eat 2 cups of cooked pasta for dinner, you've eaten 4 servings. It's easy for servings to add up quickly. One serving equals

- 1 slice of whole grain bread
- 1 cup of whole grain cereal
- ½ cup of whole grain hot cereal
- ½ cup cooked whole grain pasta
- ½ cup cooked whole grain, any variety

YOU SHOULD KNOW—

1 Serving of Pasta = 2 Ounces

Measuring out uncooked pasta is tricky.

For spaghetti: *2 ounces = a bundle the diameter of a penny;*
4 ounces (2 servings) = a bundle the diameter of a quarter.
For shaped pasta (penne, bowties): *2 ounces = ¾ cup.*

Which are the best whole grains to eat?

All whole grains offer health benefits. Expand your horizon beyond whole wheat, oatmeal, and brown rice, and try some other varieties. For times when you are in a hurry, rely on instant whole grain hot cereals, ready-to-eat whole grain cold cereals, microwave precooked whole grains, instant brown rice, popcorn, or whole grain breads and crackers.

Whole Grains from A to Z

Amaranth has a peppery taste and tiny kernels that look like brown caviar when cooked. It's high in protein and has no gluten.

Barley has a very tough hull that is difficult to remove without losing some of the bran. Because of this, hull-less barley and pearled barley are not technically whole grains, but they are far closer to whole than refined grain is. Barley is a good rice substitute, and more effective at lowering cholesterol than oats.

Buckwheat is botanically a cousin to rhubarb, not actually a grain at all, but its nutrients, nutty flavor, and appearance are grainlike. Unroasted, buckwheat is eaten as groats, and toasted, it's kasha. It is often ground into flour or made into soba (Japanese noodles).

Bulgur is wheat kernels that have been boiled, dried, and cracked. Sometimes called Middle Eastern pasta, it cooks in the same time as dry pasta and is the base for tabbouleh.

Corn has the highest antioxidant level of any grain. It can be popped into popcorn, coarsely ground into polenta, or finely ground into cornmeal. Yellow corn tastes corny and buttery, blue corn has a delicate flavor, and white corn is the sweetest. Degermed cornmeal is not whole grain, but retains more of the natural grain kernel than refined flours.

Emmer, also called *farro* or *grano farro,* is an ancient strain of wheat used to feed Roman soldiers. Semolina flour and pasta made from emmer can be found in Italian specialty stores.

Grano is lightly polished wheatberries with some of the bran removed, cutting the cooking time substantially. Grano is not technically a whole grain, but again, a better choice than refined.

Kamut is an heirloom wheat grain with a rich, buttery taste. It has more protein and vitamin E than other wheat varieties.

Millet is a tiny white, gray, yellow, or red grain with a mild flavor. It is gluten free. In the U.S. it is more likely to show up in a bird feeder than on your plate, but it is commonly eaten in China, Pakistan, South America, and Russia.

Oats almost never have the bran or germ removed, so they are always whole grain. Oats are steamed and flattened to make them cook faster as regular, quick, or instant oats. Steel-cut oats, called Irish or Scottish oats, are only sliced once or twice, making the kernel thicker so it takes longer to cook. Oats lower cholesterol and protect blood vessels against damage from bad LDL cholesterol.

Quinoa is a small light-colored, red, purple, or black kerneled grain that cooks into a fluffy dish. It is the quickest-cooking grain and is botanically related to Swiss chard and beets. Quinoa must be washed before cooking to remove a natural, bitter residue, called saponin, that wards off insects.

Rice is one of the most easily digested grains and is gluten free. Brown rice is whole grain but lower in fiber than most other whole grains. Converted rice is polished, which drives some of the B vitamins found in the bran into the endosperm, making it a better choice than regular white rice. Rice is typically white or brown, but it can also be black, red, or purple. (See "Wild rice" below.)

Rye is unusual among grains because of the high level of fiber found in the endosperm as well as in the bran. It is typically used as flour to make bread, and it helps promote a feeling of fullness after eating.

Sorghum, also called *milo,* is gluten free. It can be eaten like popcorn, cooked as hot cereal, or ground into flour.

Spelt is a high-protein type of wheat that can be used in place of regular wheat in most recipes.

Teff is the tiniest of whole grains, making it impossible to refine. It has twice the iron of other grains and is an excellent source of calcium. It can be red, brown, or white, with a sweet, molasses-like flavor. It is best known for its use in Ethiopian flatbread, *injera,* but it can also be cooked as hot cereal or ground into flour.

Triticale is our youngest whole grain and has been commercially grown for only 35 years. It is a hybrid of durum wheat and rye.

Wheat is a very versatile whole grain with high amounts of gluten, a protein needed to produce bread. Wheat is classified into hard or soft according to its protein content; winter or spring depending on when it was planted; and red or white depending on the color of the kernels. High-protein hard wheat is used to make seitan (wheat meat), and durum wheat is used to make pasta and couscous. Wheat is often milled into flour; whole wheat flour is whole grain, but white flour is refined, missing the germ and bran. Bulgur and grano (see above) are used as side dishes. Wheatberries—whole wheat kernels—need soaking and long cooking to be edible, but cracked wheat—split wheatberries—cooks faster. Wheat flakes can be used like oatmeal.

Wild rice is the seed of a water grass with twice the

protein and fiber of brown rice. It has a woodsy flavor and chewy texture that lends itself to rice blends.

How can I tell if a product is whole grain?

The label may state "100% Whole" (any grain). If it doesn't, check the ingredients list for any of the whole grains listed above. Next, check their position on the list: Is it the first ingredient? Second? If not, there is probably little whole grain in a serving. Wheat bread, multigrain cereal, or 7 grain energy bars are not always rich in whole grains. The appearance or name of a food can be deceiving. Not all dark bread is whole grain bread, because the multigrains can be refined and color can be added.

More and more foods are displaying the Whole Grain stamp, part of an awareness program developed by the Whole Grain Council. The stamp identifies foods in two ways. The Whole Grain stamp is used on foods providing

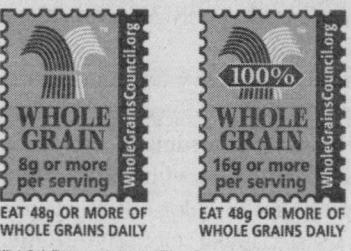

at least 8 grams of whole grain, which equals a half serving of whole grains. The 100% Whole Grain stamp is used on products providing at least 16 grams of whole grain, equal to 1 serving of whole grains. The stamps shown above have the gram value for the minimum amount required to use the stamp on labels. Companies can individualize the value to reflect the exact grams of whole grain in a serving of a specific food. These symbols will make it easier to find whole grain sources.

The following table will help you sort out whole grain label language.

WHOLE GRAIN LABEL LINGO	
Label Terms	**What do they really mean?**
Brown rice Buckwheat Oats, oatmeal (any type) Popcorn Sorghum Stoneground whole (any type of grain) Teff Wheatberries White whole wheat Whole (any type of grain) Whole wheat Whole wheat white flour Wild rice	All contain 100% whole grain
7 Grain (or any other number-grain) 100% Wheat Cracked wheat Durum wheat Multigrain Organic flour Semolina Wheat flour	Contain some whole grains but not 100% whole grain
Bran (any type) Degermed Enriched flour Honey wheat Refined flour Rice (basmati, converted, white, sticky) Stoneground (without the word whole) Wheat germ	Not whole grain foods

Is there really a whole wheat white flour?

Yes, there is. It is very common in Australia and becoming more available in the U.S. Whole wheat white flour is made from a variety of wheat that is tan or golden in color rather than the darker brown color of regular whole wheat. It is 100% whole wheat with the bran, germ, and endosperm, but has a milder flavor and texture than nutty-tasting, chewier whole wheat. It's a great whole grain alternative for diehard white bread fans and is nutritionally equivalent to whole wheat.

Can I eat whole grains if I'm allergic to wheat?

True wheat allergies are rare—and they may disappear with age. But millions of Americans can't eat gluten, the elastic protein in wheat that makes grain particles stick together while making breads, pasta, and cakes.

About 1% of the population suffers from celiac disease, a chronic inflammation of the small intestine that is triggered by eating gluten. Untreated, celiac disease causes poor absorption of nutrients because of the damage to the small intestines, and puts sufferers at higher risk for cancer, osteoporosis, gallbladder disease, and disease of the pancreas. With lifelong adherence to a gluten-free diet, the damage can be reversed.

Symptoms of gluten sensitivity can vary widely, from mild discomfort to debilitating fatigue and illness. According to experts in the field, three factors must be present for celiac disease to develop: a genetic predisposition, exposure to gluten, and a trigger such as pregnancy, a virus, or stress. Once triggered, celiac disease cannot be cured, but it can be managed by avoiding gluten. Wheat contains the most gluten, but other grains, such as barley, rye, and triticale, contain some, too, and need to be avoided as well.

Grains with Gluten	Gluten-Free Grains
Wheat, including spelt, kamut, farro, durum, semolina, and bulgur	Amaranth
	Buckwheat
Barley	Corn
Rye	Millet
Triticale	Quinoa
Oats*	Rice
	Sorghum
	Teff
	Wild Rice

* Oats are gluten free but some gluten-sensitive people may react to them; follow your doctor's advice.

Where can I find gluten-free foods?

In the past this was far more challenging, but today more and more products are labeled GLUTEN FREE, FREE OF GLUTEN, WITHOUT GLUTEN, or NO GLUTEN.

The FDA (Food and Drug Administration) is currently working on a definition for the term "gluten free" to comply with the 2004 Food Allergen Labeling and Consumer Protection Act. The proposed definition, which must be in place by August 2008, defines a gluten-free food as one with less than 20 parts per million (ppm) of gluten. This standard will help consumers identify grain foods they can eat and will help food manufacturers correctly label their products. At the moment, labeling of gluten free foods is voluntary. Stating on the label that a product contains wheat or wheat products is not voluntary. This is required as part of the allergy labeling law. For more information on allergy labeling, to go page 115.

How can I win the no-sugared-cereal battle with my kids?

The cereal aisle is a minefield and getting down it with kids in tow can be a challenge. Totally unsweetened cereals are a hard sell, and some healthier varieties are sweetened. Compromises are possible. Buy the child-selected sweetened cereal to "sweeten" the Mom-chosen, good-for-you brand—put a ¼ cup scoop into the kid choice and use that to "sweeten" the Mom-choice healthier brand.

You can also buy sweetened cereal to use as a candy substitute, giving a ½ to ¾ cup serving as an occasional sweet snack. Teaching your child that these very sweet brands are more like candy or cookies is giving a healthy eating lesson. And don't forget, all cereals, no matter how sweet, are grain based, low in fat, fortified with vitamins and minerals, and moderate in calories.

YOU SHOULD KNOW—

Healthy Cereal–Sugar Ratio

Check the nutrition facts panel and look for a total carbohydrate-to-sugar ratio of 4 to 1. For example, if a cereal has 24 grams of total carb and 6 or fewer grams of sugar, it's a good choice.

MEATY ISSUES

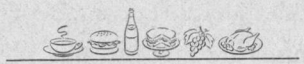

People are passionate about whether to eat meat or not. If they do eat meat, they want to know which are the healthiest, most humane choices.

Some of you have already made a decision not to eat any animal food for environmental or ethical reasons. Others eat meat, fish, and poultry, but want assurances about the food's safety and the humane treatment of animals. Still others don't give any of this a thought—you just want grassfed beef because you believe it has superior taste and quality.

Understanding Terms
So You Can Talk the Talk

Antibiotic free (no antibiotics administered, raised without antibiotics) means no antibiotics are given to the animal during its lifetime. If the animal becomes sick, it will be removed from the group and treated, but it can't be returned and then sold as antibiotic free.

Certified Humane is a certification process overseen by Humane Farm Animal Care, funded by humane societies throughout the U.S. Through inspection, it certifies that egg, dairy, meat, or poultry products were produced with the welfare of the farm animal in mind. The USDA (United States Department of Agriculture) verifies their inspection process. Under this program the producers must comply with all local, state, and federal environmental standards and with the American Meat Institute Standards for slaughtering. Growth hormones are prohibited and feed must be antibiotic free.

Downers are animals too stressed or ill to walk, that collapse during transportation or at the slaughterhouse. Downer animals have been banned from human consumption since 2004, which is another step in protecting the U.S. meat supply from mad cow disease (see page 58) and organisms that could cause foodborne illness.

Feedlots are buildings or lots where animals are confined for feeding, raising or holding. The concentration of large numbers of animals in a tight space may reduce the health of animals, promotes the spread of disease, and produces large quantities of animal waste that must be disposed of. Many feel the use of feedlots is inhumane to animals.

GMO free (no GMOs) animals are raised without feed from genetically modified organisms; see pages 13 to 14.

Grainfed animals are raised on a grain diet. Cattle are ruminants, which means they eat and use grass more effectively than grain. Grainfed cattle fatten more quickly, and grain gives meat the taste we are most accustomed to. Some people feel grassfed animals taste "gamey," which is one reason why it isn't more widely purchased by consumers.

Grain-finished cattle are fed grain before slaughter, often in feedlot situations, which many people find inhumane. Almost all cattle are grassfed earlier in life.

Grassfed (pastured or pasture raised) animals are

fed on grasses. Almost all cattle in the U.S. spend the first 12 to 18 months of their life foraging for grass. Then most grassfed cattle are moved to feedlots to be grain finished before slaughter. Cattle usually spend their last 120 to 200 days in feedlots. There is no approved definition for *grassfed*, but producers of grassfed beef, bison, dairy cows, goats, poultry, and lamb who belong to the American Grassfed Association do not use any supplemental grain. There is also no guarantee that hormones or antibiotics won't be used since members of the American Grassfed Association support both sides of this issue.

TO LEARN MORE—

About grassfed animals, go to

www.eatwild.com

and

www.americangrassfed.org.

Hormones are compounds that are given to animals to increase growth or production. The USDA has stopped the use of the term "hormone free" because all animals make natural hormones in their bodies. Animals can be raised with or without added growth hormones. Exceptions are pork, veal, and chicken, raised in the U.S., which may not be given growth hormones. The use of terms like "no hormones added" is misleading for these products. It implies the producers raised pigs, calves, and chickens without giving them added hormones when in fact the producer was not *allowed* to administer hormones.

Irradiation is when food is treated with radiant energy to reduce harmful bacteria. There is very little irradiated meat or poultry sold in the U.S. today because consumers have shown little interest in buying these products. Any that is sold must be labeled and must carry the Radura, the international irradiation symbol. Many European nations routinely use irradiation. See page 106 (When Good Foods Make You Sick) for more information about irradiation.

Mad cow disease (bovine spongiform encephalopathy, BSE) is caused in cattle by a *prion,* a protein that is folded wrong. It destroys brain tissue (encephalopathy) and leaves gaping holes (spongiform) in the animal's brain. Animals become infected only when they are given feed containing BSE-contaminated animal by-products. The human form of the disease, caused by eating infected meat, is called variant Creutzfeldt-Jakob disease (vCJD). Your risk of contracting mad cow disease is statistically very tiny, but it is not zero. Animals fed all-vegetable diets have never been exposed to BSE, therefore neither will you be if you eat only those food products.

Natural is what all fresh poultry and meat already are by definition. But when a product is labeled "natural" it cannot have any artificial color, flavor, preservatives, or synthetic ingredients added, and can only be minimally processed, such as ground beef or poultry. "Natural" does not mean the animal was pasture raised or is antibiotic free or hormone free.

Organic assures you that animals or poultry were raised on organic feed, without hormones or antibiotics, and that they spent time outdoors. Organic foods may be certified by the USDA, which allows producers to use the USDA organic seal. USDA organic certification excludes cloned animals, their offspring, and any food products from cloned sources.

Rotational grazing is the practice of moving animals between fields so that each field undergoes a grazing period and a resting period. This helps to minimize overgrazing and soil erosion. Sustainable farms often use this method.

Ruminants are animals—cows, goats, sheep, bison, deer, camels, and llamas—with four-chambered stomachs, which allows them to digest cellulose (plant fiber). All eat a vegetarian diet and are naturally grazing animals.

How do I select meat and poultry that is safe as well as animal-friendly?

Shoppers like you are driving a quiet revolution as you look for animal-friendly, hormone free, healthy meats and poultry. The market is awash with terms, claims, and certification seals, but without federal or industry oversight it can be hard to sort out choices. Supermarket chains like D'Agostino Supermarkets, Andronico's Market, and Whole Foods Market have stepped out as retail leaders, offering quality foods produced from vendors who raise their animals humanely.

But securing enough food to meet market demand is a challenge, because the stringent standards set for humane animal production are hard to replicate on a national scale. It is getting harder to meet consumers' demands for these foods. Ethically raising animals lends itself to small farms and small producers, which have a hard time competing against megafarms and large food producers. As larger retailers begin to offer more animal-friendly products, the sources will need to become global, presenting an entirely new set of challenging issues.

Restaurants have jumped on the bandwagon, too, looking for sources of natural, free range, grassfed, cage free, and humanely raised meats and poultry. The National Council of Chain Restaurants and the Food Marketing Institute have created an Animal Welfare Audit Program to support animal welfare policies for each species. They hope to strengthen food quality and food safety while ensuring animal well-being at each step in the production process. Some criticize the effort as short of ideal, with compliance and accountability challenges. But efforts by restaurants and supermarkets, backed up by consumer demand, will slowly effect change.

Until national oversight is established, you need to inform yourself about the terms and seals currently being used. But just because a cut of meat or poultry does not bear a seal doesn't mean it is unsafe or that the animals were raised in an inhumane way. Ask questions of the butcher or store manager to verify the assurances you are looking for—organic, hormone free, pasture fed. The more questions they get, the more they realize these issues are important to their customers.

How can I tell if the meat I'm buying comes from a cloned animal?

The cloning debate boils down to scientists versus consumers. Scientists are largely unified in their support of cloning, and are eager to use the techniques to enhance animal selection to achieve higher quality meat and milk. Some scientists opposed to cloning are concerned about inbreeding. Consumers who voice their opposition feel cloning is immoral and unethical.

The federal government is expected to approve the use of food from cloned animals sometime in 2008. At this point there are no special labels on cloned foods anticipated because experts say that cloned animals and the food from them are the same as those conventionally bred. Because of consumer opposition and pressure on Washington, this may change, and cloned foods may be identi-fied in some way. Cloned animals are rare and very expensive, so they are used almost exclusively for breed-ing. You'll probably never eat one, but you could eat their offspring. To avoid cloned food, buy USDA certified or-ganic. It is clone free.

Can hormones and antibiotics be given to cattle?

Cattle raised by traditional practices can be given antibiot-ics both to prevent and to treat disease. A withdrawal pe-riod is required to clear the substance from the animal's body before slaughter. Sampling conducted by the Food Safety Inspection System (FSIS) of the USDA reports a very low percentage of antibiotic residue violations.

Hormones can also be used to promote growth. Estra-diol, progesterone, and testosterone (natural hormones), and zeranol and trenbolone acetate (synthetic hormones) are given to the animal through an ear implant. Hormones are time-released and effective for 90 to 120 days, to insure a withdrawal period before slaughter. Melengestrol ace-tate, which suppresses the instinct to mate and promotes weight gain, is approved as a feed additive.

Organic beef is hormone and antibiotic free. Beef with the Certified Humane seal is hormone free and fed antibi-otic free feed. The animals can be given antibiotics to treat disease, but a withdrawal period is required to clear the substance from the animal's body before slaughter.

Should I be worried about mad cow disease?

As we have said, the risk is tiny but not zero. Mad cow dis-ease, or more correctly BSE (see page 58), is not destroyed by cooking. To keep your risk as low as possible,

- buy grassfed and organic beef
- avoid sweetbreads, bone marrow, neck bones, and beef cheeks
- buy muscle meats, preferably boneless
- buy ground beef instead of hamburger (see page 64)
- use bison, which is not susceptible to BSE

The USDA has introduced a National Animal Identification System for cattle, bison, poultry, dairy cows, and pigs that will be fully in place by 2009. Each animal will be assigned an electronic ear tag that will allow it to be traced back to its original source within days. The system is voluntary, but meat producers fully endorse it and have already begun to cooperate. The ear tags will make it quicker and easier to identify the source of an infected or sick animal, to isolate it, and facilitate quick product recalls.

Is it true that beef contains healthy fats?

Red meat gets a bad rap as a source of saturated fat, but beef and chocolate (how is that for a double good-whammy?) are the best sources of stearic acid, a beneficial saturated fat. Unlike other saturated fats, stearic acid doesn't raise your bad cholesterol and may even boost your good cholesterol.

Two other healthy fats found in meat and dairy foods are omega-3 fatty acids and conjugated linoleic acid (CLA). CLA is protective against cancer and omega-3s protect you against almost all chronic diseases. But there is a catch. Omega-3 originates in green leaves and algae. That's why fish is such a rich source—big fish eat little fish that eat algae and other sea plants. Grazing animals get omega-3 from plants and pass it on to us. But grains are low in omega-3 and rich in omega-6 (another type of fat). So meat and food products from grain fed animals don't contain as much healthy omega-3.

Why is beef called "red meat"?

Beef muscle is actually burgundy or purplish in color. Once it is exposed to air, the protein myoglobin soaks up oxygen and turns bright red. Unwrapped and stored for a few days, the color changes to brown and will eventually have an off odor and a tacky feel as the beef goes from fresh to spoiled. Beef, veal, lamb, and pork are all red meats because they contain more myoglobin protein than chicken or fish.

To help meats retain their typical red color, the FDA (Food and Drug Administration) allows a process called Modified Atmosphere Packaging (MAP). Oxygen is removed from the package and nitrogen and a small amount of carbon dioxide are introduced. The gases are harmless at the levels being used. However, using MAP to prevent color loss in beef can mislead shoppers. The beef appears bright red even when it may be past its sell-by date and is no longer fresh. MAP doesn't prevent spoilage.

Is the red liquid in the meat tray blood?

No, the animal's blood has been removed during slaughter. The red liquid you see in the package or on butcher trays is natural moisture from beef mixed with some protein. Be careful in discarding the meat tray or wrapper because this liquid may carry bacteria and could contaminate other foods.

What is the difference between hamburger and ground beef?

Hamburger comes from multiple animals, from trimmings, and from less popular cuts of beef, and it may have fat added. Older dairy cows are often used as a source for hamburger. Ground beef is made from a specific cut of meat. From highest to lowest fat content, ground beef comes from chuck, round, or sirloin.

What do the terms "lean" and "extra lean" mean on cuts of beef?

For a 3½ ounce serving of beef, nutrition labeling defines these terms as

- **Lean**—less than 10 grams of fat, 4.5 grams or less of saturated fat, and less than 95 milligrams of cholesterol.
- **Extra Lean**—less than 5 grams of fat, less than 2 grams of saturated fat, and less than 95 milligrams of cholesterol.

Extra lean cuts may have less fat and saturated fat than lean cuts, but the cholesterol value of beef is reasonably consistent, cut to cut.

Should I buy beef by brand?

Until recently very little meat or poultry was sold by brand. More and more brands of meat and poultry are appearing in the marketplace because shoppers are relying on brands to deliver the product they want—organic, grass-fed, all natural, lean, or lowfat. Brands generally fall into 3 general categories:

- breed specific—for example, certified Angus or Kobe beef
- company specific—each company offering something the shopper is looking for: grade, marbling, grassfed, grainfed, antibiotic free or hormone free
- store specific—many supermarket chains using an in-store brand to assure shoppers of the source and quality of their meat

What is Wagyu beef?

"Wagyu" refers to all Japanese beef cattle. *Wa* means "Japanese," and *gyu* means "cattle." Kobe beef, with a high degree of marbling and a very rich taste, comes from the Wagyu breed. To meet the growing demand for this type of beef, Wagyu cattle are now being raised in the U.S.

Is there any veal that is raised humanely?

More than twenty years ago, animal rights activists highlighted the inhumane treatment of commercially raised baby calves, the source of veal. Consumption of veal plummeted from 4 pounds per person per year to less than ½ pound, where it still stands today, which forced the industry to make changes.

Instead of raising calves in tiny crates that restricted movement, commercial veal producers today use individual wooden stalls or barn pens that allow interaction between animals and more normal movement and activities. Hormones have never been allowed in veal raising, but antibiotics may be given to prevent or treat disease. For those who believe the changes are not enough—and there are many, because the consumption numbers are still down—there is limited production of organic veal, which is antibiotic free.

Can hormones and antibiotics be given to pigs?

Hormones are not allowed to be used as a growth promoter in the pork industry. Antibiotics may be used to prevent or treat a disease, but a withdrawal period is required to clear the substance from the animal's body before slaughter.

Organic pork is antibiotic free. A sick organically raised pig may be treated with antibiotics, but first it must be removed from the herd, and it can't be returned once it is well. It is usually sold into nonorganic distribution channels.

Pigs are highly susceptible to disease so there has been widespread use of antibiotics, which has resulted in criticism from consumer groups. To overcome the freehanded use of antibiotics among pork producers, the National Pork Board initiated the Pork Quality Assurance (PQA) Plus program in 2007. This voluntary program offers training and guidelines in disease management and the judicious use of antibiotics. Use of antibiotics is going down.

What is the difference between pork and ham?

More pork is eaten worldwide than any other meat. Pork is meat from hogs. Young hogs are called pigs, and they are the source of most fresh pork. Cured pork—ham, bacon, and sausage—can come from either pigs or hogs.

Can hormones or antibiotics be given to lambs?

Zeronal, a synthetic hormone, administered through an ear implant, can be used as a growth promoter. It is active for 30 days and there's a mandatory 40-day withholding period before slaughter to insure clearance from the animal's system. Antibiotics can be used to prevent or treat disease, but they, too, have a mandatory withdrawal period before slaughter.

What is the difference between lamb and mutton?

Both come from sheep; lamb is less than 1 year old, and mutton—which is less tender and has a stronger flavor—is from sheep more than a year old. More than 70% of the lamb in the U.S. is imported, mostly from New Zealand and Australia. There is little USDA certified organic lamb on the market because U.S. standards prohibit the use of an antiparasitic drug that eliminates common stomach worms.

FISHY DILEMMAS

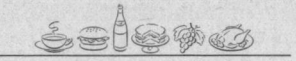

*In the child's card game Go Fish, you draw until you
get the right card. Selecting the best fish to eat often
resembles this random game of chance.*

Eat fish regularly and you reduce your risk for heart
disease, cancer, Alzheimer's, stroke, diabetes, depression,
and inflammatory disease such as rheumatoid arthritis.
Eat fish regularly and you also increase your exposure to
mercury, environmental contaminants, and microbes.

All the experts agree that we need to eat more fish. But
how much? How often? And which ones?

Which are the best fish to eat?

It's hard to make a list of "good fish" and "bad fish" because
seafood supplies change constantly and the list could become obsolete quickly. But the benefits and risks of broad
categories of seafood remain relatively consistent.

- **Lean fish** such as flounder are excellent sources
  of protein, are low in saturated fat and
  cholesterol, and offer moderate amounts of
  omega-3 fats. The levels of mercury are higher in
  larger fish and lower in smaller and farm-raised
  fish. Eat fish lower on the food chain.

- **Fatty fish** such as salmon are good sources of protein and offer the highest amounts of omega-3 fatty acids, but they also contain higher levels of saturated fat and cholesterol, and may have higher levels of pollutants like dioxin and PCBs. Their mercury level is lower than that of lean fish.
- **Shellfish and crustaceans (lobster, crab)** are high in protein and low in saturated fat, but some, like shrimp and mussels, contain a fair amount of cholesterol. If eaten raw, there is a risk of microbial infection. Children, pregnant women, and older adults should stick to cooked.

The levels of environmental contaminants in most seafood are low enough not to pose a health risk. For those particular species of fish or bodies of water that have high enough levels of contaminants to pose a public health risk, regional and local alerts are issued.

YOU SHOULD KNOW—

Environmental Protection Agency (EPA) Resources

To find out about fish and wildlife consumption advisories for the 50 states, the District of Columbia, U.S. territories, and Canada, go to:

www.epa.gov/waterscience/health/

What can I do as one shopper to help preserve marine life?

One consumer can make a difference in the fishing industry. When consumers stopped buying tuna because dolphins were being harmed by the fishing process, the fishing industry figured out how to fish dolphin safe. It's not that fishermen wanted to net dolphins—they were an unwanted and unintentional catch that wasted time and wore out equipment. But it wasn't until consumers started to vote with their food dollars that it was worthwhile for the fisherman to change the way they fished.

One in 4 animals caught in fishing gear are *bycatch*— marine life that is unwanted and unintentionally caught during normal fishing. Newer fishing methods are reducing bycatch. The use of Nordmore grates is reducing bycatch in the shrimp industry and some shrimp are now trap-caught instead of net-caught. The Turtle Excluder Device (TED) is a trapdoor that allows sea turtles to swim free instead of getting trapped. TEDs are required on U.S. shrimp boats, and the U.S. bans shrimp imports from countries that don't require TEDs. Long-liners are now using specially rigged lines that scare away seabirds so they don't get tangled in them or caught on bait hooks. And some fishing fleets are imposing bycatch allowances. If a fleet or boat exceeds the limits for unintentional catch they must stop fishing, which provides an incentive to "fish clean."

Ruining the oceans ruins the fisherman's livelihood. This becomes a great motivator to improve fishing methods. Your vote at the fish counter ultimately sends this message.

Are organic fish healthier to eat?

When the USDA Certified Organic program came into existence, fish farming was not a prominent industry. Although the Organic Food Production Act included seafood, the USDA's final rules gave no guidelines to seafood producers for organic farming. Without definite standards, seafood can't be certified, so the USDA Certified Organic label can't be used on any seafood product. That doesn't stop a supplier from using the term "organic," though, and numerous private certifying groups have popped up.

The basis of organic farming is to control the growing cycle of plants and animals to insure certain standards. However, wild fish may migrate over thousands of miles of oceans or rivers, and big fish eat smaller fish that eat marine plants. None of this can be controlled.

The National Organic Standards Board has set up a task force to draft regulations for organic production, handling, and labeling for aquatic animals. The standards will apply to animals that live in the open sea and those that are grown by aquaculture. As of the winter of 2006 the task force was completing its initial report, but it will be a lengthy process before standards are in place.

Why is there so much mercury in fish?

Most of the mercury in our environment comes from the air, as the result of the burning of coal or garbage. Many safeguards are required to keep mercury out of the environment, but some still escapes. Eventually rain dumps it into oceans, lakes, and rivers. Mercury-contaminated fish is your most likely source of mercury.

The form of mercury found in fish is methyl mercury. It is concentrated in the flesh of the fish, so there is more in older, larger fish farther up on the food chain—swordfish, tuna, shark, orange roughy, and tilefish. Sardines, salmon, and shrimp have very low levels.

Recent research from Australia suggests that the form of mercury found in fish may be less harmful than the form of mercury usually measured in standard tests for exposure. This makes it hard to set safe recommendations for intake because there are different types of mercury in the environment.

Too much mercury can be harmful to your health. It affects the nervous system, and children and unborn babies are the most vulnerable to the effects of overexposure. All experts agree that children and women who are or intend to become pregnant need to be more cautious. But the jury is still out about whether there are harmful effects from typical fish consumption. And there is no question that regular fish consumption is beneficial.

YOU SHOULD KNOW—

About an Excellent Resource:
www.GotMercury.org

Enter the type and amount of fish you will be eating, plus your weight, and the site will calculate how much mercury you'll eat.

Is canned tuna safe?

Canned tuna has no equal when it comes to affordable, lean protein that's rich in heart-healthy omega-3 fatty acids.

Still, there is no question that all canned tuna contains some mercury. The key is to keep the exposure low. Light tuna has less mercury than albacore, which comes from larger fish. Chunk light contains even less than solid light. Consumer's Union recommends adults limit intake to no more than 3 cans of chunk light or 1 can of solid light or white albacore per week.

Don't Eat Raw Shellfish

Clams, mussels, and other shellfish get food by filtering large quantities of water through their bodies. This concentrates more bacteria and viruses in their flesh, putting you at risk of getting sick. Cooking kills the harmful organisms.

Should I avoid fish if I'm pregnant?

Everything we eat can be evaluated by a risk-to-benefit ratio. So let's look at the risks and benefits of eating fish by sex and age.

Women of childbearing age, those who are pregnant or breastfeeding, and kids under 12

- will benefit from the nutrients found in seafood
- should limit consumption of white (albacore) tuna to 6 ounces a week
- should avoid large predatory fish (swordfish, tuna, shark)
- should eat 2 servings of fish a week

Teenagers, adult men, and women who do not plan on a pregnancy

- may reduce their future risk of heart disease by eating fish regularly
- should choose fish with lower levels of mercury or contaminants if they eat more than 2 servings of fish a week
- people with a known risk for heart disease should select seafood with higher amounts of

heart-healthy omega-3 fatty acids—salmon, shrimp, pollack, cod, light tuna, and catfish

Why is getting enough omega-3 fats so important?

There are two main groups of polyunsaturated fats: omega-3 and omega-6. Think of them as two different strands of beads, similar in shape but different in color sequence. Each is important to good health.

Omega-3 fats are in shorter supply in our diets. The good news is that eating as few as 2 servings of fish a week provides a rich source of omega-3 fats. It's been estimated that the ratio of omega-6 fats to omega-3 fats should range from 5:1 to 10:1. In typical American diets, the ratio is about 20:1. This means you need to make an effort to eat foods higher in omega-3 fats: fish, walnuts, canola oil, purslane, and flaxseeds. Research is showing that this imbalance in the polyunsaturated fats we eat may be contributing to higher risks for cancer, heart disease, and arthritis. Getting more omega-3 fats lowers the risk.

What is fish farming?

Fish farming is when fish are raised in tanks or in enclosures of natural bodies of water. Species typically raised in fish farms include salmon, catfish, tilapia and cod. If a fish is farm raised, it must be stated on its label.

There are pros and cons swirling around this issue. Most marine biologists agree that as the human population continues to grow, there will not be enough wild fish to meet demands. Fish farming could close this gap. But there are downsides. Some studies show fish farming is depleting wild fish reserves because fish pellets made from wild fish are often fed to farmed fish, and because some farms use wild fish eggs and wild young fish, which are then raised as farm fish for market. The waste from farms may pollute surrounding waters, and farmed fish can escape and breed with wild varieties, altering natural species. To control disease from concentrated fish populations, fish farmers use antibiotics, which can make their way into open waters and possibly into humans when we eat the farmed fish.

Many scientists feel that aquaculture, when carefully monitored and controlled, has the potential to help marine ecosystems stabilize and even rebound. Farmed oysters, clams, and mussels are good examples. Since all three must come from unpolluted waters, when farmed, they initiate efforts to clean up coastal waters. These shellfish can even improve water quality as they clear the water of excess plankton, their primary food source.

Freshwater fish farms are a good alternative to ocean farms. Catfish, trout, and tilapia can be raised inland without using wild fish as feed.

How can I tell if the fish I buy is caught wild or farm-raised?

By law, fish and shellfish must be labeled for country of origin (COOL) and method of production—wild or farm-raised. Seafood Watch, a program of the Monterey Bay Aquarium, provides national and regional seafood guides listing fish in 3 categories—best, good, avoid—along with information on whether the species was farm-raised or wild, and its place of origin.

TO LEARN MORE—

About the Seafood Watch program and to download the seafood guides go to
www.mbayaq.org/cr/seafoodwatch.asp.

Are farm-raised salmon dyed pink?

Wild salmon are pink because they eat krill, tiny shellfish loaded with pigments. Farm-raised salmon do not eat krill, so their flesh is a naturally unattractive gray. All farm-raised salmon are fed synthetic pigments to "pink up" their flesh. FDA rules require disclosure of the added color, but few retailers comply. Organically raised salmon get their pink color from eating a species of yeast that naturally contains the same pigment found in krill.

Farmed salmon are not the only fish to get a little cosmetic lift. Wild tuna steaks, which are naturally red, turn brown when exposed to air or frozen. To prevent this discoloration, seafood companies spray the steaks with carbon monoxide.

How can I tell if fish I buy is fresh?

Fresh fish and shellfish have virtually no odor. Only when seafood starts to spoil does it smell "fishy." Fresh fish has

- clean eyes that bulge a little
- firm, shiny flesh and bright red slime free gills
- flesh that springs back when pressed gently
- no darkening around the edges or brown or yellowish discoloration
- a fresh, mild smell, not "fishy" or ammonia-like

YOU SHOULD KNOW—

More nutrients are retained in fish that is baked or broiled rather than processed or fried.

HASSLES IN THE HENHOUSE

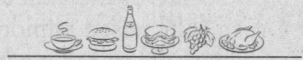

We eat more chicken than any other type of meat.
Chickens lay 72 billion eggs in the U.S. yearly.

In the good old days, you went to the store and bought a stewing hen or a broiler. Eggs were eggs—brown or white; large, medium or small. Today, neither choice is so simple anymore.

Understanding Terms
So You Can Talk the Talk

Certified Humane is a label from the Humane Farm Animal Care group. It can be displayed on egg cartons from farms that provide humane treatment of hens, cage free living space, and vegetarian feed with no added antibiotics. Eggs with this label usually cost more than regular eggs.

United Egg Producers Certified Seal is a voluntary certification program that sets standards for cleanliness, water and feed requirements, cage space allowances, beak trimming, and induced molting of laying hens. Though voluntary, most egg producers in the U.S. adhere to it and its initiation has created changes. Not only have consumers demanded change, but an unlikely ally, McDonald's, the world's largest egg buyer, told its suppliers to clean up their act or else. No one waited for the "or else," especially when Burger King, Wendy's, and others followed suit. This seal is almost always displayed on egg cartons.

USDA Certified Organic Seal can be used on either poultry products or eggs as long as the USDA organic standards have been met. The rules for organic flocks require that

- organic feed can't contain any animal by-products
- the birds must have access to the outdoors, shade, shelter, and exercise
- no antibiotics can be used; a sick bird can be removed from the flock and treated but can't later be returned and sold as organic
- beak trimming is a decision left to the farmer

For organic eggs, all requirements for poultry remain in place, but organic laying hens can't be forced into induced molting. This practice pushes the hens into a few more laying cycles after their normal productivity declines.

Both organic poultry and organic eggs cost more. The poultry may be worth it, because you know the organic poultry is free of pesticides and antibiotics. But the eggs from organic and nonorganic hens are virtually identical. Pesticides and antibiotics don't get into the egg through the shell.

EGG FACTS—

Laying hens produce 1 egg every 25 hours. Most hens produce eggs for about 18 months before naturally molting, a sort of chicken menopause.

Important Information on Your Egg Carton

It's a good thing eggs are sold by the dozen, because egg cartons have become billboards for a wide range of information—nutrition, food dating, safe handling information, animal welfare, and certification seals. Even the eggs themselves can be stamped with logos or dates. Sorting this out isn't easy, and not all the information is what it seems.

Nutrition information: Egg cartons carry the standard nutrition facts panel, usually on the inside top lid. Today we have new designer eggs to choose from, eggs that are high in vitamin E, lutein, or heart-healthy omega-3 fats. The composition of these eggs is altered by giving the chickens enhanced feed. If you do not usually eat seafood, the best source of omega-3 fats, eggs rich in this healthy fat can be a good substitute. But realize the omega-3-rich eggs are much higher in cholesterol than fish, and usually cost much more than traditional eggs.

Egg carton dating: All eggs displaying a USDA grade shield must also display a "pack" date. This is a 3-digit code that represents the day of the year, with January 1 as 001 and December 31 as 365. There may also be a *use by, sell by,* or *expiration* date. None of these are required by the federal government but may be required by state or local regulations. The locally required dating systems are in place to avoid keeping eggs in the retail system too long. Purchase eggs before the "use by," "sell by," or expiration date, but realize that eggs will be good to use for 3 to 5 weeks after that.

Safe handling information: Eggs are perishable and may contain salmonella; the handling information on the carton is meant to keep you from getting sick. Use it—don't eat raw or undercooked eggs, and refrigerate eggs in their original carton rather than on the refrigerator door. Years of production practices to produce the least expensive eggs in overcrowded situations may have contributed to the increase of salmonella found in eggs. Salmonella doesn't make chickens sick, but it can live in their bodies and get into uncracked whole eggs. Eating raw eggs, raw cookie dough or batter, Caesar salad dressing, or health drinks containing raw eggs could make you sick. Thoroughly cooking eggs kills all bacteria. In 1998, the USDA set up the Egg Safety Task Force with the goal of reducing salmonella outbreaks by 50% by the year 2010. The numbers are going down yearly.

YOU SHOULD KNOW—

The USDA inspects eggs and oversees labeling claims, but inspections are voluntary. Of the 72 billion eggs laid each year, about one-third are USDA inspected. The rest are regulated by individual states.

Are eggs healthy? I'm worried about their high cholesterol level.

Eggs are one of nature's truly remarkable products—they contain every nutrient needed to support life in a handy container. Eggs have the highest-quality protein; contain the pigments lutein and zeaxanthin, which protect your eyes; have 12 minerals and 13 vitamins; are low in overall fat and saturated fat; and average 75 calories per egg. The one downside is that eggs contain cholesterol, which is found in the yolk. But research has shown that the cholesterol in eggs is less likely to raise blood cholesterol than saturated or trans fat. If your cholesterol is within normal range, it's fine to eat 4 to 6 eggs a week.

Counting Cholesterol in Eggs

1 jumbo = 275 milligrams   *1 small = 157 milligrams*
1 extra large = 245 milligrams   *1 egg yolk = 210 milligrams*
1 large = 212 milligrams   *1 egg white = 0 milligrams*
1 medium = 186 milligrams

What do all the other terms mean that I see on fresh poultry or egg cartons, such as natural, farm fresh, cage free, and free range?

Natural and farm fresh are both very vague terms that have more to do with marketing than farming procedures. All eggs and poultry come from farms, so they all qualify as farm fresh. The term has nothing to do with how the poultry was raised, fed, or treated.

When poultry is labeled "natural" it cannot have any artificial color, flavor, preservatives, or synthetic ingredients added, and can only be minimally processed, such as ground. Natural does not mean the animal was pasture raised and is antibiotic or hormone free. By their very nature eggs in the shell are natural because nothing can be added—they come packaged in their own container.

Cage free and free range are terms that can be qualified. All chickens raised for meat are cage free, but this term can be misleading. Cage free could mean anything from being raised in an open-floor henhouse to having access to a yard. It doesn't insure the poultry were raised outdoors or that they weren't exposed to overcrowded conditions. Unless you know the supplier, you could be paying a premium for nothing.

Almost 90% of laying hens are raised in cages. Animal welfare experts feel this practice is inhumane and have lobbied against it. Cage size has been increased, and egg producers claim cages lessen stressful living conditions and salmonella, reducing the need for antibiotics. The European Union will be eliminating cages by 2012, and many hope the U.S. will follow. Be aware that cage free laying hens may still be confined indoors. And even when the barn door is open, most laying hens don't venture outside because they prefer to stay close to their nest, food, and water.

Free range or free roaming chickens are allowed to go outdoors. The USDA requires that poultry and egg producers who use this term allow the poultry to go outdoors and live more naturally for part of their lives. This does not mean the poultry are raised antibiotic-free or cruelty-free, and there are no set standards for how long the chickens remain outdoors. Realize that most broiler/fryers live for only 8 weeks, and it isn't safe to let young chicks outside for a number of weeks so free range, or free roaming, laying hens may be outside, but they are often penned to protect them against avian disease from migratory birds and from rodents and other predators.

With better standards and more comprehensive definitions, all of these terms—natural, farm fresh, cage free, free range—have value. But currently the interpretation is too broad to give you definite assurances of humane animal practices.

Are pasture-raised or grassfed poultry and eggs healthier?

Pastured poultry and eggs are from chickens raised directly on pastures, insuring that a minimum of 20% of their feed comes from pasture forage. It is impossible to produce 100% grassfed chickens because they cannot fulfill all their energy needs from grass or forage and, left to their own devices, will eat bugs for extra protein. Most farmers give grassfed chickens supplemental feed. Laying hens also need a nest and protection from predators and the weather; they can't live exclusively outdoors like cattle.

The American Pastured Poultry Producers Association sets standards for this type of farm. Pastured poultry lends itself to a sustainable model and provides a more humane and sanitary situation than larger commercial operations. It also requires a good deal more land and doesn't lend itself to large-scale production.

TO LEARN MORE—

About the American Pastured Poultry Producers Association, go to: www.apppa.org.

Can hormones or antibiotics be given to chickens?

Don't pay extra for "hormone free" chickens. Hormone use has been banned from the poultry industry for 50 years. Labels that say "No Added Hormones" are correct but also deceptive because there aren't any hormones in any chicken, turkey, goose, or duck in the store.

Antibiotics are another issue. They can be used to prevent disease and promote growth, but the same drugs you are using to fight infection are the ones poultry farmers are giving to their flocks. You don't have to worry about antibiotic residue in poultry flesh. It's the antibiotic-resistant bacteria that live in poultry flocks that are the major concern.

Bacteria harmlessly live in chickens. But in many flocks the bacteria have become antibiotic resistant. When raw chicken is improperly handled or it accidentally cross-contaminates other food, the bacteria can make you sick. Now the problem gets bigger: the antibiotics needed to treat you may not be effective because the bacteria that made you sick are antibiotic resistant.

This scenario has two culprits—the industry that freely dosed the poultry with antibiotics and the medical community that freely dosed you with antibiotics for self-limiting problems like a minor sore throat or the common cold. The result is smart bacteria that morphed into strains that could outsmart the drugs. But change is happening. The Centers for Disease Control and Prevention (CDC) is encouraging doctors to prescribe fewer antibiotics, especially for children. And they are. The CDC, FDA, and USDA have begun to monitor antibiotic use on farms and in human medicine. They are encouraging a phaseout of antibiotics as feed additives and many producers have already complied. Antibiotics will only be given to flocks to control disease. Unfortunately, it will take up to 5 years to rid flocks of some of the hardier resistant strains of bacteria, so handle raw poultry carefully.

What can I do to avoid getting sick from poultry?

Because all raw poultry can carry bacteria, the easiest precautions to take are to keep it separate from other foods and to keep it cold. Keeping it separate eliminates transferring bacteria to other foods, and the cold limits how fast the bacteria can multiply.

Buy raw poultry toward the end of your shopping trip and place it in a plastic bag so it can't drip on other foods. Don't leave chicken in a hot car, incubating while you do a round of errands on the way home. At home, store poultry covered on the bottom shelf of the refrigerator so it can't drip on other foods.

When making a chicken dish, gather and prepare all the other ingredients first, then work on the chicken. If you cut up the chicken first, it's too easy to cross-contaminate knives, countertops, or cabinet handles. Never use the same knife or cutting board for poultry and then another food without first washing it with soapy water. Always wash your hands after handling raw poultry, and cook it to an internal temperature of 165°F, which kills all bacteria present.

What are food processors doing to prevent bacteria in raw poultry?

Many are dipping raw poultry into a solution of trisodium phosphate (TSP), which can significantly reduce the level of bacteria. It's a safe product, used in many other food productions systems, and is approved by the USDA. There is even a safe way to recycle the solution so that the phosphates do not contaminate wastewater. The Center for Science in the Public Interest and other consumer groups see this as a favorable step toward lowering the incidence of foodborne illness caused by raw poultry.

Why does some of the fresh chicken I buy feel frozen?

Bacteria can grow in poultry at temperatures hovering around 40°F. To slow down growth, fresh poultry can be transported and held at temperatures as low as 26°F, which will partially freeze the meat. If the poultry was held at temperatures below this it must say *frozen* or *previously frozen* on the label.

Can you get bird flu from eating chicken?

The simple answer is no. Cooking chicken to 165°F will kill any virus. Bird, or avian, flu is more of a threat to free range poultry than to humans because it is transmitted from wild birds to domestic flocks. So if avian flu comes to the U.S., free range poultry may need to be contained to keep the birds from getting sick. Before bird flu can infect humans it would have to mutate to a different form. There has been no human-to-human transmission.

If the bones of cooked chicken are reddish pink, does that mean the meat is undercooked?

No, the best test for doneness is a meat thermometer that registers 165°F. Darkening around bones and in the meat near the bones occurs in the meat of young chickens without completely calcified bones, allowing marrow to seep out. The cooked meat is totally safe to eat.

Why does chicken have so much fat under the skin?

Unlike red meat, which is marbled with fat throughout the muscle, poultry is a leaner protein and much of the fat is found under the skin or around internal organs. That's also why skinless chicken has much less fat than chicken with the skin on. The fat is easy to remove.

Is ground chicken or turkey better than ground beef?

Generally, ground poultry is lower in fat and calories than ground beef, but the cholesterol levels in poultry may be slightly higher. That's because ground poultry contains meat, skin, and fat in proportions naturally found on the bird, about 10% to 15% fat by weight. If the label reads *ground chicken* or *ground turkey,* it will include skin and fat. If the label says *ground chicken meat* or *ground poultry meat,* no skin or fat is included, and the meat will be lower in fat and calories. The last option is ground white meat chicken or turkey, which has almost no fat and the fewest calories. If you buy a brand name ground poultry product it must have a nutrition label, which makes comparisons easier.

What's in self-basted turkey?

If a turkey is prebasted the label must clearly state "basted" or "self-basting." The bird is injected with a liquid solution of butter or oil, broth, water, spices, flavor enhancers, and preservatives. A maximum of 3% added weight is allowed from the basting solution, and the ingredients listing must include all added ingredients. The self-baster will have slightly more fat and a good deal more sodium, because salt- or sodium-containing flavor enhancers are usually part of the basting solution. Four ounces of regular roast turkey averages 70 milligrams of sodium; the same portion of prebasted turkey has about 450 milligrams.

Are brown eggs healthier than white eggs?

Eggs from all types of chickens are nutritionally equal. Eggshell color tells you nothing about the quality of the egg, the health of the chicken, or how well the animal was raised. It does tell you the breed of hen. White-shelled eggs are from white longhorn chickens, brown-shelled eggs are from Rhode Island Reds, and blue-shelled eggs are from South African Araucanas. Some breeds even produce freckled eggs. In some areas of the country you pay a premium for brown-shelled eggs; in other places, white-shelled cost more. Marketers want you to believe that the color of the shell somehow makes the egg more natural or healthier. Neither is true. And remember, you throw away the shell you may have paid a premium to buy.

Are fertilized eggs more nutritious?

Fertilized eggs are nutritionally equal to unfertilized eggs. The only differences are that the rooster got in the hen-house, and the eggs are more perishable. Fertilized eggs are not found in grocery stores because commercial egg producers and USDA and state inspectors discard them from wholesale supplies. They can be purchased from farms and at specialty ethnic food stores.

Can I use cracked eggs?

Once the eggshell is cracked, bacteria can easily enter. Don't buy cracked eggs. If you accidentally crack an egg in handling, break the egg into a clean container, cover tightly, refrigerate, and use within 2 days. If an eggshell cracks during cooking, the egg is still safe to eat.

Is the greenish tinge around the yolk of a hard-boiled egg safe to eat?

A green tinge or ring on a hard-cooked egg yolk is due to overcooking. It is caused by sulfur and iron compounds that occur naturally in the egg. It can also be caused by a high iron content in the cooking water. In either case, it does not affect taste and the egg is safe to eat.

Can you use an egg with a blood spot?

Blood spots are caused by a rupture of small blood vessels in the yolk. Though it might not look appealing, it isn't unsafe. Most eggs with blood spots are removed during inspection and are not considered kosher.

Are powdered egg whites safe to use?

Powdered egg whites are an excellent source of protein and a good substitute for raw eggs in shakes or smoothies. Powdered egg whites can be reconstituted with water and whipped like a fresh egg. They are safe to eat without cooking because they have been pasteurized to kill the bacteria.

What are pourable eggs?

Pourable eggs come in many varieties. They can be shelled, mixed whole eggs, or just egg whites sold in cardboard cartons similar to milk. They are pasteurized to reduce salmonella levels. Pourable eggs can also be egg substitutes, which are egg whites colored and flavored to more closely resemble stirred whole eggs. They are good replacements for scrambled eggs or to use in cooking, and they have no cholesterol.

DAIRY CASE—
SO MANY CHOICES

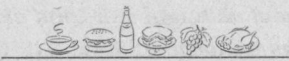

Keep it simple—aim for 2 to 3 servings a day.
Use nonfat or lowfat more often.

The dairy case may seem uncomplicated at first—milk, cheese, butter, yogurt—but look a little harder. You can buy plain milk, you can buy organic milk, you can buy milk with extra protein, extra calcium, lactose free, or hormone free. Sitting next to the cow's milk is soy milk. Both can be purchased at 4 different levels of fat and in a number of flavors. The yogurt section can be as big as a football field, with endless flavors or add-ons such as fruit, sprinkles, or granola. And there are so many varieties of cheese that some supermarkets have created a completely separate section.

Dairy foods are high in calcium, recommended to promote strong bones and prevent osteoporosis. But you need more than calcium to maintain healthy bones—you need vitamin D, potassium, and exercise, just to name a few. Focusing on just calcium may be too narrow.

Plus whole milk, cheese, and butter are high in fat, saturated fat, and cholesterol—all best avoided in large amounts. Milk contains lactose, a sugar that many people can't easily digest and that makes them sick. Some are allergic to milk protein. And then there is the ongoing debate about the use of antibiotics and hormones.

Which is the best milk to buy?

If you are only talking about nutrition, nonfat milk is the winner. It has all the nutrients with none of the fat found in whole milk, and it has far less cholesterol and fewer calories. Milk provides high-quality protein and is a good source of vitamins A, D, B_{12}, riboflavin, calcium, phosphorus, magnesium, potassium and zinc.

Are growth hormones given to cows dangerous for humans?

The FDA (Food and Drug Administration) has approved a hormone called recombinant bovine somatotropin (rBST) for use in dairy cows. Cows make natural BST in their bodies, but with injections of synthetic rBST they can produce more milk. But the more milk a cow produces, the greater the chance that her udder will become infected, requiring the use of antibiotics. Now the problem is twofold—hormones plus antibiotics.

Using rBST negatively affects the health of cows, and some believe that's reason enough to stop buying milk from treated herds. Treating cows with rBST also increases the levels of insulin-like growth factor in their milk. The good news is that this growth factor is a protein, and just like any other protein we eat, it should be broken down in the digestive tract. But some proteins we eat slip into the blood stream without being broken down, so there is a small possibility that this could happen to some of the growth factor found in milk.

There are concerns that the hormone residue in cow's milk is promoting early puberty. Puberty has been occurring earlier in all developed countries, but this is far more likely to be due to better nutrition and the increasing incidence of childhood obesity than the hormones used on dairy cows. Because of consumer pressure many dairies have stopped using rBST, and today two-thirds of all dairy cows in the U.S. are rBST-free.

How can I tell if the milk I buy comes from cows given hormones?

You can't, because there is no labeling requirement. But many dairies that do not use growth hormones proudly announce on their labels "Produced without the use of antibiotics and added growth hormones." Organic milk comes from cows that haven't been given either one.

Should I use organic milk?

Organic milk and regular milk are nutritionally equivalent. Buying organic milk assures you that cows are raised without antibiotics or added hormones, so there can be no hormone residue in the milk. But it does not mean the milk comes from a U.S. dairy. The demand for organic dairy foods is very high, and less than 2% of the current U.S. dairy herds are organic, so producers are outsourcing to foreign countries. If you are concerned about your ecological footprint and the impact of food miles on our resources, these issues need to be considered, too. But the economic incentive to change over to organic farming is persuading many dairy farmers to convert to organic production. This should make more U.S. organic milk available in the future.

Would raw milk be a better option?

The only difference between raw milk and pasteurized milk is the higher amount of bacteria in raw milk. Raw milk can be very dangerous, especially for pregnant women, children, or those with a compromised immune system. Proponents feel it's more nutritious and contains antimicrobial properties. Raw milk can't kill off bacteria naturally, and it is so likely to be contaminated that it can't be shipped across state lines.

What is the difference between pasteurization and homogenization?

Pasteurization kills most (but never all) bacteria so that milk is safe to drink. Most milk is flash pasteurized—heated to 160°F (72°C) for 15 seconds. Ultrapasteurization can also be used, heating milk to 285°F (141°C) for only 1 to 2 seconds. This method kills so many bacteria that the milk or cream remains unspoiled for weeks. During bottling, handling, and storage at home more bacteria will grow, so milk should always be kept cold and treated as a product that spoils easily.

Homogenization keeps the fat particles broken up and dispersed so they will not separate from the fluid milk. Milk processors separate the cream from the liquid milk. They then add back enough cream to make 1%, 2%, or whole milk, and then homogenize it so it will not separate. Any leftover cream is used as cream, or to make butter or other highfat dairy foods.

What is the additive palmitate that I see on my nonfat milk carton?

When the fat is removed to produce nonfat milk, the natural vitamin A is lost since it is a fat-soluble vitamin. The vitamin A is then replaced with retinyl palmitate. Retinyl is vitamin A and palmitate is palmitic acid, a palm oil fat that keeps the vitamin dissolved in nonfat milk. For every quart of vitamin A-fortified milk, you get about 2 milligrams of palmitic acid. It's a safe product.

Can I drink any milk if I am lactose intolerant?

A large number of adults can't digest *lactose,* the sugar in milk, because they don't make enough of the enzyme *lactase.* If you are *lactose intolerant,* shortly after you eat or drink dairy foods you experience gas, bloating, cramps, and possibly diarrhea. The amount of milk you can comfortably drink varies individually. It depends on the amount of enzyme you make and the kinds of bacteria you have in your intestine. Some people simply avoid dairy foods, but you don't have to.

Start with hard cheese and yogurt. Much of the lactose is lost in the cheese-making process—it's in the whey that is drained off. Yogurt is made with friendly bacteria that digest much of the lactose as the yogurt curd is formed. Try smaller amounts of milk—a ½ cup, for example—and drink it along with a meal. Chocolate milk and cooked milk—custard, pudding, creamed soups—are often better tolerated. You can also buy lactose-reduced milk or buy a lactase supplement to take with dairy foods.

If I don't drink milk, how will I get enough calcium?

Dairy foods supply 70% of the calcium in our diets, but many people avoid this food category altogether and still get enough calcium. Other strong food sources of calcium are

- soymilk, soy yogurt, soy cheese, soybeans, soynuts, and tempeh
- calcium-fortified juice, rice milk, and cereal
- dark green leafy vegetables—broccoli, collard greens, kale, turnip greens, mustard greens, and bok choy
- dried peas and beans
- canned fish with bone—salmon and sardines

If my child is allergic to milk, is he at greater risk of getting diabetes later in life?

There is a theory that cow's milk is intended to nourish calves and that when introduced to human infants it sets the stage for allergies. This has never been proven. There are some people who are truly allergic to milk protein, and even if they were not given cow's milk during infancy, the allergy will develop. If your child is allergic to milk, he does have to avoid milk and any products containing milk. Though there was some research pointing toward a link between milk allergies and autoimmune disorders such as diabetes, the evidence was circumstantial at best and a clear connection has never been made. Your child's milk allergy is not a risk for diabetes.

Which is the best cheese to buy?

The biggest concern about cheese is its saturated fat and cholesterol content. The best advice is to buy whatever you like, but eat small amounts.

Grated cheese offers a punch of flavor and is a good way to keep portions reasonable. Processed cheese, like American cheese and cheese spread, is to real cheese what margarine is to butter—not the real thing. It will contain more additives and less flavor. And the same rule applies: eat reasonable portions.

There are reduced-fat, lowfat, and no-fat cheeses available. Some, particularly the reduced-fat, are lower in fat but still taste good and melt smoothly. When you reduce the fat in cheese too low, you get too far removed from "cheese" and get closer to a cheese substitute without the characteristics of real cheese, such as the ability to melt. Some people enjoy these lower-fat varieties; others don't. As long as you keep portions small, enjoy any variety of cheese you like.

Is yogurt a healthy choice?

If you mean plain, lowfat yogurt—yes! Yogurt has become big business, with endless varieties and flavors. Here is where your label-reading skills and eating philosophy will play a role. Are you interested in limiting sugar? Do you want to avoid artificial sweeteners? Are you looking for a lowfat or whole-milk yogurt? Do you want an organic brand? Do you want a snack-sized portion? Would you prefer a nondairy, soy yogurt? All of these are available. But remember, in the end yogurt is simply a glass of milk you eat with a spoon.

Should I use yogurt drinks as a meal replacement?

Drinkable yogurt is one of the fastest-growing food categories worldwide. The drinks are similar to smoothies and can have up to 300 calories in a serving, which is far fewer than the calories in a typical meal. But yogurt drinks are less satisfying than solid food, which means you may not feel full after drinking a liquid meal. This is good if you want to gain weight, because you'll probably still be hungry and supplement the drink with some solid food. But it's not the best choice if you are hoping to lose weight by substituting a yogurt drink for a meal. Calories you chew are always more filling and satisfying than calories you drink.

What are probiotics?

Probiotics is an umbrella word for more than 30 different types of bacteria and yeasts that can provide health benefits. You can get them naturally in food or as a supplement. Kefir, buttermilk, miso, and sauerkraut are natural sources, as is yogurt that isn't pasteurized after it is cultured. Some brands of soymilk, cereal, granola bars, and yogurt are probiotic fortified. Dairy foods, especially yogurt, are excellent carriers of added probiotics because refrigeration helps to keep probiotics alive and stable.

Your digestive tract is home to live bacteria called *flora*.

Some are helpful; others are harmful. Natural probiotics are helpful. Healthy and harmful organisms are constantly jostling for the upper hand. Decreased use of fermented foods and increased use of antibiotics can upset the natural flora and give harmful bacteria the chance to grow. Eating extra probiotics can increase the amount of healthy bacteria, which helps control diarrhea, chronic constipation, irritable bowel syndrome, and inflammatory bowel disease. When eaten regularly, they may even be able to prevent some of these problems.

Are prebiotics the same as probiotics?

Prebiotics are basically food for *probiotics* and encourage probiotics to flourish. Whole grains, onions, bananas, garlic, honey, leeks, and artichokes are natural sources. Prebiotics can also be isolated from natural sources and added to foods. Inulin and fructooligosaccharides (FOS) are two of the most common and will appear on the ingredient list. Prebiotics and probiotics work together to boost your health from the inside out, creating a healthy environment in your digestive tract.

Should I use probiotic supplements?

Probiotic supplements are available without a prescription, but they also are not regulated, so there is no guarantee that the pill contains a helpful dose of live bacteria. A container of yogurt is a better bet for a substantial amount of live organisms, because of its "use by" date and limited shelf life.

To find out more about probiotics, see page 160.

WHEN GOOD FOODS
MAKE YOU SICK

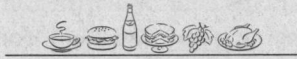

*The Centers for Disease Control and Prevention estimates
there are 76 million cases of foodborne illness each year.
More than half of these cases are caused by foods
prepared at home.*

Thoughts to consider when it comes to food safety:

- There is a risk to eating anything.
- Choosing what food to buy and eat is a series of decisions you make based on a risk-benefit ratio.
- It's not worth the risk to eat rare hamburgers, even if you prefer the taste.
- It's not wise to eat raw shellfish.
- It's probably not wise to drink unpasteurized juice.
- It doesn't seem worth the risk to eat an apple or peach without taking a few seconds to wash it off.
- It is worth the risk to continue to eat fresh fruits and vegetables. People who eat them regularly have a 15% lower chance of dying from all diseases, and the odds get even higher for specific diseases.

A Dozen Food Safety Tips

With enough warmth, moisture, and food, 1 bacterium can divide into more than 2 million in 7 hours. But there are many things you can do to prevent this from happening.

1. Wash your hands often. Half of all foodborne illness can be prevented by this one precaution. To keep it simple, wash them every time you start to prepare a different food, when you leave the kitchen, and after you go to the bathroom.

2. Don't thaw frozen food on the kitchen counter. The warm temperature in the kitchen will promote bacterial growth. Thaw foods slowly in the refrigerator, under cold running water, or quickly in the microwave.

3. Avoid cross-contamination. Wash cutting boards and knives with soap and water between cutting raw meat and preparing vegetables or cutting bread. Never place cooked food on a dish that previously held raw, unwashed food—even vegetables; remember, they grew in the dirt.

4. Don't stuff the refrigerator. Cold air needs to circulate to keep the temperature constant and low. Use a cooler for beverages if you get overloaded. And even if it's snowing, the garage isn't cold enough or clean enough to keep foods that need refrigeration.

5. Don't eat raw dough containing eggs. Don't let kids lick the bowl scraper, either; it's a leading source of food poisoning. There is no risk from baked dough, because any unhealthy organisms have been easily destroyed by heat.

6. <u>If you drop it, dump it.</u> No matter what your mother said, food that lands on the floor shouldn't be eaten.

7. <u>Travel with care.</u> If your trip is longer than a half hour—and who can predict traffic?—use a cooler or insulated bag. Microwave hot packs make great heat boosters when traveling with hot foods.

8. <u>Keep hot foods hot and cold foods cold.</u> It is better to replenish than to let foods sit out too long—2 hours at room temperature is the safe limit.

9. <u>Boil the gravy.</u> If gravy is made from pan drippings, bring it to a rolling boil. Boil it a second time if you reheat it the next day.

10. <u>Debone leftover poultry or fish.</u> The carcass can harbor bacteria.

11. <u>Refrigerate leftovers promptly.</u> Foods do not need to cool down before going in the refrigerator; counter cooling speeds up the growth of bacteria.

12. <u>Eat leftovers in 3 to 4 days or throw them out.</u> You can't see or smell bacteria, so even fine-looking food can be contaminated.

COMING TO A STORE NEAR YOU—

The Smart Label

The FreshQ label can be placed on the outside wrapper of meat and poultry, turning from bright tangerine to gray when the food is spoiled.

What are the odds that I'll get sick from food?

Actually, the odds are small. Nearly 300 million Americans eat many times a day, 365 days a year, adding up to trillions of food exposures. But the odds mean very little once you get sick. The world isn't sterile, so food will never be perfectly safe, but if everyone from the farmer to you handles food safely, the likelihood of you getting sick goes down dramatically.

If you've ever had a case of food poisoning, more correctly called "foodborne illness," you know it's no joke. Food poisoning can cause diarrhea, vomiting, stomach cramps, fever, and fatigue. Most healthy adults simply suffer for a few days, but for children, pregnant women, the elderly, or anyone with a compromised immune system, the consequences can be serious.

YOU SHOULD KNOW—

When to Call the Doctor

Children, pregnant women, the elderly, or anyone with a compromised immune system should seek immediate medical attention for food poisoning. Healthy adults should call the doctor if diarrhea doesn't resolve in 3 days or is accompanied by a fever over 101.5°F or if there is blood in the stool.

Who monitors the food supply for contamination?

Herein lies the problem—too many agencies have partial responsibility with no overall regulation, and no agency has food safety as its primary mission. There are 12 different agencies, operating under 35 health-related statutes, reporting to 28 House and Senate committees.

But this is changing. In 2007, Congress voted the FDA (Food and Drug Administration) a $10 million increase to improve food safety and appointed an Assistant Commissioner for Food Protection. Many feel this is not enough and more needs to be done. They are probably right. Congress needs to consider a complete reorganization of the U.S. food safety system.

Are cases of food poisoning on the rise?

Actually, we are seeing a continuing decline in foodborne illness because of better monitoring of the food supply and increased public awareness. The news media does a great job letting you know when there is a product recall or an outbreak. And today, the food industry responds very quickly and has put in place safe growing and processing practices to lower the overall risk of contamination. Each incidence makes us wiser about handling and eating food.

Back in the early 1980s, after many people got sick from undercooked hamburgers, the meat and poultry industry instituted safeguards to lower the chances of future contamination. The public was cautioned against eating rare meat or poultry. Many still do, but they do it knowing the risk they're taking. Some restaurant menus even carry warnings to customers who order rare meat.

Outbreaks of illness from drinking unpasteurized juice and cider resulted in a mandatory warning label to let shoppers know if the juice has not been pasteurized; 98% of our juice supply is. Knowing whether or not the cider you are buying from a local mill has been pasteurized allows you to make your own risk-benefit decision. Some feel unpasteurized juice has more healthful, living organisms, but it also has more unhealthy organisms.

Contaminated sprouts were causing a big problem not too long ago. But producers created stringent growing/handling guidelines, and there have been no headlines lately about sprouts making people sick.

More recently, we've been worried about fresh, raw

greens such as spinach. Once again the government and industry responded, first with a product recall, then with a public warning to temporarily avoid these foods, and third, with an investigation to determine the source of the contamination and prevent it in the future. The FDA has established guidelines that will be used to minimize future contamination of fresh-cut produce—bagged greens, salad mixes, peeled baby carrots, cut celery stalks, shredded cabbage, cut melons, sliced pineapple, and cup-up winter squash, to name just a few.

Are bagged greens causing more outbreaks?

No, only 6% of all foodborne illness comes from fresh produce, and bagged greens account for only a small fraction of that. The greens in the bag you buy can come from many different sources, so one bunch of contaminated spinach might wind up in many different batches, making more people sick. One contaminated leaf in many bags makes the problem more widespread.

These products undergo triple washing in chlorinated water. Additional washing at home is unnecessary and won't reduce the contamination that may have already occurred.

YOU SHOULD KNOW—

PulseNet

A network of government and public health laboratories, PulseNet helps to identify foodborne illness so that contaminated foods can be isolated and removed from supply lines and store shelves quickly.

What can I do to lower my risk of getting sick from fresh fruits and vegetables?

The prompt response by the government and industry is reassuring, but you can create the most effective "firewall" to protect yourself since most foodborne illness comes from improper handling, storage, or preparation at home. Let's look at ways to keep fresh fruits and vegetables safe.

Buying fresh fruits and vegetables

- Don't buy bruised or damaged produce.
- Buy only fresh-cut produce—half a watermelon or bagged salad greens—that is covered and refrigerated or surrounded by ice.
- Bag fresh produce separately from meat, fish, or poultry for the trip home.

Storing fresh fruits and vegetables:

- Keep them in a clean refrigerator at a temperature of 40°F or slightly below.
- Cover and refrigerate all precut or peeled produce.
- Don't put meat, fish, or poultry on open shelves above fresh produce—it might drip.

Preparing fresh fruits and vegetables:

- Wash your hands with soap and water.
- Cut away damaged or bruised areas before preparing.
- Thoroughly wash all produce before eating, including regular or organically grown—

exceptions are prewashed bagged produce. Use a vegetable brush and running water; soap or vegetable washes aren't necessary.

- Wash produce—cucumbers, apples, melons— even if you plan to peel them; bacteria on the skin can be transferred to the flesh during cutting.
- Drying washed produce with a clean paper towel further reduces bacteria.

YOU SHOULD KNOW—

Don't Let Your Guard Down

6% rarely or never wash fresh fruits and vegetables.
35% never wash fresh melons.
Over 50% never wash their hands before or after handling fresh produce.

Can irradiation make food safer?

Irradiation is a method of treating foods with gamma rays, X-rays, or high-energy electron beams to reduce the amount of harmful bacteria, mold, and insects. It does not make the food radioactive, but it reduces the need for harmful pesticides. Irradiation is used in more than 50 countries on over 40 different foods, and over the past 40 years has been proven safe. Astronauts and immune-compromised hospital patients eat irradiated food to protect them from foodborne illness. Irradiation at higher doses than those used on foods is used to sterilize hospital instruments, toothbrushes, and adhesive bandages.

You won't see many irradiated foods in the marketplace because of the negative public perception. Some exceptions are papayas from Hawaii, which are irradiated to kill fruit flies and their eggs, and spices, many of which have been irradiated for decades.

I saw an ad for a food storage container with silver nanoparticles. Do they work, and are they safe?

You are looking at a product of *nanotechnology*—small particles with big possibilities. Silver has been imbedded in these food storage containers to kill bacteria, fungi, molds, and possibly viruses, and to help fruits and vegetables stay fresher longer. The boxes aren't harmful because the silver can't migrate out of the plastic into your food. But most of us won't be rushing out to buy these new plastic storage boxes because of the price. The more important question is, how long do you want your broccoli to last?

Nanotechnology is a cutting-edge science that manipulates atoms and molecules to make *nanoparticles* that are assembled into materials, devices, or systems with desirable characteristics. Many of these new nanoproducts will have food applications. Nanosensors embedded in food packaging could alert you to the presence of bacteria, or active packaging could absorb oxygen and keep foods fresher longer. Nanoparticles could customize a functional food specific to an individual's needs or health condition. Plastics embedded with silver nanoparticles are already being used to germproof toys, air fresheners, shoe liners, washing machines, and refrigerators.

OIL YOU NEED TO KNOW

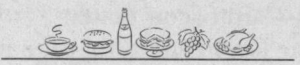

Oils are 100% fat.

Some thoughts to consider when it comes to fats and oil:

- Fats add flavor and satisfaction to eating.
- Not all fats are bad for you.
- Eat more monounsaturated fats; eat moderate amounts of polyunsaturated fats; eat small amounts of saturated (animal fats); avoid trans fat.
- A moderate amount of fats and oils should be part of a healthy diet.

For more information on fats in food, see pages 118 to 123.

You may feel like you need a chemistry degree to select the right oil from the ever-growing selection in the grocery store. Let's try to make this simple.

Oily Facts

- All varieties of oil have 120 calories in a tablespoon.
- All salad or cooking oils are from vegetable, nut, or seed sources; unidentified vegetable oils are usually from soybeans.

- All oils have 14 grams of fat per tablespoon and are mixtures of saturated, polyunsaturated, and monounsaturated fats.
- All oils are lower in unhealthy saturated fats than animal fats—lard, bacon, butter.
- Most oils are low in unhealthy saturated fats—exceptions are coconut, palm kernel, and palm oil, also called tropical oils.
- Many oils are high in healthy polyunsaturated fats—corn, cottonseed, grapeseed, poppyseed, safflower, soybean, sunflower, walnut, and wheat germ.
- Many oils are high in healthy monounsaturated fats—almond, avocado, canola, hazelnut, and olive.
- Some oils have an almost equal amount of polyunsaturated and monounsaturated fats—peanut, rice bran, and sesame.
- All liquid oils are trans fat free.

Is cold-pressed oil better?

Normal removal of oil from a plant involves pressing, heating, and treating with a solvent, usually hexane. No trace of the solvent is allowed in the finished oil. The process is similar to filtering water to get rid of dirt and bacteria. The plant is pressed to extract the oil, and the oil is then heated and treated with a solvent to get rid of plant residue. Cold-pressed oils don't go through a chemical extraction process, and little or no heat is used during the oil pressing process.

Cold-pressed oils have a reputation for being superior to normally processed oils. From a nutrition standpoint, that's not true. They may have a more robust flavor, however.

Which olive oil should I buy?

Virgin, extra virgin, light, Italian, Californian, Spanish, or flavor infused are all types of olive oil you can buy. Nutritionally, all varieties are rich in heart-healthy monounsaturated fats. The rest depends on the color and flavor you choose or how you intend to use the oil.

All extra virgin and virgin olive oil is cold or mechanically pressed, without heat or chemical solvents. Extra virgin comes from the first pressing of the olives and has the most distinct flavor. Virgin is similar but may have a less pungent flavor. Pure olive oil is produced from further pressings, is refined, and is made more flavorful by adding back a small amount of virgin or extra virgin to perk it up. Light or extra light olive oil refers to color and flavor, not fat or calories. It is a refined oil with reduced flavor and color, producing a blander olive oil. It is often used for baking.

Spain is the largest producer of olive oil in the world. California produces about 1% of all the olive oil used in the U.S. Most bottles don't list the country of origin; they just tell you where the oil was bottled or from where it was imported. Much of the Italian olive oil we use was actually produced in Spain, shipped to Italy in bulk, bottled and labeled in Italy, and then sold.

Is it true that there is a brand of oil with fat we don't absorb?

Yes. The oil is patented under the name Enova and is a blend of canola and soybean oil, manipulated so you absorb less fat. It is high in diglycerides (DAG), which the body does not absorb efficiently, and low in triglycerides (TAG), which we do absorb. Studies done on Enova show that most of the DAG slides through the intestinal tract unabsorbed. It has a bland flavor and can be used as a substitute for other oils, but it is more expensive.

How is margarine made from oil?

To harden liquid oils into margarine, the oils are sprayed with hydrogen, a process called *hydrogenation*. The hydrogen fills up or saturates the polyunsaturated oil and makes the oil hard or solid. During this process, some of the fat turns into trans fat, a fat that is twisted into an unusual shape and acts more like a saturated fat in your body. Stick margarines are more completely hydrogenated than whipped margarines.

Trans fat is listed on the nutrition label. Select margarine brands with "0" trans fat because you should eat as little as possible. For more information on trans fat, see pages 122 to 123.

How are solid shortenings made?

The original solid shortenings were butter or lard, until Crisco was introduced in 1911. It is produced in the same way as margarine, by hardening liquid oil with extra hydrogen. Solid shortenings fell out of favor once trans fats began getting bad press.

To solve the problem, companies producing solid shortening began to fully hydrogenate vegetable oil to avoid trans fat formation. The resulting oils are as solid as candle wax and need to be softened to shortening consistency by mixing back some liquid oil. Though fully hydrogenated oils become saturated fats, using the right oils in the conversion creates fats that are not as unhealthy as saturated animal fats, and they are trans fat free.

What's in nonstick cooking sprays?

These are usually canola or olive oil, atomized and mixed with a propellant to deliver a fine spray. Some are flavored, or mixed with flour to coat baking pans. Using them means using less oil than you would when pouring liquid oils or spreading solid shortenings like margarine or butter. If you'd rather not use a product with a propellant, you can buy an oil atomizer or simply use a spray bottle filled with oil to coat pans. Both of these will deliver slightly more oil per spray than the commercial sprays.

SECONDS COUNT—

Nonstick cooking sprays list "0" calories for a ⅓-second spray.

It takes 1 second or longer to cover a 10-inch pan.

A 1-second spray = 5 to 7 calories—less than 1 tablespoon of oil with 120 calories—but still, seconds count.

SHELF BY SHELF, ROW BY ROW— CONVENIENCE FOODS

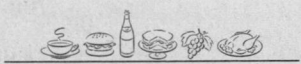

Some things to consider when it comes to convenience foods:

- Convenience foods—frozen, canned, shelf stable—come and go.
- Thousands are introduced each year and many disappear from shelves.
- Knowing how to evaluate the ingredients and use the nutrition label, you can decide for yourself which to buy and which to leave in the store.
- Voting with your buying power makes manufacturers produce the foods you want.

Frozen, canned, shelf stable—all of us buy and eat convenience foods of varying types. They can be organic or not, vegetarian, vegan, sugar free, gluten free, lactose free, trans fat free, lowfat or low calorie, or they can include full-fat ice cream, frozen tiramisu, and fettuccine Alfredo, loaded with saturated fat.

To get through the supermarket aisles, you need to take into account your individual philosophy of eating and your health needs. Do you eat mostly organic foods? Do you try to eat more plant-based products and less meat and poultry? Are you concerned about a food allergy? Are you trying to reduce fat or cholesterol? You shop for food based on these individual choices, but the choices are getting more confusing daily.

In the hope of educating shoppers about good food, there is an avalanche of healthy-eating programs popping up on store shelves and food labels. Take A Peak—an effort by the federal government, food manufacturers, and supermarket chains—is bringing the food guide pyramid to supermarket aisles. The American Heart Association allows low saturated fat, low cholesterol foods to display its heart-check symbol. The Whole Grains Council has developed a stamp to highlight good and excellent sources of whole grain foods. Individual supermarket chains are developing nutrition-friendly, in-store education programs to help you make the best choices while shopping. And major food producers, who have been accused of promoting unhealthy foods, have reformulated entire brand lines and refocused their marketing efforts toward good-for-you choices. Each company has a tag line—*Sensible Solutions, Smart Spot, Goodness Corner*—to identify these healthier options.

Instead of making food selection easier, the sheer number of these programs, stamps, seals, and promotional logos can leave you more confused. Each has been developed based on its own criteria, with no common message linking them except "make healthy food choices." Until a unified national food rating system is developed, you have to rely on what is already available.

Every food in the U.S., both imported and domestic, that is larger than a LifeSavers roll and has a food label, must display an ingredient listing and a nutrition facts panel, more commonly known as the nutrition label. Understanding and using these effectively helps you make healthy food choices.

Ingredient Listing

Ingredients are listed on labels in descending order by volume. The first ingredient is found in the largest amount, and the last ingredient in the least amount. If a food lists the first ingredient as sugar, that's a red flag. If the first ingredient is whole wheat flour, that's a totally different thing. The ingredient list can tell you a great deal. If you prefer to eat fewer additives, note how many are listed on the food you've picked. If you are trying to avoid high fructose corn syrup, see if it is listed. If you are on the lookout for allergens, the ingredient listing can help you with that, too.

Food Allergy Labeling

In compliance with the Food Allergen Labeling and Consumer Protection Act of 2004, all foods with a label sold in the U.S., even imported products, must inform you if the food contains one of the following major food allergens:

- Milk
- Egg
- Fish
- Shellfish—refers only to crab, lobster, or shrimp, which must be declared on the label (oysters, clams, mussels, and scallops are not included)
- Tree nuts—the specific type of nut must be declared on the label
- Wheat
- Peanuts

- Soybeans—soy or soya are acceptable alternative terms for soy-containing ingredients

These 8 foods account for 90% of all food allergies. Although other foods may cause a reaction in sensitive people, those ingredients are not covered under the allergy labeling law and are not required to be listed.

A "Contains" statement is required on the label immediately after or next to the ingredient listing. It must be in the same typeface and type size as the ingredient list so that it is obvious to the consumer. For example: "Contains milk, egg, peanuts." or "Contains shrimp."

Nutrition Facts Panel

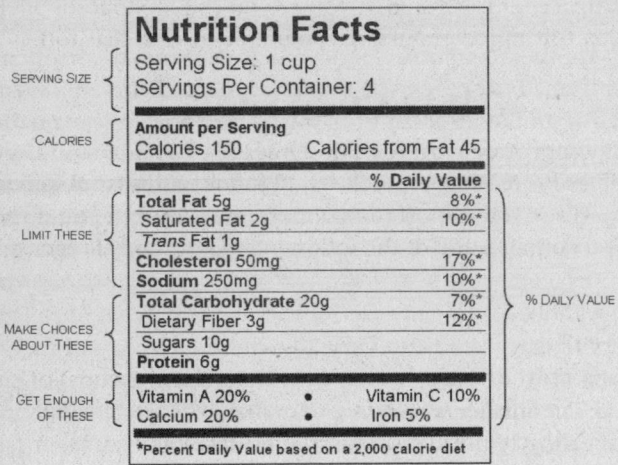

The Nutrition Facts Panel is chock-full of valuable information, but few use it effectively because it can appear complicated and confusing. Let's divide the label into 6 sections: serving size, calories, limit these, make choices about these, get enough of these, and % Daily Value (%DV). At first our sections may seem unusual, but bear with us and I think you'll see they do make sense. Look at the sample Nutrition Facts Panel as we break it down into manageable sections.

Serving Size

This one is a biggy—no pun intended. There is the serving size listed on the package, there is a standard serving size, which could be slightly smaller or larger, and there is the amount you eat. If the serving of organic, unsalted, baked potato chips is 1 ounce or 15 chips, it doesn't matter how healthy the chips are if you decide to eat the entire bag. And how many of us count out 15 chips or weigh an ounce before we dig into the bag?

Another common distortion of serving size happens with small packages. You might buy a candy bar or a small bag of sunflower seeds thinking it's one portion, but on the nutrition label a serving may be defined as only 3 squares of the candy bar or 2 tablespoons of the sunflower seeds. Once you've opened the package, are you really going to eat just the serving size listed on the label?

Servings are often unrealistically small in comparison to what you'll actually eat. A classic example is cereal. The serving size listed can vary anywhere from ½ cup to 1½ cups. Most of us eat a soup bowl full (about 2 cups) of cereal. The smaller serving size can make the food look more appealing because it seems to have less calories, sugar, fat, or sodium. And it does—*if* you eat the small amount.

Before you go any further with the nutrition label, look at the package, look at the serving size, and decide how much of the package you are going to eat. If the serving size is 1 cup and you are only going to eat 1 cup—fine. But if you know you'll be eating 2 cups or even more, you need to consider that when you look at the rest of the information.

We haven't said anything about Servings Per Container because, quite frankly, this information is usually meaningless. If the serving size is unrealistically small, the amount of servings per container has little meaning. If you eat more than 1 cup of cereal at a time, does it matter that the box says Servings Per Container 14? The amount you usually eat is all that counts.

Calories and Calories from Fat

Two calorie values are given. The first is the number of calories in one serving. Remember, if you eat more than a serving, the calorie value multiplies! The second value is Calories from Fat. This is the number of calories in one serving that comes from fat.

Calories come from protein, carbohydrate, and fat. Protein and carbohydrate have 4 calories per gram. But fat is far more calorie dense, with 9 calories per gram. If you multiply the Total Fat grams times 9, you should come up with the same number as Calories from Fat. The number may be slightly off due to rounding, but you'll be very close. You can break this down even further. If you want to know how many calories come from saturated fat, which you should try to limit, multiply the grams of saturated fat times 9. Saturated, trans fat, polyunsaturated, and monounsaturated fats are all types of fat, so they all have 9 calories per gram.

As for Total Carbohydrate or Protein, multiply either of these by 4 and you'll know how many of the calories in a serving come from carbohydrate or protein, respectively. Again, you can take this further and multiply the grams of sugar times 4 to find out how many calories come from sugar. Sugar is simply a type of carbohydrate, so it, too, has 4 calories per gram.

YOU SHOULD KNOW—

If one serving of a food equals

40 calories or less, it is a low calorie food
100 calories—it is a moderate calorie food
400 or more calories—it is a high calorie food

This shortcut can help you make a quick decision about a food without doing math.

Limit These—Fat, Cholesterol, Sodium

This is the group of nutrients you want to eat less of—less fat, less saturated fat, less trans fat, less cholesterol, and less sodium. Cutting down on these nutrients reduces your risk for high blood pressure, heart disease, stroke, and some cancers. Okay, so what are you aiming for when we say "less"?

For fat, the labeling recommendation is for less than 65 grams of total fat daily for those eating 2,000 calories. Many of us eat far less and some of us eat more. So how do you individualize this number for yourself? First, you can use the labeling recommendation as a gross benchmark.

If you would like to be more specific, consider that most health experts feel we should be eating no more than 30% to 35% of our daily calorie intake as fat. If you have a medical condition, your doctor may have made another recommendation, perhaps even lower. Regardless, the math is the same:

Step 1: Total calories per day X % fat = fat calories per day

Step 2: Fat calories ÷ 9 = fat grams per day

If you eat 1,800 calories a day:

Step 1: 1,800 X 30% = 540 fat calories per day.

Step 2: 540 fat calories ÷ 9 = 60 fat grams per day

This example shows you that the label recommendation of 65 grams of fat per day at 2,000 calories is slightly higher than the amount needed at 1,800 calories. Over time, this could add up to extra weight gain.

YOU SHOULD KNOW—

About Finding Cholesterol in Food

If a food grows in the ground, it has no cholesterol.
If a food has a face, its original source was an animal and it has cholesterol.

The recommendation for cholesterol is a little easier. Everyone is encouraged to eat fewer than 300 milligrams a day.

Now you can look at the values from 1 serving and see if the food is high in fat and cholesterol, and decide whether to buy it or eat it. Eating any food once in a while is fine. But regularly eating foods high in fat and cholesterol isn't a healthy choice.

Saturated, Trans, Polyunsaturated, and Monounsaturated Fat

Under the total fat value you will see values for saturated fat and trans fat. Both are required by law. Some manufacturers include values for monounsaturated fat and polyunsaturated fat, too. So how do you sort out fat?

We've already dealt with total fat above. Saturated, monounsaturated, polyunsaturated, and trans fat all make up portions of total fat. Each has 9 calories per gram. To find out how many calories are coming from a particular type of fat, simply multiply the grams times 9. If the food has 15 grams of saturated fat, 135 calories (15 X 9 = 135) are from saturated fat.

Within your fat allowance for the day, you want to eat more monounsaturated and polyunsaturated fats, less saturated fat, and little or no trans fat.

FOOD SOURCES OF DIFFERENT FATS

Type of Fat	Foods	Health Effects
Monounsaturated fats	Olive oil, canola oil, peanut oil, avocados, olives, cashews, peanuts, hazelnuts, macadamia nuts, pine nuts, pistachios, chicken fat	Reduce cholesterol Reduce triglycerides Reduce blood pressure Help control diabetes
Polyunsaturated fats (omega-6)	Safflower oil, sesame oil, soybean oil, corn oil, sunflower oil, nuts, seeds, soybeans, soft margarine	Reduce cholesterol Reduce heart disease risk

Type of Fat	Foods	Health Effects
Polyunsaturated fats (omega-3)	Canola oil, flaxseeds, soybean oil, walnut oil, walnuts, hempseeds, salmon, mackerel, tuna, trout, sardines, herring	Reduce triglycerides Improve immune function Reduce inflammatory diseases Protect against sudden death from heart disease Reduce tumor growth
Saturated fats	Meat, whole milk, cream, ice cream, cheese, butter, lard, palm oil, palm kernel oil, coconut, coconut oil, cocoa butter, poultry, bacon, sour cream	Raise cholesterol Increase heart disease risk Increase stroke risk May increase cancer risk
Trans fats	Cookies, crackers, cakes, pastries, shortening, stick margarine, deep-fried foods (french fries, doughnuts), partially hydrogenated oils, hydrogenated vegetable oils	Raise cholesterol Lower good HDL cholesterol Raise bad LDL cholesterol Increase heart disease risk

For more information on fats and oils in foods, go to pages 108 to 112.

Troubling Trans Fat

Many experts feel trans fat is a greater health risk than saturated fat. The good news is that you don't have to eat trans fat, and trans fat values must be listed on nutrition labels.

Almost all the trans fat found in our foods is created by passing hydrogen gas through vegetable oil, a process called *hydrogenation.* Hydrogenated fats and partially hydrogenated fats are more stable for deep-frying and are more solid, so they work well in baking and as the base for stick margarines. You'll find the most trans fat in baked goods and fried foods. It's estimated that we eat 12% to 14% of our daily calories as saturated fat, but only 1.5% to 2.5% as trans fat. Cutting down on or eliminating foods with trans fats will not eliminate any important nutrients from your diet. In fact, it may help you cut back on less healthy choices, like french fries and cakes.

Making Sense of Sodium

Nutrition labels are based on a maximum intake of 2,400 milligrams of sodium a day for the average adult. Many experts feel 1,500 milligrams a day for adults and even fewer for older adults (1,200 milligrams) would be healthier levels to aim for. In fact, most of us would do nicely on as little as 500 milligrams of sodium a day. That may be a healthy level, but would we consider this a tasty level? Giving up salt isn't easy.

When people are told to eat less sodium, their first reaction is to empty the saltshaker and stop adding salt in cooking. This may not be the most effective approach, because your daily sodium intake actually comes from

Salt and **sodium-containing food additives** added in food processing	77%
Sodium naturally occurring in food	12%
Salt added in cooking and at the table	11%

Dumping the saltshaker only reduces your salt intake slightly. Cutting down on convenience foods will make a bigger dent in your daily sodium intake.

Lighten Up on Salt

- Check the nutrition label—keep snacks and individual foods under 400 milligrams a serving; keep main dishes under 600 milligrams a serving.
- Try some "low sodium" or "no salt added" choices; you might be surprised at the taste.
- Fresh salads are naturally low in sodium; just go easy on the dressing.
- Plain frozen vegetables are lower in sodium than sauced and seasoned varieties.
- Almost all frozen vegetables are lower in sodium than canned vegetables.
- Try unsalted baldy pretzels and unsalted nuts.
- Don't add salt when cooking rice, pasta, or hot cereal.
- When you eat a high-salt/sodium choice, balance it with lower-sodium choices later in the day.

You Decide—About Carbohydrate and Protein

The amount of carbohydrate and protein you should eat depends on how you divide your calories for the day. Carb values can be as low as 30% of daily calories and as high as 70%. Protein usually stays between 10% and 20% of daily calories.

Total Carbs and Fiber

Like the section on fat, the label section on carbohydrates contains a good deal of information, but not everyone knows how to make good use of it.

Total carbohydrates are just that: the sum of all the complex carbohydrates (starch), fiber, and sugar in one serving of food. Starch and sugar can be burned for energy (calories) and both contain 4 calories per gram. Fiber has few if any calories and most passes through the digestive tract undigested. Fiber has no calories, but it has value. It helps to lower cholesterol and keeps your bowel healthy by promoting regularity.

We are generally told to eat more fiber and less sugar. Good advice. Fiber can be divided into two types, insoluble and soluble, and some labels reflect this difference. Insoluble fiber is the woody part of plants that helps promote regularity, and soluble fibers are gums and mucilages that help lower cholesterol. Most plants contain both, and many experts no longer feel the 2 categories are necessary. The total amount of fiber you eat each day is far more important than the specific type. For more information on fiber, see pages 157 to 160.

Sugar

The sugar value listed on the nutrition label is a little more confusing because it lumps together natural sugar and added sugar.

Grains, fruits, vegetables, milk, and plain yogurt all contain sugars. These are *natural* sugars and the foods come packaged with vitamins, minerals, and fiber, too. In contrast, soda, candy, fruit drinks, cakes, cookies, ice cream, jelly, and syrup offer little more than sweetness and calories, and are loaded with *added sugar.*

You can't rely on the nutrition label to distinguish between natural sugar and added sugar, but the difference is significant. The nutrition label on a quart of milk tells you that one cup has 14 grams of sugar; all of it is from naturally occurring *lactose,* or milk sugar. The label on fruit punch tells you that the same size serving has 30 grams of sugar, but almost all of that is from added sugar. How can you tell natural sugars from added sugars? Check the ingredients listing for the terms below. Ingredients on a label are listed in descending order by volume, so those ingredients listed closest to the beginning will contribute larger amounts to each serving of food.

SUGAR BY ANY OTHER NAME	
Barley malt	Honey
Beet juice	Invert sugar
Brown rice syrup	Malt syrup
Brown sugar	Maltodextrin
Cane syrup	Maple sugar
Corn sweetener	Maple syrup
Corn syrup	Molasses
Crystalline fructose	Muscavado
Dextrose	Raw sugar
Evaporated cane juice	Sorghum
Fruit juice concentrate	Sucrose
Fructose	Sugar in the raw
High fructose corn syrup (HFCS)	Turbinado

How much sugar is too much?

Americans eat 15% to 21% of their daily calories as sugar, with teenagers eating the most. The sugar itself isn't the only problem—again and again, studies have shown that as sugar intake goes up, vitamin and mineral intake goes down. We should all be eating less sugar, but there is no specific recommendation on how much to eat every day. The U.S. Dietary Reference Intakes make no specific recommendation for the amount of sugar to eat daily. It only suggests that you eat no more than 25% of your daily calories from added sugar. Obviously, people should eat less. The World Health Organization (WHO) has suggested limiting added sugars to no more than 10% of total calories, though some experts feel this amount is unrealistically low.

Without clear-cut recommendations, you need to decide for yourself how much sugar to eat. We suggest attempting to eat closer to 10% total calories as sugar, keeping in mind the 25% recommendation as the healthy upper limit.

If you eat 1,800 calories a day:

10% of 1,800 calories = 180 sugar calories per day

or

25% of 1,800 calories = 450 sugar calories per day

To figure out how many grams of sugar to eat each day, you need to know that 1 gram of sugar = 4 calories. Continuing to use the example above:

180 (10%) sugar calories per day ÷ 4 = 45 grams of sugar per day

or

450 (25%) sugar calories per day ÷ 4 = 113 grams of sugar per day

To make good sugar choices, choose foods containing natural sugars more often, choosing foods with added sugars less often.

On some labels, manufacturers also list sugar alcohols. They appear in the ingredients listing with names that end in *-ol:* mannitol, sorbitol, and xylitol. Sugar alcohols are sugar substitutes that add sweetness with fewer calories than sugar. Most sugar alcohols average 2 calories per gram; remember, sugar has 4 calories per gram.

Net Carbs

If the food label lists "net carbs" or "net effective carbs," this value was determined by subtracting the fiber and sugar alcohols from the total carb value. Your body does not digest fiber, so it provides no calories and can be subtracted from the total carbohydrate value. But subtracting sugar alcohols to arrive at "net carbs" is more creative math than sound science. Sugar alcohols do have calories (slightly less than sugar, but calories nonetheless), so subtracting them from total carbs is a little like cheating on a math test.

Protein

Your body loses millions of cells each day. They are used up, worn out, rubbed off, and even cut off, like your beard or fingernails. You need a source of protein to replace these lost cells.

When your body is stressed physically, more protein is used. When it's too hot or too cold, you need extra protein. Protein is needed to replace nitrogen lost during heavy sweating. Exercise, fever, surgery, injury, infection, and broken bones all increase your need for protein. Even emotional stress, such as losing your job or taking an exam, causes protein loss.

But protein is so plentiful in our diets, there is no concern about getting enough. Even if you are a vegetarian, you get ample protein because grains, beans, and vegetables contain protein, too. So protein is listed on the nutrition label, but no specific recommendation is made.

A quick way to estimate your daily protein need is to divide your weight by 2.2. For example, if you weigh 150 pounds, you should be eating 68 grams of protein a day.

150 pounds ÷ 2.2 = 68 grams of protein

It's estimated that many of us get more than twice the recommended amount of protein daily.

Why are beans in the protein group?

Beans are unique because they are like both vegetables and meat. They have vitamins, minerals, and phytochemicals like vegetables, but they are also high in protein, like meat. Nuts fit in the protein group for the same reason.

One ounce of protein is equal to ½ cup cooked beans or tofu, ¼ cup nuts, or 2 tablespoons of nut butter. For more information on beans, see pages 31 to 38. For more information on nuts, see pages 39 to 43.

SMART STUFF—

Top 10 Sources

Americans get most of their protein from beef, poultry, milk, yeast bread, cheese, fish, eggs, pork, ham, and pasta.

Get Enough of These—
Vitamin A, Vitamin C, Calcium, Iron

Though Americans eat a lot of calories, we often don't get enough vitamins and minerals. The nutrition label is required to list the values for vitamin A, vitamin C, calcium, and iron, but many companies provide more extensive listings. Almost all cereal brands and many natural and organic brands offer more information.

Even if they don't, the listings for these four nutrients give you an idea of whether the food is contributing micronutrients (vitamins and minerals) in addition to macronutrients (protein, fat, and carbohydrates).

Vitamins and minerals do not provide calories, and the body uses them in very small amounts. But they're still very important. They help you burn calories, build bones and tissues, and regulate the body's normal functions. Each one plays a vital role in health. They do most of their work inside cells, helping each other get a job done. You can think of them as a construction crew. Every member of the crew has a specialty—carpenter, electrician, plumber, mason—and their collective efforts build a house. The collective effort of vitamins and minerals keeps your body running smoothly.

In this book we provide values for 3 vitamins: vitamin A, vitamin C, and folic acid; and three minerals: calcium, iron, and potassium. See Looking at Vitamins and Minerals, pages 161 to 181, for more information.

% Daily Value

The % Daily Value (%DV) allows you to compare the contribution of the food you are eating to the amount you should be eating for the entire day. If the %DV for calcium is 20%, you know that you are getting 20% of your total calcium for the day by eating one serving of the food. That's the good news. The bad news is that %DV is based on a 2,000-calorie intake. As we've said before, many of us eat less, and some eat more.

You can use the %DV as a general estimate to determine if a food is rich in a nutrient. If the %DV is high for fat, saturated fat, cholesterol, or sodium, you may want to make another choice or keep your portions reasonable.

Some nutrients, like trans fat, sugar, and protein, do not have Daily Values because there isn't enough information available to set a recommendation.

DAILY VALUES USED ON NUTRITION LABELS*

Nutrient	Daily Value	Unit of Measure
Total fat	65	grams (g)
Saturated fat	20	grams (g)
Cholesterol	300	milligrams (mg)
Total Carbohydrate	300	grams (g)
Fiber	25	grams (g)
Vitamin A	5,000	International Units (IU)
Vitamin C	60	milligrams (mg)
Thiamin (B_1)	1.5	milligrams (mg)
Riboflavin (B_2)	1.7	milligrams (mg)
Niacin (B_3)	20	milligrams (mg)
Vitamin B_6 (pyridoxine)	2	milligrams (mg)
Vitamin B_{12} (cobalamin)	6	micrograms (mcg)
Sodium	2,400	milligrams (mg)
Potassium	3,500	milligrams (mg)
Calcium	1,000	milligrams (mg)
Iron	18	milligrams (mg)
Phosphorus	1,000	milligrams (mg)
Magnesium	400	milligrams (mg)
Zinc	15	milligrams (mg)

* Based on a 2,000-calorie intake for adults and children over the age of 4.

When a product is labeled "natural," what does that mean?

There is no legal definition for this term. The FDA (Food and Drug Administration) only allows it to be used on products that contain no artificial or synthetic substances, including food additives and flavors. This would exclude most convenience foods. The USDA, which regulates meat and poultry, allows "natural" to appear on a label if the product doesn't contain any artificial ingredient or added color and is only minimally processed. All products using the term "natural" must explain what it means somewhere on the label. For example, "Does not contain artificial flavor."

TODAY, TOMORROW, NEXT WEEK—FOOD DATING

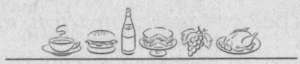

There is no uniform system of food dating in the U.S.

Almost every food you buy, even soda and water, comes with a date stamped on the package. Federal regulations only require baby food and baby formula to be dated. Twenty states have varying local rules, others have none. So what do package dates mean, and how much should you depend on them for freshness and quality?

Recent concerns about food safety have prompted many manufacturers to include "freshness dating" on packages, hence the dates on water and soda bottles. The purpose is to give the consumer a relative idea as to the age of the product, a variation on expiration dating. Shopping research has shown that in some cases this voluntary dating system is backfiring on sales. Shoppers won't buy foods that are close to the expiration date.

When asked to taste products near the end of their "dated" freshness life, consumers rated them as having poorer quality. This result was consistent whether the product was actually at the end of its freshness life, or if the researchers manipulated the date for the study. If people think a product is fresh, it tastes fresh to them. If they believe the product is not fresh, they rate the taste as poorer or stale, even when it's not.

Because dating systems vary depending on where you live and on food type, here are some tips to insure the safety and quality of foods.

- Buy foods before their *expiration, use by,* or *sell by* dates.
- Use foods by their recommended *use before* date.
- Once defrosted, use the food within 3 days regardless of the date.
- If a food is kept frozen, it is safe to eat even if the date expires.
- Every 6 months, check for "lost" items pushed to the back of your cupboard.
- All foods will lose freshness or spoil if stored improperly. Keep cold foods cold and dry foods dry.

Deciphering Dates

"Best If Used By" or **"Use Before"** are variations of freshness dating. They're found on cereal boxes, crackers, mayonnaise, and shelf-stable foods. This is not a safety date but the manufacturer's recommended time span for best flavor or quality. If the product is stored properly, eating it after the "use before" date is not an issue. A few weeks past the date is fine. If the "use before" date is months or even years past because the item landed in the back of the cupboard, throw it away.

"Use By" refers to the date after which the products will lose peak quality. Again, this is the manufacturer's recommendation. You'll find these dates on cream cheese, prepared puddings, cottage cheese, yogurt, and eggs. If stored correctly, most of these foods are completely safe to eat for a time after the date. If "Use By May 27" is stamped on a carton of eggs, you can safely use the eggs for 3 to 5 weeks after that date.

"Sell By" is a date that tells a store how long to keep a food on the shelf for sale. Bread, milk, meat, poultry, and cheese frequently have "sell by" dates. These may be a local regulation or a freshness date set by the manufacturer.

What do the number series on food packages mean?

Many foods, especially cans, jars, and boxes, display closed or coded dates. They may be a series of letters, numbers, dates and/or times, such as: 1566 12:00 PM 0F00/24/07. Regardless of what urban myth you may have heard, these are individual to the food producers and there is no universal system for decoding the numbers. They are not meant for consumer use, but as a tool for distribution, stock rotation, and in the event of a product recall.

BOTTLES, CUPS, CANS—BEVERAGES

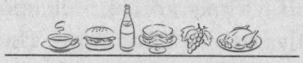

One out of every 5 calories you consume is liquid.

Americans drink an average of 3 cups of coffee a day. Our soda intake outstrips that of milk. Energy drinks are one of the fastest growing food items. And then there are the ubiquitous bottles of water we carry around.

Approximately 13% of all drinks consumed in the U.S. are alcoholic. The remaining 87% are: 28% soda, 11% bottled water, 11% milk, 9% coffee, 5% fruit drinks, and 4% tea. What's left over, the "other" category, is made up of sports drinks, vegetable juice, powdered drinks, and tap water.

We aren't going to try to encourage or to discourage you from drinking your favorite beverage. We are simply going to look at some of the issues so you can make your own decisions.

Beware of Calories in a Glass

Liquid calories may be making you fat. In fact, they may be making the entire country fat, because we don't register the calories we drink as accurately as those we chew. The two real troublemakers are alcoholic drinks and clear liquids.

Alcoholic drinks can be very calorie dense. In addition, when drunk before a meal, alcohol increases hunger while decreasing satisfaction. Some studies have shown that when alcoholic drinks are added to a meal, the calorie intake can go up as much as 40%.

Calorie-containing clear drinks—soda, fruit drinks, energy drinks, sports drinks, coffee, and tea—all have a very low satisfaction value. And the more you are offered, the more you drink. Up to 20% of our daily calories come from these, with soda being the single largest source of calories in the U.S. diet, contributing close to 300 calories daily. Interestingly, as we've consumed more calorie-containing clear drinks over the past 3 decades, there has been a sharp rise in weight gain, too.

At the same time, the portion sizes have increased. We went from an 8-ounce bottle of Coke to unlimited soda refills served in a quart-sized container. A small coffee has grown from 6 to 10 ounces. Add cream and sugar, and your small coffee equals 100 calories. And few of us ever order "small."

How much water should I drink each day?

You may have heard the 8 X 8 rule—drink 8 servings of 8 ounces each day. It sounds good, but there is no foundation for this recommendation and no scientific evidence to support it. It can go down as another urban myth.

There is no question that you do need water every day. How much? Physiologically, the answer is based on your calorie need—1 milliliter of water for each calorie. If you need 1,800 calories a day, you also need 1,800 milliliters of water. Translated into cups: 1 cup = 240 milliliters.

$$1,800 \div 240 = 7.5 \text{ cups per day}$$

But these 7½ cups a day don't all have to be water. Solid food contains a lot of water; you get 3 to 4 cups a day from food. Other liquids like juice and soup count, too. If you drink caffeinated beverages—tea, coffee, soda, energy drinks—you can count only half of your intake toward your daily fluid, since the caffeine acts as a diuretic, causing you to lose some of the water. In many cases, you can meet your fluid requirement without extra water. The exceptions would be during extremely hot weather or heavy exercise, when you need more fluids.

Drinking some water daily is a good habit. Water is calorie free and contains calcium, magnesium, and fluoride.

Should I drink bottled water?

From a nutrition standpoint, there is no advantage—water is water, as long as it is clean. But you might like the convenience, flavor, or natural carbonation of some bottled water.

Bottled water is regulated for purity. Most bottlers belong to the International Bottled Water Association. However, there are no regulations for enhancing bottled water and no oversight for some of the claims being made. Do you need vitamin- or herb-enhanced water? Should you be paying a premium price for these minuscule additions? Does your water need to travel thousands of miles before you drink it? Do you know that the sweeteners many producers put in bottled water are to mask the bitter taste of the added nutrients? If the mild taste of flavored water gets you to drink more, or if you use it in place of higher-calorie fruit drinks or soda, that's great. Paying for water with add-ons is your choice, but it may not be the best investment you'll ever make.

Bottom line: Plain or calorie free flavored water is your best thirst quencher.

Is it unsafe to refill plastic water bottles?

There are a number of misconceptions swirling around the practice of refilling plastic water bottles. The plastic—polyethylene terephthalate (PET)—is safe and will not leach into the liquid. Bottles made from PET are widely used for everything from water to fruit juice to soft drinks—even beer and wine. Harmful substances are not formed if you freeze liquids in plastic bottles, either.

You can, however, get sick from bacteria if you refill plastic bottles without cleaning and drying them between uses. The bacteria doesn't come from the bottles, but from your hands or mouth. Single-use water bottles tend to have narrow necks, making it hard to clean or rinse them thoroughly. And residual soap left in the bottle can cause diarrhea.

Bottom line: If you want a reusable water bottle, buy one with a wide neck and clean it between uses.

Which type of juice is the best to buy?

Before we go any further, let's give you the classic advice—it is better to eat the whole fruit than drink the juice. Why? The fruit comes packaged with many beneficial substances that don't make it into juice. It takes longer to eat a piece of fruit, giving you a sense of satisfaction and fullness. And you process calories you drink differently than calories you chew.

Like many other areas of the supermarket, the juice aisle seems to grow weekly—fresh, frozen, refrigerated, bottled, and boxed; and fortified with vitamins, minerals, sterols, phytochemicals, and fiber. Not to mention organic, sweetened, unsweetened, artificially sweetened, and light varieties! The options can be mind-boggling.

How much juice is recommended daily? Experts say just 8 ounces, and it should be 100% juice. That means all the other bottles, cans, and boxes could be left in the store.

Bottom line: There is no nutritional reason to drink juice except for enjoyment.

YOU SHOULD KNOW—

Some Drugs and Juice Don't Mix

Antioxidant-rich pomegranate juice may sound like a good idea, but it can interfere with blood pressure medications, antidepressants, AIDS drugs, and some narcotic pain relievers. Grapefruit juice increases the potency of cholesterol-lowering statin drugs, which could cause dangerous side effects. If you take prescription drugs and drink juice regularly, check with your pharmacist for possible interactions.

What is the difference between fruit juice and fruit drinks?

Fruit beverages come in many variations—100% juice, drinks, ades, and punches. 100% juice is just that—juice with nothing added. It is always clearly stated on the label. No other fruit beverage can make that claim, though some do state the percentage of real fruit juice in the beverage. Drinks, ades, punches, and cocktails are always less than 100% juice, and in some cases there is no real fruit juice at all. Most are sweetened and many are fortified with extra nutrients or phytochemicals.

Vitamin C is the most common addition to juice drinks. Calcium is now being added to many varieties, as well as plant sterols to lower cholesterol, glucosamine to support healthy joints, and an entire medicine chest of vitamins and minerals. Do you need juice to provide these nutrients? This question goes back to your decision to use or not use functional foods. See pages 148 to 153. Can you be well fed without fortified juices? Without a doubt, yes. Are you better off not drinking sweetened fruit drinks? Absolutely!

Bottom line: Fruit-flavored beverages in small amounts are simply a tasty drink. Drinking them regularly in large amounts, especially for children, promotes a high sugar intake and may contribute to weight gain.

100% Juice Guidelines for Children*	
Amount Daily	**Age**
No juice	*Infants under 6 months*
4 to 6 ounces	*Over 6 months to 6 years***
8 to 12 ounces	*7 to 18 years*

* Source: American Academy of Pediatrics
** Juice should always be given in a cup, not a bottle.

Do energy drinks have value?

These products are so varied—sweetened, artificially sweetened, enhanced with caffeine or herbs, vitamin and mineral fortified, artificially colored and flavored, naturally flavored—that it's hard to give a conclusive answer. But there are a few things you should consider before opting to use energy drinks.

The FDA does not allow food to be marketed as medicine. But clear beverages are exempt and they can be marketed as *nutraceuticals*—hence the exploding market for energy drinks. They claim to increase physical endurance, improve reaction time, boost mental alertness, improve well-being, enhance stamina, and eliminate waste from the body. They are marketed as healthy, fun, and youthful. Since no one regulates them, there is no way to dispute these claims.

What we do know is that they should not be used by children, pregnant women, athletes, those with heart disease, or anyone sensitive to caffeine. All contain caffeine or another stimulant compound such as guarana, kola nut, or yerba maté. How much they contain is unclear, because there are no labeling rules for these ingredients.

We can tell how much sugar there is, because of mandatory nutrition labels, and it can be anywhere from 25% to 100% of the total calories in the can. Both caffeine and sugar are dehydrating, so energy drinks have a negative effect on sports performance.

Most contain some combination of B vitamins, and the quantities can be staggering. Mixing energy drinks with alcohol may be a recipe for disaster. Whether it's the herbal content or enhanced stimulants, people have been hospitalized and some have died after drinking these cocktails.

Bottom line: Think of energy drinks as soda with a jolt.

Is natural or organic soda a better choice than regular?

Soda is soda, with little or no nutrition value except for calories. It doesn't matter if the sugar used to sweeten it is organic or the flavoring agents are natural—when it displaces more nutritious choices, or even plain water, it is not the best beverage choice.

The link between soda and cavities is undisputed. The evidence linking excess intake of high fructose corn syrup and obesity is growing. And as soda intake goes up, bone mineral density goes down.

Experts recommend no soda for children and as little as 8 ounces a day for adults. Since the average intake in the U.S. is three cans a day, we have a long way to go quitting the soda habit.

Are diet sodas any better? They don't have calories, but now you need to decide if you want to use artificial sweeteners, usually saccharin or Equal. And there is some research showing that diet soda may cause you to eat more because your body is tricked into thinking it got calories when it didn't.

Bottom line: Soda fills you up with calories, but lets you down when it comes to all other nutrients.

Is coffee bad for me?

If you are a coffee drinker, there is no need to stop. Your morning coffee may actually be good for you.

More than half of us in the U.S. drink coffee daily, averaging slightly more than three cups, and another 25% drink coffee occasionally. Most of us get more antioxidants from coffee than from any other dietary source. Coffee has 4 times the antioxidant content of green tea and more antioxidants than red wine. If you didn't know, coffee is a fruit: the beans begin as a cluster of berries on the coffee tree.

Coffee is a complex beverage containing small amounts of many vitamins and minerals. Though not a major source of these, multiple cups daily contribute to our nutrient intake.

Coffee, or more specifically the caffeine it contains, can increase alertness and stimulate performance in high-intensity, short-duration activities such as sprinting. Drinking caffeinated coffee regularly is mildly addictive, and stopping abruptly causes headaches and other annoying symptoms. But the caffeine habit is very easy to break, and symptoms can be eliminated by reducing consumption gradually. Some people carry a gene for slow caffeine metabolism; for these unusually sensitive individuals, decaf is probably a better choice.

A number of studies have shown that for men and women who regularly drank coffee, there was a significantly decreased risk for type 2 diabetes. Men who drank 4 to 5 cups a day cut their risk for Parkinson's almost in half. Women who drank at least 2 cups of decaffeinated coffee a day had over a 50% lower incidence of rectal cancer. Japanese researchers found that those who drank coffee daily had half the incidence of liver cancer of those who never or almost never drank it. All of these conclusions were drawn from studies with large numbers of subjects, making the findings reliable. Some researchers think the high antioxidant activity of coffee helps to reduce inflammation, which may be the reason for heart disease reduction seen in coffee drinkers, though this evidence is still inconclusive.

There is no question, however, that coffee can worsen anxiety and cause heartburn. For those with either, limiting intake is wise. A switch to decaf can lessen anxiety, but both decaf and caffeinated coffee irritate gastric reflux (burping and heartburn). Pregnant women have long been cautioned to go easy on coffee, and that advice still stands. A small cup or two a day is fine, but more is not wise. Heavy consumption has been linked to lower birth weight and miscarriage. Coffee has also been implicated in raising cholesterol levels, but this only occurs when the coffee is boiled and unfiltered, or made by the French press method. Filtered drip coffee, the brew of choice throughout America, does not raise cholesterol.

When the researchers talk about a cup of coffee, they

mean an 8-ounce cup, not a 20-ounce mocha grande with added syrup and whipped cream. One ounce of coffee with cream and sugar equals 10 calories, so coffee calories can add up quickly.

Bottom line: Three to five 8-ounce cups a day may have health advantages; if you order extra large, your whole day's supply might be in one serving.

Is decaf coffee safe?

Coffee roasters use many methods to remove the caffeine from coffee. All methods start with steaming coffee beans to soften them. Direct decaffeination involves soaking the beans in something that extracts the caffeine—water and solvents (methyl chloride, ethyl acetate, high-pressure carbon dioxide, or triglycerides). Indirect decaffeination, also called the Swiss water process, extracts the caffeine with water, treats the water to remove the caffeine, and then adds the water back to the beans.

Regardless of the process, decaf coffee loses some flavor and still retains a small amount of caffeine—about 1%.

Bottom line: Decaf coffee is safe to drink. Roasters no longer use harmful extraction solvents and the final product is solvent free. Water processed is a chemical free option.

Is tea a better choice than coffee?

It's really your choice: both tea and coffee contribute fluid to your body and contain antioxidants. Tea is also an excellent source of fluoride, and herbal teas have some medicinal value. Tea has about one-third the caffeine content of regular coffee, but it can be decaffeinated, too. Herbal teas have no caffeine, but yerba maté and guarana are in some herbal combinations. Regularly drinking tea can increase bone density and reduce cavities and the risk of kidney stones. All types of tea contain polyphenols—catechins, anthocyanins, and phenolic acids—which play an important role in the health of your gastrointestinal tract, most notably reducing the growth of harmful bacteria.

Is green tea the best choice?

Green, black, and oolong tea all come from the same plant. Green tea is dried, rolled, and untreated. When tea leaves are partially aged, they become oolong tea. Further aging creates black tea. As tea leaves age, caffeine develops. Green tea has a very mild flavor and is nearly caffeine free, but black tea contains significant amounts.

Because green tea is not oxidized it does have higher levels of some phytochemicals, such as catechins, and it is an excellent source of the catechin EGCG (epigallocatechin gallate), which may have cancer prevention potential. Green tea is the least popular tea in the U.S.

Bottom line: Drinking any type of tea has health benefits, but green tea may have slightly more.

What is chai?

Chai is a traditional spiced tea drink of India, where it comes in many variations. Here in the U.S., it is black tea sweetened with honey or sugar, flavored with vanilla and spices, and mixed with milk or cream. It is delicious but can add a wallop of calories and saturated fat to the otherwise calorie free, fat free tea.

Isn't alcohol healthy?

Studies have shown that people who drink moderate amounts of alcohol have a decreased risk for heart disease. And postmenopausal women who have a few drinks weekly have stronger bones than women who do not drink at all. Research has shown that red wine contains resveratrol, which has an impressive list of health benefits including cancer prevention, reducing blood clots, lowering blood pressure, and possibly slowing the aging process.

On the flip side, there is no question that too much alcohol leads to trouble. In the brain and central nervous system, alcohol acts as a depressant. In the digestive tract, it damages cells and increases the risk for cancer. The liver is seriously harmed by continued alcohol abuse over time. The organs and brains of unborn babies are affected by their mother's drinking habits. And women who regularly drink increase their risk for breast cancer.

Bottom line: Alcohol is a great example of a little can be good but a lot can be lethal.

How can alcohol have calories when it has no protein, fat, or carbohydrate?

It has alcohol calories: 1 gram of alcohol = 7 calories. Translated into alcohols that you drink: 1 shot of vodka, gin, rum, or whiskey averages 100 calories; a 12-ounce glass of beer averages 150 calories, light beer 100; and a 5-ounce glass of wine averages 110 calories. Mixed drinks can pack a real wallop of calories. A Bloody Mary has 116 calories, but drink a piña colada (263 calories), frozen daiquiri (393 calories), or mudslide (566 calories), and the calories add up quickly. A drink or two a day may be the reason why some have trouble maintaining their weight.

YOU SHOULD KNOW—

Alcohol and Cooking

There is a common misconception that when you cook with wine or spirits, the alcohol (and the calories) burn off during cooking.

Deglaze a pan and 85% of the alcohol remains.

Flambé desserts and 75% of the brandy is still there when the flame dies.

Bake a dish with sherry for 30 minutes and $1/3$ of the alcohol remains.

Stew a pot roast for more than 2 hours and 5% of the alcohol remains.

FUNCTIONAL FOODS—
HOW DO THEY FUNCTION?

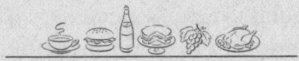

In the future, foods may be prescribed to protect or enhance a person's health.

Thoughts to consider when it comes to functional foods:

- Currently there are few well-designed research studies looking at functional foods. But there is evidence that these products may be useful.
- As our knowledge increases, the recommendations for using functional foods will become more specific.
- Right now we simply don't know enough to make population-wide recommendations.
- Wholefoods don't need to be enhanced to be good for you. They are "functional" just as they are.

Do They Function?

Water packed with vitamins. Pasta fortified with folic acid. Sodas that burn calories. Yogurts that soothe your digestive tract. Margarines and chocolate bars that lower cholesterol. Should we be eating them? Are they helpful? Do they work?

Over the past 15 years the global market for functional foods has grown to $60 billion annually, and there is no end in sight. Functional foods currently remain undefined under U.S. food regulations; the creation of these food-drug hybrids has simply outpaced the government's ability to define or regulate them or verify their health claims.

Some feel regulation is not necessary. They view these foods as simply another option for people trying to manage their health. Others see them as the Frankenstein foods of the future, destroying and gobbling up anything resembling "normal" food. As you've probably guessed, we think the answer lies somewhere in the middle. One thing is sure: Functional foods are here to stay, so each of us will have to decide whether to eat them or not. In some cases the decision will be made for us.

Folic acid has been added to bread, cereal, pasta, flour, and rice since 1998, as an extension to original regulations that require grain processors to add back three B vitamins and iron lost when grains are refined. Iodine is routinely added to table salt, and milk is fortified with vitamin D. We don't think of these as functional foods, but they are.

YOU SHOULD KNOW—

Many experts feel fortified foods are a better choice than nutrient supplements because the foods come packaged with other essential, helpful compounds, whereas supplements provide isolated sources of nutrients.

What is the difference between enriched, fortified, and functional foods?

Enrichment replaces lost nutrients, such as enriching white flour with some of the nutrients lost in milling. Most countries use grains for enrichment programs because it is an easy way to get needed nutrients to the population.

Fortification adds one or more nutrients to a food where they would not normally be found. Adding iodine to table salt was done to prevent goiter, an abnormal enlargement of the thyroid gland, a major public health issue in the early 1900s. Today, orange juice fortified with calcium or apple juice fortified with vitamin C are common examples of this same concept—delivering a nutrient in a food where it would naturally not be found. Vitamin-laced waters are recent versions of fortified foods because water does not naturally contain vitamins.

Functional foods bridge these processes and extend them. Broadly defined, a functional food is one that carries a perceived health benefit. These foods can be divided into 3 groups.

The first group consists of naturally occurring functional foods, including

- oats and oat bran, naturally high in soluble fiber, which can help reduce cholesterol and lower the incidence of heart disease
- fish, rich in omega-3 fatty acids, which can lower the risk for heart disease
- processed tomato products, such as tomato sauce, rich in lycopene, which reduces the risk of cancer when eaten regularly
- cranberry juice, which reduces bacterial levels in the urinary tract
- lutein-rich vegetables, which protect against macular degeneration

The second group is foods that have been enhanced with a nutrient or substance to protect you against disease. These include folic acid-enriched cereals, calcium-fortified orange juice, fiber-rich energy bars, yogurt with live cultures, and sterol-enhanced margarines. Eating any of these foods regularly should offer you some health benefit. For example, drinking calcium-fortified orange juice should add to your overall calcium intake and potentially reduce your future risk for osteoporosis.

The problem is that you have to eat a certain amount of these foods, usually daily, to reap the benefits. Including enough fiber-rich energy bars in your daily food intake to get enough fiber might crowd out other foods, like fruits and vegetables, which are also fiber rich but contain other valuable substances as well. Critics argue that many of these products have more marketing hype than actual value. But the other side of that argument is that if you are already eating cereal, why not eat a folic acid-enriched one to get the extra benefit? Each of us has to look at these products for ourselves and decide.

The last and fastest-growing group of functional foods is bridging the gap between foods and dietary supplements. The nutrients added may be way beyond your normal requirement. A good example is the ever-growing group of energy drinks that can provide B vitamins at levels up to 500% of your daily need. Others are antioxidant-enriched candies. Should we be looking to candy to boost our daily antioxidant intake, or should we simply eat more fruits and vegetables? And do these super-enhanced foods have the same complement of compounds that nature put into wholefoods?

There is no question that in the future we will be looking at food for much more than its calorie, vitamin, and mineral value. Phytochemicals and other active compounds will play a major role in which foods we eat. Functional foods do provide a way to eat healthier, but heavy reliance on them could push us further away from eating natural wholefoods. Evaluating the role of enhanced functional foods in our personal health will be a challenge for each of us.

YOU SHOULD KNOW—

The most popular functional foods are sodas, sports drinks, breakfast cereals, snacks, energy bars, and juice drinks.

Which functional foods currently available have the most value?

A very good example is foods with probiotics. (See pages 97–98). Others are plant sterol- and stanol-enriched foods.

Plant sterols are natural substances that reduce the absorption of cholesterol in your body. They are being added to more and more foods—margarines, orange juice, cereal bars, chocolate, and yogurt. When eaten regularly, these foods help to lower total cholesterol and bad LDL cholesterol. Studies show that getting 2 to 3 grams of plant sterols daily can reduce total cholesterol by 5% to 13% and LDL cholesterol by 6% to 24%. Couple this with other healthy habits, and the total effect could be impressive.

YOU SHOULD KNOW—

Wholefoods such as sunflower seeds, pistachios, pumpkin seeds, pine nuts, flaxseeds, almonds, macadamia nuts, walnuts, pecans, cashews, peanuts, peanut butter, hazelnuts, and Brazil nuts are also rich in natural plant sterols.

Is there any danger to eating functional foods regularly?

Danger is a strong word, but caution and common sense are wise. Let's look at some scenarios that could easily happen in families.

You regularly buy calcium-fortified orange juice, and you have a 16-year-old son. Like most boys his age, his appetite is bottomless. He drinks a quart of milk a day, eats cheese regularly, and thinks nothing of chugging down a quart of orange juice between breakfast and after school. Without any additional food sources of calcium or calcium supplementation, he's already reached the upper safe limit of 2,500 milligrams a day. Too much of anything, even a good thing, can have negative consequences.

You've decided to increase the amount of omega-3s you're eating by including many fortified products, eating fish 3 or 4 times a week, and taking fish oil supplements. Excessive amounts of heart-healthy omega-3s can cause bleeding. People taking daily low-dose aspirin, Coumadin, or Plavix should be careful about excessive intakes of omega-3s.

You've decided to have energy drinks daily to increase your stamina and drive. Does a caffeine- or guarana-laced, sugary, vitamin-enhanced, fruit-flavored drink really qualify as a healthy beverage?

Functional foods run the gamut from good ones to occasionally useful ones to really poor choices. Each of us has to make these choices for ourselves.

LOOKING AT CALORIES

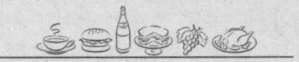

Obesity may soon replace smoking as the country's leading cause of preventable death.

Most of us eat more than we admit and exercise less than we should. The consequence is that we weigh more than we want to, and blame it on our metabolism—even if we're not quite sure what that is.

Metabolism is all the chemical changes that occur in your body. Your body takes in foods, burns some to generate power, uses some to produce new material, and routes the rest into storage for future use. The chemical changes that occur either break down large compounds into smaller units (the foods you eat are broken down into smaller units of energy) or build complex structures from smaller units (your muscles are made up of fragments that come from the protein foods you eat, like eggs). Human metabolism is the sum total of all the energy needed to keep your body alive and moving. This energy requirement can be translated into the number of calories you need each day.

Approximately 60% to 75% of your daily calories are used just to keep you alive. Energy is needed to maintain your body's temperature, allow your nerves to work, let you breathe, keep your heart beating, allow your organs to function, nourish your body tissues, and repair and replace body fluids and parts. It's a job that goes on 24 hours a day.

An interesting thing about this basic energy requirement is that different tissues in the body have different levels of activity. Fat tissue is less active and needs less energy. Muscle tissue, even at rest, is more active and uses up more energy. If you exercise and develop more muscle tissue, your body burns more calories every day just keeping your muscles healthy.

The rest of the calories you need daily are used to support your level of activity. Obviously, you need less if you are relatively inactive and more if you are very active.

To find out how many calories you need each day, you need to do two things. First, how much do you want to weigh? Not your current weight, but what is your target weight? Then select an activity factor that fits your current activity level.

1. Your target weight is _____
2. Your activity factor is _____
   20 = Very active men
   15 = Moderately active men or very active women
   13 = Inactive men, moderately active women, and people over 55
   10 = Inactive women, repeat dieters, seriously overweight people
3. Target Weight x Activity Factor = Calories needed each day.

For example, if your target weight is 130 and you are a moderately active woman (factor 13), you need about 1,600 to 1,700 calories a day.

130 pounds x 13 = 1,690 calories

Eating this number of calories each day would guarantee weight loss, because you are getting only enough calories to support your target weight, not your current heavier weight. Couple this calorie intake with some added exercise and the weight will come off even faster.

LOOKING AT FIBER

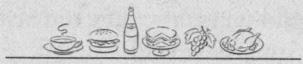

*Fiber isn't digested and provides no calories,
yet it's important.*

This is one carbohydrate all experts agree on: We need
to eat more. Why? Fiber aids in losing weight, managing
diabetes, relieving constipation, and protecting against
certain cancers. It may even lower the risk for heart disease. All this without calories!

Add a Little Fiber to Your Life

- Eat whole fruits and vegetables instead of
  drinking juices.
- Eat the fiber-rich skins of cucumbers, apples,
  pears, potatoes, and zucchini.
- Eat more berries—blueberries, blackberries,
  raspberries, strawberries.
- Choose whole grains—brown rice, cornmeal,
  barley, cracked wheat, rye, and whole wheat.
- Eat beans and lentils a few times a week.
- Use whole grain or high fiber cereals—oatmeal,
  oat flakes, bran, shredded wheat.
- Eat whole wheat bread, bagels, pasta, pretzels,
  crackers, and rolls.

- Try soybeans in every form—soynuts, tofu, tempeh, edamame.
- Snack on fig newtons, graham crackers, and popcorn.
- Enjoy vegetarian meals a few times a week.
- Eat dried fruits and raisins.
- Sprinkle ground flaxseed onto cereal or yogurt for a healthy crunch.
- Try some of the new fiber-fortified foods.

Most of us eat too little fiber. We average about 15 grams each day, far less than we should be eating.

DAILY FIBER RECOMMENDATIONS	
MEN	
19–50 years	38 grams
50 and older	30 grams
WOMEN	
19–50 years	25 grams
50 and older	21 grams
pregnant	28 grams

Slowly start adding food rich in fiber to your daily meals—beans, berries, bran, fruits, oatmeal, vegetables, and whole grains. Don't go overboard, because it takes your body a little time to adjust to the extra bulk passing through your digestive tract. And drink plenty of fluids. Fiber soaks up fluids like a sponge. This not only helps you feel fuller longer, but also helps form soft, easily passed stools.

YOU SHOULD KNOW—

High fiber foods have 5 or more grams in a serving. A good source of fiber has 2 or more grams in a serving.

How much fiber should children eat?

Kids need fiber, too, but you don't want to overdo it. A good rule to use is "Age + 5." All children 2 and older should eat the amount of fiber each day that equals their age + 5. For a 5-year-old, that would be at least 10 grams of fiber a day. The rule can be applied throughout childhood and their teen years until the age of 19, when the adult fiber recommendations would apply. Older teenage boys can eat more fiber than their age + 5, but even if they stick to that rule, they will be eating more fiber daily than most Americans.

If fiber isn't digested, how does it work in the body?

There are trillions of tiny microbes living in your digestive tract, from your mouth to your anus. These tiny helpful hitchhikers have been with you since birth. Our modern diet, high in sugar and fat, is literally starving the friendly bacteria that keeps harmful bacteria from making you sick. If they are not fed, they can't put up a good fight. Fiber is the food your friendly bacteria live on. A low fiber diet has a negative impact on your intestinal microflora and reduces your protection against infection. Eating enough fiber stimulates your natural resistance.

In addition, fiber protects you against heart disease and cancer. Fiber helps manage diabetes by reducing the amount of carbohydrate absorbed and enhancing insulin utilization. You lose weight by eating more fiber because you get the satisfaction of eating and a sense of fullness without calories.

> ## Mash It, Smash It, Break It Apart
>
> *Fiber is fiber no matter what you do in processing or cooking. Canned pureed pumpkin is a rich source of fiber, as are split-pea soup, mashed sweet potatoes, cream of broccoli soup, or a fruit smoothie.*

How can I tell if extra fiber has been added to a food?

Sometimes "fortified with fiber" is stated on the label, but your best bet is to look at the ingredient list. In addition to natural sources like whole wheat and oats, you may see inulin, fructan, FOS (fructooligosaccharides), and methylcellulose listed.

Inulin is a natural fiber found in burdock root, dandelion root, chicory root, onions, leeks, garlic, bananas, asparagus, artichokes, and wheat. Most of the inulin you find added to foods is extracted from chicory or synthesized. Inulin is a prebiotic, a fiber that acts as a food for the good bacteria present in your intestines. It is often added to fermented dairy foods, like yogurt, so it can act with the friendly bacteria in the yogurt to boost your immune protection. Inulin also boosts the absorption of calcium and magnesium, two minerals important for bone health. For more information on pre- and probiotics, see pages 97 to 98.

FOS is also a prebiotic and has many of the same benefits of inulin. It is considered a safe additive.

Methylcellulose is a synthetic fiber created by chemically altering cellulose (the cell wall of plants). It can be added to foods or used in fiber supplements as a bulking agent to prevent constipation.

LOOKING AT VITAMINS AND MINERALS

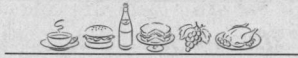

Vitamins A, C, and folic acid and the minerals calcium, iron, and potassium are called micronutrients because your body needs them in small amounts.

Vitamins

All vitamins are vital to life, even though they are needed by the body in very tiny amounts. They help you absorb, digest, and use the fats, carbohydrates, and proteins found in food.

Vitamins can be destroyed or have their shape changed. This can be both good and bad. Cooking food at high temperatures, in a lot of water, for a long time will reduce the amount of vitamins in food. But your body can also change a vitamin's shape to make it more useful in certain situations.

Vitamins are divided into two groups—fat soluble and water soluble. They are handled differently in the body. Fat soluble vitamins (like vitamin A) are carried into the body by foods containing fat and are stored in your fat tissues, waiting to be used. It isn't easy for your body to get rid of fat soluble vitamins, so they can build up if large doses are taken over time. Water soluble vitamins (like vitamin C and folic acid) are absorbed directly into the blood and travel freely around the body through the bloodstream. If high amounts of a water soluble vitamin are detected as the blood passes through the kidneys, the vitamin will be filtered out and leave your body in urine.

THE BEST SOURCES OF

Vitamin A	Vitamin C	Folic Acid
Egg yolk	Fortified fruit juices	Fortified cereal
Liver	Cabbage, raw	Asparagus
Milk	Chili peppers	Blackeyed peas
Blackeyed peas	Green leafy vegetables	Broccoli
Broccoli	Peppers	Cabbage, raw
Brussels sprouts	Potatoes	Chinese cabbage
Butternut squash	Tomatoes	Green leafy vegetables
Carrots		
Chili peppers	Tomato juice	Lentils
Green leafy vegetables	Acerola	Orange juice
Mixed vegetables	Cantaloupe	Peanuts
Peppers	Grapefruit	Spinach
Persimmon	Grapefruit juice	White beans
Romaine lettuce	Guava	Wheat germ
Sweet potatoes	Kiwis	Strawberries
Tomato juice	Mango	
Tomatoes	Orange	
Apricots	Orange juice	
Mango	Papaya	
Papaya	Persimmon	
Peach	Pineapple	
Prunes	Strawberries	
Tart cherries	Tangerine	
Watermelon	Watermelon	

Vitamin A

How much vitamin A do I need each day?

In its latest edition of the Dietary Reference Intakes (DRIs), recommendations for vitamin A are

900 REs	Men 14 and older
700 REs	Women 14 and older
770 REs	Pregnant women
1,300 REs	Breastfeeding women

VITAMIN A ARITHMETIC—

You may see vitamin A measured in IUs (international units) or as REs (retinol equivalents).

1 RE = 1 microgram vitamin A
1 RE = 3.3 IUs of active vitamin A
or
1 RE = 10 IUs of beta-carotene
or
1 RE = 5 IUs from varied sources

Using the equivalent of 1 RE = 5 IUs (because most of us get our vitamin A from varied sources), your daily need is

700 REs or 3,500 IUs for women
and
900 REs or 4,500 IUs daily for men

What does vitamin A do?

Vitamin A is crucial to maintaining healthy cells, particularly mucus, skin, and bone cells. It also boosts your immune function and helps your body fight infections. In men, vitamin A aids in the production of sperm, and in women it helps to maintain fertility. Vitamin A also maintains the health of the cornea, the clear outer window of the eye.

Provitamin A, carotenoids, may play a role in the prevention of cancer.

What's a provitamin?

Vitamin A is unique in that it comes from two sources, animal and plant foods, and in two forms, as retinoids and carotenoids.

About half of the vitamin you need comes from animal foods—liver, cod liver oil, milk, butter, margarine, and eggs—in the form of retinoids. The body easily absorbs and uses this form of vitamin A.

The other half comes as carotenoids, or provitamin A, found in dark green and deep yellow fruits and vegetables like carrots, spinach, broccoli, sweet potatoes, cantaloupe, peaches, apricots, and mangos. Your body will convert these to vitamin A as needed. There are hundreds of different carotenoids in nature, but the one that your body changes most efficiently to active vitamin A is beta-carotene. The carotenoids that are not converted to active vitamin A act as antioxidants, protecting you against harmful free radicals.

Which are richer in carotenoids, raw or cooked vegetables?

You might be surprised by this answer: it's "cooked." A few minutes of cooking breaks down chemical bonds naturally found in food, releasing carotenoids and making them easier to absorb.

> **TO HELP YOU UNDERSTAND—**
>
> *The* tolerable upper limit (UL) *is the highest average daily amount of a vitamin or mineral that you can take without causing harm. As intakes increase over the UL, the potential for harm increases.*

Can you get too much vitamin A?

The experts have set the tolerable upper limit (UL), a safe amount to take regularly, at 3,000 REs (15,000 IUs). Taking more than this amount of vitamin A regularly can cause a number of problems, including fatigue, vomiting, headache, bone and joint pain, hair loss, dry skin, loss of appetite, liver damage, and, in extreme cases, death. Recent research has shown that high intake of vitamin A weakens bones and increases the risk of broken hips. Excess vitamin A interferes with the cells that make new bone, stimulates cells that break down old bone, and disturbs the body's normal levels of calcium, a mineral essential for healthy bones. During pregnancy, high intakes of vitamin A can cause birth defects. Go easy on foods fortified with vitamin A and don't overdo supplements.

You can't overdose on carotenoids because your body will not convert it to active vitamin A unless it is needed. Overdoing carotenoids can cause a yellowing of the skin, particularly the palms of the hands and soles of the feet, but this condition *(carotenodermia)* is harmless. If you eat fewer carotenoid-containing foods, the color will fade.

Can vitamin A be used to treat acne?

Two forms of vitamin A—Retin-A and Accutane—are used to effectively treat acne. Because these medications can accumulate in the body, women should not take them if they are pregnant or planning a pregnancy.

Vitamin C

How much vitamin C do I need each day?

The Dietary Reference Intakes (DRIs) for vitamin C are

90 mg	Men 19 and older
125 mg	Men who smoke
75 mg	Women 19 and older
110 mg	Women who smoke
85 mg	Pregnant women
120 mg	Breastfeeding women

Smokers are encouraged to get an extra 35 milligrams each day because smoking produces damaging free radicals, and Vitamin C is used up as it works to remove them.

Does vitamin C cure colds?

Though the evidence is inconclusive, some studies do report a slightly lower incidence of colds in those people who regularly get enough vitamin C. The vitamin helps the immune system function properly, which in turn keeps you healthy. And vitamin C actually can shorten a cold's duration and make the symptoms more tolerable. The vitamin has antihistamine properties like those found in cold medications.

What else does vitamin C do?

Vitamin C plays a critical role in the formation of collagen, the connective tissue that holds together the structures of the body. It's found in most of the tissues throughout your body, especially in the heart, brain, pancreas, adrenal glands, thymus, lungs, pituitary gland, and lenses of the eyes.

Vitamin C also protects many other nutrients—vitamin E, folic acid, and iron—so they can work effectively in the body.

Go Red

One medium red pepper contains 2 to 3 times your daily vitamin C requirement, as well as your daily need for vitamin A.

My friend recommended I take 1,000 milligrams of vitamin C every day. Is that a good idea?

Many people firmly believe that large amounts of vitamin C are beneficial, but research has never proven this. Here are a few reasons why you may want to rethink your friend's recommendation. When you take in 100 milligrams of vitamin C, your body absorbs 80 to 90% of the vitamin. As vitamin C intake increases, absorption decreases, with most of the excess being excreted through the urine. So when you take in very large amounts at one time, the absorption can be as low as 20%. Some experts also believe that large amounts of vitamin C can reverse its normal antioxidant effect, and stimulate free radical damage instead.

Very large amounts—more than 2,000 milligrams daily—may cause nose bleeds, abdominal cramps, and diarrhea. High levels of vitamin C can also cause a false-positive result when testing for diabetes. In people prone to kidney stones, high intakes may contribute to the problem. And for people with *hemochromotosis,* a condition that causes excess accumulation of iron, too much vitamin C, which enhances iron absorption, is problematic. The UL (tolerable upper limit) for vitamin C has been set at 2,000 milligrams.

Folic Acid (B$_9$)

Why is folic acid so important?

Folic acid is important to all the cells in your body that reproduce. It's involved in making the cells' genetic material and in the production of protein and red blood cells. When you don't have enough folic acid, red blood cells develop abnormally and have a very short life span. The number of normal red blood cells goes down and the body has trouble carrying enough oxygen. A type of anemia results, with weakness, fatigue, depression, irritability, forgetfulness, and disturbed sleep. Diarrhea and a depressed immune response can also result if folic acid deficiency continues. The good news is that the body normally stores 2 to 4 months of extra folate, and if you take a supplement, a deficiency will correct itself within 24 hours.

How much folic acid do I need each day?

The Dietary Reference Intakes (DRIs) for folic acid are

400 mcg	Men 14 and older
400 mcg	Women 14 and older
600 mcg	Pregnant women
500 mcg	Breastfeeding women

The UL (tolerable upper limit) for folic acid is 1,000 micrograms from fortified foods and supplements. It is hard to take in too much folate from natural food sources.

Folate or folic acid—which is correct?

Folate is an all-encompassing term that includes naturally occurring folates in food and synthetic folic acid used in supplements and food fortification. Food sources include green leafy vegetables, orange juice, beans, liver, asparagus, broccoli, strawberries, wheat germ, and peanuts. Fortified sources are enriched bread, pasta, flour, breakfast cereal, and rice. The folic acid used to fortify foods is slightly more absorbable than what naturally occurs in foods like spinach. But that doesn't mean you should rely only on fortified foods for your folic acid needs. The natural food sources are also rich in other important nutrients and phytochemical compounds that are needed by your body. Most experts recommend getting folic acid from a variety of sources—food in which it is naturally found, fortified foods, and supplements, too.

Fragile Folate

Cooking can destroy 50 to 90% of folate. Eat folate-rich foods uncooked or cook them quickly by steaming, stir-frying, or microwaving in small amounts of water.

Do most people get too little folic acid?

Scientists estimate that 10% of Americans are folate deficient. Others are not deficient but their normal intake is below the desirable level. Based on this evidence, fortification of bread, cereal, pasta, flour, and rice was begun in

1998. Since the fortification program started, it's estimated that the average American is getting 200 micrograms more folic acid a day, but most are still falling short of their daily need.

I'm trying to get pregnant and my doctor recommended a vitamin supplement with folic acid. Why?

Because folic acid helps to make the genetic material of every cell, it's essential to support the healthy growth of an unborn child. Pregnant women who take in too little folic acid have a higher risk for miscarriage and birth defects involving the spinal cord and brain. These organs begin to develop very soon after conception, before you are even aware that you are pregnant. So most experts recommend all women of childbearing age get adequate folic acid, but unfortunately many still don't. Less than 30% of women reach the daily recommendation of 400 micrograms.

Is folic acid important for men, too?

Absolutely. Everyone needs this vitamin to ensure that new cells reproduce and develop correctly. Research has shown that men with low sperm counts and more fragile sperm have low intakes of folic acid. So when it comes to a healthy pregnancy, adequate folic acid levels are important for both parents.

Why did my cardiologist recommend more folic acid after my last checkup?

If he took blood tests, perhaps your results showed elevated levels of homocysteine (a byproduct of using protein), which is a risk factor for heart attacks and strokes. Folic acid and other B vitamins help to lower homocysteine levels by converting it to a harmless compound. As folic acid intake increases, homocysteine levels decrease, lowering your risk for heart disease.

Evolving research also shows that keeping homocysteine levels in check may slow the onset of Alzheimer's and other memory problems associated with aging. Those with high homocysteine levels were twice as likely to be diagnosed with Alzheimer's or other forms of dementia.

Is it true that folic acid can cure depression?

People who suffer from depression manage their condition with therapy and antidepressive medication. A number of studies have shown that those with depression and those who don't respond well to medication often have low folate levels. Supplemental folic acid causes improvement. Since depression is a debilitating condition affecting many, and folic acid supplementation is safe, this is worth a try.

Minerals

Minerals never change. Unlike vitamins, minerals cannot be destroyed or have their shape changed. The calcium in seashells, milk, and your bones is the same. Iron is iron, whether it's in a cast-iron frying pan or in your red blood cells. Your body absorbs most minerals in proportion to its need. Growing children absorb calcium more efficiently than adults. If you are anemic (have low iron stores), your body will absorb more iron from food than when your iron stores are adequate.

Minerals are divided into two groups—major minerals

and trace minerals. If your body needs more than 100 milligrams a day (like calcium and potassium), the mineral is classified major. Trace minerals, like iron, are needed in amounts less than 100 milligrams a day. Classification as a major or trace mineral has nothing to do with the mineral's importance in your body.

THE BEST SOURCES OF

Calcium	Potassium	Iron
Almonds	Milk	Beef
Baked beans	Molasses	Chicken
Broccoli	Salt substitutes	Clams
Cheese	Yogurt	Cocoa powder
Frozen yogurt	Artichoke	Egg
Ice cream	Bamboo shoots	Fortified cereal
Kale	Beet greens	Fortified bread
Milk	Corn on the cob	Liver
Molasses	Chinese cabbage	Molasses, blackstrap
Salmon canned w/bones	Dried beans	Oatmeal
Sardines canned w/bones	Potatoes	Oysters
Spinach	Spinach	Peanuts
Tofu	Sweet potatoes	Pork
Yogurt	Swiss chard	Red wine
	Tomatoes	Venison
	Tomato juice	Wheat germ
	Winter squash	Baked beans
	Avocado	Broccoli
	Banana	Peas
	Cantaloupe	Potatoes
	Dried fruit	Spinach
	Honeydew melon	Apricots
	Mango	Blueberries
	Papaya	
	Prune juice	

Calcium

We've all heard that calcium builds strong teeth and bones and protects us against *osteoporosis* (adult bone thinning), but it does much more than that. Calcium

- helps blood clot
- helps nerves work normally
- helps muscles work and the heart beat
- helps lower high blood pressure
- aids in weight loss
- helps prevent midlife weight gain in women
- relieves PMS (premenstrual syndrome)
- protects against complications in pregnancy
- lowers the risk for some cancers
- may help increase good HDL cholesterol in postmenopausal women
- lowers the risk for periodontal disease, a leading cause of tooth loss
- protects against infertility
- reduces the risk for kidney stones

Calcium may even influence behavior. A study with rats showed that they became frantic on a low-calcium diet, but calmed down when they were fed adequate amounts.

AND THE WINNER IS?—

Calcium

Depending on your size and weight, your body contains up to 3 pounds—more than any other mineral.

How much calcium do I need each day?

The Dietary Reference Intakes (DRIs) for calcium are

1,000 mg	Men 19 to 50
1,200 mg	Men 51 and older
1,000 mg	Women 19 to 50
1,200 mg	Women 51 and older

There is no need for calcium beyond the normal requirement during pregnancy and breastfeeding. Children between the ages of 9 and 18 should be getting slightly more—1,300 milligrams—to help them form strong bones.

SHOPPING TIPS—

Choose nonfat and lowfat milk—they have fewer calories and more calcium than whole milk.

Lowfat or nonfat ricotta cheese has twice the calcium of cottage cheese.

Lowfat chocolate milk has the same amount of calcium as regular chocolate milk.

Why do bones thin as we age?

Most of us think our bones are solid, unchanging structures. In fact, bones are living tissues that change in response to stress. Your bones and teeth contain 99% of your body's calcium. The remaining 1% is in your blood and other tissues. Your body protects that 1% at all cost because calcium has so many important functions in the body—not the least of which is to keep your heart beating!

The calcium in your bones serves as a reservoir for the

calcium needed in the rest of your body. To keep blood levels constant, your body will sacrifice bone strength. Over time, if more calcium is taken from the bones than is replaced, bones become fragile and likely to break. But because bones are living tissue, they can take up more calcium to replace the loss, and they will thicken and rebuild if you do weight-bearing exercises like walking and lifting weights. Bone loss does not have to be a standard consequence of getting older.

NOT FOR WOMEN ONLY—

Most women know they need to get enough calcium daily, but according to recent statistics, the average guy over 40 doesn't get enough.

Is all the calcium from food absorbed?

It's rare that any vitamin or mineral will be 100% absorbed. Calcium-rich foods can be divided into 3 groups, depending on how much is absorbed:

- **Excellent sources**—milk, firm tofu, dark green leafy vegetables, broccoli, and canned salmon and sardines with bones
- **Good sources**—ice cream, soft tofu, and light green leafy vegetables
- **Fair to poor sources**—cottage cheese, silken tofu, beans, almonds, and sesame seeds

Even poor sources contribute some calcium to your overall intake, and multiple servings add up.

Someone told me a high protein diet will strip my body of calcium. Is this true?

It's a complicated process for your body to turn protein into fuel, which is exactly what happens on a high protein diet. When protein is burned as fuel, an unused part of the protein is removed from your body by the kidneys. Minerals, including calcium, potassium and sodium, escort this unneeded material out of the body. In the process, they are eliminated, too.

A recent study challenged this idea, showing that high protein intakes do not deplete the body of calcium unless calcium intakes are low. So if you are considering a high protein diet, be sure to get adequate calcium.

Why does my antibiotic say, "Do Not Take with Milk"?

Many antibiotics, like Cipro, Tequin, and Levaquin, interact with the minerals calcium, iron, and zinc, causing the body to absorb less of the medication. When you get less of the drug, it could be the difference between staying sick and getting well. Drug labels often warn users not to take these medications with milk, mineral supplements, or antacids. Most labels don't say anything about calcium-fortified foods like orange juice and cereal, so be aware of those extra sources of calcium.

Should I take a calcium supplement?

Most experts would say food first, and then a supplement to make up any shortfall. Calcium supplements come in many strengths and forms—pills, liquid, and chewable. Select one with vitamin D, which aids in absorption, and take calcium with meals or with milk.

In all supplements, calcium is bound to another compound. Different combinations result in varying amounts of actual calcium in the supplement. Calcium carbonate contains the largest amount of elemental calcium—40%. A 500-milligram tablet of calcium carbonate provides approximately 200 milligrams of actual calcium.

Calcium Supplement	% Calcium
Calcium carbonate	40
Calcium phosphate (tribase)	38
Calcium phosphate (dibase)	31
Calcium citrate	21
Calcium lactate	13
Calcium gluconate	9

Can you take too much calcium?

The UL (tolerable upper limit) has been set at 2,500 milligrams a day. There is no evidence that higher levels have any benefit. High intakes of calcium will reduce the absorption of iron and zinc, cause constipation, and force the kidneys to work harder to get rid of the excess.

Iron

How much iron do I need each day?

The Dietary Reference Intakes (DRIs) for iron are

11 mg	Men 14 to 18
8 mg	Men 19 and older
15 mg	Women 14 to 18
18 mg	Women 19 to 50
8 mg	Women 50 and older
27 mg	Pregnant women
9 mg	Breastfeeding women

Iron requirements are based on growth and need. Younger people and pregnant women are growing. Women between the ages of 19 and 50 need more iron because they lose it monthly through menstruation. After menopause, the iron requirement for women is the same as it is for men.

Why is it important to get enough iron?

Iron carries oxygen in the blood as hemoglobin, and moves oxygen into muscles as myoglobin. Without enough iron, hemoglobin and myoglobin cannot be made and the body is deprived of oxygen. Besides aiding the transporting of oxygen, iron is part of hundreds of enzymes needed to make the body function, and it plays a role in brain development and immune function.

If iron is so important, does my body contain a lot of it?

No. The opposite is true. Iron is a trace mineral and most people have less than a teaspoon of iron in their body. About 80% of your body's iron is in your bloodstream, and the rest is in your muscles and enzymes. The cells in your intestines act as iron's gatekeeper. If your iron gets low, more is absorbed. When you have enough, less is absorbed and any excess is excreted.

Your body is also extremely good at recycling iron. When old red blood cells are broken down, your body recycles 95% of the iron to make new ones.

Does spinach really have a lot of iron?

Popeye was right, spinach does have iron. But the story is a little more complicated than simply gulping down a canful, as the cartoon character regularly did. Iron in food comes in two forms—heme iron and nonheme iron.

Heme iron is found only in animal tissue. You eat it in meat, fish, and poultry, and your body absorbs it efficiently. Nonheme iron is found in plants and iron-fortified foods. You eat it as green leafy vegetables (like spinach), beans, soy, and fortified breads and cereals. Your body absorbs nonheme iron less efficiently. What you eat with nonheme iron affects how your body makes use of the iron. Combine beans with tomatoes (high in vitamin C) and the iron in the beans is more easily absorbed. Have spinach with chicken (containing heme iron), and the iron from the spinach is more easily absorbed.

Easy Does It—on Antacids

Regular use of antacids can reduce the amount of iron you absorb. Absorption of iron depends on adequate stomach acids, which antacids neutralize.

Does too little iron cause anemia?

Yes. Iron deficiency is the most common nutrition deficiency in the world, affecting 500 to 600 million people. In the U.S., infants, toddlers, teenage girls, young women, and pregnant women are at risk.

Can too much iron be dangerous?

It's hard to overdose on iron in food because your body simply doesn't absorb the iron it doesn't need. Taking too much from supplements irritates the digestive tract and causes constipation. The tolerable upper limit (UL) has been set at 45 milligrams daily.

A hereditary condition, *hemochromatosis*, causes excessive iron absorption. Without treatment it can lead to organ damage and even death. It was once believed to be rare, but doctors now realize 12 of every 1,000 people of European descent may have this genetic condition.

Potassium

Why is potassium so important?

The third most abundant mineral in your body, potassium is found inside the fluid of every cell. It's important to the firing of nerves and the working of muscles. Potassium allows the heart muscle to relax—the opposite action of calcium, which makes it contract. Potassium also helps to regulate high blood pressure.

Endurance athletes, who lose potassium in sweat, especially in hot weather, often rely on bananas, orange juice, or fortified sports drinks to replenish this important mineral.

More Fruits and Vegetables = Strong Bones

Eating more fruits and vegetables increases bone mineral content. Experts believe the high potassium in fruits and vegetables encourages the body to hang on to calcium instead of excreting it—net result: stronger bones.

How much potassium do you need each day?

Potassium is so abundant in food that no Dietary Reference Intake (DRI) has been set. Experts have set an adult daily minimum requirement of 1,600 to 2,000 milligrams a day. A healthy diet supplies 2,000 to 4,000 milligrams daily, but many people's diets fall short. Some experts recommend up to 4,700 milligrams daily to lower high blood pressure. Those with high potassium intakes do have lower blood pressure.

Why did my doctor tell me to take my diuretic with orange juice?

Diuretics are used to control high blood pressure by removing water from your body. Along with the water, your body loses potassium. Orange juice is an excellent source for replacing the lost potassium. You could also drink a glass of tomato juice, eat a wedge of cantaloupe, or top your morning cereal with a banana—all high potassium sources.

Is it possible to get too little potassium?

Unlikely, but it could happen. People with eating disorders, those who abuse laxatives, people taking diuretics, endurance athletes, physical laborers, and those sick with vomiting and diarrhea could have their potassium drop too low. *Hypokalemia,* low potassium, results in muscle weakness, cramping, and fatigue, which can progress to an irregular heartbeat and paralysis. Most cases are mild and can be easily handled by eating potassium-rich foods or taking a supplement.

GO EASY—

Drinking high-sugar, high-caffeine beverages—soda, highly sweetened coffee, energy drinks—all promote fluid loss, which lowers potassium levels in the blood.

USING YOUR HEALTHY WHOLEFOODS COUNTER

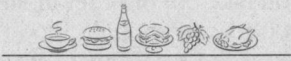

The Healthy Wholefoods Counter lists the portion size, calories, fiber, vitamin A, folic acid, vitamin C, calcium, iron, and potassium values for more than 10,000 foods. Now you can compare the values in your favorite foods and, when necessary, choose substitutes before you go out to shop or eat. This will save you time and help you decide what to buy.

In the counter section of the book, for each category, you will find nonbranded (generic) foods listed first in alphabetical order, followed by an alphabetical listing of brand name foods. The nonbranded listing will help you estimate the calorie, fiber, vitamin, and mineral values when you don't see your favorite brand. They can also help you to evaluate store brands. Large categories are divided into subcategories, such as canned, fresh, frozen, and ready-to-eat, to make it easier to find what you're looking for.

A dash (–) appears in some entries. This means no analysis was done for fiber or the specific vitamin or mineral for that food. It is not the same as a zero, which means there is no fiber or none of the specific vitamin or mineral in the food.

Because we eat out so often, more than 600 take-out foods are listed. These are found in the take-out subcategory in many categories throughout this section. Look there for foods you take out or order in, since they are not nutrition labeled.

Most foods are listed alphabetically. In some cases, though, foods are grouped by category. For example, a tuna sandwich is found in the SANDWICH category. Other group categories include:

ASIAN FOOD   **Page 198**
includes all types of Asian foods except egg rolls and sushi, which are found in separate categories.

DELI MEATS/COLD CUTS   **Page 338**
includes all sandwich meats except chicken, ham and turkey, which are found in separate categories.

DINNER   **Page 340**
includes all by brand name, except pasta dinners, which arc found in a separate category.

LIQUOR/LIQUEUR   **Page 434**
includes all alcoholic beverages and mixed drinks except beer, champagne, and wine, which are found in separate categories.

NUTRITION SUPPLEMENTS　　　**Page 459**

Includes all dieting aids, meal
replacers, and drinks, except
energy bars and energy drinks,
which are found in separate
categories.

SANDWICHES　　　**Page 551**

Includes popular sandwich,
calzone, and panini choices.

SNACKS　　　**Page 570**

Includes a variety of
miscellaneous snack items such
as trail mix, pork rinds, and
cheese puffs.

SPANISH FOOD　　　**Page 593**

Includes all types of Spanish
and Mexican foods except salsa
and tortillas, which are found in
separate categories.

Use *The Healthy Wholefoods Counter* as a guide to
help you make the best food decisions when you shop or
eat out.

Don't separate yourself from the earth that feeds you.

DEFINITIONS

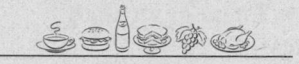

as prep (as prepared): refers to food that has been prepared according to package directions

lean and fat: describes meat with some fat on its edges that is not cut away before cooking, or poultry prepared with skin and fat as purchased

lean only: refers to lean meat that is trimmed of all visible fat, or poultry without skin

not prep (not prepared): refers to food that has not been cooked and may require the addition of other ingredients

shelf-stable: refers to prepared products found on the supermarket shelf that are ready-to-eat or are ready to be heated, and do not require refrigeration

take-out: describes prepared dishes that you purchase ready-to-eat; those included serve as a guide to the calories, fiber, vitamin A, vitamin C, folic acid, calcium, iron, and potassium in products you may purchase.

ABBREVIATIONS

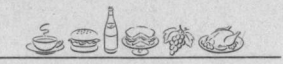

avg	=	average
diam	=	diameter
fl	=	fluid
frzn	=	frozen
g	=	gram
in	=	inch
lb	=	pound
lg	=	large
med	=	medium
mg	=	milligram
oz	=	ounce
pkg	=	package
pt	=	pint
prep	=	prepared
qt	=	quart
reg	=	regular
sec	=	second
serv	=	serving
sm	=	small
sq	=	square
tbsp	=	tablespoon
tr	=	trace
tsp	=	teaspoon
w/	=	with
w/o	=	without
<	=	less than

NOTES

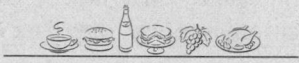

Cals = calories
Fiber = fiber
    All fiber values are given in grams (g).
Vit A = Vitamin A
    All vitamin A values are in International Units (IUs).
Folic = Folic Acid
    All folic acid values are given in micrograms (mcg).
Vit C = Vitamin C
    All vitamin C values are given in milligrams (mg).
Iron = Iron
    All iron values are given in milligrams (mg).
Calci = Calcium
    All calcium values are given in milligrams (mg).
Potas = Potassium
    All potassium values are given in milligrams (mg).
tr (trace) = less than 1 IU of vitamin A, less than 1 milligram of vitamin C, iron, calcium, or potassium, and less than 1 microgram of folic acid
– (dash) indicates data was not available
0 (zero) indicates that there is none of the nutrient in that food.

Discrepancies in figures are due to rounding, product reformulation, and reevaluation. Labeling law allows rounding of values. Because much of the data is analysis data, obtained directly from manufacturers, not from labels, in some cases our values may not be exactly the same as label information because our data have not been rounded.

Brand Name, Generic (Nonbranded) and Take-Out Food

FOOD	PORTION	CALS	FIBER	VIT A	FOLIC	VIT C	CALCI	IRON	POTAS
ABALONE									
breaded & fried	1 serv (3 oz)	162	tr	15	6	3	50	5	295
steamed	1 serv (3 oz)	127	0	135	5	3	31	3	253
ACAI JUICE									
Zola Acai									
Juice	1 box (11 oz)	170	1	300	–	15	40	3	30
ACEROLA									
fresh	1 (5 g)	2	tr	37	1	81	1	tr	7
ACEROLA JUICE									
juice	1 cup	56	1	1232	0	3872	24	1	235
ADZUKI BEANS									
canned sweetened	½ cup	351	–	7	158	0	33	2	176
dried cooked w/o salt	½ cup	147	8	7	139	0	32	2	6124
AKEE									
fresh	3.5 oz	223	–	1	–	26	40	3	–
ALFALFA									
sprouts	½ cup	40	tr	26	6	1	5	tr	13
ALLSPICE									
ground	1 tsp	5	tr	10	1	1	13	tr	20
ALMONDS									
almond butter w/ salt	2 tbsp	203	1	0	21	tr	86	1	243
almond butter w/o salt	2 tbsp	203	1	0	21	tr	86	1	243
almond paste	¼ cup	260	3	0	41	tr	98	1	178
chocolate covered	6 pieces (0.6 oz)	102	2	15	4	0	37	1	107
dry roasted w/ salt	¼ cup	206	4	0	11	0	92	2	257
dry roasted w/o salt	¼ cup	206	4	0	11	0	92	2	257
honey roasted	¼ cup	214	5	0	12	tr	95	1	202
jordan almonds	6 (0.7 oz)	99	1	0	3	0	21	tr	54
oil roasted w/ salt	¼ cup	238	4	0	11	0	114	1	274

FOOD	PORTION	CALS	FIBER	VIT A	FOLIC	VIT C	CALCI	IRON	POTAS
oil roasted w/o salt	¼ cup	238	4	0	11	0	114	1	274
praline	17 pieces (1.4 oz)	210	3	0	–	0	60	1	–
yogurt covered	6 pieces (0.8 oz)	122	1	0	4	tr	46	tr	104
American Almond									
Marzipan	2 tbsp	130	1	0		0	20	tr	–
Blue Diamond									
Almond Roca Buttercrunch	3 pieces (1.3 oz)	210	0	200	–	0	0	0	–
Honey Roasted	¼ cup	170	3	0	–	0	80	1	–
Jalapeno Smokehouse	28 pieces (1 oz)	170	3	0	–	1	80	1	180
Jordon Pastels	15 pieces (1.4 oz)	180	2	0	–	0	40	1	–
Lime 'N Chili	28 pieces (1 oz)	170	3	100	–	0	80	1	190
Maui Onion & Garlic	28 pieces (1 oz)	170	3	0	–	0	80	1	180
Milk Chocolate Covered	9 pieces (1.4 oz)	230	3	0	–	0	60	1	–
Salted	¼ cup	170	3	0	–	0	80	1	–
Smokehouse	28 pieces (1.3 oz)	170	3	0	–	0	80	1	–
Wasabi & Soy Sauce	28 pieces (1 oz)	170	3	0	–	0	60	1	180
Whole Natural	¼ cup	180	3	0	–	0	80	1	–
Yogurt Covered	12 pieces (1.4 oz)	210	0	0	–	0	60	0	–
Brach's									
Chocolate Coated	11 pieces	220	2	0	–	0	40	1	–
Eden									
Tamari	3 tbsp (1 oz)	160	4	–	–	–	60	1	230
Good Sense									
Hickory Smoked	¼ cup	180	2	0	–	30	110	1	–
Raw Whole	¼ cup	180	4	0	–	0	80	1	–
Keto									
Chocolatey Covered	1 oz	169	5	0	–	0	170	3	

FOOD	PORTION	CALS	FIBER	VIT A	FOLIC	VIT C	CALCI	IRON	POTAS
Kettle									
Butter Salted	2 tbsp	180	2	0	–	0	80	1	–
Butter Unsalted	2 tbsp	180	2	0	–	0	80	1	–
Love'n Bake									
Almond Paste	2 tbsp	140	2	0	–	0	40	1	–
Almond Schmear	2 tbsp	140	2	0	–	0	40	1	–
Roasted Butter	2 tbsp	180	3	0	–	0	100	0	–
Maisie Jane's									
Almond Butter	1 oz	184	0	0	–	0	80	1	–
Cappuccino	9 pieces (1.4 oz)	220	2	0	–	0	100	1	–
Chocolate Toffee	9 pieces (1.4 oz)	210	2	100	–	0	60	1	–
Coffee Glazed	2 tbsp (1 oz)	150	3	0	–	0	60	1	–
Cowboy BBQ	2 tbsp (1 oz)	140	3	100	–	0	80	1	–
Mint Chocolate	9 pieces (1.4 oz)	210	2	0	–	0	60	1	–
Organic Honey Glazed	2 tbsp (1 oz)	160	4	0	–	0	80	1	–
Tamari	2 tbsp (1 oz)	160	4	0	–	0	80	1	–
Mama Mellace's									
Butter Rum	1 oz	150	2	0	–	0	40	1	–
Cinnamon Roasted	1 oz	140	2	0	–	0	40	1	–
MaraNatha									
Almond Butter	2 tbsp	220	3	0	–	0	100	1	–
Raw Almond Butter	2 tbsp	190	4	0	–	0	80	1	–
Tamari Almonds	¼ cup	160	3	0	–	0	80	1	–
Odense									
Almond Paste	2 tbsp (1.4 oz)	170	0	0	–	0	100	1	–
Planters									
Chocolate Lovers Dark Chocolate	11 pieces (1.4 oz)	220	3	0	–	0	40	1	200
Dry Roasted	23 pieces (1 oz)	160	3	0	–	0	60	1	200
AMARANTH									
leaves cooked	½ cup	14	–	1828	38	27	138	1	423

FOOD	PORTION	CALS	FIBER	VIT A	FOLIC	VIT C	CALCI	IRON	POTAS
uncooked	½ cup (3.4 oz)	365	15	0	48	4	149	7	357

ANCHOVY
boneless	1 oz	60	0	15	4	0	66	1	154
canned in oil drained	1 can (2 oz)	94	0	25	6	0	104	2	245
fresh	1 (4 g)	8	0	0	1	0	9	tr	22
fresh fillets	3 (0.4 oz)	21	–	0	–	0	20	0	–
CANNED									
Brunswick									
Flat Fillets	1 can (2 oz)	25	0	0	–	0	20	0	–

ANISE
seed	1 tsp	7	tr	7	0	tr	14	1	30

ANTELOPE
roasted	4 oz	215	0	0	12	0	7	6	353

APPLE
sliced sweetened	½ cup	68	2	52	0	tr	4	tr	69
Glory									
Fried Apples	½ cup	80	1	0	–	0	0	tr	–
DRIED									
chopped	½ cup	104	4	24	0	1	6	1	192
cooked w/o sugar	½ cup	73	3	22	0	1	4	tr	134
rings	5	78	3	0	0	1	4	tr	144
Crispy Green									
Crispy Apples	1 pkg (0.36 oz)	35	1	0	–	8	0	0	–
Del Monte									
Dried Apples	¼ cup	110	3	0	–	0	100	1	180
Fruit Ripples									
Strawberry Apple	1 pkg	50	1	–	–	–	–	–	–
FRESH									
apple	1 sm	55	3	57	3	5	6	tr	113
apple	1 lg	110	5	114	6	10	13	tr	227
apple	1 med	72	3	75	4	6	8	tr	148
candied	1 med (6.5 oz)	234	4	30	6	7	66	tr	241

FOOD	PORTION	CALS	FIBER	VIT A	FOLIC	VIT C	CALCI	IRON	POTAS
candied	1 lg (9.8 oz)	357	6	40	8	10	101	tr	368
candied	1 sm (4.9 oz)	179	3	20	4	5	51	tr	185
w/ skin sliced	1 cup	57	3	59	3	5	7	tr	118
w/o skin sliced	1 cup	53	1	42	0	4	6	tr	99
Chiquita									
Apple	1 med (5.4 oz)	80	5	100	–	5	0	tr	–
Earthbound Farm									
Organic Slices	1 pkg (2 oz)	30	1	0	–	78	40	0	–
Mrs. Prindable's									
Caramel Triple Chocolate	¼ apple (1.7 oz)	120	1	0	–	1	20	tr	–
Caramel Walnut	¼ apple (2 oz)	160	1	0	–	1	40	tr	–
Rainier									
Apple	1 med (5.5 oz)	80	5	100	–	5	0	1	170
Sullivan									
McIntosh	1 (5.4 oz)	80	4	0	–	4	0	0	160
FROZEN									
sliced w/o sugar	½ cup	42	2	29	1	tr	3	tr	67
Roast Works									
Flame Roasted Fuji	1 serv (5 oz)	90	2	0	–	0	0	tr	–
TAKE-OUT									
baked	1 (6 oz)	128	4	15	3	6	10	tr	159
baked no sugar	1 (5.6 oz)	136	4	25	3	6	10	tr	167
fried apple rings	1 serv (2.7 oz)	91	2	215	2	2	5	tr	73
APPLE JUICE									
cider	1 cup	117	tr	0	0	2	17	1	295
juice + vitamin C & calcium	1 cup	117	tr	0	0	86	278	1	312
mulled cider	1 serv	265	6	122	18	37	129	4	409
unsweetened w/o vitamin C	1 cup	117	tr	2	0	2	17	1	295

FOOD	PORTION	CALS	FIBER	VIT A	FOLIC	VIT C	CALCI	IRON	POTAS
After The Fall									
Organic	8 oz	90	–	0	–	0	0	tr	240
Celestial Seasonings									
Cider Apple Caramel Kiss as prep	1 cup	80	0	0	–	66	60	0	–
Eden									
Organic Juice	8 oz	90	0	0	–	0	0	0	310
Hansen's									
100% Juice	8 oz	120	0	0	–	72	40	tr	130
Hood									
100% Juice	1 cup	120	0	0	–	72	0	0	–
Langers									
Diet Cocktail 50% Juice	8 oz	60	–	–	–	60	150	–	95
Harvest Apple 100% Juice	8 oz	120	–	6000	–	–	150	1	190
Low Carb Creations									
Apple Cider as prep	1 serv	10	0	0	–	0	0	tr	–
Minute Maid									
100% Juice	8 oz	100	–	–	–	60	0	–	0
Naked Juice									
Just Apple	8 oz	120	0	5000	–	162	20	2	280
Ocean Spray									
100% Juice	8 oz	110	0	0	–	0	–	–	240
Odwalla									
Spiced Harvest Cider	8 oz	130	0	0	–	2	20	0	–
Old Orchard									
Cider 100%	8 oz	120	–	0	–	0	0	tr	280
Healthy Balance Apple	8 oz	30	–	0	–	78	0	0	78
Organic 100% Juice	8 oz	128	–	0	–	78	100	tr	280
Phat Phruit									
Green Apple	8 oz	40	0	1000	–	60	200	–	–
Red Cheek									
100% Juice	8 oz	120	–	0	–	2	0	1	–
Seneca									
100% Juice	8 oz	110	–	–	–	72	–	–	260
Tropicana									
Orchard Style	1 bottle (14 oz)	200	0	0	–	60	0	0	500
Zeigler's									
Old Fashioned Cider	8 oz	110	1	0	–	4	0	0	170

FOOD	PORTION	CALS	FIBER	VIT A	FOLIC	VIT C	CALCI	IRON	POTAS
APPLESAUCE									
sweetened	½ cup	97	2	14	1	2	5	tr	78
unsweetened	½ cup	52	2	35	1	2	4	tr	92
Eden									
Organic	½ cup	60	2	0	–	0	0	0	100
Organic Apple Cherry	½ cup	70	3	0	–	0	0	0	130
Organic Apple Strawberry	½ cup	60	2	0	–	0	0	0	105
Organic Cinnamon	1 pkg (4 oz)	70	2	0	–	2	0	0	110
Langers									
Unsweetened	½ cup	50	2	100	–	1	0	tr	–
Musselman's									
Apple Sauce	1 pkg (4 oz)	80	2	0	–	0	0	0	–
Lite	1 pkg (4 oz)	50	2	0	–	0	0	0	–
Vermont Village									
Organic Unsweetened	½ cup	80	2	–	–	60	–	–	–
White House									
Apple Sauce	1 pkg (4 oz)	90	1	0	–	60	0	0	–
APRICOT JUICE									
nectar	6 oz	106	1	2479	2	1	13	1	215
Ceres									
Apricot	8 oz	120	0	100	–	30	20	1	190
APRICOTS									
CANNED									
heavy syrup	½ cup	91	3	3202	2	3	11	tr	157
juice pack	½ cup	59	2	2063	2	6	15	tr	201
light syrup	½ cup	80	2	1672	3	3	14	tr	175
water pack	½ cup	33	2	2380	2	4	10	tr	233
Del Monte									
Halves In Heavy Syrup	½ cup	100	1	1500	–	5	0	tr	–
Orchard Select Halves	½ cup	80	1	1500	–	60	0	tr	–
DRIED									
halves	6	51	2	757	2	tr	12	1	244
halves cooked w/o sugar	½ cup	106	3	1594	4	tr	24	1	514

FOOD	PORTION	CALS	FIBER	VIT A	FOLIC	VIT C	CALCI	IRON	POTAS
Crispy Green									
Crispy Apricots	1 pkg (0.36 oz)	40	tr	500	–	1	0	tr	–
Sunsweet									
Apricots	6 pieces (1.4 oz)	100	3	500	–	0	20	1	420
FRESH									
apricots	1	17	1	674	3	4	5	tr	91
sliced	½ cup	40	2	1589	7	8	11	tr	214
Chiquita									
Apricots	3 med (4 oz)	60	1	2250	–	12	20	tr	–
FROZEN									
sweetened	½ cup	119	3	2033	2	11	12	1	277
ARROWHEAD									
corm boiled	1 med	9	–	0	1	0	1	tr	106
ARROWROOT									
raw	1 root (1.2 oz)	21	tr	6	112	1	2	1	150
raw root sliced	1 cup	78	2	23	406	2	7	3	545
ARTICHOKE									
CANNED									
hearts in oil	1 serv (3 oz)	100	4	35	39	8	34	1	273
Gertie's Finest									
Tapenade	2 tbsp	29	tr	25	–	1	15	tr	–
Progresso									
Hearts	1 piece	15	1	100	–	–	–	tr	–
S&W									
Marinated Hearts	2 pieces (1 oz)	20	1	0	–	6	0	0	55
FRESH									
cooked	1 med	60	7	212	61	12	54	2	425
hearts cooked	½ cup	42	5	149	43	8	38	1	297
FROZEN									
cooked	1 cup	42	5	149	43	8	38	1	297
cooked w/o salt	1 pkg (9 oz)	108	11	394	286	12	50	1	634

FOOD	PORTION	CALS	FIBER	VIT A	FOLIC	VIT C	CALCI	IRON	POTAS
C&W									
Hearts	12 pieces (3 oz)	40	5	100	–	6	40	tr	–
TAKE-OUT									
stuffed	1 (8.8 oz)	397	10	175	113	17	259	4	622

ARUGULA

FOOD	PORTION	CALS	FIBER	VIT A	FOLIC	VIT C	CALCI	IRON	POTAS
fresh	1 cup	3	tr	475	19	3	32	tr	74

ASIAN FOOD

FOOD	PORTION	CALS	FIBER	VIT A	FOLIC	VIT C	CALCI	IRON	POTAS
CANNED									
chow mein chicken no noodles	1 cup	194	2	75	53	9	37	2	403
FRESH									
wonton wrappers	1	23	–	1	1	0	4	tr	7
Azumaya									
Round Wraps	10	160	1	0	–	0	20	2	–
Wrappers Large Square	8	160	1	0	–	0	20	2	–
Frieda's									
Won Ton Wrappers	4 (1 oz)	80	1	100	–	1	0	1	–
Nasoya									
Won Ton Wrappers	8	160	1	0	–	0	20	2	–
FROZEN									
Contessa									
Chow Mein Chicken w/ Sauce not prep	1¾ cups	320	3	1000	–	30	40	1	–
Curry Chicken w/ Sauce not prep	1¾ cups	240	2	400	–	9	40	2	–
Fried Rice Chicken w/ Sauce not prep	1¾ cups	260	4	750	–	12	20	2	–
General Tsao Shrimp w/ Sauce not prep	1¾ cups	270	4	2500	–	42	40	2	–
Kung Pao Shrimp w/ Sauce not prep	1¾ cups	200	3	750	–	9	60	1	–
Low Mein Shrimp w/ Sauce not prep	1¾ cups	250	2	0	–	15	40	4	–
Stir-Fry Beef w/ sauce not prep	1¾ cup	190	4	1250	–	36	60	3	–
Stir-Fry Chicken w/ Sauce not prep	1¾ cups	160	4	2500	–	4	60	2	–

FOOD	PORTION	CALS	FIBER	VIT A	FOLIC	VIT C	CALCI	IRON	POTAS
Stir-Fry Shrimp w/ Sauce not prep	1¾ cups	120	2	2000	–	1	60	2	–
Sweet & Sour Shrimp w/ Sauce not prep	1½ cups	180	3	1000	–	21	40	1	–
Tandoori Chicken w/ Sauce not prep	1⅓ cups	200	3	2500	–	12	40	1	–
Kahiki									
Beef & Broccoli	1 pkg (10.9 oz)	360	2	1250	–	9	20	4	–
Chicken Fried Rice	1 pkg (10.9 oz)	460	2	2000	–	1	40	5	–
General Tso's Chicken	1 pkg (10 oz)	400	2	1250	–	2	40	3	–
Naturals General Tso's Chicken	1 pkg (10 oz)	330	3	1500	–	9	60	2	–
Naturals Mandarin Orange Chicken	1 pkg (10 oz)	340	3	2250	–	9	40	1	–
Naturals Szechuan Peppercorn Beef	1 pkg (10 oz)	350	3	750	–	30	40	3	–
Naturals Teriyaki Mixed Vegetables	1 pkg (10 oz)	260	4	1250	–	9	100	2	–
Sesame Orange Chicken	1 pkg (10.9 oz)	420	2	1250	–	5	60	3	–
Soothing Lettuce Wraps	4 tbsp (2 oz)	90	1	200	–	1	20	tr	–
Tempura Chicken Nuggets	¾ cup (3.5 oz)	230	0	0	–	0	20	1	–
Tropical Sweet & Sour Chicken	1 pkg (10.9 oz)	490	4	1500	–	24	60	3	–
Lean Cuisine									
Cafe Classics Asian Style Beef w/ Ginger & Soy	1 pkg (9.25 oz)	210	2	750	–	4	20	1	720
Cafe Classics Bowl Chicken Fried Rice	1 pkg (10 oz)	310	3	4500	–	5	60	2	450
Cafe Classics Bowl Chicken Teriyaki	1 pkg (11 oz)	320	3	2500	–	6	80	2	580
Cafe Classics Bowl Teriyaki Steak	1 pkg (10.5 oz)	340	4	3250	–	5	40	2	790

FOOD	PORTION	CALS	FIBER	VIT A	FOLIC	VIT C	CALCI	IRON	POTAS
Cafe Classics Chicken Teriyaki Stir Fry	1 pkg (10 oz)	300	3	1250	–	4	20	1	360
Cafe Classics Hunan Beef & Broccoli	1 pkg (8.5 oz)	230	1	300	–	12	40	2	420
Cafe Classics Thai-Style Chicken	1 pkg (9 oz)	230	2	1250	–	24	60	1	650
One Dish Favorites Asian Style Pot Stickers	1 pkg (9 oz)	320	3	1500	–	4	40	2	110
One Dish Favorites Chicken Chow Mein	1 pkg (9 oz)	200	2	1250	–	2	40	1	380
Skillet Asian Style Chicken & Vegetables	1 serv	160	2	2000	–	2	20	1	320
Seeds Of Change									
Asian Stir-Fry Noodles	1 pkg (11 oz)	290	4	2250	–	12	40	4	–
Spicy Peanut Noodles	1 pkg (11 oz)	370	4	2750	–	9	100	4	–
Teriyaki Stir Fried Rice	1 pkg (11 oz)	340	6	2000	–	9	100	3	–
MIX									
Annie Chun's									
Meal Kit Chow Mein Noodles w/ Garlic Black Bean Sauce	⅓ pkg	230	2	0	–	5	0	4	–
Meal Kit Chow Mein Noodles w/ Peanut Sesame Sauce	⅓ pkg	270	2	0	–	2	0	4	–
Meal Kit Chow Mein Noodles w/ Scallion Sauce	⅓ pkg	240	2	0	–	9	0	4	–
Meal Kit Soba Noodles w/ Soy Ginger Sauce	⅓ pkg	210	3	0	–	2	0	2	–
Meal Kits Chow Mein Noodles w/ Teriyaki Sauce	⅓ box	210	2	0	–	0	20	4	–
Meal Kits Pad Thai Noodles w/ Pad Thai Sauce	⅓ pkg	210	–	0	–	1	0	2	–

FOOD	PORTION	CALS	FIBER	VIT A	FOLIC	VIT C	CALCI	IRON	POTAS
Nissin									
Chow Mein Chicken as prep	½ pkg (2 oz)	240	2	400	–	4	40	3	–
Chow Mein Thai Peanut as prep	½ pkg (2 oz)	270	tr	0	–	0	0	3	–
SHELF-STABLE									
Fantastic									
Pad Thai w/ Rice Noodles	1 pkg (7 oz)	400	5	1750	–	5	80	2	–
Thai Lemon Grass w/ Rice Noodles	1 pkg (7.4 oz)	340	5	200	–	5	40	1	–
TAKE-OUT									
beef & broccoli	1 cup	221	3	2440	67	35	46	3	436
buddha's delight w/ cellophane noodles fat choi jai	1 serv (7.6 oz)	211	2	1920	36	59	77	2	986
cha siu bao steamed buns w/ chicken filling	1 (2.3 oz)	160	tr	0	–	0	0	1	–
chow mein beef no noodles	1 cup	271	3	560	51	21	37	3	543
chow mein noodles	1 cup	237	2	0	40	0	9	2	54
chow mein pork no noodles	1 cup	284	3	570	44	21	46	2	510
chow mein shrimp no noodles	1 cup	154	2	90	44	10	59	2	394
chow mein vegetable no noodles	1 cup	224	4	65	55	38	40	1	469
dim sum meat filled	3 pieces (4 oz)	124	1	70	22	1	20	2	213
egg foo yung beef	1 patty (6 oz)	243	1	690	54	6	54	2	292
egg foo yung chicken	1 patty (3 oz)	121	1	350	27	3	28	1	141
egg foo yung pork	1 patty (3 oz)	125	1	345	26	3	28	1	162
egg foo yung shrimp	1 patty (3 oz)	153	1	575	20	2	36	1	159
filipino chicken adobo	1 serv (15 oz)	555	1	1080	15	3	56	3	366

FOOD	PORTION	CALS	FIBER	VIT A	FOLIC	VIT C	CALCI	IRON	POTAS
fried rice	1 cup	333	1	210	97	3	38	3	196
fried rice beef	1 cup	346	1	210	22	3	38	3	271
fried rice chicken	1 cup	329	1	210	143	3	38	3	246
fried rice pork	1 cup	335	1	210	91	3	40	3	269
fried rice shrimp	1 cup	323	1	44	97	4	44	3	176
general tsao's chicken	1 cup	296	1	145	23	12	26	1	251
green beans szechuan style	1 cup	176	6	315	56	26	83	2	424
kung pao beef	1 cup	410	2	75	31	2	21	3	528
kung pao chicken	1 cup	434	2	195	42	8	50	2	428
kung pao pork	1 cup	460	2	170	34	8	50	2	541
kung pao shrimp	1 cup	345	2	405	28	4	83	4	415
lo mein beef	1 cup	286	3	50	94	8	36	3	360
lo mein chicken	1 cup	262	3	70	94	8	36	2	322
lo mein meatless	1 cup	234	3	110	116	7	36	2	260
lo mein pork	1 cup	314	3	50	90	8	40	2	346
lo mein shrimp	1 cup	236	4	190	92	10	46	3	246
moo goo gai pan chicken	1 cup	272	3	520	43	34	130	2	480
moo shu pork w/o pancake	1 cup	512	1	250	21	8	32	2	337
phad thai	1 serv (9.2 oz)	232	1	505	27	21	111	6	282
sesame seed paste bun	1 (2.5 oz)	220	2	0	–	0	125	4	–
shrimp chips banh phong tom	6 med	214	tr	10	1	tr	15	1	29
shrimp w/ lobster sauce	1 cup	298	1	205	24	3	83	4	420
shu mai chicken & vegetable dumplings	6 (3.6 oz)	160	1	1000	–	5	20	1	–
spring roll	1 (3.5 oz)	112	5	–	–	–	54	3	244
sukiyaki beef	1 cup	165	1	865	62	4	68	2	454
sweet & sour chicken w/o rice	1 cup	670	2	275	40	9	53	3	441
sweet & sour pork w/ rice	1 cup	268	2	60	51	15	29	2	315
sweet & sour pork w/o rice	1 cup	231	2	18	9	21	29	1	396
sweet & sour shrimp	1 cup	480	1	95	9	6	46	3	375

FOOD	PORTION	CALS	FIBER	VIT A	FOLIC	VIT C	CALCI	IRON	POTAS
sweet red bean bun	1 (2.5 oz)	130	2	0	–	0	40	2	–
szechuan chicken	1 cup	190	2	405	16	23	28	1	300
szechuan shrimp & vegetables	1 cup	159	2	930	24	27	62	2	342
tempura vegetable	8 pieces	90	1	195	20	2	13	1	96
tempura hawaiian fish tofu vegetable	2 cups	285	2	775	34	4	81	2	237
teriyaki beef	1 cup	454	tr	10	34	16	27	6	586
teriyaki chicken plain	¾ cup	399	–	443	14	tr	39	3	511
teriyaki chicken w/ rice	1 serv (11 oz)	430	1	2000	–	12	60	4	–
teriyaki shrimp	1 cup	271	1	450	16	5	115	6	486
wonton fried meat filled	1 (0.7 oz)	54	tr	25	8	tr	5	tr	51

ASPARAGUS
CANNED

FOOD	PORTION	CALS	FIBER	VIT A	FOLIC	VIT C	CALCI	IRON	POTAS
spears	1 cup	46	4	1989	232	45	39	4	416
spears	1	3	tr	148	17	3	3	tr	31

Del Monte

Cuts & Tips	½ cup	20	1	400	–	15	0	tr	–
Spears	½ cup	20	1	400	–	15	0	tr	–
Tips	½ cup	20	1	400	–	15	0	tr	–

Gertie's Finest

White	1 oz	15	1	0	–	0	20	tr	–

S&W

Green	6 pieces (4.5 oz)	15	1	500	–	21	0	1	130

Tillen Farms

Crispy Asparagus Pickled	3 spears	10	0	100	–	2	0	0	–

FRESH

cooked	4 spears	13	1	604	89	5	14	1	134
cooked	½ cup	20	2	905	134	7	21	1	202
spears raw	4	10	1	363	25	3	12	1	97

Frieda's

White	⅔ cup	20	2	500	–	12	0	1	–

FROZEN

cooked	4 spears	11	1	484	81	15	11	tr	103
cooked	1 pkg (10 oz)	53	5	2362	396	72	53	2	504

FOOD	PORTION	CALS	FIBER	VIT A	FOLIC	VIT C	CALCI	IRON	POTAS
C&W									
Spears	7 (3 oz)	20	tr	300	–	9	0	tr	–
Europe's Best									
Spears	7 spears	15	2	400	–	9	20	2	–

AVOCADO

FOOD	PORTION	CALS	FIBER	VIT A	FOLIC	VIT C	CALCI	IRON	POTAS
california mashed	¼ cup	96	4	85	51	5	7	tr	292
california peeled & pitted	1	289	12	254	154	15	22	1	877
florida mashed	¼ cup	69	1	81	20	10	6	tr	202
florida peeled & pitted	1	365	17	426	106	53	30	1	1067
Brooks Tropical									
Lite SlimCado	1 tbsp	35	tr	0	–	2	0	0	–
Calavo									
Fresh	⅓ med (1 oz)	55	3	0	–	2	0	0	–
Chiquita									
Fresh	⅓ med (1 oz)	55	3	0	–	2	0	0	–
Earthbound Farm									
Organic Fresh	⅓ med (1 oz)	55	3	0	–	2	0	0	–
Frieda's									
Fresh Cocktail	1 (1.4 oz)	60	2	200	–	4	0	tr	–
TAKE-OUT									
guacamole	1 serv (2.2 oz)	105	2	215	38	7	9	1	378

BACON

FOOD	PORTION	CALS	FIBER	VIT A	FOLIC	VIT C	CALCI	IRON	POTAS
bacon grease	1 tbsp	116	0	0	0	0	0	0	0
beef breakfast strips cooked	3 strips	153	0	0	3	0	3	1	140
gammon lean & fat grilled	4.2 oz	274	0	0	–	0	11	2	–
pan fried	3 strips	109	0	0	1	0	2	tr	–
Boar's Head									
Sliced Fried	2 slices	70	0	0	–	0	0	0	–
Oscar Mayer									
Center Cut cooked	2 slices (0.4 oz)	50	0	0	–	0	0	0	–

FOOD	PORTION	CALS	FIBER	VIT A	FOLIC	VIT C	CALCI	IRON	POTAS
Cooked	2 slices (0.5 oz)	70	0	0	–	0	0	0	–
Wellshire									
Beef Uncured	2 oz	114	0	0	–	0	0	1	–

BACON SUBSTITUTES

FOOD	PORTION	CALS	FIBER	VIT A	FOLIC	VIT C	CALCI	IRON	POTAS
bacon bits meatless	1 tbsp	33	1	0	9	tr	7	tr	10
meatless	1 strip	16	tr	4	2	0	1	tr	9
Worthington									
Stripples	2 strips (0.5 oz)	60	tr	0	–	0	0	tr	15

BAGEL

FOOD	PORTION	CALS	FIBER	VIT A	FOLIC	VIT C	CALCI	IRON	POTAS
cinnamon raisin	1 lg (4 in)	244	2	65	99	1	17	3	132
cinnamon raisin	1 mini	71	1	19	23	tr	5	1	38
egg	1 lg (4.5 in)	364	3	143	115	1	17	5	89
low carb	1 (4 oz)	216	14	0	–	0	40	2	–
mini onion	1 (1.4 oz)	100	1	0	–	0	20	1	–
oat bran	1 lg (4 in)	227	3	4	87	tr	11	3	102
plain	1 lg (4.5 in)	360	3	0	115	0	24	5	132
plain	1 sm (3 in)	190	2	0	61	0	12	2	70
plain	1 med (3.5 in)	289	2	0	92	0	19	4	106
Alvarado Street Bakery									
Sprouted Wheat Cinnamon Raisin	1 (3.3 oz)	280	3	0	–	0	40	4	–
David's									
Deli Bagels	1 (2.8 oz)	230	2	0	–	0	100	3	–
Natural Ovens									
Blueberry	1 (3 oz)	190	4	0	160	0	200	1	–
Brainy	1 (3 oz)	170	6	1000	160	0	200	1	–
Cinnamon Raisin	1 (3 oz)	180	5	0	160	0	200	1	–
Golden Crunch	1 (3 oz)	190	8	500	120	0	200	4	–
Hearty Grains & Onion	1 (3 oz)	190	7	1000	160	0	200	1	–
Raspberry	1 (3 oz)	180	5	500	160	0	200	1	–
Whole Grain	1 (3 oz)	170	6	0	160	0	200	1	–

FOOD	PORTION	CALS	FIBER	VIT A	FOLIC	VIT C	CALCI	IRON	POTAS
Sara Lee									
Apple Cinnamon	1 (4 oz)	310	3	0	–	0	150	3	–
Banana Walnut	1 (4 oz)	350	4	0	–	2	140	2	–
Blueberry Deluxe	1 (3.3 oz)	260	2	100	–	0	100	3	–
Blueberry Junior	1 (1 oz)	70	tr	0	–	0	20	tr	–
Blueberry Toaster Size	1 (2.1 oz)	160	1	0	–	0	60	1	–
Cinnamon Raisin Deluxe	1 (3.3 oz)	260	4	0	–	0	100	3	–
Heart Healthy 100% Whole Wheat	1 (3.3 oz)	220	6	0	32	0	100	3	–
Heart Healthy Cinnamon Raisin	1 (3.3 oz)	250	7	0	40	0	150	3	–
Plain	1 (2.1 oz)	160	1	0	–	0	60	1	–
Sundried Tomato & Basil	1 (4 oz)	300	2	300	–	0	100	3	–
Whole Grain Plain	1 (3.3 oz)	240	3	0	100	0	160	3	–
Thomas'									
Carb Consider Plain	1	150	6	0	–	0	60	2	–
Carb Consider Whole Wheat	1	140	7	0	–	0	60	2	–
Weight Watchers									
Original	1 (2.8 oz)	190	10	0	60	0	80	2	–

BAKING POWDER

FOOD	PORTION	CALS	FIBER	VIT A	FOLIC	VIT C	CALCI	IRON	POTAS
baking powder	1 tsp	2	0	0	0	0	270	1	1
low sodium	1 tsp	5	tr	0	0	0	217	tr	505
Calumet									
Double Acting	⅛ tsp	0	0	–	–	–	20	–	–
Clabber Girl									
Baking Powder	1 tsp	0	–	–	–	–	84	tr	tr
Davis									
Baking Powder	1 tsp	0	0	–	–	–	80	–	–
Rumford									
Aluminum Free	⅛ tsp	0	–	–	–	–	80	–	–

BAKING SODA

FOOD	PORTION	CALS	FIBER	VIT A	FOLIC	VIT C	CALCI	IRON	POTAS
baking soda	1 tsp	0	0	0	0	0	0	0	0

BALSAM PEAR (BITTER GOURD)

FOOD	PORTION	CALS	FIBER	VIT A	FOLIC	VIT C	CALCI	IRON	POTAS
leafy tips cooked w/o salt	1 cup	20	1	1401	51	32	24	1	349

FOOD	PORTION	CALS	FIBER	VIT A	FOLIC	VIT C	CALCI	IRON	POTAS
leafy tips raw	1 cup	14	–	832	61	42	40	1	292
pods raw sliced	1 cup	16	3	438	67	78	18	tr	275
pods sliced cooked w/ salt	1 cup	24	3	140	63	41	11	tr	396

BAMBOO SHOOTS

canned sliced	½ cup	12	1	9	2	1	5	tr	52
fresh sliced cooked w/ salt	½ cup	7	1	0	1	0	7	tr	320
raw sliced	½ cup	20	2	15	5	3	10	tr	402

BANANA

banana chips	1 oz	147	2	–	4	2	5	tr	152
fresh	1 med (7 in)	105	3	76	24	10	6	tr	422
fresh	1 lg (8 in)	121	4	87	27	12	7	tr	487
fresh	1 sm (6 in)	90	3	65	20	9	5	tr	362
fresh baby	1 extra sm (< 6 in)	72	2	52	16	7	4	tr	290
fresh mashed	½ cup	100	3	72	23	10	6	tr	403
fresh sliced	1 cup	134	4	96	30	13	8	tr	537
powder	1 tbsp	21	1	15	1	tr	1	tr	92
whole dried	1 piece (1.2 oz)	130	2	100	–	0	0	tr	–

Chiquita

Fresh	1 med (4.4 oz)	110	4	–	–	9	–	–	400

Frieda's

Burro	1 (3 oz)	80	1	0	–	9	0	0	–
Dried	1 piece (1.2 oz)	130	2	100	–	12	0	tr	–

Goodniks

Nutty Bananas Crunchy Snack	⅔ cup	230	3	100	–	0	0	1	–

BARBECUE SAUCE

barbecue	2 tbsp	52	tr	82	1	tr	4	tr	73
low sodium	2 tbsp	52	tr	82	1	tr	4	tr	73

Bone Suckin'

Sauce	2 tbsp	40	0	0	–	0	0	0	–

FOOD	PORTION	CALS	FIBER	VIT A	FOLIC	VIT C	CALCI	IRON	POTAS
Cattlemen's									
Smokehouse	2 tbsp	60	tr	–	–	–	20	tr	–
Hunt's									
Hickory	2 tbsp	45	tr	0	–	0	0	0	75
Hickory & Brown Sugar	2 tbsp	70	1	0	–	0	20	tr	100
Honey Hickory	2 tbsp	50	tr	0	–	0	0	0	100
Honey Mustard	2 tbsp	50	1	0	–	0	0	tr	85
Hot & Spicy	2 tbsp	45	tr	0	–	0	0	0	90
Mesquite	2 tbsp	40	tr	0	–	0	0	0	75
Original	2 tbsp	50	tr	100	–	0	0	0	105
Original Bold	2 tbsp	45	tr	0	–	0	0	0	75
Muir Glen									
Garlic Mesquite	2 tbsp (1.3 oz)	40	tr	300	–	5	20	1	–
Hot & Smoky	2 tbsp (1.2 oz)	40	tr	300	–	5	20	1	–
Original	2 tbsp (1.2 oz)	40	tr	300	–	5	20	1	–
Wellshire									
Original	2 tbsp	39	0	150	–	2	10	tr	–
BARLEY									
flour	1 cup	511	15	0	12	0	47	4	457
pearled cooked	1 cup (5.5 oz)	193	6	11	25	0	17	2	146
pearled uncooked	¼ cup	176	8	11	12	0	15	1	140
BARRACUDA									
broiled	4 oz	239	0	245	3	4	31	2	543
cooked flaked	1 cup	287	0	290	4	5	37	2	651
poached	4 oz	227	0	80	2	2	33	2	496
TAKE-OUT									
breaded & fried	4 oz	282	tr	70	10	2	31	2	519
BASIL									
fresh chopped	1 tbsp	1	tr	140	2	1	4	tr	12
ground	1 tsp	4	–	131	–	1	30	1	48
leaves fresh	5	1	tr	132	2	1	4	tr	12
Eden									
Shiso Leaf Powder	1 tsp	0	0	0	–	0	0	0	5

FOOD	PORTION	CALS	FIBER	VIT A	FOLIC	VIT C	CALCI	IRON	POTAS
BASS									
breaded baked	4 oz	205	1	310	18	2	121	2	346
pickled mero en escabeche	2 oz	156	tr	95	2	tr	7	tr	111
striped baked	3 oz	105	0	88	8	0	16	1	279
striped bass farm raised	4 oz	110	0	100	–	0	20	1	–
BAY LEAF									
crumbled	1 tsp	2	tr	37	1	tr	5	tr	3
BEANS									
CANNED									
baked beans plain	½ cup	119	5	137	15	0	43	2	276
baked beans vegetarian	½ cup	119	5	137	15	0	43	2	276
baked beans w/ franks	½ cup	184	9	113	39	3	62	2	304
baked beans w/ pork	½ cup	134	7	225	46	3	67	2	391
baked beans w/ pork & tomato sauce	½ cup	119	5	106	19	4	71	4	373
refried beans	½ cup	134	–	–	–	8	59	2	495
B&M									
Bacon & Onion	½ cup	190	8	0	–	1	80	3	–
Maple Baked	½ cup	150	6	0	–	0	40	2	–
Vegetarian 99% Fat Free	½ cup	150	6	0	–	0	40	2	–
Bush's									
Barbecue	½ cup	150	5	1500	–	0	60	2	–
Boston Recipe	½ cup	150	5	0	–	1	80	5	–
Country Style	½ cup	170	7	0	–	1	60	2	–
Homestyle	½ cup	140	5	0	–	0	40	2	–
Maple Cured Bacon	½ cup	150	7	0	–	1	60	2	–
Onion 98% Fat Free	½ cup	140	5	0	–	0	40	2	–
Original	½ cup	150	7	0	–	0	60	2	–
Vegetarian Fat Free	½ cup	130	6	0	–	0	40	2	–
Campbell's									
Pork & Beans	½ cup	140	7	0	–	0	40	1	–
Eden									
Organic Baked w/ Sorghum	½ cup	150	7	–	–	–	100	4	460
Heinz									
Vegetarian	1 cup	250	9	200	–	0	100	3	–

FOOD	PORTION	CALS	FIBER	VIT A	FOLIC	VIT C	CALCI	IRON	POTAS
Las Palmas									
Refried	½ cup	150	2	0	–	2	40	2	–
Old El Paso									
Refried Fat Free	½ cup	100	6	0	–	0	40	2	–
Ranch Style									
Original Texas	½ cup	138	6	400	–	0	40	2	–
Read									
3 Bean Salad	½ cup	60	2	0	–	2	20	1	–
Rosarita									
Refried No Fat	½ cup	90	5	–	–	–	40	2	–
Refried Traditional 98% Fat Free	½ cup	100	5	–	–	–	40	2	–
Van Camp's									
Baked Beans w/ Chicken	1 cup	360	0	400	–	0	100	4	–
Baked Original	½ cup	140	6	0	–	0	60	2	–
Pork And Beans	½ cup	110	6	0	–	0	40	2	–
FROZEN									
Lean Cuisine									
Cafe Classics Sante Fe Style Rice & Beans	1 pkg (10.4 oz)	290	5	400	–	4	200	2	620
MIX									
Fantastic									
Instant Black Beans not prep	⅓ cup	160	7	200	–	0	60	3	–
Instant Refried Beans not prep	¼ cup	130	8	200	–	2	40	2	–
TAKE-OUT									
baked beans	½ cup	191	7	0	61	1	77	3	453
barbecue beans	3.5 oz	120	–	200	–	2	40	2	–
frijoles a la charra w/ pork tomatoes & chili peppers	1 cup	341	5	75	80	9	51	2	557
refried beans	½ cup	43	–	231	9	0	9	1	79
three bean salad	1 cup	114	5	45	56	4	34	2	252
BEAR									
simmered	3 oz	220	0	0	5	0	4	9	224
BEAVER									
roasted	4 oz	240	0	0	12	3	25	11	456

FOOD	PORTION	CALS	FIBER	VIT A	FOLIC	VIT C	CALCI	IRON	POTAS
BEECHNUTS									
dried	1 oz	163	–	0	32	4	0	1	288
BEEF									
CANNED									
corned beef	1 oz	71	0	0	3	0	3	1	39
FRESH									
arm pot roast trim 0 fat braised	3.5 oz	297	0	0	9	0	16	2	231
arm pot roast trim ⅛ in fat braised	3.5 oz	302	0	0	9	0	17	3	242
beef crumbles 70% lean pan browned	3 oz	230	0	0	11	0	35	2	279
bottom round roast trim 0 in fat braised	4 oz	253	0	0	11	0	9	3	307
bottom round roast trim 0 in fat roasted	3.5 oz	187	0	0	9	0	7	2	223
bottom round roast trim ½ in fat braised	4 oz	337	0	0	11	0	7	4	325
bottom round roast trim ⅛ in fat braised	4 oz	280	0	0	11	0	9	3	301
bottom round roast trim ⅛ in fat roasted	4 oz	247	0	0	9	0	7	2	243
bottom sirloin butt roast trim 0 in roasted	3.5 oz	182	0	0	9	0	17	2	340
brisket flat half trim ⅛ in fat braised	3.5 oz	298	0	0	9	0	16	2	227
brisket flat trim 0 fat braised	3.5 oz	221	0	0	10	0	17	3	254
brisket point half trim 0 fat braised	3.5 oz	358	0	0	7	0	8	2	233
brisket point half trim ¼ in fat braised	3.5 oz	404	0	0	6	0	9	2	221
brisket point half trim ⅛ in fat braised	3.5 oz	349	0	0	7	0	8	2	241
chuck boston cut roast trim 0 fat roasted	3.5 oz	207	0	0	9	0	7	3	367
chuck boston cut roast trim ¼ in fat roasted	3.5 oz	242	0	0	9	0	8	3	337
chuck bottom roast trim 0 fat braised	3.5 oz	334	0	0	5	0	13	3	236

FOOD	PORTION	CALS	FIBER	VIT A	FOLIC	VIT C	CALCI	IRON	POTAS
chuck bottom roast trim ¼ in fat braised	3.5 oz	345	0	0	5	0	13	3	231
chuck fillet steak trim 0 fat broiled	4 oz	181	0	0	9	0	9	3	332
chuck top roast trim 0 fat broiled	4 oz	245	0	0	9	0	8	3	339
club steak trim ½ in fat broiled	4 oz	384	0	0	8	0	10	2	381
corned beef brisket cooked	3 oz	213	0	0	8	0	7	2	123
crosscut shank trim ¼ in fat stewed	1 serv (6.8 oz)	510	0	0	17	0	58	7	784
delmonico steak trim ¼ in fat broiled	4 oz	409	0	0	8	0	15	3	372
entrecote steak trim ½ in fat broiled	4 oz	413	0	0	8	0	15	2	369
eye round roast trim 0 in fat roasted	4 oz	190	0	0	10	0	8	3	266
eye round roast trim ¼ in fat roasted	4 oz	283	0	0	8	0	4	2	415
eye round roast trim ⅛ in fat roasted	4 oz	236	0	0	10	0	6	3	257
filet mignon roast trim ¼ in fat roasted	4 oz	376	0	0	8	0	10	3	369
filet mignon roast trim ⅛ in fat roasted	4 oz	367	0	0	9	0	10	4	375
filet mignon trim 0 in fat broiled	4 oz	247	0	0	10	0	23	2	386
filet mignon trim ⅛ in fat broiled	4 oz	303	0	0	9	0	22	2	373
ground 70% lean broiled	3.5 oz	273	0	0	11	0	35	2	275
ground 75% lean broiled	2.5 oz	195	0	0	8	0	21	2	202
ground 80% lean broiled	3 oz	234	0	0	9	0	20	2	258
ground 85% lean pan fried	3 oz	197	0	0	7	0	17	2	297
ground 90% lean pan fried	3 oz	173	0	0	7	0	13	2	309

FOOD	PORTION	CALS	FIBER	VIT A	FOLIC	VIT C	CALCI	IRON	POTAS
ground 95% lean pan fried	3 oz	139	0	0	6	0	8	2	320
ground 97% fat free irradiated	4 oz	160	0	0	–	0	0	2	–
london broil trim 0 fat broiled	3.5 oz	188	0	0	9	0	20	2	339
london broil trim ¼ in fat broiled	4 oz	260	0	0	14	0	7	3	490
new york strip steak trim 0 fat broiled	4 oz	219	0	0	10	0	24	2	403
oxtails cooked	6 pieces (6.3 oz)	472	0	0	11	0	23	7	472
porterhouse steak trim 0 in fat broiled	1 lb	1252	0	0	32	0	32	13	1356
porterhouse steak trim ¼ in fat broiled	1 lb	1492	0	0	32	0	36	12	1157
porterhouse steak trim ⅛ in fat broiled	4 oz	337	0	0	8	0	9	3	364
porterhouse steak trim ⅛ in fat broiled	1 lb	1324	0	0	32	0	36	12	1455
rib eye roast trim ¼ in fat roasted	3.5 oz	365	0	0	7	0	10	2	288
rib eye steak trim ⅛ in fat broiled	4 oz	221	0	0	11	0	22	2	429
rib roast trim ¼ in fat roasted	4 oz	406	0	0	8	0	12	3	341
rib steak trim ¼ in fat broiled	4 oz	388	0	0	7	0	14	2	354
round tip roast trim 0 in fat roasted	4 oz	213	0	0	9	0	7	2	246
sandwich steaks thinly sliced	1 serv (2 oz)	173	0	0	4	0	7	1	130
shell steak trim ¼ in fat broiled	4 oz	366	0	0	8	0	10	3	392
shortribs lean & fat braised	1 serv (7.8 oz)	1060	0	0	11	0	27	5	504
skirt steak trim 0 fat broiled	4 oz	289	0	0	8	0	12	3	430
t-bone steak trim 0 fat broiled	4 oz	280	0	0	8	0	6	4	342

FOOD	PORTION	CALS	FIBER	VIT A	FOLIC	VIT C	CALCI	IRON	POTAS
t-bone steak trim ¼ in fat broiled	1 lb	1388	0	0	32	0	32	14	1279
t-bone steak trim ⅛ in fat broiled	1 lb	804	0	0	20	0	23	8	964
tip round roast trim ⅛ in fat roasted	4 oz	248	0	0	9	0	7	3	416
top loin steak boneless trim ⅛ in fat broiled	4 oz	299	0	0	9	0	22	2	372
top round roast trim 0 fat braised	4 oz	237	0	0	10	0	5	4	374
top round roast trim ¼ in fat braised	4 oz	281	0	0	10	0	6	4	357
top round roast trim ¼ in fat roasted	4 oz	265	0	0	8	0	7	3	407
top round steak trim ¼ in fat pan fried	4 oz	314	0	0	14	0	7	3	533
top sirloin steak trim ⅛ in fat broiled	4 oz	275	0	0	9	0	23	2	381
top sirloin steak trim ⅛ in fat pan fried	4 oz	355	0	0	10	0	14	4	460
tri-tip roast trim 0 fat roasted	3.5 oz	218	0	0	8	0	17	2	308
tri-tip steak trim 0 fat broiled	4 oz	300	0	0	11	0	14	4	495
Laura's Lean									
Eye Of Round	4 oz	135	0	–	–	–	–	–	–
Ground Beef 92% Lean	4 oz	160	0	–	–	–	–	–	–
Ground Beef Patties	1 (4 oz)	160	0	–	–	–	–	–	–
Ground Round 96% Lean	4 oz	140	0	–	–	–	–	–	–
Sirloin Tip	4 oz	130	0	–	–	–	–	–	–
Top Round	4 oz	135	0	–	–	–	–	–	–
Maverick Ranch									
Filet Mignon	4 oz	120	0	–	–	–	–	3	–
Ground	4 oz	130	0	–	–	–	–	2	–
Ground Round	4 oz	130	0	–	–	–	–	2	–
Ground Sirloin & Chuck	4 oz	130	0	–	–	–	–	2	–
NY Strip Steak	4 oz	150	0	–	–	–	–	2	–
Rib Eye Steak	4 oz	170	0	–	–	–	–	2	–

FOOD	PORTION	CALS	FIBER	VIT A	FOLIC	VIT C	CALCI	IRON	POTAS
Top Round Steak & Roast	4 oz	110	0	–	–	–	–	2	–
Top Sirloin	4 oz	160	0	–	–	–	–	3	–
FROZEN									
patty broiled medium	3 oz	240	0	0	8	0	9	2	250
Soy Lean									
Beef Patty	1 (2.5 oz)	90	–	0	–	0	20	2	–
READY-TO-EAT									
dried beef smoked chopped	1 oz	37	0	0	2	0	2	1	106
roast beef spread	¼ cup	127	tr	1	5	tr	13	1	148
Boar's Head									
Corned Beef Brisket	2 oz	80	0	0	–	0	0	1	–
Top Round Deluxe	2 oz	80	0	0	–	0	0	3	–
Top Round Oven Roasted No Salt Added	2 oz	90	0	0	–	0	0	3	–
Sara Lee									
Roast Beef Medium or Rare	2 oz	60	0	0	–	0	0	1	–

BEEF DISHES
CANNED
Hormel

FOOD	PORTION	CALS	FIBER	VIT A	FOLIC	VIT C	CALCI	IRON	POTAS
Corned Beef Hash 50% Reduced Fat	1 cup	290	2	0	–	0	20	2	–
Libby's									
Hash Corned Beef	1 cup	420	3	0	–	0	20	2	–
FROZEN									
Ian's									
Italian Meatballs	3 (2.2 oz)	145	1	100	–	1	20	1	–
Quaker Maid									
Sandwich Steaks Pure Beef	1 serv (1.8 oz)	120	0	0	–	0	0	40	–
REFRIGERATED									
Huxtable's									
Shepherds Pie Beef	1 pkg (10 oz)	270	3	1250	–	6	20	1	–
Morton's Of Omaha									
Beef Pot Roast w/ Gravy	1 serv (3 oz)	160	0	0	–	0	20	3	–

FOOD	PORTION	CALS	FIBER	VIT A	FOLIC	VIT C	CALCI	IRON	POTAS
Smithfield									
Beef Tips w/ Gravy	½ cup	170	tr	–	–	–	20	2	–
Tyson									
Roast Beef In Brown Gravy	1 serv + gravy (3.5 oz)	160	0	0	–	0	20	2	–
SHELF-STABLE									
TastyBite									
Beef Roganjosh	1 pkg (9.5 oz)	270	3	700	–	15	60	2	
TAKE-OUT									
beef bourguignonne	1 cup	339	1	10	29	4	44	4	766
beef curry	1 cup	432	3	1405	19	16	35	5	953
beef satay + peanut sauce	2 skewers	253	1	–	15	tr	15	–	436
bool kogi korean marinated beef ribs	4 oz	190	0	0	–	0	20	2	–
bracciola	1 roll (4.7 oz)	276	1	635	25	2	16	3	494
bubble & squeak	5 oz	186	3	180	–	10	30	1	–
bulgoghi korean grilled beef	1 serv (5.2 oz)	256	tr	125	10	3	19	3	367
chipped beef on toast	1 slice (5 oz)	226	1	600	38	0	152	2	242
cornish pasty	1 (8 oz)	847	3	0	–	0	153	4	–
goulash w/ potatoes	1 cup	298	2	50	32	18	24	3	825
greek moussaka	1 serv (8.5 oz)	450	1	960	25	4	243	2	423
irish stew	1 cup (7 oz)	280	–	10	–	11	17	2	–
kebab indian	1 (5.4 oz)	553	–	495	–	3	62	5	–
kheena	6.7 oz	781	tr	780	–	2	32	5	–
koftas	5	280	tr	250	–	2	23	2	–
meatloaf	1 lg slice (5 oz)	294	1	110	23	1	75	3	396
pepper steak	1 cup	317	1	75	26	24	28	3	542
pot roast w/ gravy	1 serv (6 oz)	320	0	0	–	0	40	5	–
samosa	2 (4 oz)	652	2	155	–	1	37	1	–

FOOD	PORTION	CALS	FIBER	VIT A	FOLIC	VIT C	CALCI	IRON	POTAS
shepherds pie	1 serv (7 oz)	282	2	110	20	4	120	3	500
steak & kidney pie w/ top crust	1 slice (5 oz)	400	1	700	–	3	52	4	–
stew w/ potatoes & vegetables	1 cup	199	3	930	35	15	35	2	630
stroganoff	1 cup	394	1	475	31	1	105	3	527
swiss steak w/ sauce	1 serv (8 oz)	234	1	285	23	7	36	3	631
toad in the hole	1 (4.7 oz)	383	1	155	–	0	117	1	–

BEEFALO
roasted	4 oz	213	0	0	20	10	27	3	520

BEER AND ALE
alcohol free beer	7 fl oz	50	–	–	15	–	5	tr	40
ale brown	10 oz	77	0	0	–	0	19	tr	–
ale pale	10 oz	88	0	0	–	0	25	tr	–
beer light	12 oz can	103	0	0	21	0	14	tr	74
beer regular	12 oz can	153	0	0	21	0	14	tr	96
black & tan	1 serv (12 oz)	146	1	–	21	–	18	tr	89
boilermaker	1 serv	216	1	–	21	–	18	tr	90
lager	10 oz	80	0	0	–	0	11	0	–
mead	1 serv	250	1	–	21	–	18	tr	90
pilsener lager	7 oz	85	–	–	6	–	4	12	55
shandy	1 serv	125	1	tr	18	1	16	tr	76
stout	10 oz	102	0	0	–	0	25	tr	–

BEET JUICE
juice	7 oz	72	–	–	–	6	–	–	484

BEETS
CANNED
harvard	½ cup	90	3	14	36	3	14	tr	202
pickled	½ cup	74	3	12	31	3	12	tr	168
sliced	½ cup	37	2	28	36	3	22	1	196

Del Monte
Pickled Sliced	½ cup	35	2	0	–	2	0	tr	–
Sliced	½ cup	35	2	0	–	2	0	tr	–

FOOD	PORTION	CALS	FIBER	VIT A	FOLIC	VIT C	CALCI	IRON	POTAS
S&W									
Julienne	½ cup (4.3 oz)	30	1	0	–	0	0	1	–
Pickled Sliced	1 oz	15	1	0	–	0	0	0	–
Pickled Whole	1 oz	15	1	0	–	0	0	0	–
Sliced	½ cup (4.3 oz)	30	1	0	–	0	0	1	–
Whole Small	½ cup (4.3 oz)	30	1	0	–	0	0	1	–
Veg-All									
Small Sliced	½ cup	40	1	0	–	0	0	0	–
FRESH									
greens cooked w/o salt	½ cup	19	2	5511	10	18	82	1	654
sliced cooked	½ cup	37	2	30	68	3	14	1	259
whole cooked	2 med (3.5 oz)	44	2	35	80	4	16	1	305
Frieda's									
Beets	½ cup	35	2	0	–	4	0	1	–
BISCUIT									
MIX									
plain as prep	1 (2 oz)	190	1	53	29	tr	105	1	107
Bisquick									
Heart Smart	⅓ cup	140	tr	–	40	–	150	1	45
Jiffy									
Buttermilk as prep	1	170	tr	0	–	0	60	2	–
King Arthur									
Whole Grain Buttermilk not prep	¼ cup	100	2	0	–	0	100	1	–
REFRIGERATED									
plain baked	1 (1 oz)	93	tr	0	22	0	5	1	42
TAKE-OUT									
buttermilk	1 lg (2.7 oz)	280	1	2	54	0	38	3	172
oatcakes	2 (4 oz)	115	1	0	–	0	14	1	–
plain	1 sm (1.2 oz)	127	1	1	25	0	17	1	78
tea biscuit	1 (3 oz)	210	1	200	–	0	150	3	–
w/ egg	1 (4.8 oz)	373	1	620	57	tr	82	3	238
w/ egg & bacon	1 (5.3 oz)	458	1	371	60	3	189	4	251
w/ egg & ham	1 (6.7 oz)	442	1	874	65	0	221	5	319

FOOD	PORTION	CALS	FIBER	VIT A	FOLIC	VIT C	CALCI	IRON	POTAS
w/ egg & sausage	1 (6.3 oz)	581	1	635	65	0	155	4	320
w/ egg & steak	1 (5.2 oz)	410	–	704	56	tr	138	5	306
w/ egg cheese & bacon	1 (5.1 oz)	477	–	648	53	2	164	3	230
w/ ham	1 (4 oz)	386	1	133	38	tr	160	3	197
w/ sausage	1 (4.4 oz)	485	1	56	46	tr	128	3	198

BITTERMELON
Frieda's
Foo Qua	1 cup	15	2	300	–	72	0	tr	–

BLACK BEANS
dried cooked	1 cup	227	15	10	256	0	47	4	611

Bean Cuisine
Pasta & Beans Mediterranean Black Beans & Fusilli	1 serv	210	4	750	–	6	60	4	–

Eden
Organic Caribbean	½ cup	90	7	–	–	–	40	3	380
Organic Refried	½ cup	110	7	–	–	–	40	3	370

BLACKBERRIES
canned in heavy syrup	½ cup	118	4	280	35	4	27	1	127
fresh	½ cup	31	4	154	18	15	21	tr	117
unsweetened frzn	½ cup	48	4	86	26	2	22	1	106

Oregon
In Light Syrup	½ cup	120	6	300	–	5	40	1	170

BLACKBERRY JUICE
canned	6 oz	65	tr	210	17	19	21	1	231

BLACKEYE PEAS
catjang dried cooked	1 cup (2.9 oz)	200	–	17	242	1	44	5	641
cowpeas canned	1 cup	184	–	32	123	7	48	2	413
cowpeas leafy tips chopped cooked	1 cup	12	–	305	–	10	36	1	186

CANNED
w/pork	½ cup	199	–	0	–	1	21	3	427

Eden
Organic	½ cup	90	4	–	24	–	20	2	210

DRIED
cooked	1 cup	198	16	26	356	1	42	4	476

FOOD	PORTION	CALS	FIBER	VIT A	FOLIC	VIT C	CALCI	IRON	POTAS
TAKE-OUT									
blackeye peas & pork	1 cup	236	8	10	252	1	36	4	501

BLINTZE

Cohen's & Wilton
Cheese	1	80	0	50	–	0	10	tr	–

Golden
Cheese	1 (2.1 oz)	80	2	0	–	0	20	0	–
Potato	1	90	2	0	–	0	0	0	–
Vegetable	1	110	0	0	–	1	20	tr	–

Ratner's
Cheese	1 (2.2 oz)	90	tr	0	–	0	0	1	–

TAKE-OUT
cheese	1 (2.7 oz)	160	tr	4500	–	0	300	1	–

BLUEBERRIES
canned in heavy syrup	½ cup	113	2	46	3	1	6	tr	51
fresh	1 pt	229	10	217	24	39	24	1	310
fresh	½ cup	41	2	39	4	7	4	tr	56
frzn unsweetened	½ cup	40	2	36	5	2	6	tr	42

A&L Farms
Bleuets Fresh	1 pt	80	5	0	–	9	0	tr	–

C&W
Ultimate	¾ cup	70	3	100	–	2	20	tr	–

De-Lite
Dried Sweetened	1 oz	86	4	9	–	22	109	tr	47

Eden
Organic Dried Wild	¼ cup	150	5	0	–	0	40	1	300

Europe's Best
Woodland frzn	¾ cup	70	4	100	–	4	20	tr	–

Frieda's
Dried	¼ cup (1.4 oz)	140	4	0	–	0	0	0	–

Hodgson Mill
Dried Wild	¼ cup	120	6	0	–	30	150	1	66

Oregon
In Light Syrup	½ cup	110	2	100	–	0	0	tr	70

Sunsweet
Dried	¼ cup (1.4 oz)	140	3	100	–	18	60	1	150

FOOD	PORTION	CALS	FIBER	VIT A	FOLIC	VIT C	CALCI	IRON	POTAS
BLUEBERRY JUICE									
Van Dyk's									
100% Juice	6 oz	74	0	0	–	0	0	0	154
BLUEFIN									
fillet baked	4.1 oz	186	0	537	2	tr	10	1	558
BLUEFISH									
fresh baked	3 oz	135	0	390	2	tr	8	1	405
BONITO									
dried	1 oz	50	0	1030	1	0	3	tr	88
fresh	3 oz	117	0	–	–	0	24	1	–
BORAGE									
fresh chopped	1 cup	19	–	3738	12	31	83	3	418
BOYSENBERRIES									
frzn unsweetened	½ cup	33	4	44	42	2	18	1	92
in heavy syrup	½ cup	113	3	51	44	8	23	1	115
BRAINS									
beef pan-fried	3 oz	167	0	0	5	3	8	2	301
beef simmered	3 oz	123	0	99	4	9	8	2	207
lamb braised	3 oz	123	0	0	4	10	10	1	174
lamb fried	3 oz	232	0	0	6	20	18	2	304
pork braised	3 oz	117	0	0	3	12	8	2	–
veal braised	3 oz	116	0	0	3	11	14	1	182
veal fried	3 oz	181	0	0	5	13	9	1	401
BRAN									
corn	1 cup (2.7 oz)	170	65	18	3	0	32	2	33
oat	½ cup (1.6 oz)	116	7	0	25	0	27	3	266
oat cooked	½ cup (3.8 oz)	44	3	0	7	0	11	1	101
rice	½ cup (2.1 oz)	187	12	0	37	0	34	11	786
wheat	½ cup (2 oz)	63	12	0	23	0	21	3	343
BRAZIL NUTS									
dried unblanched	1 oz	186	–	0	1	tr	50	1	170

FOOD	PORTION	CALS	FIBER	VIT A	FOLIC	VIT C	CALCI	IRON	POTAS
BREAD									
CANNED									
boston brown	1 slice (1.6 oz)	88	2	55	5	0	32	1	143
FROZEN									
Alexia									
Baguette Garlic	2 pieces (1.6 oz)	130	tr	200	–	2	20	tr	–
Corbi's									
Chee-Zee Bread Original	½ piece (1.8 oz)	180	1	300	–	0	100	1	–
Marie Callender's									
Cornbread & Honey Butter	1 piece + butter	210	1	100	–	0	20	tr	
Original Garlic	1 piece	190	2	200	–	0	20	1	
Parmesan & Romano Garlic	1 piece	200	2	300	–	0	200	1	
MIX									
cornbread	1 piece (2 oz)	188	1	123	33	tr	44	1	77
Buitoni									
Focaccia Italian Herb & Cheese	1 slice	110	0	0	–	0	20	tr	–
Focaccia Rosemary & Garlic	1 piece (1 oz)	110	1	0	–	2	20	1	0
Sassafras									
12 Grain & Sunflower	1 slice (1.4 oz)	150	1	0	–	0	20	1	–
READY-TO-EAT									
anadama	1 (1.1 oz)	87	1	35	27	0	26	1	100
baguette parisian	2 oz	120	tr	0	–	0	0	2	–
baguette whole wheat	2 oz	140	1	0	–	0	0	1	–
challah	1 slice (1.4 oz)	115	1	85	42	0	37	1	46
cinnamon	1 slice (0.9 oz)	69	1	0	29	0	39	1	26
cracked wheat	1 slice (1.1 oz)	78	2	0	18	0	13	1	53
cuban bread	1 slice (1.1 oz)	83	1	0	30	0	8	1	29

FOOD	PORTION	CALS	FIBER	VIT A	FOLIC	VIT C	CALCI	IRON	POTAS
french	1 slice (1.1 oz)	88	1	0	47	0	24	1	36
italian	1 loaf (1 lb)	1255	–	0	–	0	77	13	336
navajo fry	1 piece	281	–	–	104	–	48	3	65
oat bran	1 slice (1.1 oz)	71	1	2	24	0	20	1	44
oatmeal	1 slice (0.9 oz)	73	1	4	17	0	18	1	38
pan criollo	1 piece (0.9 oz)	69	tr	1	25	0	6	1	24
pannetone	1 slice (0.9 oz)	86	1	95	32	tr	14	1	51
pita	1 lg (2 oz)	165	1	0	64	0	52	2	72
pita	1 sm (1 oz)	77	1	0	30	0	24	1	34
pita whole wheat	1 sm (1 oz)	74	2	0	10	0	4	1	48
pita whole wheat	1 lg (2.2 oz)	170	5	0	22	0	10	2	109
potato scallion	1 slice (2 oz)	120	0	100	–	4	20	1	–
pumpernickel	1 slice (0.9 oz)	65	2	0	24	0	18	1	54
raisin	1 slice (1.1 oz)	88	1	0	34	0	21	1	73
rye	1 slice (1.1 oz)	83	2	0	35	tr	23	1	53
seven grain	1 slice (1.1 oz)	80	2	0	38	tr	29	1	65
wheat berry	1 slice (0.9 oz)	65	1	0	23	0	26	1	50
wheat bran	1 slice (1.3 oz)	89	1	0	38	0	27	1	82
wheat germ	1 slice (1 oz)	73	1	1	33	tr	25	1	71
white cubed	1 cup	93	1	0	39	0	53	1	35
whole wheat	1 slice (1 oz)	69	2	1	14	0	20	1	71

FOOD	PORTION	CALS	FIBER	VIT A	FOLIC	VIT C	CALCI	IRON	POTAS
Alvarado Street Bakery									
Diabetic Lifestyle	1 (1.2 oz)	80	2	0	–	0	0	1	–
Arnold									
Bakery Light 100% Whole Wheat	1 slice	80	5	0	–	0	20	1	–
Country Classics Buttermilk	1 slice	110	tr	0	–	0	60	1	–
Country Classics Wheat	1 slice	100	2	0	24	0	20	1	–
Raisin Cinnamon	1 slice (1 oz)	80	1	0	40	0	0	1	–
Smart & Healthy Omega-3 100% Whole Wheat	1 slice	80	2	0	8	0	40	1	–
Smart & Healthy Sugar Free 100% Whole Wheat	1 slice	80	2	0	8	0	60	1	–
Baker's Inn									
9 Grain	1 slice	100	2	0	32	0	150	1	–
Cracked Wheat	1 slice	100	2	0	32	0	150	1	–
Honey White Made w/ Whole Grain	1 slice	110	1	0	32	0	150	1	–
Honey Whole Wheat	1 slice	100	2	0	32	0	150	1	–
Potato Made w/ Whole Grain	1 slice	100	1	0	32	0	150	1	–
Beefsteak									
Rye Soft	1 slice	70	0	–	16	0	0	1	–
Cedar's									
Wraps Whole Wheat	1 (2 oz)	180	4	0	–	0	100	0	–
Damascus									
Roll-Up Flax	1 (2 oz)	110	9	0	–	0	40	2	–
Roll-Up Whole Wheat	1 (2 oz)	110	7	0	–	0	20	1	–
Wraps Honey Wheat	½ wrap (2 oz)	130	1	0	60	0	0	1	–
Wraps Spinach	1 (4 oz)	280	2	400	160	0	80	4	–
Earth Grains									
100% Mulit Grain Extra Fiber	1 slice	110	5	0	40	0	150	1	–
Oat & Nut	1 slice	120	1	0	40	0	100	1	–
Potato	1 slice	110	tr	0	40	0	100	1	–

FOOD	PORTION	CALS	FIBER	VIT A	FOLIC	VIT C	CALCI	IRON	POTAS
Whole Grain Honey	1 slice	110	2	0	40	0	100	1	–
Whole Wheat Honey	1 slice	110	5	0	40	0	150	1	–
Ecce Panis									
Country Wheat	1 slice (2 oz)	150	2	0	–	0	0	2	–
European Baguette	2 oz	150	1	0	–	0	0	2	–
Enjoy Life									
Rye-Less Rye	1 slice	80	1	0	80	2	80	1	–
Food For Life									
Brown Rice Bread Yeast Free	1 slice	100	1	0	–	0	0	0	–
Rice Bread Fruit & Seed Yeast Free	1 slice	140	0	0	–	0	0	0	–
Rice Bread Multi Seed Yeast Free	1 slice	120	1	0	–	0	0	0	–
White Rice Bread Yeast Free	1 slice	100	tr	0	–	0	0	tr	–
Freihofer's									
100% Whole Wheat	1 slice	90	3	0	32	0	40	2	–
Whole Wheat Light	2 slices	80	5	0	16	0	20	1	–
French Meadow Bakery									
Healthy Hemp	1 slice	92	5	–	–	–	–	–	112
Gold Medal									
100% Whole Wheat	1 slice	70	2	0	–	0	20	1	–
Home Pride									
Wheat	1 slice (1 oz)	80	1	0	16	0	20	1	–
Kangaroo									
Bread Wraps	1 (2.6 oz)	140	5	0	–	0	40	1	–
Greek Pita Flat	1 (2.6 oz)	200	3	0	–	0	70	2	–
Greek Pita Flat Wheat	1 (2.4 oz)	145	3	0	–	0	90	2	–
Pita Pockets Onion	½ (1.2 oz)	90	1	0	–	0	60	0	–
Pita Pockets Wheat N'Honey	½ (1.2 oz)	90	4	0	–	0	60	0	–
Pita Pockets White	½ (1.2 oz)	90	1	0	–	0	60	0	–
Salad Pockets	1 (1.2 oz)	90	1	0	–	0	60	0	–
Sandwich Pockets Whole Grain	1 (1.2 oz)	80	5	0	–	0	0	1	–

FOOD	PORTION	CALS	FIBER	VIT A	FOLIC	VIT C	CALCI	IRON	POTAS
Matthew's									
All Natural Cinnamon Raisin	1 slice	80	1	200	–	–	–	1	–
Milton's									
100% Whole Wheat	1 slice	110	5	0	–	0	100	1	–
Buttermilk	1 slice	90	1	0	40	0	100	2	–
Gourmet White	1 slice	110	1	0	40	0	100	2	–
Original Multi-Grain	1 slice	120	3	0	24	0	100	2	–
Potato	1 slice	90	1	0	40	0	100	2	–
Whole Grain	1 slice	90	5	0	24	0	100	1	–
Natural Ovens									
100% Whole Grain	1 slice	60	5	0	40	0	100	1	–
7 Grain Herb	1 slice	70	4	0	60	0	100	1	–
Better White	1 slice	80	2	0	40	0	100	1	–
Cracked Wheat	1 slice	80	3	0	60	0	100	1	–
English Muffin Bread	1 slice	80	2	0	40	0	100	1	–
Glorious Cinnamon Raisin	1 slice	70	2	0	40	0	100	2	–
Happiness Raisin Pecan	1 slice	70	3	0	80	0	100	2	–
Health Max	1 slice	80	3	0	60	0	100	1	–
Hunger Filler	1 slice	60	4	0	40	0	60	1	–
Lo Carb Golden Crunch	1 slice	70	4	250	60	0	100	2	–
Lo Carb Original	1 slice	60	5	50	60	0	100	2	0
Mild Rye	1 slice	70	4	0	80	0	100	2	–
Multi-Grain Stay Slim	1 slice	60	5	0	40	0	60	1	–
Nutty Natural	1 slice	70	5	0	60	0	100	1	–
Right Wheat	1 slice	60	5	0	40	0	60	1	–
Soft Wheat	1 slice	70	3	0	40	0	100	1	–
Sunny Millet	1 slice	60	4	0	40	0	100	1	–
Nature's Own									
100% Whole Wheat	1 slice	50	2	0	16	0	tr	–	–
9 Grain	1 slice	120	2	0	–	0	0	1	–
Hearty Oatmeal	1 slice	100	3	0	–	0	40	1	–
Wheat Double Fiber	1 slice	10	5	0	–	0	150	1	–
Wheat Light	2 slices	80	5	0	40	0	80	3	–
Wheat N' Fiber	1 slice	60	2	0	–	0	40	1	–
Whole Wheat w/ Organic Flour	1 slice	100	3	0	–	0	40	1	–

FOOD	PORTION	CALS	FIBER	VIT A	FOLIC	VIT C	CALCI	IRON	POTAS
Nature's Path									
Manna Carrot Raisin	1 slice	130	5	0	–	0	20	2	–
Manna Millet Rice	1 slice	130	5	0	–	0	20	2	–
Manna SunSeed	1 slice	160	7	0	–	0	30	2	–
Pepperidge Farm									
Canadian White	1 slice	100	1	0	32	0	20	1	–
Deli Rye Seedless	1 slice	80	1	0	24	0	20	1	–
Farmhouse Soft 100% Whole Wheat	1 slice	110	3	0	16	0	40	1	–
Farmhouse Soft Oatmeal	1 slice	120	1	0	32	0	20	1	–
Farmhouse Whole Grain White	1 slice	110	3	0	60	0	100	1	–
Jewish Rye Seeded	1 slice	80	2	0	24	0	20	1	–
Swirl French Vanilla	1 slice	140	tr	0	40	0	0	1	–
Whole Grain Honey Oat	1 slice	110	3	0	8	0	40	1	–
Whole Grain Honey Whole Wheat	1 slice	110	3	0	8	0	40	1	–
Whole Grain Swirl Cinnamon	1 slice	100	3	1000	80	0	200	4	–
Whole Grain Swirl Cinnamon Raisin	1 slice	100	3	1000	80	0	200	4	–
Sara Lee									
100% Whole Wheat	1 slice	70	2	0	16	0	60	1	–
Blueberry Crumble	1 slice	180	4	0	40	0	100	1	–
Cinnamon Raisin	1 slice	190	3	0	32	0	100	1	–
Classic Wheat	1 slice	70	2	0	0	0	40	1	–
Delightful 100% Whole Wheat	1 slice	90	5	0	24	0	60	1	–
Delightful Wheat	1 slice	45	2	0	16	0	20	1	–
Delightful White	1 slice	90	4	0	32	0	60	1	–
Heart Healthy 100% Whole Wheat Essentials	1 slice	80	4	0	40	0	150	1	–
Heart Healthy Multigrain	1 slice	100	2	0	16	0	40	1	–
Honey Wheat	1 slice	70	1	0	24	0	20	1	–
Honey White	1 slice	100	tr	0	40	0	40	1	–

FOOD	PORTION	CALS	FIBER	VIT A	FOLIC	VIT C	CALCI	IRON	POTAS
Multigrain	1 slice	100	2	0	8	0	60	1	–
White Whole Grain	1 slice	150	3	0	60	0	250	1	–
Stroehmann									
100% Whole Wheat	1 slice	90	3	0	8	0	40	1	–
Family Grains Twisted Bread	1 slice	70	2	0	40	0	60	1	–
Honey Cracked Wheat	1 slice	90	1	0	24	0	20	1	–
New York Rye	1 slice (1 oz)	80	1	0	24	0	20	1	–
Potato	1 slice	100	1	0	32	0	40	1	–
Soft Rye Seeded	1 slice	90	1	0	32	0	40	1	–
Super Bakery									
Athlete's Formula	1 slice (1.5 oz)	100	7	0	0	0	20	1	–
Fitness Formula	1 slice (1.5 oz)	90	7	0	40	0	20	1	–
Wrap Organic	1 (4 oz)	340	20	0	–	0	40	2	–
TastyBite									
Nan Kontos Massala	½ loaf (1.4 oz)	120	1	0	–	0	40	1	76
Nan Kontos Onion	½ loaf (1.4 oz)	120	1	0	–	0	40	1	–
Nan Kontos Roghani	½ loaf (1.4 oz)	125	1	0	–	0	20	1	–
Nan Kontos Tandoori	½ loaf (1.4 oz)	120	1	0	–	0	20	1	–
Roti Kontos Missy	½ loaf (1.4 oz)	125	2	0	–	0	20	1	–
Thomas'									
Corn	1 slice	110	1	0	–	0	40	1	–
Swirl Whole Grain Cinnamon Raisin	1 slice	110	2	0	–	0	40	1	–
Toasting Cinnamon	1 slice	130	1	0	–	0	40	1	–
Whole Grain Swirl Oatmeal Raisin	1 slice	110	2	0	–	0	20	1	–
Toufayan									
Wraps Sundried Tomato Basil	1 (2 oz)	183	2	0	–	0	50	2	–
Wraps Wheat	1 (2 oz)	183	3	0	–	0	50	1	–

FOOD	PORTION	CALS	FIBER	VIT A	FOLIC	VIT C	CALCI	IRON	POTAS
TAKE-OUT									
banana	1 slice (2 oz)	196	1	296	20	1	13	1	80
chapatis as prep w/ fat	1 (1.6 oz)	95	3	221	11	0	10	1	101
chapatis as prep w/o fat	1 (2.5 oz)	141	5	0	–	0	42	2	–
cornbread	1 piece (2.3 oz)	183	2	110	47	0	130	2	89
cornstick	1 (1.4 oz)	118	1	70	30	0	83	1	57
focaccia onion	1 piece (4.6 oz)	282	2	5	43	2	20	3	114
focaccia rosemary	1 piece (3.5 oz)	251	2	2	38	tr	13	3	68
focaccia tomato olive	1 piece (4.7 oz)	270	2	85	39	3	31	3	122
garlic bread	1 slice (1 oz)	96	1	155	37	tr	19	1	32
irish soda bread	1 slice (3 oz)	247	2	165	40	1	69	2	226
italian garlic	1 loaf (11 oz)	990	8	1590	384	1	198	7	327
naan	1 bread (3.5 oz)	286	2	1400	53	tr	54	3	107
papadums fried	2 (1.5 oz)	81	2	–	–	0	15	2	–
paratha	1 bread (2.1 oz)	201	2	1995	11	0	10	1	78
poori indian puffed bread	1 piece (1.3 oz)	112	2	0	17	tr	6	1	68
zucchini	1 slice (1.4 oz)	150	1	50	19	1	27	1	47
BREAD COATING									
Don's Chuck Wagon									
Chicken Baking Mix	¼ cup	95	1	0	–	0	0	tr	–
Fish Mix	¼ cup	95	1	0	–	0	0	1	–
Onion Ring Mix	¼ cup	100	1	0	–	0	0	1	–
Fryin' Magic									
Cornmeal	1 tbsp	30	0	0	–	0	0	0	–

FOOD	PORTION	CALS	FIBER	VIT A	FOLIC	VIT C	CALCI	IRON	POTAS
Hodgson Mill									
Vidalia Sweet Onion Mix not prep	¼ cup	100	1	0	–	0	0	1	–
Luzianne									
Cajun Chicken Coating Mix	2 tbsp (1 oz)	100	1	75	–	0	0	1	–

BREADCRUMBS

FOOD	PORTION	CALS	FIBER	VIT A	FOLIC	VIT C	CALCI	IRON	POTAS
dry seasoned	¼ cup	115	2	58	36	1	55	1	69
fresh	¼ cup	30	tr	0	12	0	17	tr	11
plain	¼ cup	107	1	0	29	0	49	1	53
4C									
Carb Careful Seasoned	⅓ cup	110	5	0	–	1	100	3	–
Salt Free Seasoned	⅓ cup	110	2	0	–	0	20	1	–
Arnold									
Italian	¼ cup	110	1	0	–	0	40	1	–
Ian's									
Panko Italian	¼ cup	70	2	0	–	0	0	1	–
Panko Original	¼ cup	71	1	0	–	0	0	0	–
Panko Whole Wheat	¼ cup	70	2	0	–	0	0	1	–
Progresso									
Italian Style	¼ cup	110	1	0	–	0	40	1	–
Rienzi									
Italian Style	¼ cup	120	2	0	–	0	100	1	–
Ronzoni									
Italian Flavored	¼ cup	120	2	0	–	1	40	1	–

BREADFRUIT

FOOD	PORTION	CALS	FIBER	VIT A	FOLIC	VIT C	CALCI	IRON	POTAS
fresh	1 sm (13.5 oz)	396	19	0	54	111	65	2	1882
fried	1 cup	379	9	0	14	39	31	1	847
raw	1 cup	227	11	0	31	64	37	1	1078

BREADNUTTREE SEEDS

FOOD	PORTION	CALS	FIBER	VIT A	FOLIC	VIT C	CALCI	IRON	POTAS
dried	1 oz	104	–	61	13	–	27	1	–

BREADSTICKS

FOOD	PORTION	CALS	FIBER	VIT A	FOLIC	VIT C	CALCI	IRON	POTAS
plain	1 lg	41	tr	0	16	0	2	tr	12
plain	1 sm	21	tr	0	8	0	1	tr	6
Angonoa									
Deli Style Sesame	3 (0.5 oz)	730	tr	0	–	0	20	tr	–

FOOD	PORTION	CALS	FIBER	VIT A	FOLIC	VIT C	CALCI	IRON	POTAS
Fattorie & Pandea									
Grissini Sesame	3	70	tr	0	–	0	0	0	–
John Wm Macy's									
CheeseSticks Original Cheddar	3 (1 oz)	130	1	0	–	0	60	1	–
Pepperidge Farm									
Snack Sticks Wheat	9 (1 oz)	130	1	0	–	0	0	1	–
Stella D'Oro									
Mini Cracked Pepper	4 (0.5 oz)	70	0	0	–	0	0	1	–
Original	1 (0.4 oz)	40	0	0	–	0	0	tr	–
Roasted Garlic	1	45	0	0	–	0	0	tr	–
Sesame	1 (0.4 oz)	50	0	0	–	0	20	1	–
BROAD BEANS									
canned	½ cup	91	–	13	42	2	33	1	310
fava fresh cooked	½ cup	94	5	13	88	tr	31	1	228
BROCCOFLOWER									
fresh raw	½ cup (1.8 oz)	16	–	76	29	44	16	tr	150
BROCCOLI									
FRESH									
chinese broccoli (gai lan) cooked	½ cup	10	1	721	44	12	44	tr	115
raab cooked	½ cup	28	2	3853	60	31	100	1	292
raw	1 bunch (1.3 lbs)	207	16	4013	383	542	286	4	1921
raw flower	1 piece	3	–	330	8	10	5	tr	36
raw flowers	1 cup	20	–	2130	50	66	34	1	231
River Ranch									
Broccoli Slaw	1 cup	25	2	2500	60	72	40	1	–
Florets	1¼ cups	25	3	2500	60	78	40	1	–
FROZEN									
chopped cooked	½ cup	26	3	1029	52	37	30	1	131
spears cooked	½ cup	26	3	1029	28	37	47	1	166
spears cooked	1 pkg (10 oz)	70	8	2795	75	100	128	2	450
Birds Eye									
Broccoli & Cheese Sauce	½ cup	90	1	0	–	24	60	tr	–
Steamfresh Cuts	1 cup	30	2	0	–	30	20	0	–

FOOD	PORTION	CALS	FIBER	VIT A	FOLIC	VIT C	CALCI	IRON	POTAS
C&W									
Broccoli & Cheddar Cheese Sauce	1⅓ cups	70	2	500	–	36	60	tr	–
Florets	1 cup	30	2	0	–	30	20	0	–
Fresh Like									
Spear	3.5 oz	26	1	2084	–	57	55	1	224
TAKE-OUT									
batter dipped & fried	4 pieces	77	1	85	23	31	40	1	144
w/ cheese sauce	1 cup	242	5	1310	164	94	315	1	538

BROWNIE
MIX
FOOD	PORTION	CALS	FIBER	VIT A	FOLIC	VIT C	CALCI	IRON	POTAS
plain low calorie	1 (0.8 oz)	84	1	0	1	0	3	tr	69
Big Train									
Low Carb Chocolate Chip as prep	1 (2 inch)	140	4	300	–	0	20	tr	–
Jiffy									
Fudge as prep	1	160	1	0	–	0	80	1	
Nature's Path									
Organic Double Fudge	¹⁄₁₀ pkg	150	3	0	–	0	20	1	
Organic HempPlus	¹⁄₁₀ pkg	140	3	0	–	0	40	1	
No Pudge!									
All Flavors	1	100	tr	0	–	0	40	1	
Sweet Rewards									
Low Fat Fudge as prep	1	130	1	–	8	0	60	tr	–
Reduced Fat Supreme as prep	1	140	–	–	8	–	60	tr	90
READY-TO-EAT									
plain	1 sm (1 oz)	115	1	20	–	–	8	1	42
plain	1 lg (2 oz)	227	1	39	–	–	16	1	84
w/ nuts	1 (1 oz)	100	–	70	–	tr	13	1	50
Joseph's									
Sugar Free	1 (1.5 oz)	150	1	100	–	1	0	1	–
Laura's Wholesome Junk Food									
Gluten Free Better Brownie	2	120	2	0	–	0	20	1	105
Sara Lee									
Brownie Bites Chocolate Dipped	1 (0.7 oz)	90	1	0	–	0	0	tr	

FOOD	PORTION	CALS	FIBER	VIT A	FOLIC	VIT C	CALCI	IRON	POTAS
TAKE-OUT									
plain	1 (2.1 oz)	243	–	11	17	3	25	1	83
BRUSSELS SPROUTS									
FRESH									
cooked	6 pieces	45	3	977	76	78	45	2	399
FROZEN									
cooked	1 cup	65	6	1435	157	71	40	1	450
C&W									
Petite	10 (3 oz)	45	3	200	–	54	20	1	–
BUCKWHEAT									
groats roasted cooked	½ cup	323	2	0	12	0	6	1	74
groats roasted uncooked	½ cup	292	9	0	26	0	9	2	391
BUFFALO									
burger	3 oz	202	0	0	13	0	11	3	290
chuck braised	4 oz	205	0	0	22	0	7	5	336
top round steak broiled	3 oz	313	0	0	34	0	9	6	688
water buffalo roasted	3 oz	111	0	–	8	–	13	2	266
BULGUR									
cooked	½ cup	76	4	2	16	0	9	1	62
uncooked	½ cup	239	13	6	19	0	25	2	287
Fantastic									
Tabouli Mix not prep	2 tbsp	70	4	100	–	1	20	1	–
Sabra									
Black Bean & Wheat Pilaf	2 oz	45	2	0	–	5	0	tr	–
Cracked Wheat Salad	2 oz	80	1	100	–	9	0	1	–
Tabouli	2 oz	70	1	400	–	24	20	1	–
TAKE-OUT									
tabbouleh	1 cup	198	4	270	30	26	30	1	250
BURBOT (FISH)									
fresh baked	3 oz	98	0	–	–	–	54	1	440
BURDOCK ROOT									
cooked w/o salt	1 cup	110	2	0	25	3	61	1	450
cooked w/o salt	1 root (5.8 oz)	146	3	0	33	4	81	1	598

FOOD	PORTION	CALS	FIBER	VIT A	FOLIC	VIT C	CALCI	IRON	POTAS
Frieda's									
Gobo Root	¾ cup	60	3	0	–	2	40	1	–
BUTTER									
clarified butter	3.5 oz	876	0	3750	–	0	tr	–	–
ghee cow's milk	1 tbsp	126	0	475	0	0	–	tr	0
stick	1 pat (5 g)	36	–	153	tr	0	1	tr	1
stick	1 stick (4 oz)	813	–	3468	3	0	27	tr	29
whipped	1 pat (4 g)	27	–	116	tr	–	1	tr	1
Cabot									
Salted	1 tbsp	100	0	400	–	0	0	0	–
Corman									
Light	1 tbsp	55	0	400	–	0	0	0	–
Crystal Farms									
Butter	1 tbsp	100	0	400	–	0	0	0	–
Whipped	1 tbsp	70	0	300	–	0	0	0	–
Horizon Organic									
European	1 tbsp	100	0	400	–	0	0	0	–
BUTTER SUBSTITUTES									
Olivio									
Spread	1 tbsp	80	0	500	–	0	0	0	–
BUTTERBUR									
canned fuki chopped	1 cup	3	–	0	–	15	42	1	15
fresh fuki	1 cup	13	–	47	–	30	97	tr	616
CABBAGE									
chinese bok choy shredded cooked w/o salt	1 cup	20	2	7223	70	44	158	2	631
chinese pe-tsai shredded cooked w/o salt	1 cup	17	2	1151	63	19	38	tr	268
green raw shredded	1 cup	19	2	69	30	26	28	tr	119
green shredded cooked w/o salt	1 cup	34	3	120	45	56	72	tr	294
japanese pickled	½ cup	22	2	142	32	1	36	tr	640
red raw shredded	1 cup	22	2	781	13	40	32	1	170

FOOD	PORTION	CALS	FIBER	VIT A	FOLIC	VIT C	CALCI	IRON	POTAS
red shredded cooked w/o salt	1 cup	44	4	250	36	52	63	1	393
savoy shredded cooked w/o salt	1 cup	35	4	1289	67	24	44	1	267
Aunt Nellie's									
Sweet & Sour Red	¼ cup	40	0	0	–	2	0	0	–
Frieda's									
Baby Bok Choy	⅔ cup	10	1	2500	–	36	80	1	–
Bok Choy	1 cup	10	1	2500	–	36	80	1	–
Gai Choy	1 cup (3 oz)	20	2	4500	–	60	80	1	–
Napa	1 cup (3 oz)	15	1	1000	–	24	60	0	–
Salad Savoy	⅔ cup (3 oz)	25	3	750	–	27	20	0	–
Tuscan	⅔ cup (3 oz)	20	2	100	–	27	40	tr	–
Glory									
Country Cabbage	½ cup	30	1	100	–	48	20	tr	–
Greenwood									
Red	½ cup	100	0	0	–	5	40	tr	–
Lohmann									
Red Cabbage Sweet & Sour	¼ cup	40	0	0	–	2	0	0	–
River Ranch									
Angel Hair	1½ cups	20	2	100	40	27	40	tr	–
TAKE-OUT									
creamed	1 cup	158	2	450	28	23	140	tr	246
kimchee	1 cup	32	2	1440	88	80	144	1	380
stuffed cabbage w/ rice & beef	1 (3.6 oz)	117	1	95	25	12	31	1	283
sweet & sour red cabbage	4 oz	61	3	170	–	14	43	1	–
CACTUS									
fresh cooked w/ fat	1 pad (1 oz)	11	1	70	1	2	47	tr	56
fresh cooked w/o fat	1 cup (5.2 oz)	22	3	165	4	8	243	1	289
pricklypear fresh	1 cup (5.3 oz)	56	4	75	–	29	–	tr	–

FOOD	PORTION	CALS	FIBER	VIT A	FOLIC	VIT C	CALCI	IRON	POTAS
Frieda's									
Cactus Pads	¾ cup (3 oz)	20	1	0	–	9	80	1	–
CAKE									
battenburg cake	1 slice (2 oz)	204	1	125	–	0	48	1	–
cream puff shell	1 (2.3 oz)	239	–	763	14	0	24	1	64
crumpet	1 (2.3 oz)	131	2	–	6	0	79	1	61
eccles cake	1 slice (2 oz)	285	1	185	–	0	47	1	–
sponge	1 piece (1.3 oz)	110	tr	59	18	0	27	1	38
sponge cake dessert shell	1 (0.8 oz)	70	0	0	–	0	30	tr	–
treacle tart	1 slice (2.5 oz)	258	1	210	–	0	43	1	–
Arnold									
Date Nut Loaf	1 slice (2 oz)	190	2	0	–	0	0	1	–
Boboli									
Mini Eclairs Custard Filled	4 (2.3 oz)	224	0	0	–	1	60	tr	–
Chudleigh's									
Apple Blossoms	1 (4 oz)	350	2	100	–	2	20	1	–
Goody Man									
Happy Birthday Cupcake Chocolate	1 (1.75 oz)	200	tr	0	16	0	40	1	–
Happy Birthday Cupcake White	1 (1.75 oz)	190	0	0	16	0	60	1	–
Guiltless Gourmet									
Dessert Bowl Bananas Foster Cake	1 pkg (2 oz)	200	tr	0	–	0	40	tr	–
Dessert Bowl Black Velvet Cake	1 pkg (2 oz)	200	3	0	–	0	40	4	–
Low Carb Creations									
Cheesecake Blueberry Swirl	1 slice (3 oz)	220	0	750	–	1	40	1	–
Cheesecake Chocolate	1 slice (3 oz)	250	0	750	–	0	60	1	–

FOOD	PORTION	CALS	FIBER	VIT A	FOLIC	VIT C	CALCI	IRON	POTAS
Cheesecake Key Lime	1 slice (3 oz)	250	0	750	–	0	40	1	–
Cheesecake New York	1 slice (3 oz)	250	0	750	–	0	60	1	–
Cheesecake Pumpkin Swirl	1 slice (3 oz)	220	0	3500	–	0	40	1	–
Nature's Path									
Organic Toaster Pastry Apple Cinnamon	1 (2 oz)	210	1	0	–	0	20	1	–
Organic Toaster Pastry Blueberry	1 (2 oz)	210	1	0	–	0	20	1	–
Organic Toaster Pastry Frosted Apple Cinnamon	1 (2 oz)	210	1	0	–	0	20	1	–
Organic Toaster Pastry Frosted Blueberry	1 (2 oz)	200	1	0	–	0	20	1	–
Organic Toaster Pastry Frosted Strawberry	1 (2 oz)	210	1	0	–	0	20	1	–
Snack & Smile									
Mini Loaf Apple Cinnamon	1 loaf (2 oz)	190	0	0	24	0	0	1	–
Mini Loaf Banana	1 loaf (2 oz)	200	0	0	24	0	0	1	–
Mini Loaf Blueberry	1 loaf (2 oz)	190	tr	0	24	0	0	1	–
Mini Loaf Carrot	1 loaf (2 oz)	200	0	100	24	0	0	1	–
Weight Watchers									
Lemon w/ Lemon Icing	1 (1 oz)	80	2	0	0	0	0	tr	–
TAKE-OUT									
angelfood	1 slice (2 oz)	143	tr	0	25	0	47	tr	75
apple crisp	1 serv (8.6 oz)	384	4	355	39	6	89	2	192
baklava	1 piece (2.7 oz)	334	2	560	27	1	30	2	134
bean cake	1 cake (1.1 oz)	130	1	0	20	0	3	1	58

FOOD	PORTION	CALS	FIBER	VIT A	FOLIC	VIT C	CALCI	IRON	POTAS
black forest chocolate cherry	1 piece (2.5 oz)	187	1	275	8	10	34	1	118
boston cream pie	1 slice (3.2 oz)	232	1	75	13	tr	21	tr	36
cannoli w/ cannoli cream	1	369	–	0	–	0	52	1	–
carrot w/ icing	1 slice (4.7 oz)	543	2	925	39	1	77	2	133
cheesecake	1 slice (4.5 oz)	410	tr	1215	17	1	63	1	116
cheesecake chocolate	1 slice (4.5 oz)	489	2	1190	38	tr	72	3	187
chinese moon cake	1 (4.8 oz)	458	4	115	116	tr	25	3	156
coconut mochiko filipino cake	1 piece (2.7 oz)	252	2	0	8	1	55	1	181
coffeecake iced	1 piece (1.6 oz)	175	1	145	34	1	34	1	52
cream puff custard filled chocolate frosted	1 (3.9 oz)	293	1	927	48	tr	71	1	131
dutch honey cake	1 slice (0.8 oz)	70	0	0	–	0	0	0	–
eclair	1 (3.5 oz)	262	1	828	43	tr	63	1	117
french apple tart	1 (3.5 oz)	302	2	345	2	3	14	1	93
fruitcake	1 slice (1.5 oz)	139	2	12	9	tr	14	1	66
funnel cake	1 (3.2 oz)	276	1	250	50	0	126	2	152
gingerbread	1 piece (2.4 oz)	213	1	40	19	tr	48	2	167
jelly roll	1 slice (1.8 oz)	146	tr	155	11	2	14	1	46
jelly roll lemon filled	1 slice (3 oz)	210	tr	100	0	1	20	1	–
napoleon	1 (3 oz)	348	1	420	29	tr	37	1	71
napoleon	1 mini (1 oz)	123	tr	150	10	0	13	tr	25
panettone	¹⁄₁₂ cake (2.9 oz)	300	2	300	–	0	40	1	–
petit fours	2 (0.9 oz)	120	0	0	–	0	20	0	–

FOOD	PORTION	CALS	FIBER	VIT A	FOLIC	VIT C	CALCI	IRON	POTAS
pineapple upside down	1 piece (4.2 oz)	387	1	365	36	2	144	2	136
pound	1 slice (1 oz)	120	–	200	–	tr	20	1	28
pound fat free	1 slice (2 oz)	160	1	54	24	0	24	1	62
strawberry shortcake	1 serv (4.1 oz)	211	1	275	21	27	32	1	117
strudel apple	1 piece (2.2 oz)	175	1	20	18	1	10	tr	95
strudel cheese	1 piece (2.2 oz)	195	tr	395	20	tr	91	1	65
strudel cherry	1 piece (2.2 oz)	179	1	245	20	3	21	1	99
tiramisu	1 piece (5.1 oz)	409	tr	1580	16	1	114	1	211
torte chocolate ganache	1 slice (3.5 oz)	400	6	100	–	0	40	1	–
trifle w/ cream	6 oz	291	1	665	–	7	119	1	–
zucchini bread	1 slice (1.4 oz)	150	1	50	19	1	27	1	47

CAKE MIX
Bob's Red Mills
Gluten Free Chocolate as prep	1/6 cake	170	2	200	–	0	250	1	–

Don's Chuck Wagon
All Purpose Batter Mix	1/4 cup	100	1	0	–	0	0	1	–

Jiffy
Devil's Food as prep	1/5 cake	220	1	0	–	0	20	2	–
Golden Yellow as prep	1/5 cake	220	tr	0	–	0	20	1	–
White Cake as prep	1/5 cake	210	tr	0	–	0	0	1	–

King Arthur
Cinnamon Buns Kit not prep	1/2 cup	240	3	0	–	2	40	1	–

CALABAZA
fresh	1/2 cup	32	–	5460	–	18	–	–	246

CANADIAN BACON
grilled	2 slices (1.6 oz)	87	0	0	2	0	5	tr	183

FOOD	PORTION	CALS	FIBER	VIT A	FOLIC	VIT C	CALCI	IRON	POTAS
Boar's Head									
Canadian Bacon	2 oz	70	0	0	–	0	0	tr	–
Celebrity									
98% Fat Free	3 slices (1.8 oz)	60	0	200	–	1	0	1	–
Wellshire									
Sliced	2 oz	20	0	0	–	0	0	1	–

CANDY

FOOD	PORTION	CALS	FIBER	VIT A	FOLIC	VIT C	CALCI	IRON	POTAS
boiled sweets	¼ lb	327	0	0	–	0	5	tr	–
butterscotch	1 piece (6 g)	24	–	8	0	0	0	0	0
candied cherries	1 (4 g)	12	–	7	–	0	tr	tr	–
candied pineapple slice	1 slice (2 oz)	179	–	59	–	13	17	tr	–
candy corn	1 oz	105	–	0	–	0	2	tr	1
caramels	1 piece (8 g)	31	–	3	0	–	11	tr	17
carob bar	1 (3.1 oz)	453	–	39	27	–	391	–	785
crisped rice bar almond	1 bar (1 oz)	130	1	750	0	–	21	2	65
crisped rice bar chocolate chip	1 bar (1 oz)	115	1	500	40	–	6	2	48
dark chocolate	1 oz	150	–	10	–	tr	7	1	86
fondant	1 piece (0.6 oz)	57	–	0	0	0	0	tr	3
fudge brown sugar w/ nuts	1 piece (0.5 oz)	56	–	11	1	tr	16	tr	52
fudge chocolate marshmallow	1 piece (0.7 oz)	84	–	66	0	0	9	tr	28
fudge chocolate w/ nuts	1 piece (0.7 oz)	81	–	38	2	tr	9	tr	30
fudge peanut butter	1 piece (0.6 oz)	59	–	6	2	0	7	tr	21
fudge vanilla w/ nuts	1 piece (0.5 oz)	62	–	30	2	tr	7	tr	17
jelly beans	10 sm (0.4 oz)	40	–	0	–	0	0	tr	4
lollipop	1 (6 g)	22	–	0	–	–	0	tr	0
marzipan	1 oz	128	2	0	16	tr	24	1	82

FOOD	PORTION	CALS	FIBER	VIT A	FOLIC	VIT C	CALCI	IRON	POTAS
milk chocolate	1 bar (1.55 oz)	226	–	82	4	tr	84	1	169
milk chocolate crisp	1 bar (1.45 oz)	203	–	23	3	tr	70	tr	141
milk chocolate w/ almonds	1 bar (1.45 oz)	215	–	30	–	tr	92	1	182
organic dark chocolate w/ raisins & pecans	1.4 oz	220	3	0	–	0	0	1	–
peanut brittle	1 oz	128	–	54	20	0	8	tr	59
peanuts chocolate covered	10 (1.4 oz)	208	–	0	3	0	42	1	201
peanuts chocolate covered	1 cup (5.2 oz)	773	–	0	12	0	155	2	748
praline	1 piece (1.4 oz)	177	–	18	6	tr	12	tr	82
pretzels chocolate covered	1 (0.4 oz)	50	–	–	–	tr	8	tr	–
taffy	1 piece (0.5 oz)	56	–	20	0	0	0	tr	1
toffee	1 piece (0.4 oz)	65	–	152	0	0	4	tr	6
truffles	1 piece (0.4 oz)	59	–	62	0	tr	19	tr	37
Bartons									
Cashew Toppers	1 (1 oz)	140	1	0	–	0	40	1	–
Brach's									
Bridge Mix	16 pieces	190	tr	0	–	0	20	1	–
Candy Corn	26 pieces	140	0	0	–	0	0	0	–
Caramel Clusters	3 pieces	210	1	0	–	0	20	1	–
Circus Peanuts	6 pieces	160	0	0	–	0	0	0	–
Fruit Slices	3 pieces	150	0	0	–	0	0	0	–
Malts	15 pieces	190	1	0	–	0	0	tr	–
Mellowcreme Pumpkins	6 pieces	130	0	0	–	0	0	0	–
Mint Patties	3 pieces	140	0	0	–	0	0	tr	–
Orange Slices	2 pieces	130	0	0	–	0	0	0	–
Peanut Butter Meltaways	3 pieces	200	1	0	–	0	40	1	–
Root Beer Barrels	3 pieces	70	0	0	–	0	0	0	–
Spearmint Leaves	5 pieces	130	0	0	–	0	0	0	–

FOOD	PORTION	CALS	FIBER	VIT A	FOLIC	VIT C	CALCI	IRON	POTAS
Spice Drops	12 pieces	130	0	0	–	0	0	0	–
Sprinkles	17 pieces	200	1	0	–	0	0	1	–
Star Brites Butterscotch	3 pieces	60	0	0	–	0	0	0	–
Stars	10 pieces	200	0	0	–	0	0	0	–
Wild'N Fruity Gummi Bears	14 pieces	140	0	0	–	0	0	0	–
Cadbury									
Milk Chocolate Roast Almond	10 blocks (1.4 oz)	220	1	0	–	0	100	tr	–
Royal Dark	10 blocks (1.4 oz)	220	3	0	–	0	0	1	–
Chargers									
Chocolate Covered Expresso Beans	1 pkg (0.5 oz)	60	tr	0	–	0	20	tr	–
Cloud Nine									
Australian Orange Peel	½ bar (1.5 oz)	220	2	0	–	1	20	2	–
Butter Nut Toffee	½ bar (1.5 oz)	230	1	100	–	1	60	1	–
Cool Mint Crisp	½ bar (1.5 oz)	220	2	0	–	1	20	2	–
Espresso Bean Crunch	½ bar (1.5 oz)	220	2	0	–	1	20	2	–
Malted Milk Crunch	½ bar (1.5 oz)	230	1	100	–	1	60	1	–
Milk Chocolate	½ bar (1.5 oz)	230	1	100	–	1	60	1	–
Oregon Red Raspberry	½ bar (1.5 oz)	230	2	0	–	2	20	2	–
Peanut Butter Brittle	½ bar (1.5 oz)	230	1	100	–	1	60	1	–
Sundried Cherry	½ bar (1.5 oz)	230	1	200	–	1	60	1	–
Toasted Coconut Crisp	½ bar (1.5 oz)	230	2	100	–	1	60	1	–
Vanilla Dark	½ bar (1.5 oz)	230	2	0	–	1	20	2	–
CocoaVia									
Chocolate	1 bar	80	1	–	40	6	250	tr	–

FOOD	PORTION	CALS	FIBER	VIT A	FOLIC	VIT C	CALCI	IRON	POTAS
Chocolate Almond	1 bar	80	1	–	1	9	250	tr	–
Chocolate Blueberry	1 bar	80	1	–	1	9	250	tr	–
Chocolate Blueberry & Almond	1 bar	100	2	–	40	6	200	tr	–
Chocolate Cherry	1 bar	80	1	–	40	6	200	tr	–
Chocolate Covered Almonds	1 bar	140	3	–	40	6	200	1	–
Crispy Chocolate	1 bar	90	2	–	40	6	200	tr	–
Original Chocolate	1 bar (0.8 oz)	100	2	–	60	9	250	1	–
Coffee Rio									
Coffee Candy All Flavors	4 pieces	60	0	0	–	0	0	0	–
Daboga									
Organic Milk Chocolate	1 bar (2 oz)	318	6	0	–	0	40	1	–
Dare									
RealFruit Gummies All Flavors	8 pieces (1.4 oz)	120	0	0	–	0	0	0	–
Endangered Species									
Dark Chocolate w/ Espresso Beans	½ bar (1.5 oz)	200	5	0	–	0	0	1	–
Dark Chocolate w/ Hazelnut Toffee	½ bar (1.5 oz)	220	4	0	–	0	0	1	–
Milk Chocolate w/ Cherries	½ bar (1.5 oz)	230	1	0	–	0	20	2	–
Organic Dark Chocolate	½ bar (0.7 oz)	100	1	0	–	0	0	1	–
Organic Dark Chocolate w/ Tangerine	½ bar (0.7 oz)	100	1	0	–	0	0	1	–
Organic Milk Chocolate w/ Key Lime	½ bar (0.7 oz)	110	0	0	–	0	0	tr	–
Ethel's									
Truffles Assorted	4	200	1	200	–	0	20	tr	–
Fauchon									
Assortment Truffles	3 pieces (1.3 oz)	160	2	0	–	0	40	1	–

FOOD	PORTION	CALS	FIBER	VIT A	FOLIC	VIT C	CALCI	IRON	POTAS
Chocolate Assortment	3 pieces (1.1 oz)	170	2	0	–	0	40	1	–
Ferrero Rocher									
Candy	3 pieces (1.3 oz)	220	1	0	–	1	60	1	–
Figamajigs									
Fig Candy Drops Dark Chocolate Covered	1 pkg (1.4 oz)	150	3	–	–	–	60	3	–
Fig Candy Drops Orange & Yellow Chocolate Covered	1 pkg (1.4 oz)	150	2	–	–	–	40	2	–
Fruitzels									
Assorted	7 pieces	120	0	0	–	30	0	0	–
Ghirardelli									
Squares Milk Chocolate w/ Caramel Filling	3 (1.6 oz)	220	tr	100	–	0	80	1	–
Squares 60% Cacao Dark Chocolate	4 (1.5 oz)	220	3	0	–	0	20	3	–
Squares 60% Cacao Dark Chocolate w/ Caramel	3 (1.6 oz)	220	3	0	–	0	20	2	–
Godiva									
Chocolatier Dark Chocolate w/ Raspberry	1 bar (1.5 oz)	220	0	0	–	2	20	2	–
Chocolatier Milk Chocolate	1 bar (1.5 oz)	230	0	0	–	0	100	2	–
Chocolatier Milk Chocolate w/ Almonds	1 bar (1.5 oz)	230	0	0	–	0	100	2	–
Sugar Free Chocolate	1 bar (1.5 oz)	190	tr	0	–	0	1000	2	–
Sugar Free Chocolate w/ Almonds	1 bar (1.5 oz)	200	1	0	–	0	900	2	–
Sugar Free Dark Chocolate	1 bar (1.5 oz)	190	4	0	–	0	0	3	–
Truffles Assorted	2 pieces (1.4 oz)	210	2	0	–	0	40	1	–
Goetze's									
Caramel Creams	3 pieces	130	tr	100	–	0	20	0	–

FOOD	PORTION	CALS	FIBER	VIT A	FOLIC	VIT C	CALCI	IRON	POTAS
Goldenberg's									
Peanut Chews	3 pieces	180	1	0	–	0	20	1	–
Guylian									
Twists Milk Chocolate Truffle	5 pieces (1.2 oz)	230	1	300	–	0	60	1	–
Twists Original Praline	4 pieces (1.2 oz)	200	1	300	–	1	80	1	–
Hershey's									
Chocolate Miniatures Sugar Free	5 pieces (1.4 oz)	170	2	0	–	0	0	tr	–
Chocolate w/ Almonds Miniatures Sugar Free	5 pieces (1.4 oz)	180	3	0	–	0	0	tr	–
Cocao Reserve 65% Cacao Extra Dark	1 block (1.3 oz)	200	4	0	–	0	0	1	–
Cocoa Reserve 35% Cacao Milk Chocolate w/ Hazelnuts	3 sq (1.3 oz)	220	1	0	–	0	60	tr	–
Dark Chocolate Miniatures Sugar Free	5 pieces (1.4 oz)	190	3	0	–	0	0	1	–
Milk Chocolate	1 bar (1.4 oz)	210	1	0	–	0	80	tr	–
Milk Chocolate w/ Almonds	1 bar (1.4 oz)	230	1	0	–	0	80	tr	–
Nuggets Cookies 'N' Creme	4	190	0	0	–	0	80	0	–
Nuggets Dark Chocolate w/ Almonds	4	220	3	0	–	0	20	1	–
Nuggets Milk Chocolate	4	230	1	0	–	0	80	tr	–
Pot Of Gold	3 pieces	130	tr	0	–	0	20	0	–
Hint Mint									
All Flavors	2 pieces	10	–	0	–	0	0	0	–
Joyva									
Halvah Chocolate Covered	1 serv (2 oz)	380	3	0	–	0	0	2	–
Halvah Marble	1 serv (2 oz)	390	2	0	–	0	0	2	–

FOOD	PORTION	CALS	FIBER	VIT A	FOLIC	VIT C	CALCI	IRON	POTAS
Lambertz									
Petits Soleils Chocolate Coated Gingerbread	1 piece (0.4 oz)	47	tr	0	–	0	7	tr	–
Landies Candies									
Sugar Free Almond Clusters	2 pieces (1.5 oz)	240	2	0	–	0	40	1	–
Sugar Free Bon Bons Peanut Butter	2 (1.5 oz)	240	tr	0	–	0	20	tr	–
Sugar Free Coconut Clusters	2 pieces (1.5 oz)	250	1	0	–	0	20	1	–
Sugar Free Cookies & Cream	2 pieces (1.5 oz)	240	tr	0	–	0	0	tr	–
Sugar Free Dark Almond Bark	1 piece (1.5 oz)	230	2	0	–	0	20	1	–
Sugar Free Dark Miniature Bars	7 pieces (1.5 oz)	230	2	0	–	0	0	1	–
Legacy Chocolates									
Truffles Assorted	1 piece (0.5 oz)	90	1	0	–	0	0	1	–
Lindt									
Dark Chocolate 70% Cocoa	4 blocks (1.4 oz)	220	2	0	–	0	40	2	–
Lindor Truffles Dark Chocolate	3 pieces	220	0	0	–	0	20	1	–
Lindor Truffles Milk Chocolate	3 pieces	220	0	100	–	0	60	tr	–
Mon Cheri									
Hazelnut	4 pieces	260	1	0	–	1	90	1	–
Mr. Goodbar									
Bar	1 (1.75 oz)	270	2	0	–	0	40	tr	–
Mrs. Fields									
Decadent Chocolates	3 pieces (1.8 oz)	240	2	100	–	0	60	1	–
Munch									
Nut Bar	1 (1.42 oz)	220	2	126	24	–	21	tr	150
Nestle									
Turtles Original	3 pieces	240	1	0	–	0	60	0	–
Nutty Ducky's									
Cashew Brittle	4 pieces (1.6 oz)	240	2	0	–	0	0	1	–

FOOD	PORTION	CALS	FIBER	VIT A	FOLIC	VIT C	CALCI	IRON	POTAS
Cashew Brittle Dark Chocolate	2 pieces (1.5 oz)	220	2	0	–	0	0	2	–
Peanut Brittle	4 pieces (1.6 oz)	230	4	0	–	0	0	0	–
Peanut Brittle Milk Chocolate	2 pieces (1.5 oz)	220	2	100	–	0	40	tr	–
Odense									
Marzipan	2 tbsp (1.4 oz)	170	0	0	–	0	100	1	–
Pearson's									
Mint Patties	1	30	tr	0	–	0	0	tr	–
Raisinets									
Candy	3 pkg (1.7 oz)	200	1	0	–	0	40	tr	–
Reese's									
Bites	16 pieces	220	1	0	–	0	20	0	–
Miniatures Peanut Butter Cups Sugar Free	5 pieces (1.4 oz)	170	5	0	–	0	0	tr	–
Nutrageous	1 bar (0.6 oz)	95	1	0	–	0	20	tr	–
Peanut Butter Cups Miniatures	5 (1.4 oz)	210	1	0	–	0	20	tr	–
Peanut Butter Cups Sugar Free	1 piece (1.5 oz)	180	5	0	–	0	0	tr	–
White Miniatures Peanut Butter Cups	4 pieces (1.4 oz)	210	tr	0	–	0	80	0	–
White Miniatures Peanut Butter Cups Sugar Free	5 pieces (1.4 oz)	180	3	0	–	0	0	0	–
Ritter Sport									
Dark Chocolate Whole Hazelnuts	6 pieces (1.3 oz)	210	7	0	–	0	20	tr	–
Russell Stover									
Assorted	3 pieces (1.4 oz)	170	1	0	–	0	20	1	–
Low Carb Pecan Delights	1 piece (1 oz)	130	2	0	–	0	0	tr	–
Pecan Delights	1 pkg (2 oz)	280	tr	100	–	1	60	1	–

FOOD	PORTION	CALS	FIBER	VIT A	FOLIC	VIT C	CALCI	IRON	POTAS
Sugar Free Peanut Butter Cups	4 pieces (1.3 oz)	200	2	0	–	0	0	tr	–
Sugar Free Pecans & Caramel	2 pieces (1.2 oz)	170	0	0	–	0	0	1	–
Scharffen Berger									
Semisweet 60% Cacao	1 bar (2 oz)	320	tr	0	–	0	20	2	–
Smucker's									
Jelly Beans	25	150	0	0		0	0	0	
The Chocolate Traveler									
Wedges Bittersweet	4 pieces	130	4	0	–	1	20	3	
Wedges Dark Chocolate Coffee	4 pieces	130	2	0	–	0	0	1	
Wedges Dark Chocolate Mint	4 pieces	130	2	0	–	0	0	1	
Wedges Dark Chocolate Orange	4 pieces	120	2	0	–	0	20	2	
Wedges Dark Chocolate Raspberry	4 pieces	120	2	0	–	0	20	2	
Wedges Dark Chocolate Tiramisu	4 pieces	120	2	1	–	0	20	2	
Wedges Milk Chocolate	4 pieces	130	0	100	–	0	20	tr	
Wedges Milk Chocolate Dulce De Leche	4 pieces	120	tr	0	–	0	40	1	–
Wedges White Chocolate	4 pieces	140	14	100	–	0	0	0	–
Wedges White Chocolate Creme Brulee	4 pieces	140	0	100	–	0	60	0	–
Tobler									
Orange Dark Chocolate	5 pieces (1.5 oz)	240	3	0	–	0	0	1	–
Toblerone									
Bittersweet Chocolate w/ Honey & Almond Nugget	⅓ bar (1.2 oz)	170	2	0	–	0	0	2	–

FOOD	PORTION	CALS	FIBER	VIT A	FOLIC	VIT C	CALCI	IRON	POTAS
Milk Chocolate w/ Honey & Almond Nougat	⅓ bar (1.76 oz)	170	tr	0	–	0	40	1	–
Tootsie Roll									
Candy	12 (1.3 oz)	130	–	0	–	0	20	tr	–
Tropical Source									
Chocolate Dairy Free California Raisin & Currant	½ bar (1.5 oz)	230	1	0	–	0	0	0	–
Chocolate Dairy Free Hazelnut Espresso Crunch	½ bar (1.5 oz)	250	1	0	–	0	0	0	–
Chocolate Dairy Free Maple Almond Granola	½ bar (1.5 oz)	230	1	0	–	0	0	0	–
Chocolate Dairy Free Mint Candy Crunch	½ bar (1.5 oz)	220	1	0	–	0	0	0	–
Chocolate Dairy Free Red Raspberry Crush	½ bar (1.5 oz)	230	1	0	–	0	0	0	–
Chocolate Dairy Free Sundried Jungle Banana	½ bar (1.5 oz)	230	2	0	–	0	0	0	–
Chocolate Dairy Free Toasted Almond	½ bar (1.5 oz)	250	1	0	–	0	0	0	–
Chocolate Dairy Free Wild Rice Crisp	½ bar (1.5 oz)	230	1	0	–	0	0	0	–
Unique Origin									
Guaranda Dark Chocolate	1 piece (0.3 oz)	54	1	0	–	0	9	1	–
Vere									
75% Chocolate Gluten Free	1 sm bar	80	2	0	–	0	20	3	–
Brownie Box Coconut Gluten Free Vegan	3 pieces (1.4 oz)	210	5	0	–	0	20	3	–
Brownie Box Peanut Butter Gluten Free	3 pieces (1.3 oz)	180	3	100	–	0	20	2	–
Brownie Box Walnut Gluten Free	3 pieces (1.3 oz)	190	3	100	–	0	20	3	–

FOOD	PORTION	CALS	FIBER	VIT A	FOLIC	VIT C	CALCI	IRON	POTAS
Clusters Chocolate Coconut Gluten Free Vegan	3 pieces (1.7 oz)	280	6	0	–	0	20	5	–
Clusters Chocolate Almond Gluten Free Vegan	2 pieces (1.3 oz)	210	4	0	–	1	60	3	–
Clusters Chocolate Rice Gluten Free Vegan	3 pieces (1.3 oz)	170	3	0	–	0	20	3	–
Clusters Chocolate Seed Gluten Free Vegan	2 pieces (1.3 oz)	210	4	0	–	1	60	3	–
Wafers Cacao Nibs Gluten Free Vegan	2 (1.1 oz)	170	4	0	–	0	20	4	–
Wafers Espresso Gluten Free Vegan	3 (1.6 oz)	250	8	0	–	0	40	6	–
Wafers Pink Peppercorn Gluten Free Vegan	3 (1.6 oz)	250	6	0	–	0	40	6	–
Wafers Spicy Pepita Gluten Free	2 (1.1 oz)	170	4	0	–	0	20	5	–
Wafers Tamari Almond Gluten Free Vegan	2 (1.2 oz)	170	5	0	–	0	40	5	–
Weight Watchers									
English Toffee Squares	3 pieces	160	6	200	–	0	40	tr	–
Mint Patties	2	100	5	0	–	0	0	tr	–
Peanut Butter Crunch	4 pieces	180	6	0	–	0	40	tr	–
Pecan Crowns	3 pieces	150	8	0	–	0	40	tr	–
Werther's									
Original	3 pieces (0.5 oz)	60	0	0	–	0	0	0	–
Whitman's									
Sampler	3 pieces (1.4 oz)	220	tr	100	–	0	40	1	–
Whoppers									
Malted Milk Balls	18 pieces	190	tr	0	–	0	80	tr	–
Yamate Chocolatier									
No Sugar Almonds & Caramel	1 piece (0.6 oz)	70	1	0	–	0	0	tr	–

FOOD	PORTION	CALS	FIBER	VIT A	FOLIC	VIT C	CALCI	IRON	POTAS
York									
Peppermint Patty	3 (1.4 oz)	150	tr	0	–	0	40	tr	–
Peppermint Patty Sugar Free	3 (1.3 oz)	110	1	0	–	0	0	tr	–

CANTALOUPE

fresh cubed	1 cup	57	1	5158	27	68	17	tr	494
fresh half	½	94	2	8608	46	113	28	1	825
Chiquita									
Wedge	¼ med (4.7 oz)	50	1	5000	–	48	20	tr	
Del Monte									
Fresh	¼ melon (4.7 oz)	50	1	5000	–	48	20	tr	–

CARAWAY

seed	1 tsp	7	–	8	–	–	14	tr	28

CARDAMOM

ground	1 tsp	6	–	–	–	–	8	tr	22

CARDOON

fresh shredded	½ cup	36	–	107	–	2	62	1	356
Frieda's									
Cardoon	1 cup	15	1	100	–	1	60	1	–

CARIBOU

roasted	3 oz	142	0	–	4	3	19	5	264

CARISSA

fresh	1	12	–	8	–	8	2	tr	52

CAROB

carob mix as prep w/ whole milk	9 oz	195	–	307	12	2	291	1	370
flour	1 tbsp	14	–	1	2	0	28	tr	66
flour	1 cup	185	–	15	30	tr	359	3	852
Sunspire									
Carob Chips Unsweetened	13 pieces (0.5 oz)	70	0	0	–	1	100	0	–
Carob Chips Vegan	13 pieces (0.5 oz)	70	0	0	–	0	0	tr	–

FOOD	PORTION	CALS	FIBER	VIT A	FOLIC	VIT C	CALCI	IRON	POTAS
CARP									
fresh cooked	1 fillet (6 oz)	276	0	54	–	3	89	3	726
fresh cooked	3 oz	138	0	27	–	1	44	1	363
roe salted in olive oil	2 tbsp (1 oz)	40	0	–	–	–	0	1	–
CARROT JUICE									
canned	6 oz	73	–	47381	7	16	44	1	538
Bolthouse Farms									
Carrot Juice	8 oz	70	tr	35000	–	15	40	tr	310
Luvli Juices									
Zingy Carrot	1 bottle (10 oz)	145	2	15000	–	120	50	1	580
Naked Juice									
Just Carrot	8 oz	80	0	34500	–	5	40	2	620
CARROTS									
CANNED									
slices	½ cup	17	1	10055	7	2	19	tr	131
slices low sodium	½ cup	17	1	10055	7	2	19	tr	131
Del Monte									
Savory Sides Honey Glazed	½ cup	70	tr	15000	–	6	40	tr	–
Sliced	½ cup	35	3	15000	–	4	20	tr	–
Glory									
Seasoned Honey	½ cup	50	2	9500	–	2	20	tr	–
S&W									
Julienne	½ cup (4.3 oz)	30	2	4500	–	0	0	0	–
Sliced	½ cup (4.3 oz)	30	2	4500	–	0	0	0	–
Whole Small	½ cup (4.3 oz)	30	2	4500	–	0	0	0	–
Tillen Farms									
Crispy Carrots Pickled	5 pieces (1 oz)	30	1	3000	–	0	0	tr	–
FRESH									
baby raw	1 (0.5 oz)	6	–	296	5	1	3	–	42
raw	1 (2.5 oz)	31	2	20253	10	7	19	tr	233
raw shredded	½ cup	24	2	15471	8	5	15	tr	178

FOOD	PORTION	CALS	FIBER	VIT A	FOLIC	VIT C	CALCI	IRON	POTAS
slices cooked	½ cup	35	–	19152	11	2	24	tr	177
Bolthouse Farms									
Baby	1 pkg (2.25 oz)	25	2	11000	–	5	20	0	230
Matchstix	3 oz	35	2	15000	–	66	20	0	310
Earthbound Farm									
Organic Tops On	1 (2.7 oz)	35	2	13500	–	6	20	0	–
Organic w/ Organic Ranch Dip	1 pkg (2.2 oz)	90	1	6500	–	4	20	tr	–
Frieda's									
Gold	⅔ cup (3 oz)	35	3	24000	–	9	20	tr	–
Grimmway									
Baby	3 oz	38	2	13500	–	6	20	0	–
Nature's Gold									
Fresh	1 med (2.7 oz)	40	3	11000	–	5	20	0	–
River Ranch									
Shredded	¾ cup	35	3	24000	8	9	20	tr	–
FROZEN									
slices cooked	½ cup	26	–	12922	8	2	21	tr	115
C&W									
Whole Baby	⅔ cup	35	2	3000	–	1	20	0	–
Fresh Like									
Carrots Sliced	3.5 oz	42	–	19856	–	5	33	1	194
CASABA									
cubed	1 cup	45	–	51	–	27	9	1	357
fresh	1/10	43	–	49	–	26	8	1	344
CASHEWS									
cashew butter w/o salt	1 tbsp	94	–	0	11	0	7	1	87
dry roasted w/ salt	18 nuts (1 oz)	160	1	0	16	–	13	2	160
dry roasted w/o salt	1 oz	163	–	0	20	0	13	2	160
oil roasted w/o salt	1 oz	163	–	0	19	0	12	1	151
oil roasted w/o salt	1 oz	163	–	0	19	0	12	1	151
Bowlby's									
Bits	½ cup	200	1	0	–	0	0	1	–
Good Sense									
Jumbo Honey Roasted	¼ cup	170	1	0	–	0	0	1	–

FOOD	PORTION	CALS	FIBER	VIT A	FOLIC	VIT C	CALCI	IRON	POTAS
Jumbo Roasted & Salted	¼ cup	190	1	0	–	0	0	1	–
Kettle									
Butter Creamy Unsalted	2 tbsp	160	1	0	–	0	20	1	–
MaraNatha									
Cashew Butter	2 tbsp	190	2	0	–	0	20	2	–
Tamari Cashews	¼ cup	160	1	0	–	0	0	2	–
Planters									
Chocolate Lovers Milk Chocolate	10 pieces (1.5 oz)	230	tr	0	–	0	60	1	210
Dry Roasted	19 pieces (1 oz)	160	tr	0	–	0	0	2	190
Organic	23 pieces (1 oz)	170	1	0	–	0	0	2	180

CASSAVA
fresh	3.5 oz	120	–	10	–	48	91	4	764

CATFISH
Simmons
Farm Raised	4 oz	140	0	0	–	0	0	0	–

CAULIFLOWER
FRESH
cooked	½ cup (2.2 oz)	14	1	19	27	28	10	tr	88
flowerets cooked	3 (2 oz)	12	1	9	24	24	9	tr	76
flowerets raw	3 (2 oz)	14	1	11	32	26	12	tr	170
green cooked	1½ cups (3.2 oz)	29	3	127	40	0	29	1	250
green raw	1 head 7 in diam (18 oz)	158	16	777	291	450	169	4	1533
green raw	1 cup (2.2 oz)	20	2	97	36	22	21	tr	192
green raw floweret	1 (0.9 oz)	8	1	38	14	22	8	tr	75
raw	½ cup (1.8 oz)	13	1	10	28	23	11	tr	151

River Ranch
Florets	1 cup	20	2	<100	40	42	<20	tr	–

FOOD	PORTION	CALS	FIBER	VIT A	FOLIC	VIT C	CALCI	IRON	POTAS
FROZEN									
cooked	½ cup	17	–	20	37	28	15	tr	125
Birds Eye									
Steamfresh Garlic Cauliflower	1 cup	40	1	0	–	21	200	tr	–
Fresh Like									
Florets	3.5 oz	26	1	23	–	52	21	1	195
CAVIAR									
black or red	2 tbsp	81	0	598	16	0	88	4	58
CELERY									
diced cooked	½ cup	13	–	99	16	5	32	tr	213
fresh	1 stalk (1.3 oz)	6	1	54	11	3	16	tr	115
raw diced	½ cup	10	1	80	17	4	24	tr	172
root raw	½ cup	31	–	0	–	6	34	1	234
seed	1 tsp	8	–	1	–		35	1	28
Dole									
Stalks	2 med (3 oz)	15	2	0	–	6	20	0	–
Earthbound Farm									
Organic Hearts	2 stalks (3.9 oz)	20	2	100	–	9	40	tr	–
Frieda's									
Celery Root	¾ cup	35	3	0	–	6	40	1	–
River Ranch									
Sticks Fresh	4 (3 oz)	15	1	100	24	6	40	tr	–
CELTUCE									
raw	3.5 oz	22	–	3500		20	39	1	330
CEREAL									
bran flakes	¾ cup	90	–	1250	–	0	14	8	180
corn flakes	1¼ cups	110	–	1250	–	15	1	2	26
farina as prep w/ water	¾ cup	88	2	0	40	0	4	1	23
granola	½ cup	285	6	23	53	1	45	3	328
oatmeal instant as prep w/ water	1 cup (8.2 oz)	138	4	1996	199	0	215	8	131

FOOD	PORTION	CALS	FIBER	VIT A	FOLIC	VIT C	CALCI	IRON	POTAS
oatmeal regular & quick as prep w/ water	¾ cup (6.1 oz)	149	3	28	7	0	14	1	98
puffed rice	1 cup	56	tr	0	3	0	1	4	16
puffed wheat	1 cup	44	1	0	4	0	3	4	42
shredded mini wheats	1 cup	107	3	0	14	0	11	1	108
shredded wheat rectangular	1 biscuit (0.8 oz)	85	2	0	12	0	10	1	77
Alpen									
Corn Flakes	1 serv (1 oz)	110	tr	0	–	0	13	1	22
Regular	1 serv (2 oz)	200	4	0	–	3	122	3	270
Alti Plano									
Hot Cereal Chai Almond	1 pkg	210	5	0	–	0	60	2	–
Hot Cereal Oaxacan Chocolate	1 pkg	170	5	0	–	0	20	3	–
Hot Cereal Orange Date	1 pkg	180	6	0	–	1	40	2	–
Hot Cereal Regular	1 pkg	190	7	0	–	0	20	2	–
Hot Cereal Spiced Apple Raisin	1 pkg	160	5	0	–	1	20	2	–
Alvarado Street Bakery									
Plain Granola	½ cup	220	4	0	–	0	40	3	–
Back To Nature									
Banana Nut Multibran	¾ cup	140	13	0	–	0	40	1	–
Flax & Fiber Crunch	1 cup	200	9	0	400	0	450	4	–
Granola Apple Blueberry	½ cup	200	4	0	–	0	20	2	–
Granola Apple Cinnamon	½ cup	180	4	0	–	0	20	2	–
Granola Classic	½ cup	180	4	0	–	0	20	2	–
Granola French Vanilla	½ cup	220	4	0	–	6	40	1	–
Hi-Protein Crunch	½ cup	150	3	0	–	0	60	2	–
Hi-Fiber Multibran	½ cup	70	8	1000	80	0	0	8	–
Muesli	¾ cup	230	6	0	–	0	40	2	–
MultiGrain Harvest	1 cup	210	9	0	–	0	60	2	–
Oat & Soy Crisp	¾ cup	180	3	0	–	0	60	2	–
Strawberry & Seven Grains	1 cup	210	5	0	–	0	0	2	–

FOOD	PORTION	CALS	FIBER	VIT A	FOLIC	VIT C	CALCI	IRON	POTAS
Barbara's Bakery									
Shredded Spoonfuls	¾ cup	120	4	0	–	5	20	1	125
Bear Naked									
Apple Cinnamon	¼ cup	140	3	0	–	0	0	1	–
Banana Nut	¼ cup	140	3	0	–	0	0	1	–
Fruit And Nut	¼ cup	140	3	0	–	0	0	1	–
Peak Protein	½ cup	200	2	0	–	0	40	3	–
CoCo Wheats									
Hot Cereal	⅓ cup	200	2	0	100	6	100	16	–
Country Choice Naturals									
Instant Oatmeal Apples 'N' Cinnamon	1 pkg	140	3	0	–	0	20	1	–
Instant Oatmeal Maple Syrup	1 pkg	170	4	0	–	0	20	1	–
Instant Oatmeal Organic Plus French Vanilla	1 pkg	180	3	0	–	0	350	2	–
Instant Oatmeal Organic Plus Golden Brown Sugar	1 pkg	180	3	0	–	0	350	2	–
Instant Oatmeal Regular	1 pkg	110	3	0	–	0	20	1	–
Oatmeal Steel Cut not prep	½ cup	150	4	0	–	0	20	2	–
Oats Old Fashioned not prep	½ cup	150	4	0	–	0	20	2	–
Oats Quick not prep	½ cup	150	4	0	–	0	20	2	–
Organic MultiGrain Hot Cereal not prep	½ cup	130	5	0	–	0	0	1	–
Deliciously Slim									
Granola Cranberry Cashew	¾ cup	230	12	0	–	0	20	2	–
Granola Strawberry Almond	¾ cup	230	12	0	–	4	20	2	–
Earthbound Farm									
Organic Granola Maple Almond	½ cup	260	4	0	–	0	40	2	–
Enjoy Life									
Cinnamon Crunch Nut & Gluten Free	¾ cup	160	5	0	140	6	350	4	–

FOOD	PORTION	CALS	FIBER	VIT A	FOLIC	VIT C	CALCI	IRON	POTAS
EnviroKidz									
Organic Orangutan O's	¾ cup	120	2	0	–	0	0	0	–
Erewhon									
Apple Stroodles	¾ cup	110	1	0	–	0	20	1	–
Aztec	1 cup	110	1	0	–	0	0	1	–
Banana O's	¾ cup	110	2	0	–	0	0	1	–
Brown Rice Cream	¼ cup	170	1	0	–	0	20	2	–
Corn Flakes	1¼ cups	210	3	500	–	1	0	3	–
Crispy Brown Rice	1 cup	110	1	0	–	1	20	tr	–
Crispy Brown Rice No Salt Added	1 cup	110	1	0	–	1	20	tr	–
Fruit'n Wheat	¾ cup	170	5	0	–	0	20	1	–
Kamut Flakes	⅔ cup	110	4	0	–	0	60	1	–
Raisin Bran	1 cup	170	6	0	–	1	40	4	–
Rice Twice	¾ cup	120	0	0	–	0	0	0	–
Whole Wheat Flakes	1 cup	180	6	0	–	1	40	5	–
Fantastic									
Oatmeal Big Cup Maple Raisin 3 Grain	1 pkg	270	8	0	–	0	40	2	–
General Mills									
Basic 4	1 cup (1.9 oz)	200	3	500	100	0	250	5	150
Cheerios	1 cup	110	3	500	200	6	100	8	200
Chex Corn	1 cup (1 oz)	110	0	500	200	6	100	9	25
Chex Multi-Bran	1 cup (2 oz)	200	8	500	400	6	100	16	220
Chex Rice	1¼ cups (1.1 oz)	120	0	500	200	6	100	9	35
Country Corn Flakes	1 cup (1 oz)	120	–	500	200	6	250	8	30
Fiber One	½ cup (1 oz)	60	14	0	100	6	100	5	180
Gold Medal Raisin Bran	1⅓ cups (1.9 oz)	170	6	500	400	0	700	18	330
Kix	1⅓ cup (1 oz)	120	1	500	200	6	150	8	35
Nature Valley Low Fat Fruit Granola	⅔ cup (1.9 oz)	210	3	0	–	0	20	1	150

FOOD	PORTION	CALS	FIBER	VIT A	FOLIC	VIT C	CALCI	IRON	POTAS
NesQuik	¾ cup (1 oz)	120	–	500	100	6	100	5	65
Oatmeal Crisp Raisin	1 cup (1.9 oz)	210	4	0	100	0	20	5	200
Raisin Nut Bran	¾ cup (1.9 oz)	200	4	0	100	0	20	5	230
Sunrise Organic	¾ cup (1 oz)	110	1	0	100	6	0	5	50
Total Brown Sugar & Oat	¾ cup (1 oz)	110	1	500	400	60	1000	18	80
Total Protein	¾ cup	120	3	500	400	60	100	18	75
Total Raisin Bran	1 cup	170	5	500	400	0	1000	18	310
Total Whole Grain	¾ cup (1 oz)	100	3	500	400	60	1000	18	90
Wheaties	1 cup (1 oz)	110	3	500	200	6	20	8	105
Wheaties Raisin Bran	1 cup (1.9 oz)	180	5	500	200	0	20	8	230
Glutino									
Gluten Free Apple Cinnamon	½ cup	120	1	0	–	0	0	tr	–
Gluten Free Honey Nut	½ cup	130	1	0	–	0	20	tr	–
Grainfield's									
Brown Rice	1 serv (1 oz)	110	tr	0	–	0	14	1	81
Crisp Rice	1 serv (1 oz)	112	tr	0	–	0	6	1	31
Raisin Bran	1 serv (1 oz)	90	2	0	–	3	16	1	130
Wheat Flakes	1 serv (1 oz)	100	2	0	–	1	28	tr	99
Grandy Oats									
Organic Granola Classic	½ cup	252	5	<50	–	1	30	3	–
Organic Granola Low Fat Cranberry Chew	½ cup	191	3	<50	–	4	<10	6	–
Organic Granola Mainely Maple	½ cup	204	4	<50	–	1	40	2	–
Hansen's									
Orange & Chocolate	½ cup	230	4	2250	340	36	700	11	60

FOOD	PORTION	CALS	FIBER	VIT A	FOLIC	VIT C	CALCI	IRON	POTAS
Strawberry & Yogurt	½ cup	230	6	2250	340	36	700	11	80
Toasted Nut Crunch	½ cup	230	7	2250	340	60	700	11	80
Tropical Cluster	½ cup	210	6	2250	340	36	700	11	60
Hodgson Mill									
Hot Cereal Bulgur Wheat w/ Soy not prep	¼ cup	115	3	0	–	0	40	2	80
Hot Cereal Oat Bran not prep	¼ cup	120	6	0	20	0	20	2	40
Kashi									
7 Whole Grain Flakes	1 cup	180	6	0	–	0	0	1	160
7 Whole Grain Honey Puffs	1 cup	120	2	0	–	0	0	1	80
7 Whole Grain Nuggets	½ cup	210	7	0	–	0	20	1	–
7 Whole Grain Pilaf as prep	½ cup	170	6	0	–	0	20	1	–
7 Whole Grain Puffs	1 cup	70	1	0	–	0	0	tr	60
GoLean	1 cup	140	10	0	–	0	60	2	480
GoLean Crunch!	1 cup	190	8	0	–	0	40	2	300
GoLean Crunch Honey Almond Flax	1 cup	200	8	0	–	0	0	1	270
GoLean Instant Hot Cereal Creamy Truly Vanilla	1 pkg	150	7	0	–	0	0	1	250
GoLean Instant Hot Cereal Hearty Honey & Cinnamon	1 pkg	150	5	0	–	0	0	1	210
Good Friends	1 cup	170	12	0	–	0	20	2	–
Heart To Heart Instant Oatmeal Golden Brown Maple	1 pkg	160	5	1250	400	30	100	2	260
Heart To Heart Instant Oatmeal Raisin Spice	1 pkg	150	4	1250	400	30	100	2	230
Heart To Heart Oat Flakes & Blueberry Clusters	1¼ cups	200	4	1250	400	30	0	2	160
Heart To Heart Toasted Oat	¾ cup	110	5	1250	400	30	0	2	100
Mighty Bites All Flavors	1 cup	110	3	500	100	15	150	8	110

FOOD	PORTION	CALS	FIBER	VIT A	FOLIC	VIT C	CALCI	IRON	POTAS
Organic Promise Autumn Wheat	1 cup	190	6	0	–	0	0	1	180
Organic Promise Cinnamon Harvest	1 cup	190	5	0	–	0	0	1	170
Organic Promise Strawberry Fields	1 cup	120	1	0	–	2	0	tr	40
Vive Probiotic	1¼ cups	170	12	0	–	0	200	1	25
Kellogg's									
All-Bran	½ cup	80	10	500	400	6	100	5	350
All-Bran Extra Fiber	½ cup	50	13	500	400	6	100	5	270
Complete Oat Bran Flakes	¾ cup	110	1	750	400	60	0	18	120
Corn Flakes	1 cup	100	1	500	100	15	0	8	25
Corn Pops	1 cup	120	tr	500	100	6	0	2	25
Cracklin' Oat Bran	¾ cup	200	6	750	100	15	20	2	220
Crispix	1 cup	110	tr	500	280	6	0	8	35
Frosted Flakes ⅓ Less Sugar	1 cup	120	tr	500	–	6	0	5	25
Fruit Loops ⅓ Less Sugar	1¼ cups	120	1	500	100	15	0	5	45
Granola Low Fat w/ Raisins	⅔ cup	230	3	750	400	1	20	2	180
Mueslix Raisins Dates & Almonds	⅔ cup	200	4	300	400	0	20	5	240
Organic Mini Wheats Frosted	24 pieces	190	5	0	100	0	0	16	160
Organic Raisin Bran	1 cup	190	8	500	100	0	0	5	220
Organic Rice Krispies	1¼ cups	120	0	500	100	6	0	2	25
Product 19	1 cup	100	1	750	400	60	0	18	50
Raisin Bran	1 cup	190	7	500	100	0	20	5	360
Rice Krispies	1¼ cups	120	0	500	–	6	0	9	40
Smart Start Antioxidants	1 cup	190	3	1250	400	15	0	18	90
Smart Start Healthy Heart	1¼ cups	230	5	500	100	6	20	5	380
Special K	1 cup	110	tr	750	400	21	0	8	60
Special K Low Carb Lifestyle Protein Plus	¾ cup	100	5	750	140	21	40	8	320

FOOD	PORTION	CALS	FIBER	VIT A	FOLIC	VIT C	CALCI	IRON	POTAS
Liquid Cereal									
Apple & Cinnamon	1 can (11 oz)	160	1	1500	–	18	300	tr	300
Chocolate	1 can (11 oz)	170	1	1500	–	18	300	1	540
Fruit	1 can (11 oz)	150	tr	1500	–	18	300	1	380
Peanut Butter	1 can (11 oz)	170	1	1500	–	18	300	1	320
Lundberg									
Purely Organic Hot'n Creamy Rice	⅓ cup	190	3	0	–	0	0	1	190
Malt-O-Meal									
Balance	¾ cup	120	3	500	200	6	0	8	115
Cinnamon Toasters	¾ cup	130	1	500	–	6	100	5	45
Colossal Crunch	¾ cup	120	0	0	100	0	0	5	30
Creamy Hot Wheat not prep	3 tbsp	130	1	0	0	0	100	11	–
Crispy Rice	1¼ cups	130	0	750	400	15	0	9	40
Frosted Flakes	¾ cup	120	1	750	100	15	0	5	20
Frosted Mini Spooners	1 cup	190	6	0	400	0	0	16	180
Honey & Oat Blenders	¾ cup	120	1	500	200	15	250	9	60
Honey Buzzers	1⅓ cup	110	1	750	100	0	0	3	35
Instant Oatmeal Apple & Cinnamon	1 pkg	130	3	1000	80	0	100	4	–
Instant Oatmeal Cinnamon & Spice	1 pkg	170	3	1000	80	0	100	4	–
Instant Oatmeal Maple & Brown Sugar	1 pkg	160	3	1000	80	0	100	4	–
Original Hot Wheat not prep	3 tbsp	130	1	0	400	0	100	11	40
Puffed Rice	1 cup	60	0	0	–	0	0	5	15
Raisin Bran	1 cup	220	7	750	100	6	20	5	380
McCann's									
Irish Oatmeal Instant Apples & Cinnamon	1 pkg (1 oz)	130	2	1250	100	0	100	5	–
Irish Oatmeal Instant Maple & Brown Sugar	1 pkg (1 oz)	160	3	1250	100	0	100	5	–
Irish Oatmeal Instant Regular	1 pkg (1 oz)	100	3	1250	100	0	200	9	–

FOOD	PORTION	CALS	FIBER	VIT A	FOLIC	VIT C	CALCI	IRON	POTAS
Mother's									
Cinnamon Oat Crunch	1 cup	230	5	0	–	0	40	2	320
Cocoa Bumpers	1 cup	120	1	0	–	0	40	1	260
Groovy Grahams	¾ cup	100	1	0	–	0	20	1	210
Honey Round-Ups	¾ cup	110	1	0	–	0	0	tr	65
Peanut Butter Bumpers	1 cup	130	1	0	–	0	20	1	210
Rolled Oats	½ cup	150	4	0	–	0	0	2	–
Toasted Oat Bran	¾ cup	120	3	0	–	0	20	1	160
Whole Wheat Hot Cereal	½ cup	130	4	0	–	0	0	1	–
Natural Ovens									
Great Granola	¼ cup	110	5	0	40	0	50	1	–
Paul's Oatmeal not prep	⅓ cup	120	3	0	40	0	30	2	–
Nature's Path									
Organic Optimum ReBound	¾ cup	190	6	0	–	1	20	3	230
Organic Zen Instant Oatmeal Cranberry Ginger	1 pkg	150	3	0	–	0	20	2	–
Perky's									
Nutty Flax	¾ cup	230	7	1250	–	0	40	1	–
PerkyO's Original	¾ cup	120	3	1000	180	2	450	5	–
Post									
Grape-Nuts	½ cup	200	6	750	200	0	20	16	260
Great Grains Raisins Dates Pecans	½ cup	210	4	750	100	0	0	9	210
Raisin Bran	1 cup (2 oz)	190	8	750	200	0	20	11	330
Shredded Wheat Original	2 biscuits (1.6 oz)	160	6	0	16	0	20	1	180
Shredded Wheat Spoon Size	1 cup	170	6	0	–	0	20	1	190
Quaker									
Instant Oatmeal Weight Control Banana Bread	1 pkg	160	6	1000	80	0	100	4	150
Instant Oatmeal Weight Control Cinnamon	1 pkg	160	6	1000	80	0	100	4	270

FOOD	PORTION	CALS	FIBER	VIT A	FOLIC	VIT C	CALCI	IRON	POTAS
Life	¾ cup	120	2	0	240	0	100	8	90
Old Fashioned Oats not prep	½ cup	150	4	0	–	0	0	2	–
Ralston									
100% Hot Wheat	⅓ cup	150	5	0	0	0	0	1	0
Apple Dapples	1 cup	120	tr	750	200	15	100	5	35
Corn Biscuits	1 cup	110	tr	500	100	6	100	9	25
Corn Flakes	1 cup	100	tr	750	100	15	0	9	25
Crisp Rice	1¼ cups	120	0	750	200	15	0	11	40
Enriched Bran Flakes	¾ cup	90	5	1250	400	15	0	9	170
Farina	3 tbsp	120	1	0	40	0	100	10	0
Grits	¼ cup	140	1	0	40	0	0	1	0
Instant Oats Bananas & Cream	1 pkg	130	2	1000	80	0	100	4	0
Oats & More w/ Almonds	¾ cup	130	1	1250	100	6	0	9	65
Oats Instant	1 pkg	100	3	1000	80	0	100	8	0
Oats Instant For Kids Cinnawow	1 pkg	140	3	1000	100	0	150	5	95
Oats Old Fashioned	½ cup	150	4	0	16	0	0	2	140
Oats Quick	½ cup	140	4	0	0	0	0	2	0
Raisin Bran	1 cup	200	8	750	100	0	20	5	340
Rice Biscuits	1¼ cups	120	0	500	200	6	100	9	35
South Beach Diet									
Toasted Wheats	1¼ cups (2 oz)	210	8	0	–	0	0	2	–
Whole Grain Crunch	¾ cup (1 oz)	110	4	750	–	0	40	2	–
Stark Sisters									
Granola Lo-Fat Raspberry Blueberry	½ cup	230	4	0	–	1	40	1	–
Granola Nutty Maple	½ cup	250	4	0	–	0	40	3	–
Granola Original Maple Almond	½ cup	240	5	0	–	0	40	1	–
Sunbelt									
Granola Low Fat Cinnamon & Raisins	½ cup	250	3	0	–	0	20	1	–
Uncle Sam									
Cereal	1 cup (1.9 oz)	190	10	0	–	1	40	2	–

FOOD	PORTION	CALS	FIBER	VIT A	FOLIC	VIT C	CALCI	IRON	POTAS
Weetabix									
Cereal	2 biscuits (1.2 oz)	100	3	0	–	1	28	2	106
Zoe's									
Granola Cinnamon Raisin	½ cup	190	7	0	–	2	40	2	280
Granola Cranberries Currants	½ cup	190	7	0	–	2	40	2	270
Granola Honey Almond	½ cup	190	7	0	–	2	40	2	270
O's Cinnamon	¾ cup	120	5	0	–	0	80	1	–
O's Honey	¾ cup	120	5	0	–	0	80	1	–
O's Natural	¾ cup	120	tr	0	–	0	80	1	–

CEREAL BARS
Attune
FOOD	PORTION	CALS	FIBER	VIT A	FOLIC	VIT C	CALCI	IRON	POTAS
Wellness Yogurt & Granola Lemon Creme	1 (1.4 oz)	180	2	0	–	0	200	1	–
Wellness Yogurt & Granola Strawberry Bliss	1 (1.4 oz)	180	5	0	–	1	200	1	–
Enjoy Life									
Caramel Apple Nut & Gluten Free	1 (1 oz)	110	2	0	240	0	150	tr	–
EnviroKidz									
Crispy Rice Panda Peanut Butter	1 (1 oz)	110	tr	0	–	0	0	tr	–
Glutino									
Gluten Free Breakfast Bar Apple	1 (1.4 oz)	120	3	0	–	15	20	1	–
Gluten Free Breakfast Bar Chocolate	1 (0.25 oz)	110	4	0	–	24	40	2	–
Kashi									
TLC Chewy Granola Honey Almond Flax	1 (1.2 oz)	140	4	0	–	0	0	1	90
TLC Chewy Granola Peanut Peanut Butter	1 (1.2 oz)	140	4	0	–	0	0	1	80
TLC Chewy Trail Mix	1 (1.2 oz)	140	4	0	–	0	0	1	100

FOOD	PORTION	CALS	FIBER	VIT A	FOLIC	VIT C	CALCI	IRON	POTAS
Kellogg's									
All-Bran Oatmeal Raisin	1	120	5	500	40	0	0	2	–
All-Bran Honey Oat	1	130	5	500	–	0	0	2	–
Crunchy Nut Sweet & Salty Chocolatey Almond	1 (1.1 oz)	160	2	500	40	0	100	2	–
Smart Start Healthy Heart Cinnamon	1 (1.4 oz)	150	2	500	40	0	0	1	350
Special K Snack Bar Chocolate Peanut	1 (0.9 oz)	110	1	1000	40	12	60	1	–
Special K Vanilla Crisp	1 (0.8 oz)	90	tr	0	–	0	0	0	–
Kudos									
Granola Chocolate Chip	1	120	1	0	–	0	250	tr	–
Granola Peanut Butter	1	130	1	0	–	0	200	0	–
Natural Ovens									
Great Granola Chocolate Almond	1	150	3	0	24	0	40	1	0
Great Granola Fruit & Lemon	1	130	3	200	60	18	60	1	0
Great Granola Mixed Fruit	1	130	3	200	60	18	60	1	0
Nature Valley									
Chewy Granola Blueberry Yogurt	1	140	1	0	–	0	100	tr	–
Chewy Granola Lemon Yogurt	1	140	1	0	–	0	100	tr	–
Chewy Granola Vanilla Yogurt	1	140	1	0	–	0	100	tr	–
Chewy Trail Mix Granola Apple Cinnamon	1	140	1	–	–	–	–	tr	–
Crunchy Granola Apple Crisp	1	140	1	0	–	0	100	tr	–
Crunchy Granola Apple Crisp	1	104	1	0	–	0	100	tr	–
Nutri-Grain									
Nutri-Grain Blueberry	1	140	tr	750	40	0	200	2	–
Nutri-Grain Mixed Berry	1	140	tr	750	40	0	200	2	–
Post									
Honey Bunches Of Oats Cranberry Almond	1 (1.2 oz)	140	1	750	–	0	100	2	70

FOOD	PORTION	CALS	FIBER	VIT A	FOLIC	VIT C	CALCI	IRON	POTAS
Quaker									
Breakfast Bar Apple Crisp	1 (1.3 oz)	130	1	1250	100	6	200	tr	–
Crunchy Granola Oats & Berries	1 (1 oz)	130	1	500	–	6	0	2	–
Oatmeal To Go Brown Sugar Cinnamon	1 (2.1 oz)	220	5	1000	80	0	200	4	135
Q-Smart Cranberry Vanilla Almond	1 (1 oz)	120	2	500	40	6	100	tr	–
Trail Mix Cranberry Raisin & Almond	1 (1.2 oz)	150	1	0	–	0	0	1	–
Rice Krispies									
Treats Original	1 (0.8 oz)	90	0	200	24	0	0	tr	–
South Beach Diet									
100 Calorie Chocolate Delight	1 (1 oz)	100	3	0	–	0	0	1	–
100 Calorie Peanut Butter Chocolate Chip	1 (1 oz)	100	3	0	–	0	0	1	–
100 Calorie Snack Bar Mixed Berry	1 (1 oz)	100	3	0	–	0	20	1	–
High Protein Chocolate	1 (1.2 oz)	140	3	750	–	0	150	2	–
High Protein Cinnamon Raisin	1 (1.2 oz)	140	3	750	–	0	150	2	–
High Protein Cranberry Almond	1 (1.2 oz)	140	3	750	–	0	150	2	–
High Protein Maple Nut	1 (1.2 oz)	140	3	750	–	0	150	2	–
High Protein Peanut Butter	1 (1.2 oz)	140	3	750	–	0	150	2	–
CHAMPAGNE									
mimosa	1 serv	117	tr	186	28	47	10	tr	186
CHAYOTE									
fresh cooked	1 cup	38	–	75	–	13	21	tr	276
CHEESE									
beaufort	1 oz	115	0	314	1	0	297	tr	33
blue	1 oz	100	–	204	10	0	150	tr	73
blue crumbled	1 cup (4.7 oz)	477	–	973	49	0	712	tr	346

FOOD	PORTION	CALS	FIBER	VIT A	FOLIC	VIT C	CALCI	IRON	POTAS
bocconcini smoked	1 oz	90	0	100	–	0	100	0	–
brick	1 oz	105	–	307	6	0	191	tr	38
brie	1 oz	95	–	189	18	0	52	tr	43
caerphilly	1.4 oz	150	0	700	–	tr	220	tr	–
camembert	1 oz	85	–	262	18	0	110	tr	53
cantal	1 oz	105	0	256	6	0	277	tr	39
chabichou	1 oz	95	0	443	36	0	86	tr	69
chaource	1 oz	83	0	486	27	0	111	tr	27
cheddar	1 oz	114	–	300	5	0	204	tr	28
cheddar low fat	1 oz	49	–	68	3	0	118	tr	19
cheddar shredded	1 cup	455	–	1197	21	0	815	1	111
cheshire	1 oz	110	–	279	–	0	182	tr	27
colby	1 oz	112	–	293	–	0	194	tr	36
comte	1 oz	114	0	319	1	0	251	tr	34
coulommiers	1 oz	88	0	280	19	0	70	tr	46
crottin	1 oz	105	0	–	–	0	33	tr	83
derby	1.4 oz	161	0	755	–	tr	272	tr	–
edam	1 oz	101	–	260	5	0	207	tr	53
emmentaler	1 oz	115	–	–	tr	tr	291	tr	31
feta	1 oz	75	–	–	–	0	140	tr	18
fontina	1 oz	110	–	333	–	0	156	tr	–
frais	1.6 oz	51	0	225	–	tr	40	0	–
gouda	1 oz	101	–	183	6	0	198	tr	34
grana padano parmesan shaved	1 tbsp	20	0	0	–	0	60	0	–
gruyere	1 oz	117	–	346	3	0	287	–	23
lancashire	1.4 oz	149	0	720	–	tr	224	tr	–
leicester	1.4 oz	160	0	730	–	tr	264	tr	–
limburger	1 oz	93	–	363	16	0	141	tr	36
lymeswold	1.4 oz	170	0	990	–	tr	108	tr	–
maroilles	1 oz	97	0	226	3	0	229	tr	37
monterey	1 oz	106	–	269	–	0	212	tr	23
morbier	1 oz	99	0	1000	6	0	217	tr	29
mozzarella	1 oz	80	–	225	1	0	147	tr	19
mozzarella fresh	1 oz	80	0	200	–	0	150	0	–
muenster	1 oz	104	–	318	3	0	203	tr	38
parmesan grated	1 tbsp	23	–	35	tr	0	69	tr	5
parmesan hard	1 oz	111	–	171	2	0	336	tr	26
pont l'eveque	1 oz	86	0	795	3	0	134	tr	39
provolone	1 oz	100	–	231	3	0	214	tr	39

FOOD	PORTION	CALS	FIBER	VIT A	FOLIC	VIT C	CALCI	IRON	POTAS
pyrenees	1 oz	101	0	915	7	0	181	tr	19
queso anego	1 oz	106	–	63	0	0	193	tr	25
queso asadero	1 oz	101	–	63	2	0	188	tr	25
queso chichuahua	1 oz	106	–	64	1	0	185	tr	15
queso fresco	1 oz	41	0	100	–	0	194	tr	–
queso manchego	1 oz	107	0	410	6	–	237	tr	57
queso panela	1 oz	74	0	70	–	0	195	1	–
raclette	1 oz	102	0	1000	15	0	157	tr	32
reblochon	1 oz	88	0	1130	7	0	179	tr	54
ricotta part skim	½ cup (4.4 oz)	171	–	536	–	0	337	1	155
romano	1 oz	110	–	162	2	0	302	–	–
roquefort	1 oz	105	–	297	14	0	188	tr	26
rouy	1 oz	95	0	790	–	0	143	tr	21
saint marcellin	1 oz	94	0	–	38	0	49	1	53
saint nectaire	1 oz	97	0	780	6	0	169	tr	36
saint paulin	1 oz	85	0	900	6	0	223	tr	23
stilton blue	1.4 oz	164	0	770	–	tr	128	tr	–
swiss	1 oz	107	–	240	2	0	272	tr	31
tilsit	1 oz	96	–	296	–	0	198	tr	18
tome	1 oz	92	0	1000	6	0	115	tr	22
triple creme	1 oz	113	0	1925	3	tr	28	tr	46
vacherin	1 oz	92	0	90	3	0	200	tr	34
wensleydale	1.4 oz	151	0	635	–	tr	224	tr	–
whey cheese	1 oz	126	0	356	–	1	97	tr	–
Athenos									
Feta	1 oz (1 in cube)	80	0	200	–	0	60	0	–
Back To Nature									
Organic American Slices	1 slice (0.7 oz)	80	0	200	–	0	100	0	–
Organic Cheddar Cubes	8 pieces (1.1 oz)	130	0	400	–	0	200	0	–
Organic Cheddar Shredded	¼ cup	110	0	300	–	0	200	0	–
Organic Mozzarella Shredded	¼ cup	80	0	200	–	0	200	0	–
Organic White Cheddar Slices Reduced Fat	1 slice (0.7 oz)	60	0	200	–	0	100	0	–

FOOD	PORTION	CALS	FIBER	VIT A	FOLIC	VIT C	CALCI	IRON	POTAS
Cabot									
American	1 slice (0.7 oz)	80	0	300	–	0	100	0	–
Cheddar	1 oz	110	0	300	–	0	200	0	25
Cheddar Smoked	1 oz	110	0	300	–	0	200	0	–
Colby Jack	1 oz	110	0	300	–	0	200	0	–
Monterey Jack	1 oz	110	0	300	–	0	200	0	20
Mozzarella Shredded	¼ cup	80	0	200	–	0	200	0	–
Pepper Jack	1 oz	110	0	300	–	0	200	0	–
Cantare									
Baked Brie En Croute	1 oz	100	0	300	–	0	40	tr	–
Cedar Grove									
Organic Tomato Basil Cheddar	1 oz	110	0	400	–	0	200	0	–
Chavrie									
Goat's Milk	2 tbsp	50	0	100	–	0	20	0	–
Connoisseur									
Asiago Spread	1 tbsp	90	0	300	–	0	150	0	–
Brie Spread	2 tbsp	90	0	400	–	0	150	0	–
Gorgonzola Spread	1 tbsp	90	0	300	–	0	150	0	–
Wheel Asiago Pesto	2 tbsp	90	0	300	–	0	150	0	–
Wheel Swiss Bacon	2 tbsp	90	0	200	–	0	150	0	–
Crystal Farms									
American Singles	1 slice (0.7 oz)	70	0	200	–	0	100	0	–
American Singles 2%	1 slice (0.7 oz)	50	0	400	–	0	250	0	–
American Singles Fat Free	1 slice (0.7 oz)	30	0	0	–	0	150	0	–
Blue Crumbled	2 tbsp	100	0	300	–	0	200	0	–
Cheese Curds	8 pieces (1 oz)	110	0	500	–	0	150	0	–
Cheezoids Sticks	1 piece (0.8 oz)	70	0	400	–	0	150	0	–
Danish Havarti	1 oz	110	0	400	–	0	200	0	–
Deli Slices Muenster	1 slice (0.8 oz)	80	0	200	–	0	150	0	–
Deli Slices Swiss	1 slice (0.7 oz)	80	0	200	–	0	200	0	–
Feta Crumbled	¼ cup	90	tr	300	–	0	80	0	–

FOOD	PORTION	CALS	FIBER	VIT A	FOLIC	VIT C	CALCI	IRON	POTAS
Gorgonzola Crumbled	2 tbsp	100	0	300	–	0	200	0	–
Marble Jack	1 oz	110	0	400	–	0	200	0	–
Parmesan Grated	2 tsp	25	0	100	–	0	60	0	–
Pepper Jack	1 oz	110	0	300	–	0	200	0	–
Ricotta	¼ cup	90	0	200	–	0	100	0	–
Smoked Gouda	1 oz	100	0	200	–	0	150	0	–
String	1 piece (1 oz)	80	0	400	–	0	200	0	–
Fage									
Feta	1 oz	80	0	500	–	0	80	0	–
Finlandia									
Muenster	1 slice (1.1 oz)	120	0	400	–	0	200	0	–
Formaggio									
Fresh Mozzarella	1 oz	90	0	200	–	1	150	tr	–
Heluva Good Cheese									
Cheddar Extra Sharp	1 oz	110	0	300	–	0	200	0	–
Horizon Organic									
American	1 slice (0.7 oz)	60	0	100	–	0	100	0	–
Cheddar	1 oz	110	0	300	–	0	200	0	–
Monterey Jack	1 oz	100	0	300	–	0	200	0	–
Shred Mexican	¼ cup	110	0	300	–	0	200	0	–
Shred Parmesan	1 tbsp	20	0	0	–	0	60	0	–
Slice Provolone	1 slice (0.7 oz)	70	0	200	–	0	150	0	–
Sticks Colby	1 (1 oz)	110	0	300	–	0	200	0	–
String Mozzarella	1 stick (1 oz)	80	0	200	–	0	200	0	–
Jordan's									
Provolone	1 slice (1 oz)	100	0	200	–	0	200	0	–
Kraft									
LiveActive Cheddar Sticks	1 (1 oz)	120	0	300	–	0	200	0	–
Land O Lakes									
Cheddar Mild	1 slice (1 oz)	110	0	300	–	0	200	tr	–
Swiss	1 slice (1 oz)	110	0	200	–	0	250	0	–

FOOD	PORTION	CALS	FIBER	VIT A	FOLIC	VIT C	CALCI	IRON	POTAS
Laughing Cow									
Cheese Bites Light	6 pieces (0.8 oz)	35	0	200	–	0	70	0	–
Creamy Swiss Light Original	1 wedge (0.7 oz)	35	0	200	–	0	60	0	–
Creamy Swiss Original	1 wedge (0.7 oz)	50	0	100	–	0	60	0	–
Mini Babybel Bonbel	1 piece (0.7 oz)	70	0	300	–	0	150	0	–
Mini Babybel Gouda	1 piece (0.7 oz)	80	0	100	–	0	100	0	–
Mini Babybel Original	1 piece (0.7 oz)	70	0	300	–	0	150	0	–
Meza									
Baked Brie In Pastry w/ Cranberries & Spiced Almonds	1 oz	110	tr	200	–	0	40	tr	–
Miller's									
Mozzarella	1 slice (1 oz)	81	0	200	–	0	230	0	–
Mont Chevre									
Assorted Crottins	1 oz	70	0	0	–	0	20	0	–
Mt Vikos									
Feta Sheep & Goat Milk	1 oz	80	0	300	–	0	80	0	–
Polly-O									
Mozzarella Part Skim	1 oz	70	0	100	–	0	100	0	–
Ricotta Part Skim	¼ cup	90	0	200	–	0	250	0	–
Ricotta Lite	¼ cup	70	0	300	–	0	250	0	90
President									
Feta	1 oz	90	0	300	–	0	60	0	–
Sargento									
String	1 piece (0.8 oz)	70	0	200	–	0	150	0	–
Smart Balance									
Cheddar Shredded	1 oz	80	0	0	–	0	200	0	–
Mozzarella Shredded	1 oz	80	0	0	–	0	200	0	–
Sorrento									
Mozzarella Fresh	1 oz	90	0	200	–	0	100	0	–

FOOD	PORTION	CALS	FIBER	VIT A	FOLIC	VIT C	CALCI	IRON	POTAS
CHEESE DISHES									
FROZEN									
Alexia									
Mozzarella Stix	2 pieces	120	tr	200	–	0	100	tr	–
TAKE-OUT									
fondue	½ cup (3.8 oz)	247	–	447	5	0	514	tr	113
fried mozzarella sticks	3 (4.6 oz)	503	1	840	28	0	855	2	168
souffle	1 serv (7 oz)	504	1	1000	38	tr	446	2	274
welsh rarebit	1 slice	228	1	825	–	tr	204	1	–
CHERIMOYA									
fresh	1	515	–	55	–	49	126	3	–
CHERRIES									
CANNED									
maraschino	1 (4 g)	7	tr	0	0	0	2	tr	1
maraschino	¼ cup (1.4 oz)	66	1	0	0	0	22	tr	8
sour in light syrup	½ cup	94	1	915	10	3	13	2	120
sour water packed	½ cup	44	1	920	10	3	13	2	120
sour in heavy syrup	½ cup	116	1	914	10	3	13	2	119
sweet juice pack	½ cup	68	2	156	5	3	18	1	164
sweet pitted in heavy syrup	½ cup	105	2	195	5	5	11	tr	183
sweet water pack	½ cup	57	2	198	5	3	14	tr	162
Del Monte									
Sweet Dark Pitted In Heavy Syrup	½ cup	100	tr	0	–	4	0	tr	–
DRIED									
bing unsulfured	¼ cup	130	2	1000	–	0	20	1	–
montmorency tart pitted	⅓ cup	160	2	1250	–	0	20	1	–
rainier unsulfured	⅓ cup	140	2	200	–	6	20	tr	–
tart	½ cup	200	2	2250	–	0	20	1	–
yogurt covered	¼ cup	170	5	300	–	0	40	tr	–
De-Lite									
Tart	1 oz	95	1	189	–	2	10	tr	103

FOOD	PORTION	CALS	FIBER	VIT A	FOLIC	VIT C	CALCI	IRON	POTAS
Eden									
Montmorency	¼ cup	140	3	500	–	–	40	tr	350
Frieda's									
Bing	¼ cup (1.4 oz)	120	3	100	–	0	20	tr	–
Tart	⅓ cup (1.4 oz)	150	2	1500	–	0	0	1	–
Good Sense									
Cherries	⅓ cup	145	2	1500	–	0	20	1	–
Sunsweet									
Tart & Sweet	¼ cup (1.4 oz)	100	2	750	–	0	20	tr	115
FRESH									
sour	1 cup	52	2	1321	8	10	16	tr	178
sour pitted	1 cup	78	3	1989	12	16	25	1	268
sweet	20	86	3	87	5	10	18	tr	302
Chiquita									
Cherries	21	90	9	100	–	9	20	tr	–
Rainier									
Sweet Premium Northwest	1 cup	90	3	100	–	9	20	tr	300
Super Cherry									
Rainier	21	90	3	0	–	6	20	0	–
FROZEN									
sour unsweetened	½ cup	36	1	674	4	1	10	tr	96
sweet sweetened	½ cup	115	3	245	5	1	16	tr	258
CHERRY JUICE									
tart cherry concentrate	1 cup	140	0	0	–	0	20	1	–
Eden									
Organic Montmorency	8 oz	140	0	200	–	0	20	1	370
Ocean Spray									
Black Cherry	8 oz	140	0	0	–	60	–	–	0
Old Orchard									
100% Pure Tart Cherry	8 oz	140	–	0	–	0	20	0	360
CHESTNUTS									
chinese steamed	3 (1 oz)	43	–	39	13	7	3	tr	87
creme de marrons	1 oz	73	1	0	9	0	4	tr	49
japanese roasted	1 oz	57	–	21	17	8	10	1	121

FOOD	PORTION	CALS	FIBER	VIT A	FOLIC	VIT C	CALCI	IRON	POTAS
ready-to-eat vacuum packed	5 (1 oz)	40	0	0	–	0	0	0	–
roasted	3 (1 oz)	70	1	0	20	7	8	tr	168

CHEWING GUM
bubble gum	1 block (8 g)	27	–	0	–	0	–	–	0
stick	1 (3 g)	10	–	0	–	0	–	–	0

Brach's
Abra Cabubble	1 piece	45	0	0	–	0	0	0	–

CHIA SEEDS
dried	1 oz	134	–	10	–	–	150	3	–

CHICKEN
CANNED
breast meat in water	2 oz	70	0	0	–	0	0	0	–
w/ broth	½ can (2.5 oz)	117	0	–	–	1	10	1	98

Valley Fresh
Chunk White	2 oz	70	0	0	–	0	0	0	–
White & Dark Chunk	2 oz	80	0	0	–	0	0	tr	–

FRESH
broiler/fryer breast w/ skin batter dipped & fried	½ breast (4.9 oz)	364	–	94	8	0	28	1	282
broiler/fryer breast w/ skin roasted	½ breast (3.4 oz)	193	0	91	3	0	14	1	240
broiler/fryer breast w/ skin stewed	½ breast (3.9 oz)	202	0	90	3	0	14	1	195
broiler/fryer breast w/o skin fried	½ breast (3 oz)	161	–	20	4	0	14	1	237
broiler/fryer breast w/o skin roasted	½ breast (3 oz)	142	0	18	3	0	13	1	220
broiler/fryer drumstick w/ skin batter dipped & fried	1 (2.6 oz)	193	–	62	6	0	12	1	134
broiler/fryer drumstick w/ skin floured & fried	1 (1.7 oz)	120	–	41	4	0	6	1	112
broiler/fryer drumstick w/ skin roasted	1 (1.8 oz)	112	0	52	4	0	6	1	119

FOOD	PORTION	CALS	FIBER	VIT A	FOLIC	VIT C	CALCI	IRON	POTAS
broiler/fryer drumstick w/ skin stewed	1 (2 oz)	116	0	52	4	0	7	1	105
broiler/fryer drumstick w/o skin fried	1 (1.5 oz)	82	0	26	4	0	5	1	105
broiler/fryer drumstick w/o skin roasted	1 (1.5 oz)	76	0	26	4	0	5	1	108
broiler/fryer drumstick w/o skin stewed	1 (1.6 oz)	78	0	26	4	0	5	1	92
broiler/fryer leg w/ skin batter dipped & fried	1 (5.5 oz)	431	–	144	14	0	28	2	299
broiler/fryer leg w/ skin floured & fried	1 (3.9 oz)	285	–	103	9	0	15	2	261
broiler/fryer leg w/ skin roasted	1 (4 oz)	265	0	154	8	0	14	2	256
broiler/fryer leg w/ skin stewed	1 (4.4 oz)	275	0	156	8	0	14	2	220
broiler/fryer leg w/o skin fried	1 (3.3 oz)	195	–	62	8	0	12	1	239
broiler/fryer leg w/o skin roasted	1 (3.3 oz)	182	0	60	8	0	12	1	230
broiler/fryer leg w/o skin stewed	1 (3.5 oz)	187	0	60	8	0	11	1	192
broiler/fryer neck w/ skin stewed	1 (1.3 oz)	94	0	61	1	0	10	1	41
broiler/fryer neck w/o skin stewed	1 (.6 oz)	32	0	22	tr	0	8	tr	25
broiler/fryer skin floured & fried	from ½ chicken (2 oz)	281	–	130	2	0	8	1	70
broiler/fryer skin roasted	from ½ chicken (2 oz)	254	0	146	1	0	8	1	76
broiler/fryer skin stewed	from ½ chicken (2.5 oz)	261	0	143	1	0	9	1	84
broiler/fryer thigh w/ skin batter dipped & fried	1 (3 oz)	238	–	82	8	0	16	1	165

FOOD	PORTION	CALS	FIBER	VIT A	FOLIC	VIT C	CALCI	IRON	POTAS
broiler/fryer thigh w/ skin floured & fried	1 (2.2 oz)	162	–	61	5	0	8	1	147
broiler/fryer thigh w/ skin roasted	1 (2.2 oz)	153	0	102	4	0	8	1	137
broiler/fryer thigh w/ skin stewed	1 (2.4 oz)	158	0	103	4	0	8	1	115
broiler/fryer thigh w/o skin fried	1 (1.8 oz)	113	–	37	4	0	7	1	134
broiler/fryer thigh w/o skin roasted	1 (1.8 oz)	109	0	34	4	0	6	1	124
broiler/fryer thigh w/o skin stewed	1 (1.9 oz)	107	0	34	4	0	6	1	101
broiler/fryer w/ skin floured & fried	½ chicken (11 oz)	844	–	280	20	0	52	4	735
broiler/fryer w/ skin fried	½ chicken (16.4 oz)	1347	–	434	35	0	97	6	863
broiler/fryer w/ skin roasted	½ chicken (10.5 oz)	715	0	482	16	0	45	4	667
broiler/fryer w/ skin stewed	½ chicken (11.7 oz)	730	0	488	16	0	44	4	556
broiler/fryer w/ skin neck & giblets batter dipped & fried	1 chicken (2.3 lbs)	2987	–	6202	241	4	218	18	1951
broiler/fryer w/ skin neck & giblets roasted	1 chicken (1.5 lbs)	1598	–	4340	201	4	105	11	1447
broiler/fryer w/ skin neck & giblets stewed	1 chicken (1.6 lbs)	1625	–	4350	200	4	104	12	1224
broiler/fryer w/o skin fried	1 cup	307	–	82	10	0	24	2	360
broiler/fryer w/o skin roasted	1 cup (5 oz)	266	0	74	8	0	21	2	340
broiler/fryer w/o skin stewed	1 cup (5 oz)	248	0	70	8	0	19	2	252
broiler/fryer wing w/ skin batter dipped & fried	1 (1.7 oz)	159	–	55	3	0	10	1	68

FOOD	PORTION	CALS	FIBER	VIT A	FOLIC	VIT C	CALCI	IRON	POTAS
broiler/fryer wing w/ skin floured & fried	1 (1.1 oz)	103	–	40	1	0	5	tr	57
broiler/fryer wing w/ skin roasted	1 (1.2 oz)	99	0	54	1	0	5	tr	62
broiler/fryer wing w/ skin stewed	1 (1.4 oz)	100	0	53	1	0	5	tr	56
capon w/ skin neck & giblets roasted	1 chicken (3.1 lbs)	3211	–	10408	367	6	211	25	3439
cornish hen w/ skin roasted	1 hen (8 oz)	595	0	241	5	1	31	2	562
cornish hen w/o skin & bone roasted	1 hen (3.8 oz)	144	0	70	2	1	14	1	268
cornish hen w/o skin & bone roasted	½ hen (2 oz)	72	0	35	1	tr	7	tr	134
cornish hen w/skin roasted	½ hen (4 oz)	296	0	120	3	1	15	1	280
roaster dark meat w/o skin roasted	1 cup (5 oz)	250	0	76	9	0	15	2	313
roaster light meat w/o skin roasted	1 cup (5 oz)	214	0	35	5	0	18	2	330
roaster w/ skin neck & giblets roasted	1 chicken (2.4 lbs)	2363	–	6400	251	4	136	17	2183
roaster w/ skin roasted	½ chicken (1.1 lbs)	1071	0	399	22	0	58	6	1014
roaster w/o skin roasted	1 cup (5 oz)	469	0	57	7	0	25	2	321
stewing dark meat w/o skin stewed	1 cup (5 oz)	361	0	203	12	0	17	2	285
stewing w/ skin neck & giblets stewed	1 chicken (1.3 lbs)	1636	–	5487	211	3	78	11	1052
stewing w/ skin stewed	½ chicken (9.2 oz)	744	0	343	13	0	33	4	476

Amish Select

Boneless Skinless Breast w/ Honey Dijon Mustard	1 serv (4 oz)	130	0	0	–	0	40	1	–

Murray's

Breast Boneless & Skinless	4 oz	110	0	0	–	0	0	1	–

FOOD	PORTION	CALS	FIBER	VIT A	FOLIC	VIT C	CALCI	IRON	POTAS
Ground	3 oz	130	0	–	–	–	–	tr	–
Whole Lean	4 oz	170	0	0	–	0	0	1	–
Perdue									
Boneless Skinless Breasts Cooked	3 oz	110	0	–	–	–	–	1	–
Boneless Breast Roasted Garlic Herb	1 piece (3 oz)	90	–	–	–	1	–	1	–
Breaded Breast Strips Barbecue	3 oz	120	–	–	–	–	80	1	–
Breaded Breast Strips Hot & Spicy	3 oz	110	–	200	–	2	80	1	–
Breaded Breast Strips Original	3 oz	120	–	–	–	–	100	1	–
Burger Cooked	1 (3 oz)	160	0	–	–	–	–	1	–
Chicken Breast Seasoned Italian Cooked	1 piece (3 oz)	90	–	200	–	1	–	1	–
Chicken Breast Seasoned Teriyaki Cooked	1 piece (3 oz)	90	–	–	–	0	–	1	–
Ground Cooked	3 oz	170	0	–	–	–	40	1	–
Ground Breast Cooked	3 oz	80	0	–	–	–	–	tr	–
Honey Rotisserie Dark Meat	3 oz	200	–	0	–	2	–	1	–
Honey Rotisserie White Meat	3 oz	140	–	0	–	0	–	1	–
Oven Stuffer Dark Meat Roasted	3 oz	210	0	100	–	–	–	1	–
Oven Stuffer Drumstick Roasted	1 (3.6 oz)	190	0	100	–	–	–	1	–
Oven Stuffer White Meat Roasted	3 oz	170	0	0	–	–	–	0	–
Oven Stuffer Wingette Roasted	3 (3.4 oz)	220	0	200	–	–	–	1	–
Ovenables Breast Lemon Pepper Cooked	1 piece (3 oz)	90	–	–	–	1	–	1	–
Seasoned Roasting Chicken Toasted Garlic Dark Meat	3 oz	190	–	–	–	–	20	1	–

FOOD	PORTION	CALS	FIBER	VIT A	FOLIC	VIT C	CALCI	IRON	POTAS
Seasoned Roasting Chicken Toasted Garlic White Meat	3 oz	160	–	–	–	–	0	1	–
Seasoned Strips Parmesan Garlic cooked	3 oz	100	–	–	–	1	20	1	–
Seasoned Strips Savory Classic cooked	3 oz	90	–	–	–	0	–	1	–
Seasoned Strips Spicy Fiesta cooked	3 oz	140	–	300	–	4	–	1	–
Split Breast Cooked	1 piece (6.8 oz)	370	0	200	–	–	20	1	–
Whole Dark Meat cooked	3 oz	150	0	100	–	–	–	1	–
Whole White Meat Cooked	3 oz	170	0	0	–	–	–	1	–
Wings Roasted	2 (3.2 oz)	210	0	100	–	–	–	1	–
FROZEN									
Barber									
Buffalo Fingers	1 (3.3 oz)	160	tr	0	–	0	0	0	–
Nuggets 4 Cheese Stuffed	3 (3 oz)	230	tr	300	–	1	80	1	–
Nuggets Cheddar & Bacon Stuffed	3 (3 oz)	240	tr	300	–	1	60	1	–
Potato Chip Sticks	2 pieces (4.5 oz)	350	tr	0	–	1	20	1	–
Bell & Evans									
Breaded Breast Nuggets	1 serv (4 oz)	190	1	0	–	0	20	1	–
Breaded Whole Breast Tenders	1 (4 oz)	190	1	0	–	0	20	1	–
Burgers	1 (3 oz)	120	0	0	–	0	0	1	–
Chicken Sandwich Steaks	1 serv (2 oz)	60	0	0	–	0	0	0	–
Country Skillet									
Bites	5	270	1	0	–	0	20	1	–
Breast Tenders	3	240	1	0	–	0	20	1	–
Chunks	5	270	1	0	–	0	20	1	–
Fried	3 oz	270	1	0	–	4	80	1	–
Nuggets	10	280	1	0	–	0	20	1	–

FOOD	PORTION	CALS	FIBER	VIT A	FOLIC	VIT C	CALCI	IRON	POTAS
Patties	1	190	1	0	–	0	0	1	–
Southern Fried Chunks	5	270	1	0	–	0	20	1	–
Southern Fried Patties	1	190	1	0	–	1	0	1	–
Ian's									
Fingers	3 pieces	190	0	0	–	1	0	1	–
Nuggets	5 pieces	190	0	0	–	3	0	1	–
Nuggets Allergy Free	5 pieces	190	0	0	–	4	0	1	–
Patties	1 (3.4 oz)	220	0	0	–	1	0	1	–
Weaver									
Breast Strips	3 pieces	230	1	–	–	–	–	–	–
Breast Tenders	5 pieces	240	0	–	–	–	–	–	–
Buffalo Popcorn Chicken	7 pieces	230	1	–	–	–	0	0	–
Crispy Breast Strips	2 pieces	220	2	–	–	–	–	–	–
Crispy Mini Drums	5 pieces	250	1	–	–	–	20	1	–
Croquettes	2 + gravy	230	0	–	–	–	80	–	–
Honey Batter Breast Tenders	5 pieces	220	2	–	–	–	–	–	–
Hot Wings Buffalo Style	3 pieces	190	0	–	–	0	20	1	–
Nuggets	4 pieces	210	1	–	–	–	–	–	–
Patties Italian	1	210	1	0	–	0	60	1	–
Patties Breast	1	170	1	–	–	–	20	1	–
Patties Original	1	180	1	–	–	–	20	1	–
Wings Honey BBQ	3	200	–	100	–	–	20	tr	–
Wellshire									
Chicken Bites Dinosaur Shaped Gluten Free	5 pieces	160	2	–	–	–	–	1	–
READY-TO-EAT									
chicken salad sandwich spread	¼ cup	104	0	72	3	1	5	tr	95
Boar's Head									
Breast Hickory Smoked	2 oz	60	0	0	–	0	0	tr	–
Breast Oven Roasted	2 oz	60	0	0	–	0	0	tr	–
Butterball									
Crispy Baked Breasts Italian Style Herb	1 piece (0.5 oz)	190	1	0	–	1	0	1	–
Crispy Baked Breasts Lemon Pepper	1 piece (0.5 oz)	200	tr	0	–	1	0	1	–

FOOD	PORTION	CALS	FIBER	VIT A	FOLIC	VIT C	CALCI	IRON	POTAS
Crispy Baked Breasts Original	1 piece (0.5 oz)	180	1	0	–	0	0	1	–
Crispy Baked Breasts Parmesan	1 piece (0.5 oz)	200	tr	0	–	1	20	1	–
Crispy Baked Breasts Southwestern	1 piece (0.5 oz)	170	2	100	–	1	0	1	–
Tenders Baked Breast	3 pieces	170	1	0	–	0	0	tr	–
Tenders Hickory Smoked Grilled	4 pieces + sauce	160	1	0	–	2	20	1	–
Tenders Oriental Grilled	4 pieces + sauce	160	1	0	–	1	0	1	–
Hillshire Farm									
Smoked Breast	6 slices (2 oz)	60	0	0	–	0	0	0	–
Perdue									
Breast Cutlets Italian Style	1 (2.9 oz)	120	–	–	–	1	–	1	–
Breast Filets In Barbecue Sauce	1 piece + 3 tbsp sauce (5.9 oz)	200	–	–	–	9	–	2	–
Breast Strips In Garlic & Herb Sauce	1 serv (5 oz)	100	2	–	–	–	–	1	–
Breast Strips In Marinara Sauce	1 serv (5 oz)	120	–	200	–	9	20	1	–
Cutlets Cooked	1 (3.5 oz)	220	–	100	–	–	–	1	–
Nuggets	5 (3.4 oz)	210	–	100	–	–	–	1	–
Nuggets Chicken & Cheese	5 (3.4 oz)	230	–	200	–	–	60	1	–
Short Cuts Chicken Strips Fajita Style	½ cup	90	–	200	–	4	20	1	–
Short Cuts Grilled Italian	½ cup	90	–	100	–	4	10	1	–
Sara Lee									
Breast Oven Roasted	2 slices (1.6 oz)	45	0	0	–	0	0	0	–
Tyson									
Grilled Breast Strips	1 serv (3 oz)	120	0	0	–	0	0	0	–
Roasted Whole Chicken w/ Skin	1 serv (3 oz)	160	0	0	–	0	0	1	–

FOOD	PORTION	CALS	FIBER	VIT A	FOLIC	VIT C	CALCI	IRON	POTAS
TAKE-OUT									
oven roasted breast of chicken	2 oz	60	0	–	–	–	–	tr	–

CHICKEN DISHES
FROZEN
Barber

FOOD	PORTION	CALS	FIBER	VIT A	FOLIC	VIT C	CALCI	IRON	POTAS
Broccoli & Cheese Reduced Fat	1 piece (5.5 oz)	250	tr	300	–	12	150	1	–
Cordon Bleu	1 piece (6 oz)	370	0	300	–	1	150	1	–
Cordon Bleu Reduced Fat	1 piece (5.5 oz)	260	0	200	–	1	100	1	–
Creme Brie & Apple	1 piece (6 oz)	350	tr	300	–	1	150	1	–
Kiev	1 piece (6 oz)	430	tr	300	–	1	40	1	–
Mashed Potato Stuffed	1 piece (6 oz)	340	tr	500	–	6	20	tr	–
Skinless Breast Stuffed	1 piece (6 oz)	280	tr	1000	–	2	20	1	–

Maple Leaf Farms

FOOD	PORTION	CALS	FIBER	VIT A	FOLIC	VIT C	CALCI	IRON	POTAS
Chicken Breast Stuffed Broccoli & Cheese	1 serv (6 oz)	340	0	0	–	0	100	1	–

REFRIGERATED
Lloyd's

FOOD	PORTION	CALS	FIBER	VIT A	FOLIC	VIT C	CALCI	IRON	POTAS
Barbecue Shredded Chicken	¼ cup (2 oz)	90	–	100	–	–	–	1	–

Old El Paso

FOOD	PORTION	CALS	FIBER	VIT A	FOLIC	VIT C	CALCI	IRON	POTAS
For Tacos Shredded Chicken	¼ cup	60	1	200	–	0	20	tr	–

Tyson

FOOD	PORTION	CALS	FIBER	VIT A	FOLIC	VIT C	CALCI	IRON	POTAS
Chicken Breast Medallions In Tomato & Herb Sauce	1 serv (5 oz)	120	0	0	–	0	0	0	–

Wellshire

FOOD	PORTION	CALS	FIBER	VIT A	FOLIC	VIT C	CALCI	IRON	POTAS
Shredded Chicken In BBQ Sauce	¼ cup	70	0	200	–	0	0	tr	–

FOOD	PORTION	CALS	FIBER	VIT A	FOLIC	VIT C	CALCI	IRON	POTAS
SHELF-STABLE									
TastyBite									
Chicken Moglai	1 pkg (9.5 oz)	300	3	200	–	9	100	3	–
TAKE-OUT									
boneless breast w/ apple stuffing	1 serv (5 oz)	260	1	0	–	1	30	1	–
breast & wing breaded & fried	2 pieces (5.7 oz)	494	–	192	9	0	60	1	566
chicken & dumplings	¾ cup	256	tr	233	10	4	61	2	163
chicken & noodles	1 cup	365	–	430	–	tr	26	2	149
chicken a la king	1 cup	470	–	1130	–	12	127	3	404
chicken cacciatore	¾ cup	394	2	1586	18	40	45	4	149
chicken paprikash	1½ cups	296	–	–	–	–	99	–	–
chicken pie w/ top crust	1 slice (5.6 oz)	472	1	800	–	0	122	1	–
chicken cordon bleu	1 serv (5 oz)	280	0	50	–	1	30	1	–
chicken curry ½ breast	1 serv	160	1	405	10	7	22	1	321
chicken curry boneless	1 serv (6.2 oz)	219	2	560	14	9	30	2	441
chicken curry leg & thigh	1 serv	180	1	455	12	7	25	1	361
chicken meatloaf	1 lg slice (5 oz)	243	1	230	29	5	73	2	312
chicken satay + peanut sauce	2 skewers	239	1	–	12	tr	24	–	346
drumstick breaded & fried	2 pieces (5.2 oz)	430	–	222	10	0	36	2	446
grilled breast strips	4 strips (3 oz)	100	0	0	–	0	0	1	–
groundnut stew hkatenkwan	1 serv (15.7 oz)	576	4	1535	51	21	79	3	973
jamaican jerk wings	4 wings (9.9 oz)	709	tr	580	10	4	51	3	402
sancocho de pollo dominican chicken stew	1 serv	702	1	2735	52	49	72	5	1324
thigh breaded & fried	2 pieces (5.2 oz)	430	–	222	10	0	36	2	446

FOOD	PORTION	CALS	FIBER	VIT A	FOLIC	VIT C	CALCI	IRON	POTAS
CHICKEN SUBSTITUTES									
Boca									
Chik'n Nuggets	1 serv (3 oz)	180	3	100	–	0	40	1	–
Chik'n Patties	1 (2.5 oz)	160	2	100	–	0	40	2	–
Lightlife									
Smart Cutlet Seasoned Chicken	1 (4 oz)	180	4	–	–	–	–	–	310
Smart Menu Chick'n Nuggets	4 pieces	220	2	–	–	–	–	–	130
Smart Menu Chick'n Patties	1 patty	160	2	–	–	–	–	–	110
Smart Menu Chick'n Strips	1 serv (3 oz)	80	3	–	–	–	–	–	470
Loma Linda									
Fried Chik'n w/ Gravy	2 pieces (2.8 oz)	150	2	0	–	0	20	2	70
Morningstar Farms									
Chik'n Roasted Herb	1 pattie (2.2 oz)	110	2	0	–	0	20	1	210
Meal Starters Chik'n Strips	12 pieces (3 oz)	140	1	0	–	0	40	5	110
Quorn									
Cutlets	1 (3.5 oz)	200	4	0	–	0	60	1	–
Gruyere Cutlet	1 (4 oz)	260	3	0	–	0	110	0	–
Naked Cutlet	1 (2.4 oz)	80	2	0	–	0	50	tr	–
Nuggets	3–4 pieces (3 oz)	180	3	0	–	0	40	1	–
Patties	1 patty (2.6 oz)	160	3	0	–	0	20	1	–
Tenders	1 cup (3 oz)	90	3	0	–	0	40	tr	–
Viana									
Veggie Chickin Fillets	1 (3.7 oz)	260	4	0	–	0	60	4	–
Veggie Chickin Nuggets	3 pieces (2.6 oz)	200	2	0	–	0	40	1	–
Worthington									
FriChik Original	2 pieces (3.2 oz)	140	1	0	–	0	20	2	90

FOOD	PORTION	CALS	FIBER	VIT A	FOLIC	VIT C	CALCI	IRON	POTAS
Meatless Chicken Style	1 slice (2 oz)	90	1	0	–	0	100	1	240

CHICKPEAS
CANNED
| chickpeas | 1 cup | 285 | – | 58 | 160 | 9 | 78 | 3 | 413 |

Eden
| Organic Garbanzo | ½ cup | 130 | 5 | – | – | – | 60 | 1 | 250 |

DRIED
| cooked | 1 cup | 269 | – | 44 | 282 | 2 | 80 | 5 | 477 |

REFRIGERATED
Sabra
| Balela Vinaigrette | 2 oz | 100 | 3 | 200 | – | 9 | 20 | 0 | – |
| Spicy Armenian Salad | 2 oz | 50 | 1 | 400 | – | 21 | 20 | 1 | – |

CHICORY
endive fresh chopped	½ cup	4	–	513	36	2	13	tr	79
greens raw chopped	½ cup	21	–	3600	–	22	90	1	378
root raw	1 (2.1 oz)	44	–	4	–	3	25	tr	174
roots raw cut up	½ cup (1.6 oz)	33	–	3	–	2	18	tr	131
witloof head raw	1 (1.9 oz)	9	–	15	20	2	10	tr	112
witloof raw	½ cup (1.6 oz)	8	–	13	17	1	9	tr	95

Frieda's
| Belgian Endive | 2 cups | 115 | 3 | 1750 | – | 6 | 40 | 1 | – |

CHILI
| chili w/ beans | 1 cup | 286 | – | 860 | – | 4 | 119 | 9 | 932 |
| powder | 1 tsp | 8 | – | 908 | – | 2 | 7 | tr | 50 |

Amy's
Chili & Cornbread	1 pkg (10.5 oz)	320	8	–	–	–	–	–	–
Organic Black Bean	1 cup	200	15	–	–	–	–	–	–
Organic Medium	1 cup	190	7	–	–	–	–	–	–
Organic Medium w/ Vegetables	1 cup	190	8	–	–	–	–	–	–

Boca
| Chili w/ Ground Burger | 1 pkg (9.4 oz) | 150 | 12 | 2250 | – | 2 | 100 | 4 | – |

FOOD	PORTION	CALS	FIBER	VIT A	FOLIC	VIT C	CALCI	IRON	POTAS
Bush's									
ChiliMagic Chili Starter as prep	1 cup	250	4	500	–	15	80	5	–
Original No Beans	1 cup	240	3	750	–	6	80	3	–
Carroll Shelby's									
Original Texas Chili Kit	2 tbsp	60	0	1500	–	0	40	2	
Del Monte									
Sauce	1 tbsp	20	0	0	–	0	0	0	
Fantastic									
3 Bean	1 pkg (8 oz)	180	5	2000	–	6	100	4	–
Vegetarian Mix not prep	¼ cup	100	4	1000	–	5	60	2	–
Hunt's									
Family Favorites Chili	¼ cup (2.2 oz)	25	1	500	–	4	20	tr	
Instant India									
Chili Ginger Paste	2 tbsp (1 oz)	90	0	0	–	0	0	0	–
Lean Cuisine									
Cafe Classics Three Bean Chili	1 pkg (10 oz)	260	8	1000	–	5	150	3	710
Lightlife									
Smart Chili	1 pkg	200	12	–	–	–	–	–	870
Marie Callender's									
Chili & Cornbread	1 meal (16 oz)	560	7	500	–	0	80	2	–
McCormick									
Mexican Style Chili Powder	¼ tsp	0	0	–	–	–	–	–	–
Nature's Entree									
Texas Chili	1 pkg (12 oz)	320	11	3000	–	2	200	5	–
Pacific Foods									
Beef Steak w/ Beans	1 cup	250	8	1250	–	0	60	5	–
Ro-Tel									
Chili Fixin's	½ cup	35	3	750	–	4	40	1	–
Soy7									
Chili Mix as prep	1 cup	150	7	–	–	–	–	–	–

FOOD	PORTION	CALS	FIBER	VIT A	FOLIC	VIT C	CALCI	IRON	POTAS
Spice Hunter									
Powder Blend Salt Free	¼ tsp	0	0	100	–	–	–	–	–
Stagg									
Chunkero w/ Beans	1 cup	300	5	1000	–	1	40	3	–
Classic w/ Beans	1 cup	330	5	750	–	1	60	3	–
Country Blend	1 cup	330	6	200	–	0	40	3	–
Country Blend w/ Beans	1 cup	33	6	200	–	0	40	3	–
Ranch House Chicken w/ Beans	1 cup	290	6	500	–	2	60	3	–
Silverado Beef w/ Beans	1 cup	230	6	750	–	2	60	3	–
Turkey Ranchero w/ Beans	1 cup	240	6	500	–	4	60	2	–
Vegetable Garden Four Bean	1 cup	200	7	2000	–	1	60	3	–
Wick Fowler's									
2 Alarm Chili Kit	3 tbsp	60	0	5000	–	0	20	2	–
False Alarm Chili Kit	2 tbsp	50	0	4500	–	0	20	1	–
Worthington									
Vegetarian	1 cup	280	8	0	–	0	40	4	330
TAKE-OUT									
chiles rellenos cheese filled	1 (5 oz)	365	1	860	29	111	399	2	376

CHINESE PRESERVING MELON

cooked	½ cup	11	–	0	–	9	16	tr	5

CHIPS

apple chips	10	101	2	5	0	tr	3	tr	100
corn	1 oz	153	1	27	6	0	36	tr	40
corn barbecue	1 oz	148	1	173	–	1	37	tr	67
potato	1 oz	152	–	0	13	9	7	tr	361
potato sour cream & onion	1 oz	150	–	48	18	11	20	tr	377
potato sticks	½ cup (0.6 oz)	94	1	0	7	9	3	tr	223
taro	10 (0.8 oz)	115	–	0	–	1	14	tr	174
tortilla	1 oz	142	2	56	–	0	44	tr	56

FOOD	PORTION	CALS	FIBER	VIT A	FOLIC	VIT C	CALCI	IRON	POTAS
Bachman									
Potato Golden Crisp	1 pkg (1 oz)	150	0	0	–	12	8	1	–
Bravos!									
Tortilla Nacho Cheese	1 oz	150	1	0	–	0	20	tr	–
Cape Cod									
Potato 40% Reduced Fat	19	130	1	0	–	6	0	tr	–
Potato Beachside BBQ	19	150	1	0	–	6	0	tr	–
Potato Classic	19	150	1	0	–	6	0	tr	–
Potato Fresh Garden Herb Reduced Fat	19	130	1	0	–	18	0	tr	–
Potato Jalapeno & Cheddar	19	140	3	0	–	9	20	tr	–
Potato No Salt	19	150	tr	0	–	9	0	tr	–
Potato Robust Russet	19	150	1	0	–	6	0	tr	–
Potato Salt & Vinegar	19	150	1	0	–	6	0	tr	–
Potato Sea Salt & Cracked Pepper	19	140	1	0	–	6	0	tr	380
Tortilla Reduced Carb	10	140	2	0	–	0	40	1	–
Tortilla Veggie	12	140	1	0	–	0	80	tr	–
Corazonas									
Tortilla Jalapeno Jack	1 oz	140	3	100	–	0	20	1	–
Tortilla Original	1 oz	140	3	0	–	0	20	1	–
Tortilla Salsa Picante	1 oz	140	3	200	–	1	20	1	–
Deliciously Slim									
Tortilla Black Bean & Sour Cream	1 oz	140	5	0	–	0	40	1	–
Tortilla Lightly Salted	1 oz	140	5	0	–	1	20	1	–
Tortilla Ranch	1 oz	140	5	0	–	0	40	1	–
Doritos									
Baked Cooler Ranch	15 (1 oz)	120	2	0	–	0	40	1	–
Baked Nacho Cheesier	15	120	2	100	–	0	40	1	–
Cooler Ranch	12	140	1	0	–	0	40	tr	–
Four Cheese	12	140	1	100	–	0	40	0	–
Guacamole	12	150	1	100	–	0	0	tr	–
Light Nacho Cheesier	11	90	1	0	–	0	40	0	–
Natural White Nacho Cheese	11	150	1	0	–	0	20	0	–
Ranchero	12	150	1	300	–	5	0	tr	–
Rollitos Cooler Ranch	17	140	1	100	–	0	20	tr	–

FOOD	PORTION	CALS	FIBER	VIT A	FOLIC	VIT C	CALCI	IRON	POTAS
Rollitos Zesty Taco	17	150	1	0	–	0	20	tr	–
Toasted Corn	13	140	1	0	–	0	40	0	–
Eatsmart									
Cafe Fries Malt Vinegar & Sea Salt	1 oz	150	–	100	–	0	0	0	–
Cafe Fries Tangy Tomato & Spices	1 oz	150	–	200	–	0	0	0	–
CheddAirs	1 oz	135	–	0	–	0	20	0	–
Soy Crisps Parmesan Garlic & Olive Oil	1 oz	160	–	0	–	0	0	1	–
Soy Crisps Tomato Romano & Olive Oil	1 oz	160	–	0	–	0	0	1	–
Veggie Crisps	1 oz	140	–	0	–	0	0	tr	–
Veggie Crisps Cheddar & Jalapeno	1 oz	130	–	100	–	0	0	tr	–
Veggie Crisps Sundried Tomato & Pesto	1 oz	140	–	0	–	0	0	0	–
Eden									
Brown Rice Chips	25	150	0	0	–	0	0	0	35
Sea Vegetable Chips	25	140	0	0	–	0	20	tr	35
Vegetable	25	130	0	0	–	0	0	tr	35
Wasabi	25	130	0	0	–	0	0	tr	35
Flat Earth									
Baked Fruit Crisps Apple Cinnamon Grove	14 (1 oz)	130	2	0	–	6	20	1	105
Baked Fruit Crisps Peach Mango Paradise	14 (1 oz)	130	1	0	–	6	20	1	95
Baked Fruit Crisps Wild Berry Patch	14 (1 oz)	130	1	0	–	6	20	1	100
Baked Veggie Crisps Farmland Cheddar	14 (1 oz)	130	2	1000	–	6	20	tr	170
Baked Veggie Crisps Garlic & Herb Field	14 (1 oz)	130	2	1000	–	6	20	tr	170
Baked Veggie Crisps Tangy Tomato Ranch	14 (1 oz)	130	2	1000	–	6	20	tr	180
French's									
Potato Sticks Barbecue	¾ cup	160	1	0	–	0	40	1	–

FOOD	PORTION	CALS	FIBER	VIT A	FOLIC	VIT C	CALCI	IRON	POTAS
Potato Sticks Cheddar	¾ cup	170	tr	0	–	0	150	tr	–
Potato Sticks Original	¾ cup	190	1	0	–	0	80	tr	–
Garden Of Eatin'									
Organic Pita Baked Brown Sugar & Cinnamon	8	120	1	0	–	0	0	tr	–
Organic Tortilla Blue Corn	7	140	2	0	–	0	20	tr	–
Organic Tortilla Blue No Salt Added	16	140	2	0	–	0	20	tr	–
Organic Tortilla White Corn	7	140	2	0	–	0	40	1	–
GeniSoy									
Soy Crisps	1 oz	110	2	0	–	0	80	2	–
Soy Crisps Apple Cinnamon Crunch	1 oz	120	2	100	–	1	80	2	–
Soy Crisps Creamy Ranch	1 oz	110	2	100	–	1	100	2	–
Soy Crisps Deep Sea Salt	1 oz	110	2	0	–	0	80	2	–
Soy Crisps Rich Cheddar Cheese	1 oz	110	2	100	–	0	80	2	–
Soy Crisps Roasted Garlic & Onion	1 oz	100	2	100	–	1	80	2	–
Soy Crisps Zesty Barbeque	1 oz	110	2	100	–	1	80	2	–
Glenny's									
Organic Soy Barbeque	1 oz	110	3	–	–	–	–	–	–
Organic Soy Creamy Ranch	1 oz	110	3	–	–	–	–	–	–
Soy Crisps Apple Cinnamon	½ pkg (0.6 oz)	70	2	–	–	–	–	–	–
Soy Crisps Caramel	½ pkg (1.3 oz)	70	1	–	–	–	–	–	–
Soy Crisps Low Fat Lightly Salted	½ pkg (0.6 oz)	70	2	–	–	–	–	–	–
Soy Crisps No Salt	½ pkg (0.6 oz)	70	2	–	–	–	–	–	–
Soy Crisps Salt & Pepper	½ pkg (0.6 oz)	70	2	–	–	–	–	–	–

FOOD	PORTION	CALS	FIBER	VIT A	FOLIC	VIT C	CALCI	IRON	POTAS
Soy Crisps White Cheddar	½ pkg (0.6 oz)	70	2	–	–	–	–	–	–
Spud Delites Sea Salt	1 pkg (1.1 oz)	100	1	–	–	–	–	–	–
Veggie Fries	½ pkg (0.6 oz)	70	0	–	–	–	–	–	–
Zen Health Tortilla Crisps Original	1 oz	110	tr	–	–	–	–	–	–
Guiltless Gourmet									
Potato Au Gratin	1 oz	100	3	0	–	2	60	2	–
Potato Pico De Gallo	1 oz	100	3	0	–	2	40	2	–
Potato Sea Salt	1 oz	90	3	0	–	2	40	2	–
Tortilla Chili Lime	18 (1 oz)	110	2	0	–	0	60	tr	–
Tortilla Chili Verde	18 (1 oz)	120	2	100	–	5	60	tr	–
Tortilla Chipotle	18 (1 oz)	120	2	0	–	0	60	tr	–
Tortilla Red Corn	18 (1 oz)	110	2	0	–	0	60	tr	–
Tortilla Spicy Black Bean	18 (1 oz)	110	2	0	–	0	60	tr	–
Tortilla Sweet White Corn	18 (1 oz)	110	2	0	–	0	60	tr	–
Tortilla Yellow Corn Unsalted	18 (1 oz)	110	2	0	–	0	60	tr	–
Herr's									
Potato	1 oz	140	1	0	–	6	0	tr	–
Husman's									
Deli Style Tortilla	11	150	1	0	–	0	20	tr	–
Potato	18 (1 oz)	160	1	0	–	9	0	tr	–
Potato Sour Cream & Onion	18 (1 oz)	150	1	0	–	5	20	tr	–
Potato Sweet N' Sassy	18 (1 oz)	155	1	100	–	9	0	tr	–
Jay's									
Potato	1 oz	150	1	0	–	5	0	tr	–
Kettle									
Bakes Potato Aged White Cheddar	1 oz	120	2	0	–	9	20	1	430
Bakes Potato Hickory Honey Barbeque	1 oz	120	2	100	–	9	0	1	420
Bakes Potato Lightly Salted	1 oz	120	2	0	–	9	0	1	450

FOOD	PORTION	CALS	FIBER	VIT A	FOLIC	VIT C	CALCI	IRON	POTAS
Krinkle Cut Potato Barbeque	1 oz	150	2	100	–	0	150	tr	420
Krinkle Cut Potato Dill & Sour Cream	1 oz	150	2	100	–	9	20	tr	420
Krinkle Cut Potato Lightly Salted	1 oz	150	2	0	–	9	0	tr	430
Krinkle Cut Potato Salt & Fresh Ground Pepper	1 oz	150	2	0	–	9	0	tr	420
Organic Tortilla Blue Corn	1 oz	140	2	0	–	0	40	1	25
Organic Tortilla Brown Rice & Black Bean w/ Garlic & Onions	1 oz	120	2	0	–	0	150	1	20
Organic Tortilla Fire Roasted Chili	1 oz	140	2	100	–	1	60	1	5
Organic Tortilla Five Grain Yellow Corn	1 oz	140	2	0	–	0	40	1	35
Organic Tortilla Lightly Salted Yellow Corn	1 oz	140	2	0	–	0	40	1	25
Organic Tortilla Little Dippers	1 oz	140	2	0	–	0	40	1	25
Organic Tortilla Sesame Blue Moons	1 oz	150	2	0	–	0	30	1	25
Potato Cheddar Beer	1 oz	150	1	0	–	9	0	tr	430
Potato Honey Dijon	1 oz	150	1	0	–	9	0	tr	410
Potato Sea Salt & Vinegar	1 oz	150	1	0	–	9	0	1	410
Potato Spicy Thai	1 oz	150	1	0	–	9	0	tr	430
Potato Unsalted	1 oz	150	2	0	–	9	0	tr	430
Potato Yogurt & Green Onion	1 oz	150	1	0	–	9	20	tr	430
Lundberg									
Rice Chips Original Sea Salt	1 oz	140	tr	0	–	0	0	0	35
Rice Chips Sesame & Seaweed	1 oz	140	tr	0	–	0	0	0	35
Rice Chips Wasabi	1 oz	140	1	0	–	1	20	tr	–

FOOD	PORTION	CALS	FIBER	VIT A	FOLIC	VIT C	CALCI	IRON	POTAS
Madhouse Munchies									
Potato Creamy French Onion	16	150	1	0	–	6	0	tr	–
Potato Sea Salted	16	150	1	0	–	6	0	tr	–
Tortilla White	9	140	1	0	–	0	0	tr	–
Manny's									
Organic Tortilla Blues	1 oz	150	3	0	–	0	0	0	–
Tortilla No Salt Added	1 oz	150	3	0	–	0	0	0	–
Maui									
Shrimp Chips	17	140	tr	0	–	0	0	0	–
Met-Rx									
Pro Chips Bar-B-Que	1 pkg (2 oz)	260	0	–	–	–	–	–	–
Pro Chips Nacho	1 pkg (2 oz)	260	0	–	–	–	–	–	–
Moore's									
Corn Chips	1 oz	160	1	0	–	0	20	tr	–
New York Deli									
Potato Kettle Cooked	1 oz	150	1	0	–	6	0	tr	–
Pita-Snax									
Cheddar Cheese	34 (1 oz)	110	tr	0	–	0	20	tr	–
Chili & Lime	34 (1 oz)	120	tr	200	–	0	0	tr	–
Cinnamon	34 (1 oz)	120	tr	0	–	0	0	tr	–
Dill Ranch	34 (1 oz)	120	tr	0	–	0	20	tr	–
Garlic	34 (1 oz)	120	tr	200	–	0	0	tr	–
Lightly Salted	34 (1 oz)	110	tr	0	–	0	0	tr	–
Popchips									
Corn Hint Of Butter	23 (1 oz)	120	2	0	–	0	0	tr	–
Potato Barbeque	19 (1 oz)	120	1	100	–	1	20	tr	–
Potato Original	22 (1 oz)	120	1	0	–	0	20	tr	–
Rice Sea Salt	19 (1 oz)	120	1	0	–	0	0	tr	–
Rice Wasabi	20 (1 oz)	120	1	100	–	1	0	tr	–
Revival									
Baked Soy Pasta Chips Lightly Salted Sunshine	1 bag (0.9 oz)	100	0	–	–	–	14	1	<2
Baked Soy Pasta Chips Naturally Nice	1 bag (0.9 oz)	80	0	–	–	–	13	1	<2
Baked Soy Pasta Chips Rev It Up Ranch	1 bag (0.9 oz)	105	0	–	–	–	17	1	7

FOOD	PORTION	CALS	FIBER	VIT A	FOLIC	VIT C	CALCI	IRON	POTAS
Skinny									
BBQ	1½ cups	90	1	100	–	0	0	0	–
Corn	1½ cups	90	1	200	–	0	0	0	–
Nacho Cheese	1½ cups	90	1	200	–	0	0	0	–
Sour Cream & Onion	1½ cups	90	1	200	–	0	0	0	–
Sticks Garden Veggie	1 oz	140	1	0	–	4	60	1	–
Sticks Island Lime Chili	1 oz	140	1	0	–	4	60	1	–
Sticks Maui Wowie	1 oz	140	1	0	–	4	60	1	–
Sticks Original Spud	1 oz	140	1	0	–	4	60	1	–
Snyder's Of Hanover									
Kosher Dill	1 oz	140	4	0	–	9	0	tr	–
MultiGrain Sunflower	1 oz	140	2	0	–	0	0	0	–
MultiGrain Sunflower Southwestern Cheddar	1 oz	140	2	0	–	9	0	0	–
MultiGrain Tortilla Lightly Salted	1 oz	130	3	0	–	0	0	tr	–
MultiGrain Tortilla Strips Flaxseed Gold	1 oz	140	2	0	–	9	40	1	–
Organic Veggie Crisps	1 oz	140	2	0	–	0	0	tr	–
Potato Original	1 oz	150	3	0	–	9	0	tr	–
Sweet Potato Baked	1 oz	110	1	500	–	0	40	1	–
Tortilla White Corn	1 oz	140	2	0	–	0	0	1	–
Tortilla Pounder MultiGrain	1 oz	130	2	0	–	9	0	tr	–
Solea									
Polenta Corn	1 oz	120	0	0	–	0	40	tr	–
Potato Olive Oil Sea Salt	1 oz	120	1	0	–	12	20	tr	–
Stacy's									
Pita Chips Multigrain	1 pkg	140	2	0	–	0	0	1	–
Pita Chips Parmesan Garlic & Herb	1 oz	140	2	0	–	0	0	1	–
Pita Chips Texarkana Hot	1 oz	130	2	500	–	0	0	1	–
Soy Thin Chips Sticky Bun	18 (1 oz)	130	3	0	–	0	20	1	–
Soy Thin Crisps Simply Cheese	18 (1 oz)	130	3	0	–	0	40	1	–
Sunchips									
French Onion	10	140	2	0	–	0	0	0	–
Harvest Cheddar	10	140	2	0	–	0	0	0	–

FOOD	PORTION	CALS	FIBER	VIT A	FOLIC	VIT C	CALCI	IRON	POTAS
Tastee									
Potato Yukon Gold	1 oz	130	1	0	–	0	0	1	–
Terra									
Parsnip Chips	12	150	5	0	–	5	60	tr	–
Potato Unsalted Au Natural	18	150	2	0	–	4	0	tr	–
Potato Unsalted Hickory BBQ	16	150	1	0	–	5	20	1	–
Potato Unsalted Lemon Pepper	16	150	1	0	–	2	0	1	–
Spiced Sweet Potato	1 pkg (0.5 oz)	190	3	3000	–	3	40	1	–
Torengos									
Chips	13 (1 oz)	140	1	0	–	0	20	1	–
Utz									
No Salt Added	20 (1 oz)	150	1	0	–	9	0	tr	370

CHITTERLINGS

FOOD	PORTION	CALS	FIBER	VIT A	FOLIC	VIT C	CALCI	IRON	POTAS
pork cooked	3 oz	258	0	0	3	0	23	3	–

CHIVES

FOOD	PORTION	CALS	FIBER	VIT A	FOLIC	VIT C	CALCI	IRON	POTAS
freeze-dried	1 tbsp	1	–	137	–	1	2	tr	6
fresh chopped	1 tbsp	1	–	131	3	2	3	tr	9
fresh chopped	1 tsp	0	–	44	1	1	1	tr	3

CHOCOLATE
BAKING

FOOD	PORTION	CALS	FIBER	VIT A	FOLIC	VIT C	CALCI	IRON	POTAS
baking	1 oz	145	–	10	–	0	22	2	235
grated unsweetened	¼ cup	165	6	0	9	0	99	6	274
liquid unsweetened	1 oz	134	5	3	5	0	15	1	331
mexican	1 sq (0.7 oz)	85	1	0	1	0	7	tr	79
squares unsweetened	1 square (1 oz)	145	5	0	8	0	59	5	241

Love'n Bake

FOOD	PORTION	CALS	FIBER	VIT A	FOLIC	VIT C	CALCI	IRON	POTAS
Chocolate Schmear	2 tbsp	140	2	0	–	0	40	1	–

CHIPS

FOOD	PORTION	CALS	FIBER	VIT A	FOLIC	VIT C	CALCI	IRON	POTAS
milk chocolate	1 cup (6 oz)	862	–	312	14	1	321	2	646
semisweet	60 pieces (1 oz)	136	–	6	1	0	9	1	104

FOOD	PORTION	CALS	FIBER	VIT A	FOLIC	VIT C	CALCI	IRON	POTAS
semisweet	1 cup (6 oz)	804	–	35	4	0	54	5	614
Baker's									
Chocolate Chunks	13 pieces (0.5 oz)	70	tr	0	–	0	0	1	–
Cloud Nine									
Double Dark Chocolate	13 pieces (0.5 oz)	80	0	0	–	0	0	tr	–
Ghirardelli									
Semi-Sweet	33 pieces (0.5 oz)	70	tr	0	–	0	0	1	–
Sunspire									
Chocolate Sundrops	47 pieces (1.4 oz)	190	1	100	–	0	80	tr	–
Dark Chocolate Grain Sweetened	13 pieces (0.5 oz)	70	1	0	–	0	0	tr	–
Organic	13 pieces (0.5 oz)	70	0	0	–	0	20	tr	–
Tropical Source									
Espresso Roast Dairy Free	13 pieces (1.5 oz)	70	1	0	–	0	0	tr	–
Semi-Sweet Dairy Free	13 pieces (1.5 oz)	80	0	0	–	0	0	tr	–
MIX									
powder	2–3 heaping tsp	75	–	4	–	tr	8	1	128
powder as prep w/ whole milk	9 oz	226	–	312	12	3	300	1	498

CHOCOLATE SPREAD
Twist

FOOD	PORTION	CALS	FIBER	VIT A	FOLIC	VIT C	CALCI	IRON	POTAS
Sugar Free Chocolate Spread	2 tbsp	170	0	–	–	–	–	–	–

CHOCOLATE SYRUP

FOOD	PORTION	CALS	FIBER	VIT A	FOLIC	VIT C	CALCI	IRON	POTAS
chocolate fudge	1 cup (11.9 oz)	1176	–	306	–	–	340	4	731
chocolate fudge	1 tbsp (0.7 oz)	73	–	19	–	–	21	tr	45
syrup	1 cup	653	–	89	12	1	42	6	672
syrup	2 tbsp	82	–	11	2	tr	5	1	84

FOOD	PORTION	CALS	FIBER	VIT A	FOLIC	VIT C	CALCI	IRON	POTAS
syrup as prep w/ whole milk	9 oz	232	–	319	14	2	297	1	455
Colac									
Chocolate Topping	1 tbsp	37	0	–	–	–	–	–	–
DaVinci Gourmet									
Sugar Free	2 tbsp	15	1	–	–	–	–	–	–
Walden Farms									
Sugar Free	2 tbsp	0	0	–	–	–	–	–	–

CHUTNEY

FOOD	PORTION	CALS	FIBER	VIT A	FOLIC	VIT C	CALCI	IRON	POTAS
apple	1.2 oz	68	1	5	–	1	9	tr	
coconut	¼ cup	74	2	–	–	–	–	–	–
mango	1 tbsp	54	tr	207	–	0	4	tr	11
tomato	1 tbsp	32	tr	–	2	1	5	tr	62
Patak's									
Major Grey	1 tbsp	60	0	0	–	0	0	0	–
Mango Hot	1 tbsp	60	0	0	–	0	0	0	–
Mango Sweet	1 tbsp	60	0	0	–	0	0	0	–
Wild Thyme Farms									
Apricot Cranberry Walnut	1 tbsp	15	–	300	–	5	–	–	–
Pineapple Peach Lime	1 tbsp	14	–	100	–	5	–	tr	–

CILANTRO
Dorot

FOOD	PORTION	CALS	FIBER	VIT A	FOLIC	VIT C	CALCI	IRON	POTAS
Chopped Cube frzn	1 cube (4 g)	5	tr	–	–	–	–	–	–

CINNAMON

FOOD	PORTION	CALS	FIBER	VIT A	FOLIC	VIT C	CALCI	IRON	POTAS
cinnamon sugar	1 tsp	16	tr	0	0	tr	3	tr	1
ground	1 tsp	6	–	6	–	1	28	1	11
sticks	0.5 oz	39	3	20	–	4	175	5	–

CISCO

FOOD	PORTION	CALS	FIBER	VIT A	FOLIC	VIT C	CALCI	IRON	POTAS
smoked	1 oz	50	0	264	1	–	7	tr	82

CLAMS
CANNED

FOOD	PORTION	CALS	FIBER	VIT A	FOLIC	VIT C	CALCI	IRON	POTAS
meat only	3 oz	126	–	484	–	–	78	24	534
meat only	1 cup	236	–	912	158	–	148	45	1005
Brunswick									
Baby	2 oz	50	0	100	–	4	40	13	–

FOOD	PORTION	CALS	FIBER	VIT A	FOLIC	VIT C	CALCI	IRON	POTAS
Bumble Bee									
Baby	¼ cup	50	0	0	–	0	60	16	–
Chopped Or Minced	¼ cup	25	0	0	–	0	0	tr	–
Smoked	¼ cup	130	0	100	–	0	60	11	–
Chicken Of The Sea									
Chopped	¼ cup	30	0	0	–	0	0	tr	–
Whole Baby	¼ cup	30	0	0	–	0	0	1	–
Orleans									
Clam Juice	1 tbsp	0	0	0	–	0	0	1	–
FRESH									
cooked	20 sm	133	–	513	–	–	83	25	565
cooked	3 oz	126	–	–	–	–	78	24	534
raw	3 oz	63	–	255	–	–	39	12	267
raw	20 sm (6.3 oz)	133	–	540	–	–	83	25	565
raw	9 lg (6.3 oz)	133	–	540	–	–	83	25	565
TAKE-OUT									
breaded & fried	20 sm	379	–	568	–	–	119	26	612

CLEMENTINES
FOOD	PORTION	CALS	FIBER	VIT A	FOLIC	VIT C	CALCI	IRON	POTAS
Haddon House									
In Light Syrup	½ cup	80	1	1250	–	4	20	tr	–
Sunkist									
Fresh	2	80	4	100	60	174	40	tr	400
Tina									
Fresh	1	50	3	0	–	30	40	0	–

CLOVES
FOOD	PORTION	CALS	FIBER	VIT A	FOLIC	VIT C	CALCI	IRON	POTAS
ground	1 tsp	7	–	11	–	2	14	tr	23

COCOA
FOOD	PORTION	CALS	FIBER	VIT A	FOLIC	VIT C	CALCI	IRON	POTAS
powder unsweetened	1 cup (3 oz)	197	29	17	27	0	110	12	1310
powder unsweetened	1 tbsp (5 g)	11	2	1	2	0	6	1	76
Ah!Laska									
Organic	2 tbsp	100	5	0	–	0	80	tr	–
Organic Bakers Cocoa	1 tbsp	20	1	–	–	–	–	1	–

COCONUT
FOOD	PORTION	CALS	FIBER	VIT A	FOLIC	VIT C	CALCI	IRON	POTAS
dried sweetened flaked	1 cup	351	–	0	–	0	10	1	234

FOOD	PORTION	CALS	FIBER	VIT A	FOLIC	VIT C	CALCI	IRON	POTAS
dried sweetened flaked canned	1 cup	341	–	0	–	–	11	1	249
dried sweetened shredded	1 cup	466	–	0	–	1	14	2	313
dried toasted	1 oz	168	–	–	–	–	8	1	157
dried unsweetened	1 oz	187	–	0	3	tr	7	1	154
fresh	1 piece (1.5 oz)	159	4	0	12	2	6	1	160
fresh shredded	1 cup	283	7	0	21	3	12	2	285
Frieda's									
White	¼ cup (1.4 oz)	140	4	0	–	1	0	1	–

COCONUT JUICE

FOOD	PORTION	CALS	FIBER	VIT A	FOLIC	VIT C	CALCI	IRON	POTAS
coconut water fresh	1 cup	552	5	0	38	7	38	4	631
milk canned	1 cup	445	–	0	32	2	41	7	497
milk frozen	1 cup	485	–	0	34	3	10	2	557
A Taste Of Thai									
Coconut Milk	⅓ cup	140	0	0	–	–	0	–	–
Lite Coconut Milk	⅓ cup	45	0	0	–	–	0	–	–
Amy & Brian									
Juice	8 oz	76	–	–	–	–	20	1	–
Goya									
Coconut Water	1 can (11.8 oz)	120	tr	0	–	0	80	1	–
O.N.E.									
Natural Coconut Water	1 box (11 oz)	60	0	–	–	–	40	–	670
Thai Kitchen									
Milk	2 oz	124	0	–	–	–	–	–	–
Vita Coco									
Coconut Water	1 box (11 oz)	65	–	–	–	–	50	–	630
Coconut Water w/ Fruit Juice All Flavors	1 box (11 oz)	110	5	200	–	2	40	1	160
Zico									
Coconut Water Mango	11 oz	60	0	–	–	–	40	–	670
Coconut Water Natural	11 oz	60	0	–	–	–	40	–	670
Coconut Water Passion Fruit + Orange Peel	11 oz	60	0	–	–	–	40	–	670

FOOD	PORTION	CALS	FIBER	VIT A	FOLIC	VIT C	CALCI	IRON	POTAS
COD									
atlantic canned	1 can (11 oz)	327	0	144	–	1	66	2	1647
atlantic canned	3 oz	89	0	39	–	1	18	tr	449
atlantic dried	3 oz	246	0	120	–	3	136	2	1239
atlantic fresh cooked	1 fillet (6.3 oz)	189	0	83	–	2	25	1	440
atlantic fresh cooked	3 oz	89	0	39	–	1	12	tr	208
atlantic fresh raw	3 oz	70	0	34	–	1	13	tr	351
pacific fresh baked	3 oz	95	0	29	–	–	8	tr	465
roe canned	1 oz	34	–	–	–	–	4	tr	–
roe tarama	3.5 oz	547	–	–	–	–	29	2	111
TAKE-OUT									
roe baked w/ butter & lemon juice	1 oz	36	–	–	–	–	43	tr	38
COFFEE									
INSTANT									
decaffeinated as prep	8 oz	2	0	0	0	0	5	tr	128
decaffeinated powder	1 rounded tsp	4	0	0	0	0	3	tr	63
powder	1 rounded tsp	4	0	0	0	0	3	tr	319
REGULAR									
brewed	8 oz	2	0	0	5	0	5	tr	116
roasted beans	1 oz	64	2	–	–	–	42	1	–
Flavia									
English Breakfast	1 bag	0	0	0	–	0	0	0	–
Espresso Roast	1 bag	0	0	0	–	0	0	0	–
French Roast	1 bag	0	0	0	–	0	0	0	–
French Vanilla	1 bag	0	0	0	–	0	0	0	–
Revival									
Soy Caramal Corn	1 cup (8 oz)	0	0	–	–	–	–	–	–
Soy Hazelnut	1 cup (8 oz)	0	0	–	–	–	–	–	–
Soy Original Roast	1 cup (8 oz)	0	0	–	–	–	–	–	–
Soy Java									
All Flavors	1 tbsp	20	0	–	–	–	–	–	–

FOOD	PORTION	CALS	FIBER	VIT A	FOLIC	VIT C	CALCI	IRON	POTAS
COFFEE BEVERAGES									
AchievONE									
All Flavors	1 bottle (9.5 oz)	120	–	1250	180	15	250	5	–
America's Best Brew									
Iced Coffee All Flavors	8 oz	110	–	–	–	–	80	–	–
Big Train									
Low Carb Blended Ice Mocha as prep	1 serv (16 oz)	90	1	0	–	1	150	tr	340
Cafe Sepia									
House Blend	1 bottle (6.2 oz)	80	0	0	–	0	60	0	–
Mocha	1 bottle (6.2 oz)	70	0	0	–	–	40	0	–
Cinnabon									
Latte Caramel Nut	1 can (8 oz)	170	1	200	–	1	80	0	–
Latte Cinnamon Vanilla	1 can (8 oz)	170	1	200	–	1	80	0	–
Lattes All Flavors	1 can (9.5 oz)	190	1	200	–	2	200	0	–
Cool Java									
Cappuccino Dark Roast	1 bottle (11 oz)	190	0	100	–	0	150	tr	–
Cappuccino French Vanilla	1 bottle (11 oz)	190	0	100	–	0	150	1	–
Cappuccino Mocha	1 bottle (11 oz)	190	0	100	–	0	150	1	–
Flavour Creations									
Coffee Flavoring Tablets All Flavors	1 tablet	0	0	–	–	–	–	–	–
Frappio									
Iced Coffee Energy Drink	1 can (15 oz)	260	0	200	–	0	200	0	–
Froid									
Original or French Vanilla	1 bottle (11 oz)	180	1	100	–	0	200	tr	–
Godiva									
Latte French Vanilla	1 bottle (12 oz)	200	0	0	–	0	200	0	–

FOOD	PORTION	CALS	FIBER	VIT A	FOLIC	VIT C	CALCI	IRON	POTAS
Mocha Dark Chocolate	1 bottle (16 oz)	200	1	0	–	0	200	1	–
Iced 'Spresso									
Ultra Light American Vanilla	1 bottle (9.5 oz)	90	0	100	–	0	200	tr	–
Ultra Light Expresso Latte	1 bottle (9.5 oz)	70	0	0	–	0	250	tr	–
Jakada									
Latte Mocha	1 bottle (10.5 oz)	180	0	100	–	0	150	0	–
Latte Vanilla	1 bottle (10.5 oz)	180	0	100	–	0	150	0	–
Loco-Joe									
Iced Coffee	1 box (8.25 oz)	160	0	250	–	0	200	0	–
Low Carb Creations									
Cappuccino	1 cup	30	0	0	–	0	0	tr	–
Shock									
Latte	8 oz	150	tr	–	–	–	–	–	–
Triple Latte	1 can (8 oz)	125	0	0	–	0	30	0	–
Triple Mocha	1 can (8 oz)	125	0	0	–	0	30	0	–
Silk									
Coffee Soylatte	1 bottle (11 oz)	220	0	400	24	0	400	1	100
Sipper Sweets									
Sugar Free Low Carb Cappuccino	1 serv	50	0	–	–	–	–	–	–
Starbucks									
DoubleShot	1 (6.5 oz)	140	–	–	–	–	150	–	–
Frappuccino	1 bottle (9.5 oz)	190	0	100	–	0	220	0	–
Frappuccino Mocha	1 bottle (9.5 oz)	190	0	100	–	0	220	0	–
Frappuccino Vanilla	1 bottle (9.5 oz)	190	0	100	–	0	220	0	–
Stomping Grounds									
Latte Caramel not prep	⅓ cup	70	0	0	–	0	0	0	–
Latte Espresso not prep	⅓ cup	35	0	0	–	0	0	0	–

FOOD	PORTION	CALS	FIBER	VIT A	FOLIC	VIT C	CALCI	IRON	POTAS
Latte Mocha not prep	⅓ cup	60	0	–	–	0	0	tr	–
Latte Vanilla not prep	⅓ cup	60	0	–	–	0	0	0	–
Tully's Coffee									
Bellaccino All Flavors	1 bottle (9.5 oz)	210	0	–	–	–	250	–	–
Wolfgang Puck									
Gourmet Heated Lattes All Flavors	1 can (10 oz)	100	0	200	–	0	200	–	–
TAKE-OUT									
cafe amaretto w/ alcohol	1 serv	192	0	337	1	tr	25	tr	197
cafe au lait	1 cup (8 oz)	77	–	230	6	1	148	tr	249
cafe brulot	1 cup	48	–	0	tr	0	2	tr	64
cafe brulot w/ alcohol	1 serv	130	3	82	12	24	55	1	162
cappuccino	1 cup (8 oz)	77	–	230	6	1	148	tr	249
coffee con leche	1 cup (6 oz)	104	0	125	6	0	103	tr	171
espresso	1 cup (4 oz)	2	0	0	1	tr	2	tr	138
irish coffee	1 serv (8 oz)	209	0	580	4	tr	19	tr	89
latte w/ skim milk	1 serv (13 oz)	88	0	750	13	2	304	tr	470
latte w/ whole milk	1 serv (14 oz)	143	0	610	12	tr	310	tr	555
mocha	1 serv (17 oz)	403	2	730	15	1	335	2	739
turkish	1 cup (4 oz)	50	0	0	2	0	1	tr	53

COFFEE SUBSTITUTES
Pixie

FOOD	PORTION	CALS	FIBER	VIT A	FOLIC	VIT C	CALCI	IRON	POTAS
Mate Latte Chai	½ cup (4 oz)	80	tr	0	–	0	20	tr	–
Mate Latte Dark Roast	½ cup (4 oz)	70	tr	0	–	0	20	tr	–
Mate Latte Mocha	½ cup (4 oz)	70	0	0	–	0	0	0	–

FOOD	PORTION	CALS	FIBER	VIT A	FOLIC	VIT C	CALCI	IRON	POTAS
Mate Latte Original	½ cup (4 oz)	70	0	0	–	0	0	1	–
Teeccino									
Herbal Coffee All Flavors	1 cup	15	1	0	–	0	0	0	65

COFFEE WHITENERS
Farmland

FOOD	PORTION	CALS	FIBER	VIT A	FOLIC	VIT C	CALCI	IRON	POTAS
Nondairy Creamer	2 tbsp	40	0	100	–	0	40	0	–

Hood

FOOD	PORTION	CALS	FIBER	VIT A	FOLIC	VIT C	CALCI	IRON	POTAS
Country Creamer Non Dairy	1 tbsp	20	0	0	–	0	0	0	–

International Delight

FOOD	PORTION	CALS	FIBER	VIT A	FOLIC	VIT C	CALCI	IRON	POTAS
Amaretto	1 tbsp	40	0	0	–	0	0	0	–
Fat Free Amaretto	1 tbsp	30	0	0	–	0	0	0	–
Fat Free French Vanilla	1 tbsp	30	0	0	–	0	0	0	–
Fat Free Irish Creme	1 tbsp	30	0	0	–	0	0	0	–
French Vanilla	1 tbsp	45	0	0	–	0	0	0	–
Sugar Free French Vanilla	1 tbsp	20	0	0	–	0	0	0	–

Silk

FOOD	PORTION	CALS	FIBER	VIT A	FOLIC	VIT C	CALCI	IRON	POTAS
Creamer	1 tbsp	15	0	0	–	0	0	0	–
Creamer French Vanilla	1 tbsp	20	0	0	–	0	0	0	–
Creamer Hazelnut	1 tbsp	15	0	0	–	0	0	0	–

COLESLAW
Dole

FOOD	PORTION	CALS	FIBER	VIT A	FOLIC	VIT C	CALCI	IRON	POTAS
Classic Cole Slaw	1½ cups (3 oz)	25	2	1500	–	36	40	0	–

Fresh Express

FOOD	PORTION	CALS	FIBER	VIT A	FOLIC	VIT C	CALCI	IRON	POTAS
3 Color Deli	1½ cups	20	2	750	–	27	40	tr	–
Cole Slaw Kit as prep	2 cups	120	2	1250	–	24	40	tr	–

River Ranch

FOOD	PORTION	CALS	FIBER	VIT A	FOLIC	VIT C	CALCI	IRON	POTAS
Country Homestyle Kit	1 cup	140	2	2000	32	24	40	tr	–
Honey Dijon Peppercorn Kit	1 cup	120	2	2000	32	24	40	1	–
Mix	1¼ cups	25	2	2250	32	27	40	tr	–

TAKE-OUT

FOOD	PORTION	CALS	FIBER	VIT A	FOLIC	VIT C	CALCI	IRON	POTAS
coleslaw w/ dressing	¾ cup	147	–	338	39	8	34	1	177
vinegar & oil coleslaw	3.5 oz	150	–	500	–	30	20	–	–

FOOD	PORTION	CALS	FIBER	VIT A	FOLIC	VIT C	CALCI	IRON	POTAS
COLLARDS									
fresh cooked	½ cup	17	–	1745	4	8	15	tr	84
frzn chopped cooked	½ cup	31	–	5084	65	23	179	1	214
raw chopped	½ cup	6	–	599	2	4	5	tr	30
Allens									
Seasoned Southern Style	½ cup	35	1	2500	–	6	150	1	–
Glory									
Green Fresh	2 cups	25	3	3000	–	27	100	0	–
Seasoned canned	½ cup	35	2	5000	–	12	80	1	–
Sensibly Seasoned canned	½ cup	20	2	5500	–	12	100	1	–
COOKIES									
MIX									
chocolate chip	1 (0.56 oz)	79	–	–	–	0	7	tr	34
oatmeal	1 (0.6 oz)	74	tr	–	–	–	5	tr	30
oatmeal raisin	1 (0.6 oz)	74	tr	–	–	–	5	tr	30
Aunt Paula's									
Low Carb Chef Chocolate Chip as prep	1	66	1	–	–	–	–	–	–
Low Carb Chef Peanut Butter as prep	1	66	1	–	–	–	–	–	–
Big Train									
Low Carb Chocolate Chip as prep	2	140	4	300	–	0	20	tr	–
Low Carb Peanut Butter as prep	2	140	4	308	–	0	20	tr	–
Bob's Red Mill									
Gluten Free Chocolate Chip as prep	2	260	2	200	–	0	20	2	–
Keto									
Chocolate Chip as prep	1	47	1	–	–	–	–	–	–
Oatmeal Raisin as prep	2	59	1	–	–	–	–	–	–
King Arthur									
Chocolate Chip Whole Grain not prep	2 tbsp	90	1	0	–	0	20	1	–
MiniCarb									
All Flavors as prep	1	110	5	–	–	–	–	–	–

FOOD	PORTION	CALS	FIBER	VIT A	FOLIC	VIT C	CALCI	IRON	POTAS
Nature's Path									
Organic Chocolate Chip	¹⁄₁₀ pkg	150	3	0	–	0	20	3	–
Pillsbury									
Ready To Bake Chocolate Chip Sugar Free	1	90	3	–	–	–	–	–	–
READY-TO-EAT									
animal	11 (1 oz)	126	–	–	4	0	12	1	28
animal crackers	1 box (2.4 oz)	299	–	27	22	tr	11	1	57
animal crackers	1 (2.5 g)	11	–	–	0	0	1	tr	2
butter	1 (5 g)	23	tr	0	0	0	1	tr	6
chocolate chip	1 (0.4 oz)	48	tr	–	1	0	2	tr	14
chocolate w/ creme filling	1 (0.35 oz)	47	tr	0	0	0	3	tr	18
cream cheese	1 (1.1 oz)	141	tr	447	4	0	12	1	24
digestive biscuits plain	2	141	1	0	–	0	28	1	–
fig bars	1 (0.56 oz)	56	1	–	2	–	10	tr	33
fortune	1 (0.28 oz)	30	tr	–	1	0	1	tr	3
gingersnaps	1 (0.24 oz)	29	–	–	–	0	5	tr	24
graham	1 square (0.24 oz)	30	–	0	1	0	2	tr	9
graham chocolate covered	1 (0.49 oz)	68	–	–	–	0	8	1	29
graham honey	1 (0.24 oz)	30	tr	0	1	0	2	tr	9
hermits	1 (1 oz)	117	1	178	5	tr	16	1	76
jumbles coconut	1 (1 oz)	121	1	264	4	tr	5	tr	31
ladyfingers	1 (0.38 oz)	40	–	61	4	tr	5	tr	12
macaroons	1 (0.8 oz)	97	–	0	1	0	12	tr	38
madeleines	1 (0.8 oz)	86	tr	258	5	tr	7	tr	17
peanut butter soft-type	1 (0.5 oz)	69	tr	0	1	0	2	tr	16
pinenut cookies	1 (1.1 oz)	134	1	0	7	tr	29	1	130
reginette queen's biscuit	1 (0.8 oz)	86	tr	129	8	tr	27	1	32
spritz	1 (0.4 oz)	42	tr	66	2	tr	4	tr	11
toll house original	1 (0.8 oz)	105	tr	162	4	tr	15	1	57
vanilla sandwich	1 (0.35 oz)	48	tr	0	0	0	3	tr	9
zeppole	1 (0.8 oz)	78	tr	8	3	0	3	tr	9

FOOD	PORTION	CALS	FIBER	VIT A	FOLIC	VIT C	CALCI	IRON	POTAS
Alex & Dani's									
Original Hazelnut	3 (1 oz)	130	1	100	24	0	0	1	–
Annie's Homegrown									
Bunny Grahams All Flavors	26	130	tr	0	–	0	20	tr	–
Archway									
Fruit Filled Apricot	1 (0.8 oz)	90	0	0	–	0	0	tr	–
Fruit Filled Raspberry	1 (0.8 oz)	90	0	0	–	0	0	tr	–
Oatmeal Raisin	1	120	tr	0	–	0	20	1	–
Windmill	1	90	0	0	–	0	0	1	–
Arico									
Gluten Free Casein Free	1 bar	150	3	0	–	0	250	1	–
Gluten Free Casein Free Almond Cranberry	1 bar	150	3	0	–	0	250	1	–
Gluten Free Casein Free Double Chocolate	1 bar	150	3	0	–	0	250	1	–
Arnott's									
Raspberry Tartlets	2	100	tr	0	–	0	40	tr	–
Back To Nature									
Chocolate Chunk	2	130	tr	0	–	0	0	1	–
Crispy Oatmeal	2	120	tr	0	–	0	0	1	–
Sandwich Chocolate & Mint Creme	2	130	tr	0	–	0	0	1	–
Sandwich Classic Creme	2	130	tr	0	–	0	0	1	–
Bahlsen									
Butter Leaves	7 (1 oz)	140	tr	0	–	0	0	tr	–
Delice	6 (1 oz)	140	tr	0	–	0	0	0	–
Hanover Waffelin	5 (1 oz)	160	0	0	–	0	0	0	–
Nuss Dessert	3 (1.1 oz)	170	0	0	–	0	20	tr	–
Baker's Breakfast Cookie									
Apple Pie	1 (3 oz)	204	6	0	–	0	60	2	–
Banana Walnut	1 (3 oz)	274	5	0	–	0	0	2	–
Chocolate Chunk Raisin	1 (3 oz)	260	5	0	–	0	0	2	–
Double Chocolate Chunk	1 (3 oz)	250	5	0	–	0	40	3	–
Fruit & Nut	1 (3 oz)	270	5	0	–	0	40	2	–
Lemon Poppy Seed	1 (3 oz)	230	5	0	–	0	80	2	–
Mocha Chocolate Chunk	1 (3 oz)	250	5	0	–	0	40	4	–

FOOD	PORTION	CALS	FIBER	VIT A	FOLIC	VIT C	CALCI	IRON	POTAS
Oatmeal Raisin	1 (3 oz)	250	5	0	–	0	40	2	–
Peanut Butter	1 (3 oz)	290	6	0	–	0	0	2	–
Peanut Butter & Jelly	1 (3 oz)	320	6	0	–	5	40	1	–
Pumpkin Spice	1 (3 oz)	230	5	3100	–	2	180	3	–
Vegan Chocolate Chunk	1 (3 oz)	260	5	0	–	0	0	2	–
Vegan Peanut Butter Chocolate Chunk	1 (3 oz)	310	6	0	–	0	0	2	–
Carbolite									
Chocolate Chip	1 (1 oz)	120	4	–	–	–	–	–	–
Peanut Butter	1 (1 oz)	120	4	–	–	–	–	–	–
Shortbread	1 (1 oz)	180	5	–	–	–	–	–	–
Cookie Lover's									
Chocolate Chip	1 (0.8 oz)	90	0	100	–	0	20	1	–
Creme Supremes	2 (0.9 oz)	120	1	0	–	0	20	tr	–
Creme Supremes Mint	2 (0.9 oz)	120	1	0	–	0	20	tr	–
Grahams	2 (1 oz)	100	1	0	–	0	0	0	–
Grahams Cinnamon	2 (1 oz)	110	1	0	–	0	0	0	–
Peanut Butter	1 (0.8 oz)	100	0	100	–	0	20	1	–
Shortbread	1 (0.8 oz)	120	0	200	–	0	20	1	–
Country Choice Naturals									
Chocolate Chip Walnut	1	100	tr	0	–	0	0	tr	–
Double Fudge Brownie	1 (0.8 oz)	90	tr	0	–	0	0	tr	–
Ginger	1	90	tr	0	–	0	0	tr	–
Ginger Snaps	5	120	2	0	–	0	0	1	–
Lemon	1	90	tr	0	–	0	0	tr	–
Oatmeal Chocolate Chip	1 (0.8 oz)	100	1	0	–	0	0	tr	–
Oatmeal Raisin	1 (0.8 oz)	100	1	0	–	0	0	tr	–
Old Fashioned Oatmeal	1 (0.8 oz)	100	1	0	–	0	0	tr	–
Peanut Butter	1	100	tr	0	–	0	0	tr	–
Sandwich Cremes Chocolate	1	130	0	0	–	0	0	1	–
Sandwich Cremes Duplex	2	130	0	0	–	0	0	1	–
Sandwich Cremes Ginger Lemon	2	130	0	0	–	0	0	1	–

FOOD	PORTION	CALS	FIBER	VIT A	FOLIC	VIT C	CALCI	IRON	POTAS
Sandwich Cremes Mint Creme	2	130	0	0	–	0	0	1	–
Sandwich Cremes Vanilla	2	130	0	0	–	0	0	1	–
Vanilla Wafers	7	120	2	0	–	0	0	1	–
Crummy									
Organic Chocolate Chip	1 (2 oz)	240	0	200	–	0	40	1	–
Organic Lavender Chocolate Chip	1 (2 oz)	240	0	200	–	0	40	1	–
Dare									
Breaktime Coconut	4	140	1	0	–	0	0	1	–
Breaktime Ginger	4	130	0	0	–	0	0	1	–
Creme Chocolate Fudge	1	100	0	0	–	0	0	tr	–
Maple Leaf Creme	1	80	0	0	–	0	0	tr	–
Whipper	2	130	0	0	–	0	0	1	–
David's									
Hamantash Raspberry	1 (0.7 oz)	85	7	100	–	0	20	1	–
De Beukelaer									
Pirouline	8 (1 oz)	130	tr	0	–	0	0	0	–
DiCamillo									
Biscotti DiPrato	5 (1 oz)	130	tr	0	24	0	20	1	–
Doritos									
Barras De Coco	5	120	tr	200	40	0	0	1	–
Dove									
Beyond Chocolate Chunk	1 (0.7 oz)	110	1	–	–	–	–	tr	–
Milk Chocolate Moment	3 (1.1 oz)	160	1	–	–	–	20	tr	–
Earthbound Farm									
Organic Ginger Snaps	2	120	0	200	–	0	40	1	–
Elite									
Tea Biscuits Chocolate	4	80	0	0	–	0	0	3	–
English Bay									
Strawberry Fruit Bar	1 (1.2 oz)	120	1	0	–	0	0	1	–
Enjoy Life									
Gingerbread Spice Nut & Gluten Free	2 (1 oz)	100	1	0	–	0	20	1	–

FOOD	PORTION	CALS	FIBER	VIT A	FOLIC	VIT C	CALCI	IRON	POTAS
No-Oat Oatmeal Nut & Gluten Free	2 (1 oz)	110	1	0	–	0	20	1	–
Snickerdoodle Nut & Gluten Free	2 (1 oz)	130	1	0	–	0	20	1	–
Entenmann's									
Original Chocolate Chip	3	140	tr	0	–	0	0	0	–
Soft Baked Chocolate Chunk	1 (1.3 oz)	190	0	0	–	0	0	1	–
Estee									
Fructose Sweetened Chocolate Chip	4	160	1	–	–	–	–	–	–
Fructose Sweetened Lemon	4	160	2	–	–	–	–	–	–
Fructose Sweetened Sandwich Chocolate	3	170	tr	–	–	–	–	–	–
Fructose Sweetened Sandwich Original	3	170	0	–	–	–	–	–	–
Fructose Sweetened Sandwich Peanut Butter	3	190	tr	–	–	–	–	–	–
Fructose Sweetened Vanilla	4	160	1	–	–	–	–	–	–
Fructose Sweetened Vanilla Sandwich	3	170	0	–	–	–	–	–	–
Sugar Free Chocolate Chip	3	110	1	–	–	–	–	–	–
Sugar Free Lemon	3	110	1	–	–	–	–	–	–
Sugar Free Wafer Chocolate Creme	4	150	0	–	–	–	–	–	–
Sugar Free Wafer Lemon Creme	4	150	0	–	–	–	–	–	–
Sugar Free Wafer Peanut Butter Creme	4	150	0	–	–	–	–	–	–
Sugar Free Wafer Strawberry Creme	4	150	0	–	–	–	–	–	–
Sugar Free Wafer Vanilla Creme	4	150	0	–	–	–	–	–	–
Fauchon									
Assorted Chocolate	4 (2 oz)	330	5	250	–	0	0	1	–
Frieda's									
Asian Almond	2 (1 oz)	170	0	0	–	0	0	0	–

FOOD	PORTION	CALS	FIBER	VIT A	FOLIC	VIT C	CALCI	IRON	POTAS
Gamesa									
Animalitos	14	110	tr	200	60	0	0	2	–
Arcoiris Marshmallow	6	220	1	300	60	0	20	1	–
Arcoiris Merengue	6	200	1	0	–	0	0	2	–
Emperador Chocolate	2	120	tr	100	32	0	0	2	–
Emperador Fresa	2	120	tr	100	32	0	0	1	–
Emperador Limon	6	270	1	400	100	0	20	4	–
Emperador Vanilla	2	120	0	200	32	0	0	2	–
Hawaianas	3	130	tr	200	40	0	0	2	–
Marias	8	120	tr	200	60	0	0	2	–
Ricanelas	8	140	2	200	60	0	0	2	–
Roscas	3	130	1	0	–	0	0	1	–
Sugar Wafers Chocolate	3	160	0	0	–	0	0	tr	–
Sugar Wafers Strawberry	3	160	0	0	–	0	0	tr	–
Sugar Wafers Vanilla	3	160	0	0	–	0	0	tr	–
Girl Scout									
Cafe Cookies	5	150	1	0	–	0	0	1	–
Lemon Cooler Reduced Fat	5	130	0	0	–	0	0	tr	–
Samoas	2	150	tr	0	–	0	20	tr	–
Tagalongs	2	130	1	0	–	0	0	tr	–
Thin Mints	4	140	tr	0	–	0	20	1	–
Trefoils	4	130	0	0	–	0	0	1	–
Gluten-Free Pantry									
Gluten Free Buckwheat Raisin	1 (1 oz)	140	1	0	–	0	0	tr	–
Gluten Free Chocolate Chunk	1 (1 oz)	140	1	0	–	0	0	tr	–
Glutino									
Gluten Free Wafers Chocolate	4	160	3	0	–	0	40	1	–
Gluten Free Wafers Lemon	3	150	0	0	–	0	0	0	–
Godiva									
Biscotti Dipped In Milk Chocolate	1 (0.9 oz)	120	0	100	–	0	20	1	–
Gol D Lite									
Low Carb Pizzelle	1 (0.3 oz)	46	1	–	–	–	–	–	–

FOOD	PORTION	CALS	FIBER	VIT A	FOLIC	VIT C	CALCI	IRON	POTAS
Golightly									
Fabulous Tastes Caramel Dulce De Leche	4	100	5	100	–	0	20	tr	–
Goody Man									
Marshmallow Crispy Squares	1 (1.17 oz)	130	0	100	–	0	0	1	–
Grandma's									
Homestyle Big Chocolate Chip	1 (1.4 oz)	190	tr	0	–	0	0	1	75
Homestyle Big Fudge Chocolate Chip	1 (1.4 oz)	170	1	0	–	0	0	2	–
Homestyle Big Oatmeal Raisin	1 (1.4 oz)	180	1	0	–	0	100	1	–
Homestyle Big Peanut Butter	1 (1.4 oz)	200	1	0	–	0	0	1	–
Mini Vanilla Creme	9	150	tr	0	–	0	0	1	–
Peanut Butter Sandwich	5	210	1	0	–	0	0	1	–
Rich N'Chewy Chocolate Chip	1 pkg	270	2	0	–	0	0	1	–
Vanilla Creme Sandwich	5	210	tr	0	–	0	20	1	–
Granny Oats									
Low Carb Oatmeal	4	98	3	–	–	–	–	–	–
Healthy Handfuls									
Organic Crocodile Cookies	1 pkg (1 oz)	130	7	0	–	0	20	1	–
Organic Koala Krackers	1 pkg (1 oz)	120	2	100	–	0	0	1	–
Joseph's									
Almond Sugar Free	4	100	1	0	–	0	0	1	–
Chocolate Chip Sugar Free	4	95	1	100	–	1	0	1	–
Lemon Sugar Free	4	95	0	200	–	0	0	1	–
Oatmeal Chocolate Chip w/ Pecans Sugar Free	4	100	1	100	–	0	0	1	–
Peanut Butter Sugar Free	4	95	0	100	–	0	0	tr	–

FOOD	PORTION	CALS	FIBER	VIT A	FOLIC	VIT C	CALCI	IRON	POTAS
Karen's									
Fabulous Tastes Heavenly Chocolate Chip	4	90	5	100	–	0	20	1	–
Fabulous Tastes Luscious Raspberry Almond	4	110	5	100	–	0	20	1	–
Fabulous Tastes Pecan Vanilla Pralines	4	120	6	100	–	0	10	1	–
Kashi									
TLC Happy Trail Mix	1 (1 oz)	130	4	0	–	0	0	0	–
TLC Oatmeal Raisin Flax	1 (1 oz)	130	4	0	–	0	0	0	–
TLC Oatmeal Dark Chocolate	1 (1 oz)	130	3	0	–	0	0	0	–
Kedem									
Tea Biscuits Chocolate	2	32	tr	0	–	0	0	0	–
Tea Biscuits Orange	2	32	tr	0	–	0	0	0	–
Keebler									
100 Calorie Pack Sandies Shortbread	1 pkg	100	tr	0	–	0	0	tr	–
Chips Deluxe	1 (0.5 oz)	80	tr	0	–	0	0	1	–
Graham Honey	8 (1.1 oz)	140	0	0	–	0	100	tr	–
Sandies Fruit Delights Lemon	1 (0.6 oz)	80	0	0	–	0	0	0	–
Soft Batch Chocolate Chip	1 (0.6 oz)	80	tr	0	–	0	0	tr	–
Keto									
Low Carb Biscotti Chocolate	1 (1.2 oz)	157	3	–	–	–	–	–	–
Low Carb Biscotti Lemon Nut	1 (1.2 oz)	157	3	–	–	–	–	–	–
Low Carb Biscotti Vanilla Almond	1 (1.2 oz)	157	3	–	–	–	–	–	–
La Dolce Vita									
Biscotti Chocolate Passion	1 (1.2 oz)	130	1	200	–	0	40	1	–
Landies Candies									
Sugar Free Dark Royal Pecan Shortbread	2	167	1	50	–	0	0	4	–

FOOD	PORTION	CALS	FIBER	VIT A	FOLIC	VIT C	CALCI	IRON	POTAS
Sugar Free Milk Chocolate Chip	2	173	tr	50	–	1	0	2	–
Sugar Free Milk Chocolate Peanut Butter	2	171	tr	50	–	0	0	2	–
Sugar Free White Chocolate Lemon	2	177	0	150	–	0	0	1	–
Laura's Wholesome Junk Food									
Anna Banana Split	1	105	1	0	–	1	10	1	90
Gluten Free Charlotte's Chocolate Chip	2	120	1	0	–	0	20	1	85
Gluten Free Sally's Raisin	2	110	tr	0	–	0	20	1	110
Lemon Vanilla	2	120	1	0	–	1	20	1	110
Oatmeal Chocolate Chip	2	110	1	0	–	0	10	1	53
Oatmeal Raisin	2	100	1	0	–	0	10	1	88
Wheat Free X-Treme Chocolate Fudge	2	110	2	–	–	–	20	1	95
Lee's									
Dreamy Mallows	2	150	0	0	–	0	0	0	–
Leibniz									
Butter Biscuits	6	130	1	0	–	0	0	tr	–
Liz Lovely									
Vegan Cowboy	½ cookie (1.3 oz)	190	2	0	–	0	0	2	–
Vegan Cowgirl	½ cookie (1.5 oz)	210	0	0	–	0	0	1	–
Vegan Ginger Snapdragons	½ cookie (1.5 oz)	190	0	0	–	0	0	1	–
Low Carb Creations									
Chocolate Chip	1 (1 oz)	140	1	–	–	–	–	–	–
Coconut	1 (1 oz)	140	1	–	–	–	–	–	–
Lemon	1 (1 oz)	140	1	–	–	–	–	–	–
Snickerdoodle	1 (1 oz)	140	1	–	–	–	–	–	–
LU									
Chocolatier	3 (1 oz)	150	1	0	–	0	0	0	–
Le Bastogne	2 (0.8 oz)	120	0	0	–	0	0	0	–
Le Fondant	4 (1.1 oz)	170	1	0	–	0	0	0	–
Le Petit Beurre	4 (1.2 oz)	150	tr	0	–	0	0	0	–
Le Petit Ecolier Dark Chocolate	2 (0.9 oz)	130	1	0	–	0	0	0	–

FOOD	PORTION	CALS	FIBER	VIT A	FOLIC	VIT C	CALCI	IRON	POTAS
Le Petit Ecolier Extra Dark Chocolate	2	120	2	0	–	0	0	0	–
Le Petit Fruit Strawberry	5 (1.2 oz)	110	0	0	–	0	0	0	–
Pim's Orange	2 (0.9 oz)	90	tr	0	–	0	0	0	–
Pim's Sensation Bar Chocolate	1	110	tr	0	–	0	0	0	–
Pim's Sensation Bar Hazelnut	1	110	tr	0	–	0	0	0	–
Shortbread	2	140	tr	300	–	0	20	0	–
Mamma Says'									
Biscotti Almond Pistachio	1 (0.5 oz)	50	1	0	–	0	10	tr	–
Biscotti Chocolate Macadamia	1 (0.5 oz)	45	1	0	–	0	10	tr	–
Biscotti Orange Citrine	1 (0.5 oz)	60	1	200	–	0	10	1	–
Miss Meringue									
Chocolatette Strawberry Vanilla	4	130	1	0	–	0	0	0	–
Chocolettes Crunchy Chocolate	4	110	21	1	–	0	0	1	–
Classiques Cappuccino	4	110	0	0	–	0	0	0	–
Classiques Chocolate Chip	4	120	1	0	–	0	0	tr	–
Classiques Dulce De Leche Artisan	4	110	0	0	–	0	0	0	–
Macaroons Traditional	1 (1.3 oz)	180	1	0	–	0	0	0	–
Madeleines Traditional	2 (1.2 oz)	160	0	0	–	0	0	tr	–
Minis Vanilla	13 (1.1 oz)	110	0	0	–	0	0	0	–
Minis Vanilla Sugar Free	13	35	3	0	–	0	0	0	–
MoonPie									
Chocolate	1 (2.75 oz)	330	0	0	–	0	0	1	–
Nabisco									
100 Calorie Pack Lorna Doone	1 pkg	100	0	0	–	0	0	1	–
Biscos Sugar Wafers	8 (1 oz)	140	0	0	–	0	0	tr	–

FOOD	PORTION	CALS	FIBER	VIT A	FOLIC	VIT C	CALCI	IRON	POTAS
Honey Maid Cinnamon Sticks	1 pkg (1 oz)	120	tr	0	–	0	0	1	–
Lorna Doone	4 (1 oz)	140	0	0	–	0	0	1	–
Mallomars	2	120	tr	0	–	0	0	tr	–
Social Tea	6	140	1	0	–	0	0	1	–
Nana's									
No Gluten Berry Vanilla	1 bar (1.2 oz)	130	tr	0	–	1	20	tr	55
No Gluten Chocolate	1 (3.5 oz)	360	2	200	–	2	40	1	–
No Gluten Ginger	1 (3.5 oz)	360	2	0	–	2	40	1	–
No Gluten Nana Banana	1 bar (1.2 oz)	130	0	100	–	1	20	tr	50
No Wheat Oatmeal Raisin	1 (3.5 oz)	280	6	0	–	0	80	2	–
Vegan Chocolate Chip	1 (4 oz)	320	6	0	–	2	80	3	–
Vegan Peanut Butter	1 (4 oz)	360	4	0	–	2	40	2	–
Vegan Sunflower	1 (3.5 oz)	380	6	0	–	0	40	2	–
Natural Ovens									
Carob Chip	1	90	3	–	60	–	60	1	–
Chocolate Raspberry	1	120	3	–	60	–	60	1	–
Oatmeal Raisin	1	90	3	500	60	–	60	1	–
Nature's Path									
Organic Signature Lemon Poppyseed	4	130	tr	0	–	0	0	tr	–
Organic Animal Vanilla	9	120	tr	0	–	0	0	0	–
Newman's Own									
Organic Champion Chip Chocolate Chocolate Chip	4	160	1	–	–	–	–	–	–
Organic Champion Chip Chocolate Chip	4	160	1	–	–	–	–	–	–
Organic Champion Chip Double Chocolate Mint Chip	4	160	1	–	–	–	–	–	–
Organic Champion Chip Expresso Chocolate Chip	4	150	1	–	–	–	–	–	–
Organic Champion Chip Orange Chocolate Chip	4	160	1	–	–	–	–	–	–

FOOD	PORTION	CALS	FIBER	VIT A	FOLIC	VIT C	CALCI	IRON	POTAS
Organic Champion Chip Wheat Free Dairy Free	4	160	0	–	–	–	–	–	–
Organic Fig Newmans Fat Free	2	120	1	–	–	–	–	–	–
Organic Fig Newmans Low Fat	2	140	1	–	–	–	–	–	–
Organic Fig Newmans Wheat Free Dairy Free	2	120	1	–	–	–	–	–	–
Organic Newman-O's Chocolate Creme	2	130	1	–	–	–	–	–	–
Organic Newman-O's Ginger-O's	2	120	0	–	–	–	–	–	–
Organic Newman-O's Mint Creme	2	130	1	–	–	–	–	–	–
Organic Newman-O's Original	2	130	1	–	–	–	–	–	–
Organic Newman-O's Tops & Bottoms	6	120	1	–	–	–	–	–	–
Organic Newman-O's Wheat Free Dairy Free	2	130	0	–	–	–	–	–	–
Nonni's									
Biscotti Decadence	1 (1.1 oz)	130	1	200	–	0	20	1	–
Biscotti Original	1 (1 oz)	100	1	200	–	0	20	1	–
Pepperidge Farm									
Brussels	2	100	tr	0	–	0	0	tr	–
Chessmen	3	120	tr	100	–	0	0	tr	–
Chocolate Chunk Minis Nantucket	1 pkg (1.75 oz)	260	0	100	–	0	0	1	–
Goldfish Grahams Cinnamon	1 pkg (1.75 oz)	240	2	0	–	0	0	1	–
Soft Baked Chocolate Chunk Dark Chocolate	1	140	0	0	–	1	0	1	–
Soft Baked Chocolate Chunk Milk Chocolate Caramel	1	140	tr	0	–	0	0	1	–
Soft Baked Sugar	1	140	0	0	–	0	0	1	–
Whims Chocolate Cashew	9 (1 oz)	150	tr	0	–	0	0	tr	–

FOOD	PORTION	CALS	FIBER	VIT A	FOLIC	VIT C	CALCI	IRON	POTAS
Pure De-Lite									
High Protein Chocolate Fudge	1 (2.2 oz)	210	5	–	–	–	–	–	–
High Protein Peanut Butter Crunch	1 (2.2 oz)	210	5	–	–	–	–	–	–
Quaker									
Breakfast Cookie Oatmeal Raisin	1	180	5	750	–	0	300	6	–
Right Direction									
Chocolate Chip	1	60	5	–	–	–	–	–	–
SnackWell's									
Creme Sandwich	1 pkg (1.7 oz)	210	tr	0	–	0	20	1	–
Mint Creme	2	110	tr	0	–	0	0	1	–
Sugar Free Chocolate Chip	3 (1.2 oz)	150	tr	0	–	0	0	1	–
Sugar Free Oatmeal	1 (0.8 oz)	90	tr	0	–	0	0	1	–
South Beach Diet									
Oatmeal Chocolate Chip	1 pkg	100	3	0	–	0	0	tr	–
Peanut Butter	1 pkg	100	4	0	–	0	0	tr	–
Soybite									
All Flavors	1	79	1	–	–	–	–	–	–
Stella D'Oro									
Lady Stella	3	130	tr	0	–	0	0	1	–
Margherite	2	130	0	0	–	0	0	1	–
Super Chip									
Chocolate Chip	2 (0.9 oz)	100	3	–	–	–	–	–	–
Temptations									
Chocolate Alps	1 bar (1.6 oz)	170	1	0	–	0	0	1	–
Chocolate Mocha	1 bar (1.6 oz)	170	1	0	–	0	0	1	–
No Gluten Chocolate Rush	1 bar (1.6 oz)	170	1	0	–	0	0	0	–
TAKE-OUT									
biscotti w/ nuts chocolate dipped	1 (1.3 oz)	117	1	100	–	1	10	1	–
black & white	1 lg (3 oz)	302	1	465	11	tr	32	2	68
finikia	1 (1.2 oz)	171	1	312	6	tr	8	1	26

FOOD	PORTION	CALS	FIBER	VIT A	FOLIC	VIT C	CALCI	IRON	POTAS
koulourakia butter cookie twist	1 (0.9 oz)	113	tr	278	5	0	15	1	16
linzer tart	1 (2.4 oz)	280	0	100	–	1	20	tr	–

CORIANDER

FOOD	PORTION	CALS	FIBER	VIT A	FOLIC	VIT C	CALCI	IRON	POTAS
cilantro fresh	1 tsp (2 g)	tr	tr	98	1	1	1	tr	8
cilantro fresh	1 cup (1.6 oz)	11	1	2820	29	1	31	1	235
leaf dried	1 tsp	2	–	–	–	3	7	tr	27
leaf fresh	¼ cup	1	–	111	–	–	4	tr	22
seed	1 tsp	5	–	–	–	–	13	tr	23

Instant India

FOOD	PORTION	CALS	FIBER	VIT A	FOLIC	VIT C	CALCI	IRON	POTAS
Tomato Coriander Paste	2 tbsp (1 oz)	90	0	0	–	0	0	0	–

CORN
CANNED

FOOD	PORTION	CALS	FIBER	VIT A	FOLIC	VIT C	CALCI	IRON	POTAS
cream style	½ cup	93	–	124	57	6	4	tr	172
w/ red & green peppers	½ cup	86	–	265	–	10	5	1	174
white	½ cup	66	–	tr	–	–	–	1	–
yellow	½ cup	66	1	128	–	–	–	1	–

Del Monte

FOOD	PORTION	CALS	FIBER	VIT A	FOLIC	VIT C	CALCI	IRON	POTAS
Cream Style	½ cup	60	2	0	–	2	0	tr	–
Cream Style No Salt Added	½ cup	60	2	0	–	2	0	tr	–
Fiesta	½ cup	50	2	200	–	4	0	tr	–
Gold & White	½ cup	80	2	0	–	4	0	tr	–
Savory Sides In Butter Sauce	½ cup	90	tr	300	–	5	0	tr	–
Savory Sides Santa Fe	½ cup	70	1	500	–	9	0	1	–
Summer Crisp	½ cup	70	3	0	–	4	0	1	–
White	½ cup	60	3	0	–	4	0	tr	–

Green Giant

FOOD	PORTION	CALS	FIBER	VIT A	FOLIC	VIT C	CALCI	IRON	POTAS
Mexicorn	⅓ cup	70	1	0	–	4	0	0	–
Yellow & White	⅓ cup	60	1	0	–	2	0	0	–

S&W

FOOD	PORTION	CALS	FIBER	VIT A	FOLIC	VIT C	CALCI	IRON	POTAS
Cream Style	½ cup (4.4 oz)	60	2	0	–	2	0	tr	–
Whole Kernel	⅓ cup (3 oz)	70	2	0	–	2	0	0	–

FOOD	PORTION	CALS	FIBER	VIT A	FOLIC	VIT C	CALCI	IRON	POTAS
Veg-All									
Whole Kernel	½ cup	80	2	0	–	4	0	0	–
FRESH									
white cooked	½ cup	89	–	tr	38	5	2	1	204
white raw	½ cup	66	–	tr	35	5	2	tr	208
yellow cooked	1 ear (2.7 oz)	83	–	167	36	5	2	tr	192
yellow cooked	½ cup	89	–	178	38	5	2	1	204
yellow raw	½ cup	66	–	216	35	5	2	tr	208
yellow raw	1 ear (3 oz)	77	–	253	41	6	2	tr	243
FROZEN									
cooked	½ cup	67	–	204	19	2	2	tr	114
on the cob cooked	1 ear (2.2 oz)	59	–	133	19	3	2	tr	158
Birds Eye									
Steamfresh Southwestern	⅔ cup	90	1	100	–	6	0	0	–
Steamfresh Super Sweet	⅔ cup	70	2	100	–	6	0	tr	–
Steamfresh Sweet Mini Corn On The Cob	1	90	1	0	–	5	0	0	–
C&W									
Cheddar Bacon	½ cup	130	3	0	–	2	40	tr	–
Early Harvest Supersweet Petite	⅔ cup	70	2	100	–	6	0	tr	–
Salsa Corn	1 cup	90	3	0	–	12	20	1	–
Europe's Best									
Baby Sweet	⅔ cup	50	2	100	–	4	0	tr	–
Fresh Like									
Cut	3.5 oz	85	1	242	–	5	5	1	196
On The Cob	1 ear (3 in)	96	1	208	–	6	4	1	304
Glory									
Savory Accents Fried Corn	½ cup	110	2	100	–	5	20	tr	–
Green Giant									
Niblets & Butter Sauce Low Fat	⅔ cup	110	2	0	–	2	0	0	–

FOOD	PORTION	CALS	FIBER	VIT A	FOLIC	VIT C	CALCI	IRON	POTAS
Pictsweet									
Cut Corn	⅔ cup	100	1	0	–	4	0	0	–
Roast Works									
Flame Roasted Cob Corn	1 cob (3 oz)	130	4	750	–	9	0	1	–
TAKE-OUT									
fritters	1 (1 oz)	62	1	66	3	1	21	tr	47
on the cob w/ butter cooked	1 ear	155	–	391	44	7	5	tr	360
scalloped	1 cup	257	3	715	54	6	92	1	417

CORNMEAL

FOOD	PORTION	CALS	FIBER	VIT A	FOLIC	VIT C	CALCI	IRON	POTAS
cornmeal mush as prep w/ water	1 cup	223	5	35	98	0	12	3	98
cornmeal yellow	1 cup	505	10	295	322	0	7	6	224
harina de maize con leche	1 cup	295	7	295	45	1	234	1	306
Expert Foods									
Low Carb Grits Mix	1½ tsp	15	2	–	–	–	–	–	–
Indian Head									
Stone Ground	¼ cup	100	2	–	40	–	–	1	–
Quaker									
Old Fashioned Grits not prep	¼ cup	140	2	–	60	–	–	1	–
Quick Grits not prep	¼ cup	130	2	–	40	–	–	1	–
Yellow	3 tbsp (1 oz)	90	2	100	40	–	–	1	–
TAKE-OUT									
corn pone	1 piece (2.1 oz)	128	2	0	5	0	70	1	87
fritter puerto rican style	1 (1.4 oz)	109	1	115	16	0	59	tr	27
harina de maiz con coco	½ cup	383	4	5	41	3	18	2	320
hush puppies	1 (0.8 oz)	74	1	45	20	0	61	1	32
johnnycake	1 piece (1.7 oz)	134	2	80	56	tr	51	1	105

CORNSTARCH

FOOD	PORTION	CALS	FIBER	VIT A	FOLIC	VIT C	CALCI	IRON	POTAS
cornstarch	1 cup (4.5 oz)	488	1	0	0	0	3	1	4

FOOD	PORTION	CALS	FIBER	VIT A	FOLIC	VIT C	CALCI	IRON	POTAS
COTTAGE CHEESE									
creamed	1 cup (7.4 oz)	217	–	342	26	tr	126	tr	177
creamed	4 oz	117	–	184	14	tr	68	tr	95
creamed w/ fruit	4 oz	140	–	139	11	tr	54	tr	76
dry curd	4 oz	96	–	34	17	0	36	tr	37
dry curd	1 cup (5.1 oz)	123	–	44	21	0	46	tr	47
lowfat 1%	1 cup (7.9 oz)	164	–	84	28	tr	138	tr	193
lowfat 1%	4 oz	82	–	42	14	tr	69	tr	97
lowfat 2%	4 oz	101	–	79	15	tr	77	tr	109
lowfat 2%	1 cup (7.9 oz)	203	–	158	30	tr	155	tr	217
Breakstone's									
Fat Free	½ cup	80	0	200	–	0	150	0	–
Cabot									
Cottage Cheese	½ cup	100	0	300	–	0	100	0	–
No Fat	½ cup	70	0	300	–	0	100	0	–
Hood									
4% Fat w/ Pineapple	½ cup	130	0	200	–	2	80	0	–
Fat Free	½ cup	80	0	200	–	0	100	0	–
Low Fat	½ cup	90	0	200	–	0	100	0	–
Low Fat No Salt Added	½ cup	90	0	200	–	0	80	0	–
Low Fat w/ Peaches	½ cup	110	0	200	–	6	80	0	–
Horizon Organic									
Lowfat	½ cup	100	0	200	–	0	150	0	–
Regular	½ cup	120	0	200	–	0	150	0	–
Light N'Lively									
Lowfat	½ cup	80	0	200	–	0	200	0	–
COTTONSEED									
kernels roasted	1 tbsp	51	–	–	–	1	10	1	135
COUSCOUS									
cooked	1 cup (5.5 oz)	176	2	0	24	0	13	1	91
dry	1 cup (6.1 oz)	650	9	0	35	0	42	2	287
Hodgson Mill									
Whole Wheat not prep	⅓ cup	210	5	0	–	0	20	2	–

FOOD	PORTION	CALS	FIBER	VIT A	FOLIC	VIT C	CALCI	IRON	POTAS
Marrakesh Express									
Mango Salsa as prep	1 cup	190	1	0	–	0	20	1	–
Mushroom as prep	1 cup	190	1	0	–	0	0	1	–
Plain as prep	1 cup	270	2	0	–	0	0	1	–
Near East									
Broccoli & Cheese as prep	1 cup	230	3	300	–	9	60	1	–
Curry as prep	1 cup	220	3	200	–	1	20	1	–
Herbed Chicken as prep	1 cup	220	3	200	–	0	20	1	–
Original as prep	1 cup	230	2	100	–	0	0	1	–
Parmesan as prep	1 cup	220	2	100	–	0	60	1	–
Roasted Garlic Olive Oil as prep	1 cup	230	2	0	–	0	0	1	–
Toasted Pine Nut as prep	1 cup	230	2	0	–	0	0	1	–
Tomato Lentil as prep	1 cup	220	3	300	–	1	20	1	–
Wild Mushroom Herb as prep	1 cup	230	3	100	–	0	20	1	–
CRAB									
CANNED									
blue	½ cup	67	0	5	29	2	68	1	252
blue drained	1 can (6.5 oz)	124	0	9	54	3	126	1	468
Brunswick									
Crabmeat 15% Leg	2 oz	40	0	0	–	0	40	0	–
Fancy Lump	2 oz	45	0	0	–	0	40	1	–
Bumble Bee									
Lump	¼ cup	40	0	0	–	0	20	tr	–
Pink	¼ cup	35	0	0	–	0	20	tr	–
White	¼ cup	40	0	0	–	0	20	tr	–
Chicken Of The Sea									
Fancy	½ can (2 oz)	40	0	0	–	0	60	tr	–
Lump	½ can (2 oz)	35	0	0	–	0	20	tr	–
Madam									
Crab Meat	½ cup	40	0	0	–	0	60	tr	–

FOOD	PORTION	CALS	FIBER	VIT A	FOLIC	VIT C	CALCI	IRON	POTAS
Terry's									
Crabmeat	¼ cup	40	0	0	–	0	60	tr	–
FRESH									
alaska king meat only steamed	3 oz	82	0	25	43	7	50	1	223
blue cooked flaked	1 cup (4 oz)	120	0	8	60	4	123	1	382
dungeness steamed	3 oz	94	0	88	36	3	50	tr	347
queen steamed	3 oz	98	0	147	36	6	28	2	170
TAKE-OUT									
alaska king leg steamed	1 leg (4.7 oz)	130	0	39	68	10	79	1	351
baked	1 (3.8 oz)	160	–	78	20	3	415	1	598
cakes	2 (4.2 oz)	186	0	302	64	3	126	1	389
crab imperial	1 crab (6.8 oz)	289	0	765	80	10	182	2	508
crab salad	1 serv (5.5 oz)	285	1	140	62	4	120	1	402
crab thermidor	1 serv (6.4 oz)	456	tr	1840	37	2	185	2	401
deviled	1 serv (4.5 oz)	254	1	695	56	9	110	2	355
dungeness steamed	1 crab (4.5 oz)	140	0	132	53	5	75	1	518
empanada de jueyes	1 (4.4 oz)	341	2	165	42	22	154	1	557
fried crab puffs	4 (3.2 oz)	323	1	800	47	0	52	2	147
kenagi korean crab cooked	1 serv (3 oz)	71	0	–	–	0	60	tr	170
salmorejo de jueyes (in tomato sauce)	1 serv (4.5 oz)	215	tr	30	52	9	109	1	404
soft-shell breaded & fried	1 med (2.3 oz)	216	1	60	43	1	76	1	207
taco de jueyes	1 (4.2 oz)	266	2	280	47	11	160	2	317
CRACKER CRUMBS									
cracker meal	1 cup	440	3	0	156	0	26	5	132
graham cracker crumbs	1 cup	355	2	0	39	0	20	3	113
Kellogg's									
Corn Flake Crumbs	6 tbsp (1.2 oz)	120	tr	500	100	6	0	9	–

CRACKERS

FOOD	PORTION	CALS	FIBER	VIT A	FOLIC	VIT C	CALCI	IRON	POTAS
melba toast round	1	12	tr	0	4	0	3	tr	6
oyster cracker	¼ cup	48	tr	0	16	0	8	1	17
saltines	1	13	tr	0	4	0	2	tr	5
water biscuits	3	92	1	0	–	0	25	tr	–
zwieback	1 oz	107	1	–	–	–	12	tr	46
American Vintage									
Wine Biscuits All Flavors	5	140	tr	–	–	–	20	1	–
Andre's									
CarboSave Crackerbread All Flavors	1 oz	140	4	–	–	–	–	–	–
Annie's Homegrown									
Cheddar Bunnies BBQ	50	130	2	0	–	0	0	1	–
Cheddar Bunnies Original	50	150	1	0	–	0	20	tr	–
Cheddar Bunnies Ranch	50	130	2	0	–	0	0	1	–
Cheddar Bunnies Whole Wheat	50	130	2	0	–	0	0	1	–
Back To Nature									
Classic Rounds	5	70	0	0	–	0	20	1	–
Crispy Wheats	17	130	1	0	–	0	20	1	–
Rice Thin Sesame Ginger	16	120	0	0	–	0	0	0	–
Rice Thin White Cheddar	16	120	0	0	–	0	0	0	–
Blue Diamond									
Nut-Thins Almond	16	130	1	0	–	0	200	tr	–
Nut-Thins Hazelnut	16	130	tr	0	–	0	0	0	–
Nut-Thins Pecan	16	130	tr	0	–	0	0	0	–
Bran-A-Crisp									
Low Carb Wheat Bran	1	20	2	–	–	–	–	–	–
Bremner Wafers									
Cracked Wheat	7	70	0	0	–	0	0	1	–
Low Sodium	7	70	0	0	–	0	0	1	–
Original	7	70	0	0	–	0	0	1	–
Cheeters									
Low Carb All Flavors	1 pkg (1 oz)	104	2	–	–	–	–	–	–
Dare									
Breton Minis	13	80	0	0	–	0	0	0	–
Breton Multigrain	3 (0.5 oz)	80	1	0	–	0	0	1	–
Breton Original	3	60	0	0	–	0	0	1	–

FOOD	PORTION	CALS	FIBER	VIT A	FOLIC	VIT C	CALCI	IRON	POTAS
Breton Reduced Fat & Sodium	7	120	2	0	–	0	150	1	–
Cabaret	3	70	0	0	–	0	0	1	–
Crispy Baguettes Original	9	110	1	0	–	0	0	1	–
Crispy Baguettes Three Cheese	8	130	tr	0	–	0	20	1	–
Grainsfirst	4	90	2	0	–	0	20	tr	–
Vinta	2 (0.5 oz)	70	0	0	–	0	0	tr	–
Vivant	3	60	0	0	–	0	0	1	–
Water Crackers Original	5	60	0	0	–	0	0	0	–
Dr. Kracker									
Flatbread Klassic 100% Whole Wheat 3 Seed	1	90	5	0	–	0	30	1	–
Flatbread Klassic Seed	1	100	3	0	–	0	30	1	–
Flatbread Pumpkin Seed	1	100	3	0	–	0	30	1	–
Flatbread Seeded Spelt	1	110	3	0	–	0	30	1	–
Flatbread Seedlander	1	100	2	0	–	0	10	tr	–
Flatbread Spelt Sunflower Cheese	1	100	3	0	–	0	50	1	–
Kribbons Krispy Graham	5	120	3	0	–	0	0	1	–
Kribbons Muesli	5	120	5	0	–	0	30	1	–
Eden									
Brown Rice	8 (1.1 oz)	120	2	0	–	0	20	1	110
Nori Nori Rice	15 (1 oz)	110	2	0	–	0	40	tr	25
Foods Alive									
Golden Flax Maple & Cinnamon	5	150	8	0	32	0	60	2	170
Golden Flax Mexican Harvest	5	150	9	100	32	0	60	1	280
Golden Flax Onion Garlic	5	140	9	100	32	0	60	1	310
Golden Flax Organic Hemp	5	130	11	0	32	0	80	2	240
Golden Flax Regular	5	150	11	0	32	0	80	2	240
Gamesa									
Sabrisas	11	150	0	200	–	0	0	1	–
Glutino									
Gluten Free	4 (0.5 oz)	70	0	0	–	0	0	0	–
Gluten Free Rusks	2 (0.7 oz)	80	2	0	–	0	0	0	–
Gold'n Krackle									
Cheese	0.5 oz	65	0	0	–	0	0	1	–

FOOD	PORTION	CALS	FIBER	VIT A	FOLIC	VIT C	CALCI	IRON	POTAS
Cheese & Oregano	0.5 oz	65	0	0	–	0	0	1	–
Hot & Spicy	0.5 oz	58	0	0	–	0	0	1	–
Onion & Garlic	0.5 oz	58	0	0	–	0	0	1	–
Plain	0.5 oz	58	0	0	–	0	0	1	–
Healthy Handfuls									
Lucky Duckies Cheddar Cheese	1 pkg (1 oz)	100	1	0	–	0	20	tr	–
Heavenly									
All Flavors Cholesterol Free Sugar Free	1	16	0	–	–	–	–	–	–
Jacob's									
Table Cracker Bran	1	33	tr	–	–	–	–	–	–
Kashi									
TLC Country Cheddar	18 (1 oz)	130	tr	0	–	0	0	0	270
TLC Honey Sesame	15 (1 oz)	130	2	0	–	0	20	1	–
TLC Natural Ranch	15 (1 oz)	130	2	0	–	0	20	tr	–
TLC Original 7 Grain	15 (1 oz)	130	2	0	–	0	20	1	–
Keebler									
Sandwich Cracker Wheat & Cheddar	1 pkg	200	tr	0	–	0	40	1	–
Toasteds Buttercrisp	5 (0.6 oz)	80	0	0	–	0	0	tr	–
Toasteds Sesame	5 (0.6 oz)	80	tr	0	–	0	0	1	–
Toasteds Wheat	5 (0.6 oz)	80	tr	0	–	0	0	1	–
Kitchen Table Bakers									
Aged Parmesan	3	80	0	100	–	0	200	tr	–
Caraway Cheese	3	80	1	100	–	0	150	tr	–
Sesame Cheese	3	80	1	100	–	0	150	tr	–
Milton's									
Multi-Grain	2	70	0	0	–	0	60	tr	–
Nabisco									
Vegetable	4	90	tr	0	–	0	0	1	–
Water Original	4	60	0	0	–	0	0	1	–
Water Pepper & Poppy	4	60	tr	0	–	0	0	tr	–
Wheat	4	90	tr	0	–	0	0	1	–
Nature's Path									
Signature Tamari Flax	15	110	tr	0	–	0	20	tr	–
New York Style									
Panetini Garlic Parmesan	5	130	1	0	–	0	20	1	–
No-Carb Kitchen									
Cheese	1	25	0	–	–	–	–	–	–

FOOD	PORTION	CALS	FIBER	VIT A	FOLIC	VIT C	CALCI	IRON	POTAS
Old London									
Mediterranean Toast	3	60	0	0	–	0	0	tr	–
Pepperidge Farm									
Giant Goldfish Peanut Butter Sandwich	1 pkg (1.4 oz)	190	1	0	–	0	150	1	–
Giant Goldfish Wheat	14	140	1	0	–	0	20	1	–
Goldfish Cheddar	55	140	tr	0	–	0	40	tr	–
Goldfish Colors On The Go	1 pkg	170	1	0	–	0	40	1	–
Goldfish Original	55	140	tr	0	–	0	20	1	–
Goldfish Pizza	55 (1 oz)	140	tr	0	–	0	20	1	–
Goldfish Pretzel	43	130	tr	0	–	0	0	2	–
Goldfish w/ Whole Grain	55	140	2	–	–	–	–	–	–
Peter Pan									
Peanut Butter Cheese	1 pkg	210	1	0	–	0	80	1	–
Peanut Butter Toast	1 pkg	210	1	0	–	0	80	1	–
Premium									
Saltine Fat Free	5	60	0	0	–	0	20	1	–
Saltine Unsalted Tops	5	60	0	0	–	0	20	1	–
Ritz									
Reduced Fat	5	70	0	0	–	0	20	1	–
Rykrisp									
Seasoned	2	60	3	0	–	0	0	tr	–
San-J									
Brown Rice Black Sesame	5	140	1	–	–	–	–	2	–
Brown Rice Sesame	5	130	1	–	–	–	–	1	–
Brown Rice Tamari	6	170	1	–	–	–	–	1	–
Sara Lee									
Cracked Pepper Trio	7	130	tr	0	–	0	0	1	–
English Water	7	130	tr	0	–	0	0	1	–
Harvest Vegetable	6	140	tr	100	–	0	0	1	50
SnackWell's									
Cracked Pepper	5	60	0	0	–	0	20	tr	–
South Beach Diet									
Whole Wheat	1 pkg	100	3	0	–	0	20	1	–
Wasa									
Crisp'N Light 7 Grain	3	60	2	0	–	0	0	0	–
Fiber Rye	1	30	2	0	–	0	0	1	–
Hearty Rye	1	45	2	0	–	0	0	tr	–

FOOD	PORTION	CALS	FIBER	VIT A	FOLIC	VIT C	CALCI	IRON	POTAS
Oats	1	60	2	0	–	0	0	tr	–
Sourdough Rye	1	35	2	0	–	0	0	0	–
Wheat Thins									
Harvest Crisps Five-Grain	13	140	1	0	–	0	20	1	–
Wheatsworth									
Crackers	5	80	tr	0	–	0	0	1	–
Wisecrackers									
Low Fat Roasted Garlic	10	110	tr	0	–	0	0	1	–

CRANBERRIES

FOOD	PORTION	CALS	FIBER	VIT A	FOLIC	VIT C	CALCI	IRON	POTAS
cranberry sauce sweetened	½ cup	209	–	28	–	3	5	tr	35
dried organic	⅓ cup	120	2	0	–	0	0	0	–
fresh chopped	1 cup	54	–	50	2	15	8	tr	78
De-Lite									
Dried Sweetened	1 oz	92	1	22	–	tr	2	tr	–
Earthbound Farm									
Organic Dried	⅓ cup	130	2	0	–	2	0	0	–
Eden									
Organic Dried	⅓ cup	140	2	0	–	0	20	tr	115
Frieda's									
Dried	⅓ cup (1.4 oz)	110	2	0	–	0	0	0	–
Good Sense									
Cranberries 'N More	¼ cup	170	2	0	–	4	20	1	–
Dried Sweetened	½ cup	130	4	0	–	0	0	0	–
Lollipop Tree									
Cranberry Curd	1 tbsp	50	–	0	–	0	0	0	–
Mariani									
Dried Sweetened	⅓ cup	130	2	0	–	0	0	0	20
Newman's Own									
Organic Dried	¼ cup	130	2	–	–	–	–	–	–
Ocean Spray									
Craisins	⅓ cup	130	2	0	–	0	–	–	–
Cranberry Sauce Jellied	¼ cup	110	tr	0	–	0	–	–	0
Cranorange	¼ cup	120	1	0	–	0	–	–	0
Whole Berry Sauce	¼ cup	110	1	0	–	0	–	–	0
Steel's									
Spiced Cranberry Sauce	⅓ cup	20	1	–	–	–	–	–	–

FOOD	PORTION	CALS	FIBER	VIT A	FOLIC	VIT C	CALCI	IRON	POTAS
Sunsweet									
Dried	⅓ cup (1.5 oz)	140	2	0	–	0	0	0	25
Wild Thyme Farms									
Cranberry Sauce	1 tbsp	19	–	50	–	2	–	–	–
CRANBERRY BEANS									
canned	½ cup	108	8	0	100	1	44	2	338
dried cooked w/o salt	½ cup	120	9	0	183	0	44	2	342
CRANBERRY JUICE									
cranberry juice cocktail	6 oz	108	–	7	1	67	7	tr	34
cranberry juice cocktail low calorie	6 oz	33	–	–	–	57	16	tr	39
cranberry juice cocktail frzn	12 oz can	821	–	148	0	148	48	1	213
cranberry juice cocktail frzn as prep	6 oz can	102	–	18	0	18	9	tr	27
Keto									
Kooler	½ tsp	0	0	–	–	–	–	–	–
Langers									
Cranberry 100	8 oz	140	–	500	–	60	100	–	–
Nantucket Nectars									
Big Cran	8 oz	140	0	0	–	60	0	0	–
Northland									
100% Juice	8 oz	130	–	–	–	78	–	–	230
Ocean Spray									
Cocktail	8 oz	140	0	0	–	60	–	–	–
Cocktail Reduced Calorie	8 oz	50	0	0	–	60	–	–	45
Cocktail Light Low Calorie	8 oz	40	0	0	–	60	–	–	45
Cranberry Drink	8 oz	130	–	0	–	60	–	–	0
Crantastic	8 oz	100	0	0	–	60	–	–	0
White Cranberry	8 oz	120	–	0	–	60	–	–	0
White Cranberry Peach	8 oz	120	–	0	–	60	–	–	0
White Cranberry Strawberry	8 oz	120	–	0	–	60	–	–	0
Old Orchard									
Cocktail	8 oz	140	–	0	–	78	0	0	–

FOOD	PORTION	CALS	FIBER	VIT A	FOLIC	VIT C	CALCI	IRON	POTAS
CRAYFISH									
cooked	3 oz	97	0	–	–	3	26	3	298
raw	3 oz	76	0	–	–	3	20	2	233
raw	8	24	0	–	–	1	6	1	74
CREAM									
clotted cream	2 tbsp (1 oz)	164	0	985	2	0	10	tr	15
creme fraiche	2 tbsp (1 oz)	100	0	400	–	0	20	0	–
half & half	1 tbsp (0.5 oz)	20	–	65	tr	tr	16	tr	19
half & half	1 cup (8.5 oz)	315	–	1050	6	2	254	tr	314
heavy whipping	1 tbsp (0.5 oz)	52	–	220	1	tr	10	tr	11
heavy whipping whipped	1 cup (4.1 oz)	411	–	3499	9	1	77	tr	179
light coffee	1 cup (8.4 oz)	496	–	1728	6	2	14	tr	292
light coffee	1 tbsp (0.5 oz)	29	–	108	tr	tr	14	tr	18
light whipping	1 tbsp (0.5 oz)	44	–	169	1	tr	10	tr	15
light whipping cream whipped	1 cup (4.2 oz)	345	–	2694	9	1	83	tr	231
Cabot									
Whipped	2 tbsp	30	0	0	–	0	0	0	–
Hood									
Half & Half	2 tbsp	40	0	100	–	0	40	0	–
Light	1 tbsp	30	0	100	–	0	0	0	–
Simply Smart Fat Free Half & Half	2 tbsp	15	0	100	–	0	40	0	–
Whipping Cream	1 tbsp	45	0	200	–	0	0	0	–
Horizon Organic									
Half & Half	2 tbsp	35	0	100	–	0	40	0	–
Heavy Whipping	1 tbsp	50	0	200	–	0	0	0	–
CREAM CHEESE									
cream cheese	1 oz	99	–	405	4	0	23	tr	34

FOOD	PORTION	CALS	FIBER	VIT A	FOLIC	VIT C	CALCI	IRON	POTAS
cream cheese	1 pkg (3 oz)	297	–	1213	11	0	68	1	101
Boar's Head									
Cream Cheese	2 tbsp (1 oz)	100	0	300	–	0	20	0	–
Connoisseur									
Wheel Mango Peach	2 tbsp	110	0	300	–	0	20	0	–
Wheel Wild Blueberry	2 tbsp	100	0	300	–	0	20	0	–
Crystal Farms									
Regular	1 oz	90	0	300	–	0	20	0	–
Tub	2 tbsp	100	0	300	–	0	20	0	–
Whipped	2 tbsp	70	0	400	–	0	20	0	–
Horizon Organic									
Reduced Fat	2 tbsp	70	0	400	–	0	20	0	–
Spreadable	2 tbsp	110	0	400	–	0	20	0	–
Philadelphia									
⅓ Less Fat	1 oz	70	0	300	–	0	20	0	–
Fat Free	1 oz	30	0	400	–	0	150	0	–

CREAM CHEESE SUBSTITUTE
WholeSoy & Co.

FOOD	PORTION	CALS	FIBER	VIT A	FOLIC	VIT C	CALCI	IRON	POTAS
Soy Cream Cheese Organic Original & Flavored	2 tbsp	70	1	0	–	0	10	0	–

CREAM OF TARTAR

FOOD	PORTION	CALS	FIBER	VIT A	FOLIC	VIT C	CALCI	IRON	POTAS
cream of tartar	1 tsp	8	0	0	0	0	0	tr	495

CREPES

FOOD	PORTION	CALS	FIBER	VIT A	FOLIC	VIT C	CALCI	IRON	POTAS
basic crepe unfilled	1 (7 in)	112	tr	190	21	0	46	1	80
Frieda's									
Ready-To-Use	1 (0.5 oz)	30	0	0	–	0	0	0	–

CROAKER

FOOD	PORTION	CALS	FIBER	VIT A	FOLIC	VIT C	CALCI	IRON	POTAS
atlantic breaded & fried	3 oz	188	–	–	–	–	27	1	289
atlantic raw	3 oz	89	0	–	–	–	13	tr	293

CROCODILE

FOOD	PORTION	CALS	FIBER	VIT A	FOLIC	VIT C	CALCI	IRON	POTAS
cooked	3 oz	78	0	15	–	0	9	1	–

CROISSANT

FOOD	PORTION	CALS	FIBER	VIT A	FOLIC	VIT C	CALCI	IRON	POTAS
apple	1 (2 oz)	145	1	–	7	–	17	1	51
cheese	1 (2 oz)	236	2	–	19	–	30	1	76

FOOD	PORTION	CALS	FIBER	VIT A	FOLIC	VIT C	CALCI	IRON	POTAS
plain	1 mini (1 oz)	115	1	–	8	–	10	1	34
plain	1 (2 oz)	232	2	–	16	–	21	1	67
Sara Lee									
Croissant	1 (1.5 oz)	170	1	200	–	0	20	1	–
Petite	2 (2 oz)	230	1	200	–	0	40	1	–
TAKE-OUT									
w/ egg & cheese	1 (4.5 oz)	368	–	1001	47	tr	244	2	174
w/ egg cheese & bacon	1 (4.5 oz)	413	–	472	45	2	151	2	201
w/ egg cheese & ham	1 (5.3 oz)	474	–	451	46	11	144	2	272
w/ egg cheese & sausage	1 (5.6 oz)	523	–	422	43	tr	144	3	283

CROUTONS

FOOD	PORTION	CALS	FIBER	VIT A	FOLIC	VIT C	CALCI	IRON	POTAS
plain	1 cup (1 oz)	122	2	0	7	0	23	1	37
seasoned	1 cup (1.4 oz)	186	2	–	16	–	38	1	72
Cardini's									
Italian	2 tbsp	30	0	0	–	0	0	0	–
Pepperidge Farm									
Whole Grain Caesar	6	35	0	–	–	–	–	–	–
Whole Grain Seasoned	6	30	tr	–	–	–	–	–	–
Rothbury Farms									
Seasoned	2 tbsp	30	0	0	–	0	0	tr	–

CUCUMBER

FOOD	PORTION	CALS	FIBER	VIT A	FOLIC	VIT C	CALCI	IRON	POTAS
fresh peeled	1 med (7 oz)	24	1	145	28	6	28	tr	273
fresh sliced	1 cup	14	1	86	17	4	17	tr	162
fresh w/ peel sliced	½ cup	34	tr	55	4	2	8	tr	76
Chiquita									
Cucumber	⅓ med (3.5 oz)	15	1	200	–	6	20	tr	–
Frieda's									
Japanese	⅔ cup	10	1	200	–	5	0	0	–
Seedless Hothouse	⅔ cup	110	1	200	–	5	0	0	–

FOOD	PORTION	CALS	FIBER	VIT A	FOLIC	VIT C	CALCI	IRON	POTAS
TAKE-OUT									
cucumber & onion salad w/ vinegar	1 cup	52	1	25	10	4	22	tr	196
cucumber salad w/ oil & vinegar	1 cup	183	1	30	10	4	21	tr	176
cucumber salad w/ sour cream dressing	1 cup	68	1	255	17	4	45	tr	184
kimchee	½ cup (1.8 oz)	36	tr	158	6	6	10	tr	79
tzatziki	½ cup (3.4 oz)	72	1	83	10	3	59	tr	146
CUMIN									
seed	1 tsp	8	–	27	–	tr	20	1	38
CURRANT JUICE									
black currant nectar	7 oz	110	–	tr	tr	60	30	tr	196
red currant nectar	7 oz	108	–	tr	tr	12	14	tr	220
CurrantC									
Black Currant Juice	8 oz	130	0	–	–	108	20	tr	159
CURRANTS									
black fresh	½ cup	36	–	129	–	101	31	1	180
zante dried	½ cup	204	–	52	7	3	62	2	642
Sun-Maid									
Zante	¼ cup	130	2	–	–	–	20	1	310
CURRY									
curry powder	1 tsp	7	1	20	3	tr	10	1	31
A Taste Of Thai									
Curry Paste Green	1 tsp	15	1	0	–	–	0	–	–
Curry Paste Panang	1 tsp	25	0	0	–	–	0	–	–
Curry Paste Red	1 tsp	20	0	0	–	–	0	–	–
Curry Paste Yellow	1 tsp	30	1	0	–	–	0	–	–
Instant India									
Curry Paste Cilantro Garlic	2 tbsp (1 oz)	110	0	0	–	0	0	0	–
Curry Paste Ginger Garlic	2 tbsp (1 oz)	90	0	0	–	0	0	0	–
Patak's									
Curry Paste Biryani	2 tbsp	180	3	0	–	0	0	2	–
Garam Masala Paste	2 tsp	130	0	950	–	0	0	2	–

FOOD	PORTION	CALS	FIBER	VIT A	FOLIC	VIT C	CALCI	IRON	POTAS
Tandoori Paste	2 tbsp	30	1	0	–	0	0	2	–
Vandaloo Paste	2 tbsp	160	0	1250	–	0	0	3	–
Spice Hunter									
Curry Seasoning Salt Free	¼ tsp	0	0	0	–	–	–	–	–

CUSK

FOOD	PORTION	CALS	FIBER	VIT A	FOLIC	VIT C	CALCI	IRON	POTAS
fillet baked	3 oz	106	0	–	–	–	12	1	477

CUSTARD
MIX

FOOD	PORTION	CALS	FIBER	VIT A	FOLIC	VIT C	CALCI	IRON	POTAS
as prep w/ 2% milk	½ cup (4.7 oz)	148	–	296	10	1	197	tr	287
as prep w/ whole milk	½ cup (4.7 oz)	163	–	200	–	1	194	tr	–
flan as prep w/ 2% milk	½ cup (4.7 oz)	135	–	249	3	1	153	tr	194
flan as prep w/ whole milk	½ cup (4.7 oz)	150	–	183	5	1	150	tr	191

READY-TO-EAT
Kozy Shack

FOOD	PORTION	CALS	FIBER	VIT A	FOLIC	VIT C	CALCI	IRON	POTAS
Flan	1 pkg (4 oz)	145	0	200	–	0	129	tr	141

TAKE-OUT

FOOD	PORTION	CALS	FIBER	VIT A	FOLIC	VIT C	CALCI	IRON	POTAS
baked	½ cup (5 oz)	148	–	313	44	1	158	tr	216
flan	½ cup (5.4 oz)	220	–	314	–	1	132	1	185
flan de calabaza	1 piece (3.5 oz)	225	tr	1200	24	3	38	1	186
tocino del cielo heaven's delight	1 cup	856	0	0	85	0	106	2	114
zabaione	½ cup (57.2 g)	135	0	485	24	0	23	1	16

CUTTLEFISH

FOOD	PORTION	CALS	FIBER	VIT A	FOLIC	VIT C	CALCI	IRON	POTAS
steamed	3 oz	134	–	–	–	7	153	9	542

DANDELION GREENS

FOOD	PORTION	CALS	FIBER	VIT A	FOLIC	VIT C	CALCI	IRON	POTAS
fresh cooked	½ cup	17	–	6084	–	9	73	1	121
raw chopped	½ cup	13	–	3920	–	10	52	1	111

FOOD	PORTION	CALS	FIBER	VIT A	FOLIC	VIT C	CALCI	IRON	POTAS
Frieda's									
Dandelion Greens	2 cups	40	3	12000	–	30	150	3	–
DANISH PASTRY									
TAKE-OUT									
cheese	1 (2.5 oz)	266	1	91	43	tr	25	1	70
cinnamon	1 (5 oz)	572	2	34	97	tr	101	3	178
fruit	1 (5 oz)	527	3	72	67	6	65	3	118
lemon	1 (2.5 oz)	263	1	124	11	3	33	1	59
raisin nut	1 (2.3 oz)	280	1	23	54	1	61	1	62
DATES									
deglet noor dried	10	240	–	–	–	–	40	–	–
dried chopped	1 cup	489	–	89	22	0	58	2	1161
dried whole	10	228	–	42	10	0	27	1	541
jujube dried	1 oz	75	2	5	–	4	18	1	149
jujube fresh	1 oz	30	–	tr	–	17	9	tr	80
jujube preserved in sugar	1 oz	91	–	2	tr	tr	7	tr	18
medjool	2–3 (1.4 oz)	120	3	0	–	0	20	tr	–
Earthbound Farm									
Organic Dried	6 (1.4 oz)	120	3	0	–	0	20	tr	–
Frieda's									
Medjool	2–3 (1.4 oz)	120	3	0	–	0	20	tr	–
SunDate									
Fancy Medjool	3	120	3	0	–	0	0	tr	170
Sunsweet									
California Pitted	5 to 6 (1.4 oz)	120	3	0	–	0	20	0	270
DELI MEATS/COLD CUTS									
barbecue loaf pork & beef	1 slice (0.8 oz)	40	0	16	2	0	13	tr	76
beerwurst beef	2 oz	155	1	6	3	tr	15	1	137
beerwurst beef	1 slice (4 in x ⅛ in)	75	–	–	1	3	2	tr	42
berliner pork & beef	1 slice (0.8 oz)	53	0	0	1	0	3	tr	65
blood sausage	1 slice (0.9 oz)	95	0	0	1	0	2	2	10

FOOD	PORTION	CALS	FIBER	VIT A	FOLIC	VIT C	CALCI	IRON	POTAS
bologna beef	1 slice (1 oz)	88	0	20	3	4	9	tr	48
bologna beef low fat	1 slice (1 oz)	57	0	0	1	tr	3	tr	41
bologna beef reduced sodium	1 slice (1 oz)	88	0	0	1	0	3	tr	43
bologna beef & pork	1 slice (1 oz)	87	0	24	2	tr	24	tr	89
bologna beef & pork low fat	1 slice (1 oz)	64	0	0	1	0	3	tr	44
braunschweiger pork	1 slice (1 oz)	92	0	3938	12	0	3	3	56
dutch brand loaf pork & beef	1 slice (1.3 oz)	104	tr	59	5	1	3	tr	82
headcheese pork	1 slice (1.6 oz)	71	0	0	1	0	7	1	14
honey loaf pork & beef	1 slice (1 oz)	35	0	0	2	8	5	tr	96
lebanon bologna beef	2 slices (1 oz)	105	0	22	3	1	11	1	188
mortadella beef & pork	1 slice (0.5 oz)	47	0	0	0	0	3	tr	24
olive loaf pork	2 slices (2 oz)	134	0	114	1	0	62	tr	169
pastrami beef	1 slice (1 oz)	41	tr	187	2	tr	3	1	66
peppered loaf pork & beef	1 slice (1 oz)	41	0	0	1	0	15	tr	110
pepperoni pork & beef	15 slices (1 oz)	135	tr	0	2	tr	6	tr	91
picnic loaf pork & beef	1 slice (1 oz)	65	0	0	1	0	13	tr	75
salami cooked beef & pork	1 slice (0.8 oz)	58	0	0	0	0	3	1	46
salami hard pork	3 slices (0.9 oz)	14	0	0	1	0	2	tr	102
salami hard pork & beef less sodium	1 slice (1 oz)	113	tr	3	2	tr	27	tr	389
sandwich spread pork & beef	¼ cup	141	tr	52	1	0	7	tr	66

FOOD	PORTION	CALS	FIBER	VIT A	FOLIC	VIT C	CALCI	IRON	POTAS
summer sausage thuringer cervelat	2 oz	203	0	0	1	9	5	1	146
Boar's Head									
Abruzzese Hot & Sweet	1 oz	100	0	0	–	0	0	tr	–
Bologna 25% Lowered Sodium	2 oz	150	0	0	–	0	0	1	–
Bologna Beef	2 oz	150	0	0	–	0	0	1	–
Bologna Garlic	2 oz	150	0	0	–	0	0	1	–
Bologna Lebanon	2 oz	100	0	0	–	0	0	1	–
Bologna Pork & Beef	2 oz	150	0	0	–	0	0	1	–
Braunschweiger Lite	2 oz	120	0	11000	–	0	0	5	–
Capocollo Hot & Sweet	1 oz	80	0	0	–	0	0	tr	–
Dutch Loaf	2 oz	150	0	0	–	0	0	tr	–
Liverwurst Smoked	2 oz	170	0	11000	–	0	0	5	–
Mortadella	2 oz	160	0	0	–	0	0	1	–
Olive Loaf	2 oz	130	0	0	–	0	20	1	–
Pastrami	2 oz	70	0	0	–	0	0	2	–
Pickle & Pepper Loaf	2 oz	150	0	0	–	0	0	1	–
Prosciutto	1 oz	60	0	0	–	0	0	0	–
Salami Beef	2 oz	120	0	0	–	0	0	1	–
Salami Cooked	2 oz	130	0	0	–	0	0	1	–
Salami Hard	1 oz	110	0	0	–	0	0	tr	–
Sopressata Hot & Sweet	1 oz	100	0	0	–	0	0	tr	–
Spiced Ham	2 oz	120	0	0	–	0	0	tr	–
Hebrew National									
Bologna Beef	1 slice (1 oz)	80	0	–	–	–	0	tr	–
Bologna Lean Beef	4 slices (2 oz)	90	–	–	–	–	0	1	–
Salami Beef	3 slices (2 oz)	150	0	–	–	–	0	–	–
Salami Lean Beef	4 slices (2 oz)	90	–	–	–	–	0	1	–
Russer									
Turkey Breast Honey Roasted	1 slice (1 oz)	25	0	0	–	0	0	0	–
Sara Lee									
Corned Beef	1 slice (2 oz)	50	0	0	–	15	0	1	–

FOOD	PORTION	CALS	FIBER	VIT A	FOLIC	VIT C	CALCI	IRON	POTAS
Pastrami	2 slices (1.6 oz)	60	0	0	–	0	0	1	–
Salami Genoa	4 slices (1 oz)	110	0	0	–	0	0	1	–
Salami Hard	4 slices (1 oz)	120	0	200	–	0	0	1	–
Wellshire									
Salami Genoa	1 oz	100	0	0	–	0	0	tr	–
Salami Hard	1 oz	100	0	0	–	0	0	tr	–
Sopressata Sliced	1 oz	100	0	0	–	0	0	tr	–
TAKE-OUT									
corned beef brisket	2 oz	90	0	–	–	12	–	2	–

DILL

FOOD	PORTION	CALS	FIBER	VIT A	FOLIC	VIT C	CALCI	IRON	POTAS
seed	1 tsp	6	–	1	–	–	32	tr	25
sprigs fresh	1 cup	4	–	0	13	–	18	–	66
sprigs fresh	5	0	–	–	1	–	2	–	7
weed dry	1 tsp	3	–	–	–	–	18	tr	33

DINNER

FOOD	PORTION	CALS	FIBER	VIT A	FOLIC	VIT C	CALCI	IRON	POTAS
Birds Eye									
Voila! Pasta Primavera w/ Chicken	1⅔ cups	250	7	100	–	9	40	1	–
Voila! Shrimp Scampi	1¾ cups	190	3	300	–	15	40	2	–
Voila! Southwestern Chicken	2 cups	250	2	1000	–	21	100	1	–
Boston Market									
Glazed Rotisserie Chicken w/ Mashed Potatoes Gravy Vegetables	1 pkg (16 oz)	390	4	4500	–	12	100	1	–
Meatloaf w/ Mashed Potatoes & Gravy	1 pkg (16 oz)	880	3	300	–	0	150	3	–
C&W									
Stir Fry Feast Pot Sticker + Sauce	2 cups	200	4	2500	–	36	60	3	–
Stir Fry Feast Ultimate + Sauce	1½ cups	190	3	3000	–	15	40	2	–
Contessa									
Beef Goulash not prep	1¾ cups	210	3	3000	–	15	40	3	–

FOOD	PORTION	CALS	FIBER	VIT A	FOLIC	VIT C	CALCI	IRON	POTAS
Chicken Cacciatore not prep	1¾ cups	230	6	1000	–	36	40	1	–
Chicken Alfredo not prep	1¾ cups	330	2	1000	–	24	100	2	–
Fantastic									
Ginger Shitake w/ Rice Noodles	1 pkg (7.4 oz)	340	4	1000	–	5	80	2	–
Glory									
Savory Singles Chicken & Dumplings	1 pkg	290	6	0	–	1	60	3	–
Savory Singles Chicken Smoked Sausage & Rice Casserole	1 pkg	440	1	0	–	1	60	3	–
Savory Singles Ham & Sausage Jambalaya	1 pkg	400	2	300	–	12	60	3	–
Savory Singles Turkey & Gravy w/ Cornbread Stuffing	1 pkg	440	2	100	–	2	60	3	–
Golden Cuisine									
Beef Stew	1 pkg	350	9	3606	185	26	112	4	354
Boneless Pork Patty	1 pkg	504	13	13370	245	42	159	4	399
Breaded Baked Fish w/ Rice Pilaf	1 pkg	300	6	6262	119	37	58	2	280
Chicken Cacciatore	1 pkg	417	10	826	230	26	152	3	252
Chicken & Noodles	1 pkg	331	8	5952	203	17	89	2	411
Chicken Parmesan	1 pkg	430	14	1556	213	51	157	2	310
Chicken w/ Marinara Sauce	1 pkg	329	15	11391	158	21	137	3	430
Meatloaf Patty & Gravy	1 pkg	340	7	3141	157	19	163	3	271
Mesquite Chicken	1 pkg	320	10	7531	123	9	119	3	274
Pot Roast w/ Gravy	1 pkg	343	10	0	158	13	59	3	282
Salisbury Steak & Mushroom Sauce	1 pkg	350	7	900	158	24	111	3	312
Swedish Meatballs	1 pkg	440	9	3466	164	39	106	4	351
Turkey Tetrazzini	1 pkg	304	11	682	173	56	79	2	323
Healthy Choice									
Beef Merlot	1 pkg	240	6	2500	–	0	40	2	1070
Beef Pot Roast	1 pkg	320	6	1250	–	18	20	2	–
Beef Stroganoff	1 pkg	320	6	500	–	18	60	2	–
Beef Teriyaki	1 pkg	310	5	500	–	2	20	1	–

FOOD	PORTION	CALS	FIBER	VIT A	FOLIC	VIT C	CALCI	IRON	POTAS
Beef Tips Portabello	1 pkg	280	3	500	–	12	20	2	–
Blackened Chicken	1 pkg	300	5	500	–	30	20	1	–
Boneless Beef Ribs w/ Classic BBQ Sauce	1 pkg	360	8.	1000	–	0	20	2	1040
Charbroiled Beef Patty	1 pkg	310	6	750	–	4	40	2	–
Cheesy Rice & Chicken	1 pkg	250	4	1250	–	15	200	tr	700
Chicken Carbonara	1 pkg	290	2	0	–	0	100	1	–
Chicken Margherita	1 pkg	340	6	500	–	6	20	2	–
Chicken Parmigiana	1 pkg	320	6	300	–	6	80	2	–
Chicken Breast & Vegetables	1 pkg	260	6	500	–	6	40	1	–
Chicken Broccoli Alfredo	1 pkg	300	2	100	–	12	100	2	–
Chicken Piccata	1 pkg	260	2	500	–	6	20	tr	–
Chicken Teriyaki	1 pkg	270	6	500	–	27	20	1	–
Chicken Tuscany	1 pkg	340	4	750	–	0	60	2	–
Country Breaded Chicken	1 pkg	370	5	1000	–	0	60	1	–
Country Glazed Chicken	1 pkg	230	3	0	–	0	0	tr	–
Country Herb Chicken	1 pkg	280	5	500	–	12	40	1	–
Creamy Herb Roasted Chicken	1 pkg	240	5	1500	–	18	60	1	–
Grilled Basil Chicken	1 pkg	330	5	750	–	0	60	1	–
Grilled Chicken Breast & Pasta	1 pkg	250	4	1250	–	6	100	1	–
Grilled Chicken Breast w/ Mashed Potatoes	1 pkg	190	3	300	–	0	20	1	–
Grilled Chicken Caesar	1 pkg	300	5	2000	–	05	80	1	–
Grilled Chicken Marinara	1 pkg	270	5	400	–	18	80	2	–
Grilled Steak w/ Roasted Garlic Sauce	1 pkg	220	5	400	–	9	40	1	–
Grilled Turkey Breast	1 pkg	250	5	1250	–	30	40	2	–
Grilled Whiskey Steak	1 pkg	280	6	0	–	6	40	3	–
Herb Baked Fish	1 pkg	360	6	500	–	6	20	1	–
Homestyle Chicken & Pasta	1 pkg	250	5	1000	–	1	60	1	–
Honey Glazed Chicken	1 pkg	320	6	1250	–	9	40	1	940

FOOD	PORTION	CALS	FIBER	VIT A	FOLIC	VIT C	CALCI	IRON	POTAS
Lemon Pepper Fish	1 pkg	280	4	500	–	30	20	tr	–
Mandarin Chicken	1 pkg	250	4	1000	–	15	20	1	–
Mesquite Chicken BBQ	1 pkg	300	5	1250	–	6	20	1	–
Mixed Grills Chicken Honey BBQ w/ Dipping Sauce	1 pkg	380	8	500	–	15	80	2	–
Mixed Grills Chicken Honey Mustard w/ Dipping Sauce	1 pkg	360	10	3500	–	6	80	4	–
Mixed Grills Chicken Teriyaki w/ Dipping Sauce	1 pkg	340	9	3500	–	18	100	2	–
Mixed Grills Chicken Tomato Garlic w/ Dipping Sauce	1 pkg	370	10	3500	–	0	60	2	–
Mixed Grills Steak BBQ Sauce	1 pkg	420	7	300	–	6	100	3	–
Mixed Grills Steak Teriyaki w/ Dipping Sauce	1 pkg	350	11	3500	–	30	80	4	–
Mixed Grills Steak w/ Zesty Steak Sauce	1 pkg	350	8	3500	–	6	80	3	–
Oriental Style Beef	1 pkg	310	5	1500	–	12	20	2	–
Oriental Style Chicken	1 pkg	240	4	1250	–	5	20	1	–
Oven Roasted Beef	1 pkg	280	5	0	–	6	20	2	–
Princess Chicken	1 pkg	310	5	1250	–	0	20	tr	–
Roast Turkey Breast	1 pkg	220	3	1250	–	0	20	tr	–
Roasted Chicken Breast	1 pkg	280	7	1000	–	9	20	2	–
Roasted Chicken Chardonnay	1 pkg	290	4	400	–	6	40	1	–
Salisbury Steak	1 pkg	360	5	500	–	21	80	3	–
Salisbury Steak w/ Red Skin Mashed Potatoes	1 pkg	200	4	0	–	0	40	2	–
Sesame Chicken	1 pkg	260	4	1500	–	12	20	1	–
Slow Roasted Turkey Breast w/ Mashed Potatoes	1 pkg	210	4	0	–	0	20	tr	–
Sweet & Sour Chicken	1 pkg	340	3	1000	–	30	20	1	–
Traditional Meatloaf	1 pkg	300	6	100	–	18	80	2	–

FOOD	PORTION	CALS	FIBER	VIT A	FOLIC	VIT C	CALCI	IRON	POTAS
Traditional Turkey Breast	1 pkg	330	4	4000	–	0	40	2	–
Tuna Casserole	1 pkg	270	5	0	–	0	100	1	–
Ian's									
Chicken Finger Meal Allergen Free	1 pkg (7 oz)	368	3	0	–	9	40	4	–
Chicken Nugget Meal	1 pkg (8 oz)	440	2	100	–	6	0	3	–
Fish Stick Meal	1 pkg (8.4 oz)	480	4	100	–	9	100	5	–
Hamburger Meal	1 pkg (7 oz)	296	3	100	–	6	20	4	–
Pizza Meal	1 pkg (6.7 oz)	340	4	100	–	5	40	1	–
Popcorn Turkey Dog Meal Allergen Free	1 pkg (7 oz)	442	1	0	–	2	20	3	–
Kashi									
Black Bean Mango	1 pkg (10 oz)	340	7	7500	–	60	40	2	430
Lemon Rosemary Chicken	1 pkg (10 oz)	330	5	100	–	60	40	2	360
Lime Cilantro Shrimp	1 pkg (10 oz)	250	6	6000	–	5	60	2	300
Southwest Style Chicken	1 pkg (10 oz)	240	6	300	–	24	40	3	540
Sweet & Sour Chicken	1 pkg (10 oz)	320	6	300	–	42	60	2	600
Lean Cuisine									
Cafe Classics Baked Chicken Florentine	1 pkg (8 oz)	200	3	4500	–	15	200	1	820
Cafe Classics Baked Lemon Pepper Fish	1 pkg (9 oz)	220	7	500	–	18	200	1	700
Cafe Classics Beef Peppercorn	1 pkg (8.75 oz)	220	3	400	–	12	100	1	890
Cafe Classics Beef Portabello	1 pkg (9 oz)	200	2	0	–	0	60	1	1080
Cafe Classics Beef Pot Roast	1 pkg (9 oz)	190	2	500	–	0	60	1	850

FOOD	PORTION	CALS	FIBER	VIT A	FOLIC	VIT C	CALCI	IRON	POTAS
Cafe Classics Bowl Creamy Basil Chicken	1 pkg (10.5 oz)	310	3	1000	–	12	150	2	490
Cafe Classics Bowl Grilled Chicken Caesar	1 pkg (9 oz)	270	3	500	–	15	100	1	400
Cafe Classics Chicken Carbonara	1 pkg (9 oz)	280	2	200	–	4	100	1	650
Cafe Classics Chicken & Vegetables	1 pkg (10.5 oz)	240	2	1250	–	2	150	2	630
Cafe Classics Chicken L'Orange	1 pkg (9 oz)	230	2	2000	–	12	20	tr	380
Cafe Classics Chicken Marsala	1 pkg (8.1 oz)	140	3	2000	–	2	40	1	200
Cafe Classics Chicken Parmesan	1 pkg (10.9 oz)	280	3	500	–	12	150	1	830
Cafe Classics Chicken Tuscan	1 pkg	300	5	1000	–	4	60	3	620
Cafe Classics Chicken w/ Almonds	1 pkg (8.5 oz)	260	3	100	–	5	40	1	330
Cafe Classics Chicken w/ Basil Cream Sauce	1 pkg (8.5 oz)	270	2	300	–	12	100	1	310
Cafe Classics Fiesta Grilled Chicken	1 pkg (9.5 oz)	250	3	400	–	24	100	1	520
Cafe Classics Garlic Beef & Broccoli	1 pkg (9 oz)	170	3	4500	–	27	80	1	530
Cafe Classics Glazed Chicken	1 pkg (8.5 oz)	220	2	0	–	2	20	1	500
Cafe Classics Glazed Turkey Tenderloins	1 pkg (9 oz)	260	4	4500	–	0	100	1	540
Cafe Classics Grilled Chicken	1 pkg (9.4 oz)	160	4	1000	–	42	40	1	540
Cafe Classics Grilled Chicken w/ Teriyaki Glaze	1 pkg (10 oz)	270	0	1250	–	2	20	1	510
Cafe Classics Herb Roasted Chicken	1 pkg (8 oz)	190	3	300	–	24	60	1	790
Cafe Classics Honey Dijon Grilled Chicken	1 pkg (8 oz)	220	2	300	–	5	60	1	660

FOOD	PORTION	CALS	FIBER	VIT A	FOLIC	VIT C	CALCI	IRON	POTAS
Cafe Classics Honey Mustard Chicken	1 pkg (8 oz)	250	1	750	–	0	60	tr	370
Cafe Classics Honey Roasted Pork	1 serv (9.5 oz)	230	5	3500	–	5	60	1	370
Cafe Classics Mandarin Chicken	1 pkg (9 oz)	270	2	1500	–	4	40	2	290
Cafe Classics Meatloaf w/ Gravy & Whipped Potatoes	1 pkg (9.4 oz)	280	3	0	–	0	80	3	850
Cafe Classics Orange Peel Chicken	1 pkg (12 oz)	390	3	2250	–	15	80	1	430
Cafe Classics Oven Roasted Beef	1 pkg (9.25 oz)	210	2	500	–	18	150	1	760
Cafe Classics Roasted Garlic Chicken	1 pkg (8.8 oz)	200	2	2500	–	6	150	1	530
Cafe Classics Roasted Turkey & Vegetables	1 pkg (8 oz)	150	3	500	–	6	60	1	510
Cafe Classics Roasted Turkey Breast	1 pkg (12 oz)	280	4	200	–	0	100	1	780
Cafe Classics Roasted Turkey Breast w/ Dressing	1 pkg (9.75 oz)	270	3	0	–	54	40	1	360
Cafe Classics Salisbury Steak	1 pkg (12.5 oz)	310	8	2000	–	0	100	4	1470
Cafe Classics Salisbury Steak w/ Mac & Cheese	1 pkg (9.5 oz)	280	3	0	–	0	100	3	750
Cafe Classics Sesame Chicken	1 pkg (9 oz)	330	2	100	–	1	40	1	250
Cafe Classics Southern Beef Tips	1 pkg (8.75 oz)	250	3	400	–	5	40	1	1130
Cafe Classics Steak Tips Portabello	1 pkg (7.5 oz)	180	3	750	–	24	40	1	520
Cafe Classics Steak Tips Dijon	1 pkg (12 oz)	320	5	750	–	15	150	4	1040
Cafe Classics Stuffed Cabbage	1 pkg (9.5 oz)	200	4	100	–	0	80	1	710
Cafe Classics Swedish Meatballs	1 pkg (9.1 oz)	290	2	0	–	0	100	2	570

FOOD	PORTION	CALS	FIBER	VIT A	FOLIC	VIT C	CALCI	IRON	POTAS
Cafe Classics Sweet & Sour Chicken	1 pkg (10 oz)	290	1	1500	–	6	20	tr	710
Cafe Classics Three Cheese Chicken	1 pkg (8 oz)	230	2	1250	–	24	150	1	590
Comfort Classics Baked Chicken	1 pkg (8.6 oz)	230	2	200	–	0	60	1	600
Dinnertime Selects Balsamic Glazed Chicken	1 pkg (12 oz)	400	4	500	–	54	100	2	510
Dinnertime Selects Chicken Florentine	1 pkg (13.25 oz)	420	6	3500	–	0	350	2	700
Dinnertime Selects Chicken Portabello	1 pkg (12 oz)	370	3	1250	–	15	40	1	580
Dinnertime Selects Lemon Garlic Shrimp	1 pkg (12 oz)	350	5	1000	–	24	60	1	420
Skillet Beef Teriyaki & Rice	1 serv	190	2	1750	–	12	20	tr	500
Spa Cuisine Chicken Mediterranean	1 pkg (10.5 oz)	240	6	500	–	9	60	2	730
Spa Cuisine Chicken In Peanut Sauce	1 pkg (9 oz)	280	2	500	–	5	100	2	460
Spa Cuisine Chicken Pecan	1 pkg (9 oz)	260	4	1000	–	5	40	1	440
Spa Cuisine Lemon Chicken	1 pkg (9 oz)	290	1	200	–	6	60	1	300
Spa Cuisine Lemongrass Chicken	1 pkg (9.4 oz)	240	4	2500	–	12	40	1	500
Spa Cuisine Pork w/ Cherry Sauce	1 pkg (8.25 oz)	260	4	400	–	2	40	1	290
Spa Cuisine Rosemary Chicken	1 pkg (8.25 oz)	230	3	2000	–	6	60	1	460
Spa Cuisine Salmon w/ Beef	1 pkg (9.5 oz)	360	5	4500	–	5	150	2	510
Luzianne									
Cajun Creole Dirty Rice	1 serv	160	0	300	–	0	40	1	–
Cajun Creole Etouffee	1 serv	200	1	400	–	2	20	3	–
Cajun Creole Gumbo	1 serv	160	1	200	–	2	20	3	–
Cajun Creole Jambalaya	1 serv	200	1	1000	–	2	20	2	–

FOOD	PORTION	CALS	FIBER	VIT A	FOLIC	VIT C	CALCI	IRON	POTAS
Nature's Choice									
Broccoli Parmesan Alfredo	1 pkg (12 oz)	270	5	1250	–	36	250	3	–
Nature's Entree									
Hearty Stew	1 pkg (12 oz)	290	3	1500	–	2	40	2	–
Tuscany White Bean	1 pkg (12 oz)	330	4	6000	–	9	450	5	–
Pacific Foods									
Beef Steak Stew	1 cup	250	8	1250	–	–	60	5	–
Chicken Stew	1 cup	200	2	1000	–	9	60	1	–
Patak's									
Vegetable Curry w/ Rice Rich Creamy Coconut	1 pkg	400	5	500	–	0	20	1	–
Vegetable Curry w/ Rice Rich Tomato & Onion	1 pkg (10.5 oz)	290	5	300	–	0	20	1	–
Vegetable Curry w/ Rice Tangy Lemon & Cilantro	1 pkg	300	5	1000	–	0	40	1	–
Quorn									
Meat Free Simply Saute Indian	½ pkg	240	9	0	–	0	100	1	–
Meat Free Simply Saute Mexican	½ pkg	340	7	0	–	0	30	1	–
Meat Free Simply Saute Thai	½ pkg	240	8	0	–	0	60	2	–
Savvy Faire									
Baja Jack Scramble	1 pkg (8.2 oz)	370	2	4000	–	21	300	4	–
Braised Beef	1 pkg (9.4 oz)	320	3	3000	–	21	60	4	–
Herb Crusted Chicken	1 pkg (9.7 oz)	430	6	1250	–	42	250	3	–
Seeds Of Change									
Chicken Teriyaki	1 pkg (10 oz)	300	4	1250	–	15	60	2	–
Mushroom Wild Pilaf	1 pkg (11 oz)	350	5	3000	–	9	160	3	–

FOOD	PORTION	CALS	FIBER	VIT A	FOLIC	VIT C	CALCI	IRON	POTAS
Seven Grain Pilaf	1 pkg (11 oz)	390	10	3000	–	12	300	3	–

South Beach Diet

FOOD	PORTION	CALS	FIBER	VIT A	FOLIC	VIT C	CALCI	IRON	POTAS
Beef & Broccoli & Asian Style Noodles	1 pkg	320	9	2000	–	15	60	3	–
Caprese Style Chicken w/ Cauliflower & Broccoli	1 pkg	250	3	750	–	15	200	2	–
Cashew Chicken w/ Sugar Snap Peas	1 pkg	360	8	750	–	9	40	3	–
Chicken Alfredo A La Roma	1 pkg	270	8	2000	–	18	200	2	–
Chicken Basilico w/ Rotini	1 pkg	280	7	1750	–	15	100	2	–
Garlic Herb Chicken w/ Green Beans Almondine	1 pkg	250	4	400	–	6	80	2	–
Garlic Parmesan Chicken w/ Penne	1 pkg	290	8	2000	–	24	150	2	–
Garlic Sesame Beef w/ Cauliflower Sugar Snap Peas & Peppers	1 pkg	250	4	300	–	30	60	3	–
Kung Pao Chicken Breast Strips w/ Peppers & Broccoli	1 pkg	300	5	1500	–	42	60	3	–
Orange Beef Slices & Brown Rice In Sauce w/ Broccoli & Carrots	1 pkg	260	4	1750	–	12	60	3	–
Savory Beef w/ Cheesy Broccoli	1 pkg	240	3	1750	–	15	150	2	–
Savory Pork w/ Pecans & Green Beans	1 pkg	260	4	300	–	9	80	2	–
Szechwan Pork & Asian Noodles In Sauce	1 pkg	270	9	1750	–	6	80	3	–

Tamarind Tree

FOOD	PORTION	CALS	FIBER	VIT A	FOLIC	VIT C	CALCI	IRON	POTAS
Alu Chole	1 pkg (9.25 oz)	320	7	500	0	6	80	4	430
Channa Dal Masala	1 pkg (9.25 oz)	290	90	4500	8	15	80	4	480

FOOD	PORTION	CALS	FIBER	VIT A	FOLIC	VIT C	CALCI	IRON	POTAS
Dal Makhani	1 pkg (9.25 oz)	350	11	750	80	9	100	5	770
Navratan Korma	1 pkg (9.25 oz)	370	7	4500	32	12	100	4	450
Palak Paneer	1 pkg (9.25 oz)	350	8	8500	120	36	200	5	640
Saag Chole	1 pkg (9.25 oz)	330	9	6000	120	27	150	6	830
Vegetable Jalfrazi	1 pkg (9.25 oz)	280	7	5000	40	27	60	3	400

DIP

FOOD	PORTION	CALS	FIBER	VIT A	FOLIC	VIT C	CALCI	IRON	POTAS
spinach sour cream	¼ cup	155	1	7955	29	5	52	1	115
Bravos!									
Salsa	2 tbsp	15	0	0	–	0	0	0	–
Cabot									
Bac'n Horseradish	2 tbsp	50	0	200	–	0	40	0	–
Clam	2 tbsp	50	0	200	–	0	20	0	–
French Onion	2 tbsp	50	0	200	–	0	20	0	–
Ranch	1 tbsp	50	0	200	–	0	40	0	–
Salsa Grande	2 tbsp	50	0	200	–	1	40	0	–
Veggie	2 tbsp	50	0	300	–	0	20	0	–
Eatsmart									
Flame Roasted Salsa Con Queso	2 tbsp	35	–	100	–	1	20	0	–
Garden Style Sweet Salsa	2 tbsp	20	–	200	–	1	20	0	–
Jalapeno & Lime Tres Bean	2 tbsp	25	–	100	–	5	0	tr	–
Guiltless Gourmet									
Black Bean Mild	2 tbsp	30	2	0	–	0	20	1	–
Roasted Red Pepper Salsa	2 tbsp	15	0	100	–	0	20	0	–
Southwestern Grill Salsa	2 tbsp	15	0	100	–	0	20	0	–
Marzetti									
Veggie Fat Free Ranch	2 tbsp	35	0	100	–	1	0	0	–
Veggie Dip Light Veggie	1 pkg (3.25 oz)	170	0	0	–	0	0	0	–
Snyder's Of Hanover									
Three Bean	2 tbsp	25	1	100	–	5	0	tr	–

DOCK

FOOD	PORTION	CALS	FIBER	VIT A	FOLIC	VIT C	CALCI	IRON	POTAS
fresh cooked	3½ oz	20	–	3474	–	26	38	2	321
raw chopped	½ cup	15	–	2680	–	32	29	2	261

DOUGHNUTS

FOOD	PORTION	CALS	FIBER	VIT A	FOLIC	VIT C	CALCI	IRON	POTAS
cake type unsugared	1 (1.6 oz)	198	1	27	4	–	21	1	60
chocolate glazed	1 (1.5 oz)	175	1	–	–	–	89	1	–
chocolate sugared	1 (1.5 oz)	175	1	–	–	–	89	1	–
chocolate coated	1 (1.5 oz)	204	1	–	–	–	15	1	–
creme filled	1 (3 oz)	307	–	–	–	–	22	2	68
french cruller glazed	1 (1.4 oz)	169	–	–	–	–	11	–	32
frosted	1 (1.5 oz)	204	1	–	–	–	15	1	–
honey bun	1 (2.1 oz)	242	1	–	13	–	26	1	65
jelly	1 (3 oz)	289	–	–	–	–	21	2	67
old fashioned	1 (1.6 oz)	198	1	27	4	–	21	1	60
sugared	1 (1.6 oz)	192	1	4	–	–	27	tr	46
wheat glazed	1 (1.6 oz)	162	–	–	–	–	22	1	66
wheat sugared	1 (1.6 oz)	162	–	–	–	–	22	1	66
yeast glazed	1 (2.1 oz)	242	1	–	13	–	26	1	65
Entenmann's									
Crumb	1	260	tr	100	–	0	40	1	–
Frosted Devil's Food	1	310	2	0	–	0	40	1	–
Glazed	1	260	tr	100	–	0	40	1	–
Glazed Popems	4	220	0	200	–	0	40	1	–
Mini Frosted	1 (1 oz)	150	tr	0	–	0	0	tr	–
Plain Old Fashion	1	230	tr	100	–	0	0	1	–
Rich Chocolate Frosted	1	280	1	0	–	0	0	1	–
Snack & Smile									
Mini Donuts Chocolate	6	370	2	500	40	0	20	3	–
Mini Donuts Glazed	6	340	tr	0	40	0	80	1	–
Mini Donuts Powdered Sugar	6	320	1	500	40	0	20	3	–
Super Bakery									
Daily Donut	1 (2.2 oz)	250	tr	750	140	30	150	7	–
Proballs Slam Powdered Baseballs	1 (1.3 oz)	130	0	1000	60	12	80	4	–

DRINK MIXERS

FOOD	PORTION	CALS	FIBER	VIT A	FOLIC	VIT C	CALCI	IRON	POTAS
whiskey sour mix not prep	1 pkg (0.6 oz)	64	–	5	0	1	45	tr	3
whiskey sour mix	2 oz	55	0	14	0	2	1	tr	18

FOOD	PORTION	CALS	FIBER	VIT A	FOLIC	VIT C	CALCI	IRON	POTAS
Baja Bob's									
Pina Colada	4 oz	30	1	0	–	60	0	0	–
DRUM									
freshwater baked	3 oz	130	0	–	–	–	65	1	300
DUCK									
w/ skin roasted	1 cup (4.9 oz)	472	0	294	8	0	15	4	286
w/ skin w/ bone leg roasted	3 oz	184	0	–	–	1	9	2	–
w/ skin w/o bone breast roasted	3 oz	172	0	–	–	2	7	3	–
w/o skin roasted	1 cup (4.9 oz)	281	0	108	14	0	17	4	353
w/o skin w/ bone leg braised	1 cup (6.1 oz)	310	0	–	–	4	17	4	–
w/o skin w/o bone breast broiled	1 cup (6.1 oz)	244	0	–	–	6	16	8	–
wild w/ skin raw	½ duck (9.5 oz)	571	0	–	–	14	12	11	672
wild w/o skin breast raw	½ breast (2.9 oz)	102	0	44	–	5	3	4	222
Maple Leaf Farms									
Breast Filet	4 oz	360	0	100	–	–	–	2	–
Leg Quarters	4 oz	420	0	200	–	–	–	1	–
Orange Breast Filet	4 oz	320	–	100	–	–	–	3	–
DUMPLING									
Kahiki									
Potstickers Chicken	5 (3.3 oz)	230	1	0	–	5	20	2	–
Samosas Coconut Curry Chicken	4 (2.8 oz)	170	1	0	–	5	20	2	–
Traveling Chef									
Potstickers Chicken + Dipping Sauce	5 pieces + 1 tbsp sauce	285	1	1000	–	5	20	2	–
DURIAN									
fresh	3.5 oz	141	–	tr	–	42	12	1	601

FOOD	PORTION	CALS	FIBER	VIT A	FOLIC	VIT C	CALCI	IRON	POTAS
EEL									
fresh cooked	1 fillet (5.6 oz)	375	0	6021	–	–	41	1	555
fresh cooked	3 oz	200	0	3219	–	–	22	1	297
raw	3 oz	156	0	2954	–	–	17	tr	232
smoked	3.5 oz	330	0	–	–	–	–	–	–
EGG									
CHICKEN									
hard or soft cooked	1	77	0	420	22	0	25	1	63
pickled	1	72	0	395	21	0	24	1	59
poached	1	73	0	350	18	0	26	1	66
scrambled plain	2	199	0	836	53	3	54	2	138
sunny side up	2	155	0	770	30	0	46	2	116
white cooked	1	17	0	0	1	0	2	tr	53
yolk cooked	1	55	0	320	19	0	22	tr	19
Crystal Farms									
In Shell Pasteurized	1	70	0	300	–	0	20	1	–
Peeled Hard Cooked	1	70	0	300	–	0	20	tr	–
Davidson's									
Pasteurized Shell Eggs	75	0	–	–	–	–	–	–	–
Egg-Land's									
Extra Large	1 (2 oz)	80	0	400	24	0	20	1	–
Large	1	70	0	300	24	0	20	1	–
Organic Brown	1	70	0	300	–	0	20	1	–
Eggology									
100% Organic Egg Whites	¼ cup	30	0	–	–	–	–	–	–
Gold Circle Farms									
Cage Free	1 large	70	–	300	–	0	20	1	–
Horizon Organic									
Jumbo	1 (2.2 oz)	90	0	400	–	0	40	1	–
Land O Lakes									
Brown Extra Large	1 (2 oz)	80	–	400	–	0	20	1	–
Pete And Gerry's									
Organic	1	70	–	300	–	0	20	1	–
Sunny Fresh									
Eggs ASAP!	2	140	0	500	–	0	40	1	–

FOOD	PORTION	CALS	FIBER	VIT A	FOLIC	VIT C	CALCI	IRON	POTAS
OTHER POULTRY									
duck 100 year old	1 (1 oz)	49	–	305	–	–	18	1	43
duck cooked	1 (2.5 oz)	129	0	675	42	0	45	3	155
duck preserved hard core	1 (1.8 oz)	80	0	100	–	0	0	1	–
duck preserved soft core	1 (1.8 oz)	80	0	500	–	0	0	1	–
duck salted	1 (1 oz)	54	–	190	–	–	34	1	52
goose cooked	1 (5 oz)	265	0	1340	82	0	86	5	301
quail canned	1 (0.3 oz)	14	0	70	6	0	6	tr	12
turkey raw	1 (2.8 oz)	135	0	438	56	0	78	3	112
EGG DISHES									
TAKE-OUT									
deviled	1 half	62	0	250	13	0	15	tr	37
eggs benedict	2	825	2	2620	119	4	182	4	441
omelet cheese	3 eggs	387	0	1675	52	0	342	3	356
omelet mushroom	3 eggs	251	1	1175	50	0	125	3	293
omelet mushroom & onion	3 eggs	294	1	1390	57	1	146	3	326
omelet plain	3 eggs	338	0	1670	64	0	154	3	312
omelet spanish	3 eggs	496	3	2500	79	45	175	3	767
omelet spinach	3 eggs	279	1	2065	108	22	177	4	438
omelet western	3 eggs	355	tr	1205	48	11	127	3	381
salad	½ cup	353	0	800	37	0	46	1	110
scotch egg	1 (4.2 oz)	301	2	180	–	–	60	2	–
tortilla de amarillo omelet w/ plantain	3 eggs	536	3	1055	55	17	64	3	742
EGG ROLLS									
egg roll wrapper fresh	1	83	–	4	5	0	13	1	23
Chun King									
Chicken Mini	6	210	2	100	–	0	20	1	–
Chicken Restaurant Style	1 (3 oz)	190	2	500	–	1	20	1	–
Pork & Shrimp Mini	6	210	2	100	–	0	20	1	–
Shrimp Mini	6	190	2	500	–	0	20	1	–
Shrimp Restaurant Style	1 (3 oz)	180	2	100	–	0	40	1	–
Frieda's									
Egg Roll Wrappers	2 (1.6 oz)	130	1	0	–	0	0	1	–

FOOD	PORTION	CALS	FIBER	VIT A	FOLIC	VIT C	CALCI	IRON	POTAS
Kahiki									
Chicken	1 (3 oz)	160	1	300	–	5	20	tr	–
Chipotle Lime Chicken	1 (3 oz)	170	2	750	–	5	40	1	–
Lemongrass Chicken Stix	3 (2.6 oz)	100	tr	0	–	6	20	1	–
Pork & Shrimp	1 (3 oz)	140	1	1500	–	6	20	tr	–
Vegetable	1 (3 oz)	90	1	750	–	9	20	0	–
La Choy									
Chicken Mini	6	210	2	100	–	0	20	1	–
Chicken Restaurant Style	1 (3 oz)	210	2	500	–	1	20	1	–
Pork Restaurant Style	1 (3 oz)	220	2	300	–	0	20	1	–
Pork & Shrimp Bite Size	12	210	2	100	–	0	20	1	–
Pork & Shrimp Mini	6	210	2	100	–	0	20	1	–
Shrimp Mini	6	190	2	500	–	0	20	1	–
Shrimp Restaurant Style	1 (3 oz)	180	2	200	–	0	40	1	–
Sweet & Sour Chicken Restaurant Style	1 (3 oz)	220	2	100	–	2	20	1	–
Vegetable w/ Lobster Mini	6	190	2	0	–	1	0	1	–
Lean Cuisine									
Cafe Classics Vegetable	1 pkg (9 oz)	310	3	2000	–	9	40	1	230
Loompya									
Lumpia Chicken & Vegetables	2	170	2	400	–	4	20	2	–
Nasoya									
Egg Roll Wrapper	3	170	1	0	–	0	20	2	–
Pagoda									
Sweet & Sour Chicken	1 (2.7 oz)	170	2	1000	–	6	40	1	–
TAKE-OUT									
chicken	1 (3 oz)	140	4	200	–	1	40	2	–
lobster	1 (4.8 oz)	270	6	0	–	2	20	1	–
lumpia vegetable & shrimp	2 (3 oz)	120	2	400	–	2	0	1	–
meat & shrimp	1 (4.8 oz)	320	4	100	–	5	20	1	–
pork & shrimp	1 (5 oz)	300	7	400	–	0	40	2	–
shrimp	1 (3 oz)	170	5	100	–	0	20	1	–

FOOD	PORTION	CALS	FIBER	VIT A	FOLIC	VIT C	CALCI	IRON	POTAS
spicy pork	1 (3 oz)	200	3	400	–	0	20	1	–
vegetable	1 (3 oz)	170	4	750	–	0	20	1	–

EGG SUBSTITUTES
Better'n Eggs
All Whites	¼ cup	30	0	0	–	0	0	0	100
Ham & Cheese	¼ cup	45	0	500	60	0	100	1	–
Original	¼ cup (2 oz)	30	0	400	–	0	100	1	80
Plus	¼ cup	35	0	750	–	0	100	1	100
Three Cheese	¼ cup	45	0	500	60	0	100	1	–

Deb-El
Just Whites	2 tsp	12	0	–	–	–	–	–	–

Egg Beaters
Original	¼ cup	30	0	750	60	0	20	1	–

Fantastic
Tofu Scrambler not prep	1 tbsp	35	1	100	–	1	0	tr	–

Horizon Organic
Liquid Egg	¼ cup	35	0	300	32	0	40	1	–

Land O Lakes
Liquid Egg	¼ cup	30	0	1000	40	0	40	1	–

Quick Eggs
Fat Free Cholesterol Free	¼ cup	30	0	300	40	0	100	1	–

EGGNOG
eggnog	1 qt	1368	–	3576	9	15	1321	2	1678
eggnog	1 cup	342	–	894	2	4	330	1	420
eggnog flavor mix as prep w/ milk	9 oz	260	–	307	12	2	291	tr	369

Farmland
Egg Nog	½ cup	180	0	300	–	0	150	0	–

Hood
Fat Free Sugar Free	1 cup	110	0	500	–	0	300	0	–
Golden	½ cup	180	0	300	–	0	150	0	–
Light	½ cup	140	0	300	–	0	150	0	–

Horizon Organic
Lowfat	½ cup	140	0	400	–	0	200	tr	–

TAKE-OUT
eggnog	1 cup	306	0	690	3	tr	49	tr	93

FOOD	PORTION	CALS	FIBER	VIT A	FOLIC	VIT C	CALCI	IRON	POTAS
EGGNOG SUBSTITUTES									
Silk									
Nog	½ cup	90	0	0	–	0	20	1	–
EGGPLANT									
cubed cooked w/ oil	1 cup	133	5	410	27	3	12	1	240
pickled	½ cup	33	2	34	14	0	17	1	8
slices grilled	1 (2 oz)	36	1	110	7	1	3	tr	64
Celentano									
Eggplant Parmigiana	1 serv (7 oz)	330	5	1250	–	27	100	1	–
Frieda's									
Chinese	⅔ cup (3 oz)	20	2	0	–	1	0	0	–
Japanese Nasu	⅔ cup (3 oz)	20	2	0	–	1	0	0	–
Peloponnese									
Baba Ganoush	2 tbsp	40	1	0	–	0	0	tr	63
Sabra									
Baba Ghanoush	2 oz	50	1	0	–	1	20	1	–
Stonewall Kitchen									
Eggplant Spread	1 tbsp	25	–	–	–	1	–	–	–
TastyBite									
Punjab Eggplant	½ pkg (5 oz)	130	4	0	–	0	50	4	–
TAKE-OUT									
caponata	2 tbsp (1 oz)	30	–	–	–	4	–	–	–
iman bayildi eggplant w/ onion & tomato	1 serv (15.6 oz)	345	2	497	59	29	43	2	773
indian eggplant runi	1 serv	180	1	378	13	15	30	1	527
moussaka	1 serv (9 oz)	372	5	415	46	15	119	3	611
papoutsaki little shoes	1 serv (15.5 oz)	245	1	461	37	12	144	2	669
ELDERBERRIES									
fresh	1 cup	105	–	870	–	52	55	2	406
ELDERBERRY JUICE									
elderberry	7 oz	76	–	–	12	52	10	–	576

FOOD	PORTION	CALS	FIBER	VIT A	FOLIC	VIT C	CALCI	IRON	POTAS
ELK									
roasted	4 oz	215	0	0	12	0	7	6	353
ENERGY BARS									
Activex									
Organic All Flavors	1 (1.6 oz)	200	2	0	–	0	20	2	–
All In One									
All Flavors	1 bar (1.8 oz)	180	5	1250	60	21	350	3	–
Amino Vital									
Fit Apple Pie	1 bar (1.76 oz)	150	2	2510	203	30	303	5	210
Fit Chocolate Peanut	1 bar (1.76 oz)	190	2	2509	203	30	224	5	85
Fit Toasted Nut Cranberry	1 bar (1.76 oz)	180	2	2502	208	32	290	4	70
Atkins									
Advantage Almond Brownie	1 bar (1.6 oz)	220	7	1250	100	15	300	3	330
Advantage Chocolate Coconut	1 bar (1.6 oz)	230	9	1250	100	15	300	3	230
Advantage Chocolate Decadence	1 bar (1.6 oz)	220	11	1250	100	15	300	3	320
Advantage Chocolate Mocha Crunch	1 bar (1.6 oz)	220	10	1250	100	15	350	3	340
Advantage Chocolate Peanut Butter	1 bar (1.6 oz)	240	10	1250	100	15	300	3	260
Advantage Cookies 'N Creme	1 bar (1.6 oz)	220	11	1250	100	15	300	3	230
Advantage S'mores	1 bar (1.6 oz)	220	11	1250	100	15	350	3	190
Attune									
Wellness Chocolate Crisp	1 (0.7 oz)	100	1	0	–	2	200	1	–
Wellness Cool Mint Chocolate	1 (0.7 oz)	100	1	0	–	2	200	1	–
Balance									
Big Bar Honey Peanut	1 bar	310	tr	3500	140	90	150	6	180
Chocolate Banana + Antioxidants	1 bar	200	1	5000	100	120	100	5	95

FOOD	PORTION	CALS	FIBER	VIT A	FOLIC	VIT C	CALCI	IRON	POTAS
Chocolate Mint + Antioxidants	1 bar	200	0	5000	100	120	100	5	80
Gold Caramel Nut Blast	1 bar	210	tr	2500	100	60	100	5	115
Gold Chocolate Peanut Butter	1 bar	210	tr	2500	100	60	100	5	125
Gold Rocky Road	1 bar	210	1	2500	100	60	100	5	135
Gold Triple Chocolate Chaos	1 bar	200	tr	2500	100	60	100	5	90
Gold Crunch Chocolate Chocolate	1 bar	210	tr	2500	100	60	100	5	105
Gold Crunch Chocolate Mint Cookie	1 bar	210	tr	2500	100	60	100	5	90
Gold Crunch S'mores	1 bar	210	0	2500	100	60	100	5	100
Honey Peanut + Ginseng	1 bar	200	tr	2500	100	60	100	5	110
Lemon Meringue + Calcium	1 bar	190	0	2500	100	60	400	5	80
Original Almond Brownie	1 bar	200	2	2500	100	60	100	5	220
Original Chocolate	1 bar	200	tr	2500	100	60	100	5	160
Original Chocolate Raspberry Fudge	1 bar	200	1	2500	100	60	100	5	170
Original Honey Peanut	1 bar	200	tr	2500	100	60	100	5	115
Original Mocha Chip	1 bar	200	tr	2500	100	60	100	5	70
Original Peanut Butter	1 bar	200	1	2250	100	60	100	5	130
Original Yogurt Honey Peanut	1 bar	200	tr	2500	100	60	100	5	150
Outdoor Chocolate Crisp	1 bar	200	3	–	–	–	80	3	260
Outdoor Crunchy Peanut	1 bar	200	2	–	–	–	80	1	250
Outdoor Honey Almond	1 bar	200	3	–	–	–	100	1	250
Outdoor Nut Berry	1 bar	200	2	–	–	–	100	1	250
Satisfaction Apple Cinnamon Oatmeal	1 bar	280	6	2500	100	60	150	5	140
Satisfaction Chocolate Crisp	1 bar	280	6	2500	100	60	150	5	210

FOOD	PORTION	CALS	FIBER	VIT A	FOLIC	VIT C	CALCI	IRON	POTAS
Satisfaction Chocolate Peanut	1 bar	280	6	2500	100	60	150	5	120
Satisfaction Peanut Butter Crisp	1 bar	280	6	2500	100	60	150	5	140
Yogurt Berry + Antioxidants	1 bar	200	0	5000	100	120	100	5	160
Be Natural									
Almond & Apricot	1 bar	218	4	0	–	1	40	1	–
Almond & Coconut	1 bar	248	1	0	–	0	60	1	–
Banana & Wheat Bran	1 bar	201	4	0	–	0	0	1	–
Fruit & Nut Delight	1 bar	225	3	0	–	0	40	1	–
Macadamia & Apricot	1 bar	224	3	0	–	0	10	1	–
Nut Delight	1 bar	266	3	0	–	0	50	1	–
Sesame Nut Split	1 bar	256	2	0	–	0	40	1	–
Walnut & Date	1 bar	147	1	0	–	0	10	1	–
Yogurt Coated Almond & Apricot	1 bar	233	2	0	–	0	90	1	–
Yogurt Coated Fruit & Nut	1 bar	190	1	100	–	0	60	tr	–
Belly-bar									
Baby Needs Chocolate	1 bar	170	2	750	800	21	250	18	–
Berry Nutty Cravings	1 bar	170	2	750	800	21	250	18	35
Mellow Oat	1 bar	180	2	750	800	21	250	18	40
Boomi Bar									
Almond Protein Plus	1	270	4	0	–	0	110	1	–
Cashew Almond Delicacy	1	260	1	0	16	9	60	2	250
Cranberry Apple	1	210	4	0	–	1	60	1	–
Merry Macadamia	1	220	3	0	–	2	80	–	–
Pistachio Pineapple	1	200	3	200	–	6	20	1	–
Boost									
Chocolate Crunch	1 bar (1.5 oz)	190	tr	750	60	9	150	1	105
Bora Bora									
Organic Cranberry Crunch	1 (1.4 oz)	170	2	0	–	0	20	1	–
Organic Peanut Peanut	1 (1.4 oz)	230	2	0	–	0	0	1	–
Organic Sesame Raisin	1 (1.4 oz)	170	3	0	–	0	10	2	–

FOOD	PORTION	CALS	FIBER	VIT A	FOLIC	VIT C	CALCI	IRON	POTAS
Carb Options									
Chocolate Chip	1 bar	200	tr	1750	140	21	300	3	400
Chocolate Peanut	1 bar	200	tr	1750	140	21	300	3	400
Cinnamon Delight	1 bar	200	0	1750	60	21	300	3	400
CarbWise									
Chocolate S'Mores Crunch	1 bar	240	1	1250	120	15	250	3	40
Centrum									
Energy Chocolate Nougat	1 (1.98 oz)	220	tr	1250	40	1	300	5	135
Energy Chocolate Peanut Butter	1 (1.98 oz)	220	tr	1250	40	1	300	5	135
Choice									
Berry Almond Crispy	1 bar	50	0	–	–	60	100	–	15
Fudge Brownie	1 bar	140	3	750	60	30	150	4	105
Peanut Butter Crispy	1 bar	60	tr	–	–	–	60	–	30
Peanutty Chocolate	1 bar	140	3	750	60	30	150	4	105
Clif									
Banana Nut Bread	1 bar (2.4 oz)	250	5	1500	80	60	250	5	310
Builders Chocolate Mint	1 bar (2.4 oz)	270	4	1500	80	60	250	5	200
Builders Peanut Butter	1 bar (2.4 oz)	270	4	1500	80	60	250	5	210
Carrot Cake	1 bar (2.4 oz)	240	5	1500	80	60	250	5	250
Chocolate Brownie	1 bar (2.4 oz)	240	5	1500	80	60	250	5	370
Chocolate Chip	1 bar (2.4 oz)	250	5	1500	80	60	250	5	250
Cool Mint Chocolate	1 bar (2.4 oz)	250	5	1500	80	60	250	5	240
Crunchy Peanut Butter	1 bar (2.4 oz)	250	5	1500	80	60	250	5	230
Mojo Mixed Nuts	1 bar (1.6 oz)	220	3	0	–	0	40	1	–
Mojo Mountain Mix	1 bar (1.6 oz)	200	2	0	–	0	40	1	–
Nectar Cinnamon Pecan	1 bar (1.6 oz)	170	6	0	–	0	20	1	205

FOOD	PORTION	CALS	FIBER	VIT A	FOLIC	VIT C	CALCI	IRON	POTAS
Nectar Lemon Vanilla Cashew	1 bar (1.6 oz)	180	6	100	–	0	20	1	310
Oatmeal Raisin Walnut	1 bar (2.4 oz)	240	5	1500	80	60	250	5	310
ZBar Peanut Butter	1 bar (1.3 oz)	140	3	300	80	21	300	2	160
Deliciously Slim									
Chocolate Fudge Cake	1 bar (2.1 oz)	200	tr	750	60	9	100	4	100
DrSoy									
Double Chocolate	1 bar (1.76 oz)	180	1	5000	400	60	350	18	80
Ensure									
All Flavors	1 bar (2.1 oz)	230	1	1250	–	30	300	4	–
Fast Fuel Up									
Natural Chocolate Espresso	1 bar (2.3 oz)	300	3	0	–	1	40	2	–
Natural Chocolate Crunch	1 bar (2.3 oz)	300	3	0	–	1	40	2	–
Organic Chocolate Espresso	1 bar (1.8 oz)	230	2	0	–	0	20	1	–
Organic Chocolate Crunch	1 bar (1.8 oz)	230	2	0	–	0	20	1	–
Gatorade									
All Flavors	1 bar (2.3 oz)	260	2	750	–	18	20	1	–
GeniSoy									
Soy Protein Arctic Frost Crispy Chocolate Mint	1 bar (2.2 oz)	230	2	1250	400	15	250	5	290
Soy Protein Dutch Crunch Sour Apple Crisp	1 bar (2.2 oz)	230	1	1250	400	15	250	5	160
Soy Protein Fair Trade Arabica Cafe Mocha Fudge	1 bar (2.2 oz)	220	1	1250	400	15	250	5	200
Soy Protein New York Style Blueberry Cheesecake	1 bar (2.2 oz)	220	1	1250	400	15	250	5	130

FOOD	PORTION	CALS	FIBER	VIT A	FOLIC	VIT C	CALCI	IRON	POTAS
Soy Protein Obsession Fudge Cookies & Cream	1 bar (2.2 oz)	230	2	1250	400	15	250	5	170
Soy Protein Pure Golden Honey Creamy Peanut Yogurt	1 bar (2.2 oz)	230	1	1250	400	15	250	5	200
Soy Protein Southern Style Chunky Peanut Butter Fudge	1 bar (2.2 oz)	240	1	1250	400	15	250	5	270
Soy Protein Ultimate Chocolate Fudge Brownie	1 bar (2.2 oz)	230	2	1250	400	15	250	5	250
Xtreme Carrot Cake Quake	1 bar (1.6 oz)	190	1	1250	100	15	150	5	150
Xtreme Peanut Butter Fix	1 bar (1.6 oz)	200	2	1250	100	15	200	5	190
Xtreme Raspberry Rush	1 bar (1.6 oz)	190	2	1250	100	15	100	5	190
Xtreme Rocky Roadtrip	1 bar (1.6 oz)	190	2	1250	100	15	150	5	180
Glucerna									
All Flavors	1 bar (1.3 oz)	140	4	750	–	60	250	3	60
Gnu									
Flavor & Fiber Banana Walnut	1 (1.4 oz)	130	12	200	–	3	30	1	–
Flavor & Fiber Orange Cranberry	1 (1.4 oz)	130	12	150	–	4	40	1	–
Hansen's									
Chocolate Banana Crunch	1 bar	180	2	5000	–	60	20	1	–
Chocolate Orchard Crunch	1 bar	170	2	5000	–	60	20	1	–
Natural Bar Tropical Fruit Crunch	1 bar	170	1	5000	–	60	20	1	–
Natural Bar Yogurt Strawberry Crunch	1 bar	190	1	5000	–	60	20	1	–

FOOD	PORTION	CALS	FIBER	VIT A	FOLIC	VIT C	CALCI	IRON	POTAS
Hi-Lo									
Chocolate Caramel	1 bar (1.76 oz)	200	0	1000	80	12	100	tr	–
Chocolate Mint	1 bar (2.1 oz)	200	tr	650	60	9	100	4	90
Chocolate Peanut Butter	1 bar (2.1 oz)	210	0	750	60	9	100	4	80
Chocolate Raspberry	1 bar (2.1 oz)	200	tr	750	60	9	100	4	100
Hooah!									
Chocolate Crisp	1 bar (2.29 oz)	280	2	–	200	21	40	2	180
Ideal									
Mixed Berry Tart	1 bar (1.7 oz)	200	0	1250	120	15	300	1	20
Kashi									
GoLean Chocolate Almond Toffee	1 (2.7 oz)	290	6	0	–	0	80	2	250
GoLean Cookies 'N Cream	1 (2.7 oz)	290	6	0	–	0	80	1	250
GoLean Crunchy Chocolate Peanut	1 (1.8 oz)	180	6	0	100	9	200	2	–
GoLean Malted Chocolate Chip	1 (2.7 oz)	290	6	200	–	1	80	1	270
GoLean Oatmeal Raisin Cookie	1 (2.7 oz)	280	6	0	–	0	100	1	250
GoLean Peanut Butter & Chocolate	1 (2.7 oz)	290	6	0	–	0	80	2	250
GoLean Roll Caramel Peanut	1 (1.9 oz)	200	6	0	100	9	200	2	120
TLC Chewy Granola Cherry Dark Chocolate	1 (1.2 oz)	120	4	0	–	0	0	1	–
TLC Crunchy Granola Honey Toasted 7 Grain	1 (1.4 oz)	180	4	0	–	0	0	1	–
TLC Crunchy Granola Pumpkin Spice	1 (1.4 oz)	180	4	0	–	0	0	1	–
TLC Crunchy Granola Roasted Almond	1 (1.4 oz)	180	4	0	–	0	0	1	–

FOOD	PORTION	CALS	FIBER	VIT A	FOLIC	VIT C	CALCI	IRON	POTAS
LaraBar									
Apple Pie	1	190	4	0	8	1	60	1	270
Banana Cookie	1	210	5	0	8	0	60	1	450
Cashew Cookie	1	230	3	0	24	0	20	2	290
Cherry Pie	1	190	4	400	–	0	80	2	240
Chocolate Coconut Chew	1	220	5	0	16	0	60	1	340
Cocoa Mule	1	200	5	200	8	0	60	1	350
Ginger Snap	1	220	5	0	8	0	60	1	340
Lean Body For Her									
Chocolate Honey Peanut	1 bar (1.76 oz)	190	tr	2500	200	30	250	7	150
Living Harvest									
Organic Hemp Protein Forbidden Fruit	1 (1.6 oz)	170	4	0	–	1	20	3	–
Luna									
Caramel Nut Brownie	1 bar (1.7 oz)	190	4	1250	400	60	350	6	180
Chai Tea	1 bar (1.7 oz)	180	3	1250	400	60	350	6	115
Dulce De Leche	1 bar (1.7 oz)	180	3	1250	400	60	350	6	160
Iced Oatmeal Raisin	1 bar (1.7 oz)	180	3	1250	400	60	350	6	190
Key Lime Pie	1 bar (1.7 oz)	180	2	1250	400	60	350	6	105
LemonZest	1 bar (1.7 oz)	180	3	1750	400	60	350	6	115
Nutz Over Chocolate	1 bar (1.7 oz)	180	3	1250	400	60	350	6	105
Met-Rx									
Big 100 Gram Bar Peanut Butter	1 bar (3.5 oz)	340	2	4500	400	60	700	9	–
Source/One Chocolate Cheesecake	1 bar (2.1 oz)	160	tr	2250	400	78	600	7	400
Momentum									
Chocolate Caramel Nut	1 bar	150	3	750	120	4	250	2	–
Chocolate Peanut Butter	1 bar	150	2	750	120	4	250	2	–
Double Chocolate	1 bar	150	2	750	120	4	250	2	–

FOOD	PORTION	CALS	FIBER	VIT A	FOLIC	VIT C	CALCI	IRON	POTAS
Mommy Munchies									
Chocolate Mint	1 bar (1.8 oz)	180	5	2500	320	48	500	16	400
Cinnamon Bun	1 bar (1.8 oz)	180	5	2500	320	48	500	16	390
Moto Bar									
Bodacious Banana Split	1 bar	300	6	0	–	0	40	2	–
Charming Cherry Almond	1 bar (2.9 oz)	300	3	0	–	1	20	1	–
Cozy Pumpkin Pie	1 bar	300	6	0	–	0	40	2	–
Jazzy Peanut Butter & Jelly	1 bar	300	4	0	–	0	40	2	–
Kooky Cappuccino	1 bar	300	8	0	–	0	40	1	–
Luscious Lemon Blueberry	1 bar	300	4	0	–	1	20	1	–
Saucy Apple Cinnamon	1 bar	280	6	0	–	0	20	1	–
Zany Cranberry Orange	1 bar	300	4	0	–	0	20	2	–
Nature's Path									
Optimum Blueberry Flax & Soy	1 bar (2 oz)	200	5	0	–	0	250	3	–
Optimum Cranberry Ginger & Soy	1 bar (2 oz)	200	5	0	–	0	250	3	–
Optimum Peanut Butter	1 bar (2 oz)	230	4	100	–	0	250	3	–
Optimum ReBound	1 bar (2 oz)	190	4	100	–	0	250	3	–
New You									
Chocolate Crisp	1 bar (1.65 oz)	180	3	5000	400	100	380	2	90
NuGo									
Banana Chocolate Protein	1 bar	190	3	2000	160	24	300	1	–
Blue Berry Boom	1 bar	180	3	2000	160	24	300	1	–
Chocolate Blast	1 bar	180	3	2000	160	24	300	1	–
Coffee Break	1 bar	180	3	2000	160	24	300	1	–
Orange Smoothie Protein	1 bar	190	1	2000	160	24	300	1	–
Peanut Butter Pleaser	1 bar	180	3	2000	160	24	300	1	–
Nutiva									
Organic Flax & Raisin	1 (1.4 oz)	200	4	0	–	0	80	2	–

FOOD	PORTION	CALS	FIBER	VIT A	FOLIC	VIT C	CALCI	IRON	POTAS
Organic Flaxseed Flax Chocolate	1 (1.4 oz)	200	5	0	–	0	80	3	–
Original Organic Hempseed	1 (1.4 oz)	210	5	0	–	0	0	1	–
Nutribar									
Chocolate Covered Belgian Chocolate	1 bar (2.3 oz)	252	2	2000	140	15	350	6	375
Chocolate Covered Caramel	1 bar (2.3 oz)	261	tr	2000	140	15	350	6	375
Chocolate Covered Chocolate Fudge	1 bar (2.3 oz)	267	2	2000	140	15	350	6	380
Chocolate Covered Hazelnut	1 bar (2.3 oz)	261	1	2000	140	15	350	6	400
Chocolate Covered Mocha Almond	1 bar (2.3 oz)	261	tr	2000	140	15	350	6	375
Chocolate Covered Peanut	1 bar (2.3 oz)	262	1	2000	140	15	350	6	375
Yogurt Covered Peach Apricot	1 bar (2.3 oz)	261	tr	2000	140	15	350	6	375
Yogurt Covered Raspberry	1 bar (2.3 oz)	261	tr	2000	140	15	350	6	375
Yogurt Covered Wildberry	1 bar (2.3 oz)	261	tr	2000	140	15	350	6	375
Oh Mama!									
Chocolate Peanut Butter	1 bar (1.8 oz)	190	3	0	400	60	500	9	–
Frosted White Lemon	1 bar (1.8 oz)	180	3	0	400	60	500	9	–
Frosted White Raspberry	1 bar (1.8 oz)	180	3	0	400	60	500	9	–
Peacekeeper									
Nuts About Peace All Flavors	1 bar (1.4 oz)	180	2	0	–	0	60	1	–
Perfect 10									
Bliss Apricot	1 (1.8 oz)	215	5	1750	–	2	78	2	506
Bliss Cranberry	1 (1.8 oz)	215	4	50	–	2	72	1	256
Natural Apricot	1 (1.8 oz)	205	4	1250	–	2	80	2	506
Natural Cranberry	1 (1.8 oz)	164	4	50	–	2	72	1	238
Natural Lemon	1 (1.8 oz)	210	5	0	–	2	80	1	340

FOOD	PORTION	CALS	FIBER	VIT A	FOLIC	VIT C	CALCI	IRON	POTAS
PermaLean									
Protein Crunch Chocoholic Chocolate	1 bar (1.8 oz)	170	tr	1000	400	90	200	tr	100
Protein Crunch Chocolate Raspberry	1 bar (1.8 oz)	180	0	5000	400	90	200	tr	90
Protein Crunch Stark Raving Peanutz	1 bar (1.8 oz)	180	0	5000	400	90	200	tr	80
PowerBar									
Harvest Apple Cinnamon Crisp	1 bar (2.3 oz)	240	4	0	200	60	150	3	–
Harvest Chunky Cherry Crunch	1 bar (2.3 oz)	240	4	0	200	60	150	3	–
Harvest Dipped Double Chocolate Crisp	1 bar (2.3 oz)	250	3	0	200	60	150	3	–
Harvest Dipped Oatmeal Raisin Cookie	1 bar (2.3 oz)	250	3	0	200	60	500	5	–
Harvest Dipped Toffee Chocolate Chip	1 bar (2.3 oz)	250	3	0	200	60	150	3	–
Harvest Peanut Butter Chocolate Chip	1 bar (2.3 oz)	240	4	0	200	60	150	3	–
Harvest Strawberry Crunch	1 bar (2.3 oz)	230	4	0	200	60	150	3	–
Performance Apple Cinnamon	1 bar (2.3 oz)	230	3	0	400	60	300	6	125
Performance Banana	1 bar (2.3 oz)	230	3	0	400	60	300	6	190
Performance Cappuccino	1 bar (2.3 oz)	230	3	0	400	60	300	6	115
Performance Chocolate	1 bar (2.3 oz)	230	3	0	400	60	300	6	200
Performance Chocolate Peanut Butter	1 bar (2.3 oz)	240	3	0	400	60	300	6	170
Performance Cookies & Cream	1 bar (2.3 oz)	240	2	0	400	60	300	6	170
Performance Malt Nut	1 bar (2.3 oz)	230	3	0	400	60	300	6	110
Performance Oatmeal Raisin	1 bar (2.3 oz)	230	3	0	400	60	300	6	160

FOOD	PORTION	CALS	FIBER	VIT A	FOLIC	VIT C	CALCI	IRON	POTAS
Performance Peanut Butter	1 bar (2.3 oz)	230	3	0	400	60	300	6	130
Performance Strawberry Cream	1 bar (2.3 oz)	230	2	0	400	60	300	6	105
Performance Vanilla Crisp	1 bar (2.3 oz)	230	3	0	400	60	300	6	110
Performance Wild Berry	1 bar (2.3 oz)	230	3	0	400	60	300	6	110
Protein Plus Carb Select Chocolate	1 bar (2.5 oz)	260	1	0	120	27	200	4	–
Protein Plus Carb Select Chocolate Caramel Crunch	1 bar (2.6 oz)	270	2	0	120	36	200	3	–
Protein Plus Carb Select Chocolate Peanut Butter	1 bar (2.5 oz)	270	2	0	100	27	200	3	–
Protein Plus Carb Select Peanut Caramel	1 bar (2.6 oz)	270	1	0	120	36	200	3	–
Protein Plus Chocolate Fudge Brownie	1 bar (2.7 oz)	270	2	0	400	60	400	8	–
Protein Plus Chocolate Peanut Butter	1 bar (2.7 oz)	290	1	0	400	60	400	8	–
Protein Plus Cookies & Cream	1 bar (2.7 oz)	290	1	0	400	60	400	8	–
Protein Plus Vanilla Yogurt	1 bar (2.7 oz)	290	1	0	400	60	450	8	–
Triple Treat Caramel Peanut Crisp	1 bar (1.9 oz)	220	4	0	200	60	150	3	–
Triple Treat Caramel Peanut Fusion	1 bar (1.9 oz)	230	4	0	200	60	150	3	–
Triple Treat Chocolate Caramel Fusion	1 bar (1.9 oz)	230	4	0	200	60	150	3	–
Triple Treat Chocolate Peanut Butter Crisp	1 bar (1.9 oz)	220	4	0	200	60	150	5	–
Prana Bar									
Apricot Goji	1 (1.7 oz)	220	3	750	–	0	40	2	–
Coconut Acai	1 (1.7 oz)	220	3	0	–	0	60	1	–
Pear Ginseng	1 (1.7 oz)	220	4	0	–	0	150	2	–

FOOD	PORTION	CALS	FIBER	VIT A	FOLIC	VIT C	CALCI	IRON	POTAS
Pria									
Carb Select Caramel Nut Brownie	1 bar (1.7 oz)	170	2	750	240	36	300	4	–
Carb Select Chocolate Mocha Crisp	1 bar (1.7 oz)	130	4	750	240	36	300	4	–
Carb Select Chocolate Peanut Butter Crisp	1 bar (1.7 oz)	130	4	750	240	36	300	4	–
Carb Select Cookies N' Caramel	1 bar (1.7 oz)	170	2	750	240	36	300	4	–
Carb Select Peanut Butter Caramel Nut	1 bar (1.7 oz)	170	2	750	240	36	300	4	–
Chocolate Peanut Crunch	1 bar (1 oz)	110	1	750	240	36	300	4	–
Complete Nutrition Chocolate Mint Crisp	1 bar (1.6 oz)	170	5	1000	280	42	400	5	–
Complete Nutrition Chocolate Peanut Butter Crisp	1 bar (1.6 oz)	170	5	1000	280	42	400	5	–
Complete Nutrition French Vanilla Crisp	1 bar (1.6 oz)	170	5	1000	280	42	400	5	–
Creme Caramel Crisp	1 bar (1 oz)	110	1	750	240	36	300	4	–
Double Chocolate Cookie	1 bar (1 oz)	110	1	750	240	36	300	4	–
French Vanilla Crisp	1 bar (1 oz)	110	1	750	240	36	300	4	–
Mint Chocolate Cookie	1 bar (1 oz)	110	1	750	240	36	300	4	–
Strawberry Shortcake	1 bar (1 oz)	110	1	750	240	36	300	4	–
Pure Protein									
Blueberry Cheesecake	1 bar	190	0	2500	200	30	500	tr	130
PureFit									
Almond Crunch	1 (2 oz)	230	3	0	–	0	80	3	180
Peanut Butter Crunch	1 (2 oz)	240	2	0	–	0	60	3	160
Revival									
Soy Apple Cinnamon Celebration	1 bar	200	1	–	–	–	60	3	40
Soy Autumn Frost Low Carb	1 bar	200	1	–	–	–	60	3	40

FOOD	PORTION	CALS	FIBER	VIT A	FOLIC	VIT C	CALCI	IRON	POTAS
Soy Chocolate Raspberry Zing Low Carb	1 bar	200	2	–	–	–	40	3	30
Soy Chocolate Temptation	1 bar	220	tr	–	–	–	40	3	60
Soy Marshmallow Krunch	1 bar	220	tr	–	–	–	40	3	40
Soy Peanut Butter Chocolate Pal	1 bar	240	1	–	–	–	40	3	35
Soy Peanut Butter Pal	1 bar	240	tr	–	–	–	40	3	35
Slim-Fast									
Classic Meal Bar Chocolate Cookie Dough	1 bar	220	2	1750	60	21	300	3	70
Classic Meal Bar Milk Chocolate Peanut	1 bar	220	2	1750	60	21	300	3	160
High Protein Granola Bar Chocolate Chip	1 bar	190	2	780	60	21	300	3	300
High Protein Granola Bar Peanut	1 bar	200	2	750	60	21	300	3	270
Low Carb Breakfast Bar Apple Cobbler	1 bar	180	3	1750	60	21	300	3	340
Low Carb Breakfast Bar Peanut Butter	1 bar	190	3	1750	60	21	300	3	330
Low Carb Snack Bar Caramel Nut	1 bar	120	1	750	60	6	250	3	–
Low Carb Snack Bar Coconut Almond	1 bar	120	2	750	60	9	250	3	–
Low Carb Snack Bar Peanut Butter Crunch	1 bar	120	1	750	60	6	200	3	–
Optima Meal Bar Apple Crisp	1 bar	180	3	750	60	21	300	3	270
Optima Meal Bar Caramel Crispy Peanut	1 bar	220	2	1750	60	21	300	3	400
Optima Meal Bar Chewy Granola Trail Mix	1 bar	210	2	750	60	21	300	3	400
Optima Snack Bar Banana Nut Muffin	1 bar	150	1	750	–	–	250	3	–

FOOD	PORTION	CALS	FIBER	VIT A	FOLIC	VIT C	CALCI	IRON	POTAS
Optima Snack Bar Blueberry Muffin	1 bar	140	1	750	–	–	250	3	–
Optima Snack Bar Chocolate Peanut Nougat	1 bar	120	1	750	60	6	250	3	–
Optima Snack Bar Oatmeal Raisin Cookie	1 bar	120	1	750	–	–	250	3	–
Snickers Marathon									
Chewy Chocolate Peanut	1 (1.9 oz)	210	5	1750	400	60	450	6	120
SoBe									
Milk Chocolate	1 bar (1.75 oz)	240	tr	200	–	–	60	tr	–
Solo GI									
Berry Bliss	1 bar (1.6 oz)	190	3	500	40	6	150	tr	80
Chocolate Charger	1 bar (1.6 oz)	190	4	500	40	6	200	1	170
Mint Mania	1 bar (1.6 oz)	190	4	500	40	6	200	1	170
Peanut Power	1 bar (1.6 oz)	200	3	500	40	6	150	1	160
South Beach Diet									
Meal Replacement Chocolate Crisp	1 bar	210	5	2500	–	60	100	5	–
Meal Replacement Chocolate Peanut Butter	1 bar	210	6	2500	–	60	100	5	–
Meal Replacement Cinnamon & Creme	1	220	5	2500	–	60	100	5	–
Meal Replacement Peanut Crisp	1 bar	210	5	2500	–	60	100	5	–
Meal Replacement Vanilla Creme	1 bar	210	5	2500	–	60	100	5	–
Strive									
Crunchy Chocolate Smores	1 bar (2.1 oz)	200	0	1250	140	15	250	3	–
T.H.E. Bar									
Granola Raisin	1 (1.8 oz)	200	1	1500	–	36	–	–	–

FOOD	PORTION	CALS	FIBER	VIT A	FOLIC	VIT C	CALCI	IRON	POTAS
Zoe's									
Chocolate Delight	1 bar (1.7 oz)	190	5	0	–	0	50	3	235
Chocolate Peanut Butter Bliss	1 bar (1.7 oz)	200	5	0	–	0	20	2	165
Heavenly Apple	1 bar	180	5	0	–	0	30	1	150
Peanut Butter Paradise	1 bar (1.7 oz)	190	5	0	–	0	20	2	150

ENERGY DRINKS

FOOD	PORTION	CALS	FIBER	VIT A	FOLIC	VIT C	CALCI	IRON	POTAS
1In3 Trinity									
Energy Drink	1 can (8.4 oz)	10	0	–	–	60	0	0	–
Accelerade									
All Flavors	8 oz	80	0	0	–	1	0	0	15
Amino Vital									
Amino Acid Supplement All Flavors	8 oz	35	–	–	–	–	20	–	35
Pro Fruit Punch	8 oz	35	–	–	–	–	20	–	35
Pro Tropic Fruit	8 oz	40	–	–	–	–	18	–	35
Puredge All Flavors	8 oz	50	–	–	–	–	29	–	70
Arizona									
Diet Green Tea Energy Drinks	8 oz	10	–	0	–	60	0	0	–
Green Tea Energy Drink	8 oz	100	–	0	–	60	0	0	–
Pomegranate Lite	8 oz	70	–	0	–	30	0	0	–
Balance									
Chocolate as prep w/ 2% milk	1 serv	310	2	3000	120	60	600	5	870
Vanilla as prep w/ 2% milk	1 serv	310	2	3000	120	60	600	5	850
Black Hole									
Citrus	8 oz	110	–	–	–	1	100	–	–
Bliss									
Energy Drink	1 can (8.4 oz)	110	–	–	–	96	–	–	–
Low Carb	1 can (8.4 oz)	26	–	–	–	96	–	–	–
Blox									
Orange Rush	8 oz	103	–	–	–	24	79	–	–

FOOD	PORTION	CALS	FIBER	VIT A	FOLIC	VIT C	CALCI	IRON	POTAS
Boost									
High Protein Vanilla	8 oz	240	0	1250	140	60	330	5	380
Bossa Nova									
Acai Juice Mango	1 bottle (10 oz)	132	1	2000	–	60	30	1	–
Acai Juice Original	1 bottle (10 oz)	138	1	3500	–	102	80	3	–
Acai Juice Passion Fruit	1 bottle (10 oz)	132	1	2000	–	60	30	1	–
Brain Twist									
Flu & Cold Defense All Flavors	8 oz	70	–	–	–	84	–	–	–
Celsius									
All Flavors	1 bottle (12 oz)	10	–	–	–	60	50	–	–
Choice									
Chocolate	1 can (8 oz)	220	3	1250	100	60	350	5	430
Chocolate Fudge Sugar Free	1 pkg (11 oz)	125	9	1000	80	–	250	4	340
French Vanilla Sugar Free	1 pkg (11 oz)	100	6	1000	80	–	250	4	110
Strawberries'n Cream Sugar Free	1 pkg (11 oz)	100	6	1000	80	–	250	4	110
Vanilla	1 can (8 oz)	220	3	1250	100	60	350	5	430
Cintron									
Citrus Mango	8 oz	110	0	–	–	–	–	–	tr
Cytomax									
Sport Drinks All Flavors	1 bottle (20 oz)	130	tr	–	–	66	–	–	75
Defcon3									
Healthy Energy Soda	1 can (12 oz)	45	2	750	–	84	12	–	–
Defense									
Effervescent Supplement	1 can	150	–	1500	–	400	320	–	160
Everlast									
High Energy Citrus Blast	1 can (8.3 oz)	140	–	1000	–	–	–	–	–

FOOD	PORTION	CALS	FIBER	VIT A	FOLIC	VIT C	CALCI	IRON	POTAS
Freedom									
Energy Drink	1 can (12 oz)	160	–	–	–	90	–	–	–
Fuze									
Energize Blackberry Grape	8 oz	100	–	–	–	60	–	–	–
Energize Exotic Punch	8 oz	100	–	–	–	60	–	–	–
Energize Mojo Mango	8 oz	100	–	–	–	60	–	–	–
Essential Cranberry Grapefruit	8 oz	90	–	1250	–	30	–	–	–
Focus Orange Carrot	8 oz	90	–	1250	–	30	–	–	–
Refresh Banana Colada	8 oz	90	–	1250	–	30	250	–	–
Refresh Mixed Berry	8 oz	90	–	1250	–	30	10	–	–
Refresh Peach Mango	8 oz	90	–	1250	–	30	100	–	–
Replenish Agave Cactus	8 oz	90	–	–	–	60	–	–	–
Stamina Grape & Aronia Punch	8 oz	80	–	–	–	60	–	–	–
Vitaboost Citrus Starfruit Punch	8 oz	90	–	5000	–	90	–	–	–
Gatorade									
Nutrition Shake All Flavors	1 can (11 oz)	370	1	1000	–	60	300	4	740
GeniSoy									
Soy Protein Shake Chocolate	1 scoop (1.2 oz)	120	2	1250	100	15	250	5	230
Soy Protein Shake Vanilla	1 scoop (1.2 oz)	130	0	1250	100	15	250	5	70
Soy Protein Shake Strawberry Banana	1 scoop	130	1	1250	100	15	250	5	70
Gleukos									
Preformance All Flavors	8 oz	70	0	–	–	–	–	–	50
Guayaki									
Organic Empower Mint	8 oz	38	tr	–	–	–	–	–	–
Organic Raspberry Revolution	8 oz	50	tr	–	–	–	–	–	–
Organic Unsweetened	8 oz	15	tr	–	–	–	–	–	–
Hansen's									
Energy Kiwi Strawberry	8 oz	120	–	0	–	60	100	0	–
Energy Peach	8 oz	130	–	0	–	60	100	0	–
Energy Punch	8 oz	120	–	0	–	60	100	0	–

FOOD	PORTION	CALS	FIBER	VIT A	FOLIC	VIT C	CALCI	IRON	POTAS
Healthy Start Carrot Orange Antioxidant Blend	8 oz	130	–	7000	–	120	20	tr	–
Healthy Start Cranberry Grape Defense Blend	8 oz	110	–	–	–	60	100	–	–
Healthy Start Tropical Orange Vitamix Blend	8 oz	110	–	5000	–	60	100	–	100
Her Energy									
Pink Lemonade	1 can (8.4 oz)	130	0	0	–	54	<20	0	–
Pink Lemonade Sugar Free	1 can (8.4 oz)	0	0	0	–	54	<20	0	–
High Voltage									
Sugar Free	8 oz	5	–	1250	–	60	–	–	–
Hooah!									
Soldier Fuel All Flavors	1 can (12 oz)	160	–	–	–	30	–	–	–
Hype									
Classic Energy	1 can (8.3 oz)	110	–	1250	100	9	–	–	–
Invigor8									
Energy Boost	1 can	110	1	2500	–	60	100	0	–
Nutrition Boost	1 can	110	1	2500	–	60	100	0	–
Iron Energy									
All Flavors	8 oz	90	–	–	–	60	–	–	65
KaBoom									
All Flavors	8 oz	105	0	0	240	48	0	0	–
Krank'd									
All Flavors	1 bottle (16 oz)	80	–	400	–	16	–	–	44
Liv Natural									
Hydrate Restore	8 oz	70	0	–	–	–	–	–	45
Lolli's Pop									
Cheery Energy Drink	1 bottle	170	–	–	–	60	–	–	–
Passion Stimulating Elixir	1 bottle	140	–	–	–	60	–	–	–
Lost									
Five-O	8 oz	70	–	200	–	12	–	–	–
Monster									
Energy Assault	8 oz	100	–	–	–	60	–	–	–

FOOD	PORTION	CALS	FIBER	VIT A	FOLIC	VIT C	CALCI	IRON	POTAS
Energy Drink	8 oz	100	–	–	–	60	–	–	–
Khaos Energy Juice	8 oz	90	–	300	–	60	30	–	–
Lo Carb	8 oz	10	–	–	–	60	–	–	–
Mr. Re									
Restorative	1 can (11 oz)	80	0	5000	4	60	0	–	–
Natural Ovens									
Ultra Omega Balance	1 tbsp	75	4	250	200	30	50	1	–
Zesty Flax Energy Mix	1 tbsp	40	3	0	40	0	60	1	–
New York Minute									
Energy Drink	1 can (8.4 oz)	130	–	–	100	105	–	–	–
Nitro2Go									
High Energy	1 can	110	–	–	–	60	–	–	–
High Energy Lite	1 can	20	0	–	–	60	–	–	–
NOS									
High Performance	8 oz	110	–	–	100	60	–	–	–
Odwalla									
C Monster	8 oz	150	2	2250	–	600	150	4	–
Femme Vitale	8 oz	130	1	1500	400	180	100	5	360
Glorious Morning	8 oz	130	3	1000	–	282	300	tr	370
Mango Tango	8 oz	150	0	4000	–	60	20	0	–
Mo Beta	8 oz	140	1	25000	–	300	40	1	370
Serious Energy	8 oz	150	1	100	–	9	0	1	–
Strawberry C Monster	8 oz	150	tr	2000	–	600	20	1	330
Super Protein	8 oz	170	2	100	–	90	350	2	460
Superfood	8 oz	140	2	4500	–	36	0	1	440
Wellness	8 oz	150	1	750	–	150	20	tr	350
Peep One									
Erotic Drink	1 can (8.3)	109	–	–	–	–	24	–	10
Pickle Juice									
Sport	8 oz	7	–	–	–	18	–	–	70
Pimpjuice									
Energy Drink	1 can (8 oz)	140	–	–	–	60	–	–	–
PJ Tight	1 can (8 oz)	20	–	–	–	60	–	–	–

FOOD	PORTION	CALS	FIBER	VIT A	FOLIC	VIT C	CALCI	IRON	POTAS
Piranha									
Phunky Fruit Punch	1 can (8.4 oz)	140	0	0	–	0	0	0	–
Pit Bull									
Energy Drink	1 can (8.4 oz)	110	–	–	–	60	–	–	–
Sugar Free	1 can (8.4 oz)	0	0	–	–	60	–	–	–
Rehab									
Recovery Supplement	1 can (12 oz)	150	–	–	–	45	50	–	20
Resurrect									
Daily Detox & Anti-Hangover Elixir	1 can (12 oz)	5	–	–	400	60	–	–	–
Rip It									
Citrus X	8 oz	130	–	–	100	60	–	–	–
Citrus X Sugar Free	8 oz	0	0	–	400	60	–	–	–
Energy Fuel	8 oz	130	–	–	400	60	–	–	–
Energy Lite	8 oz	0	0	–	400	60	–	–	–
Rockstar									
Energy Cola	8 oz	120	–	–	–	60	–	–	–
Energy Drink	8 oz	110	–	–	–	60	–	–	–
Juiced	8 oz	90	0	–	–	60	30	–	–
Ronin									
Diet	1 can (16 oz)	15	–	1250	400	300	40	–	–
Original	1 can (16 oz)	180	–	1250	400	300	40	–	–
Rumba									
Energy Juice	8 oz	120	–	400	–	60	40	tr	100
Slim-Fast									
Classic Ready-To-Drink Creamy Milk Chocolate	1 can	220	5	1750	120	60	400	3	600
Classic Ready-To-Drink French Vanilla	1 can	220	5	1750	120	60	400	3	600
High Protein Ready-To-Drink All Flavors	1 can	190	5	1750	120	60	500	3	550

FOOD	PORTION	CALS	FIBER	VIT A	FOLIC	VIT C	CALCI	IRON	POTAS
Low Carb Diet Ready-To-Drink All Flavors	1 can	190	4	1750	120	60	400	3	550
Snapple A Day									
Meal Replacement All Flavors	1 bottle (11.5 oz)	210	5	5000	240	60	250	3	400
SoBe									
Adrenaline Rush	1 can (8.3 oz)	140	–	–	400	60	–	–	22
Black & Blue Berry Brew	8 oz	120	–	–	–	60	–	–	–
Courage Cherry Citrus	8 oz	110	–	–	–	60	–	–	–
Elixir Cranberry Grapefruit	8 oz	110	–	–	–	60	40	–	–
Elixir Pomegranate Cranberry	8 oz	100	–	–	–	60	40	–	–
Fuerte	8 oz	130	–	–	–	60	–	–	–
Lean Diet Citrus	8 oz	5	–	–	–	60	–	–	–
Long John Lizard's Grape Grog	8 oz	120	–	–	–	60	–	–	–
Power	8 oz	120	–	–	–	60	–	–	–
Synergy All Flavors	1 can (11.5 oz)	120	–	700	–	60	140	–	–
Tsunami	8 oz	110	–	500	–	60	–	–	–
Wisdom	8.5 oz	110	–	–	–	60	–	–	–
Zen Blend	8.5 oz	90	–	–	–	60	–	–	–
Source Burn									
2	8 oz	130	–	1250	–	15	–	–	65
Sugar Free	8 oz	10	0	2500	–	60	–	–	–
Vipa									
Energy Drink	1 can (12 oz)	0	0	0	–	132	0	0	–
Who's Your Daddy									
Original	8 oz	110	–	–	–	60	–	–	–
Wide Open Performance									
Energy Drink	1 can (8.3 oz)	120	–	1250	–	30	–	–	–
Xcyto									
Sugar Free	1 can (12.5 oz)	10	0	0	–	60	–	–	–

FOOD	PORTION	CALS	FIBER	VIT A	FOLIC	VIT C	CALCI	IRON	POTAS
XO									
Balance	8 oz	50	–	500	–	24	>20	–	–
Berry	1 bottle	90	–	–	–	18	–	–	–
Citrus	1 bottle	90	–	–	–	15	–	–	–
Defense	8 oz	40	–	–	–	60	–	–	–
Diet	1 bottle	15	–	–	–	18	–	–	–
Endurance	8 oz	50	–	500	–	36	–	–	–
Energy	8 oz	40	–	1250	–	60	–	–	–
Essential	8 oz	40	–	2500	9	–	20	1	50
Focus	8 oz	40	–	1250	–	60	–	–	–
Grape	1 bottle	90	–	–	–	18	–	–	–
Multi-V	8 oz	40	–	5000	–	60	20	–	–
Original	1 bottle	110	–	–	–	60	–	–	–
Peach	1 bottle	90	–	–	–	18	–	–	–
Power-C	8 oz	40	–	1250	–	150	–	–	–
Rescue	8 oz	40	–	–	–	60	–	–	–
Revive	8 oz	50	–	500	–	36	–	–	–
Stress-B	8 oz	40	–	–	–	36	–	–	–
Vanilla	1 bottle	90	–	–	–	15	–	–	–
XS Energy									
Electric Lemon Blast	1 can (8.4 oz)	16	–	0	–	0	0	0	25
Xtazy									
All Flavors	1 can	160	–	–	–	360	–	–	–
YET									
Your Energy Drink	1 can	8	0	0	–	60	0	0	25
ENGLISH MUFFIN									
READY-TO-EAT									
apple cinnamon	1	138	–	–	–	–	84	1	119
granola	1	155	–	–	–	0	129	2	103
mixed grain	1	155	–	–	–	0	129	2	103
plain	1	134	–	–	–	–	99	1	75
plain toasted	1	133	–	–	–	–	99	1	74
raisin cinnamon	1	138	–	–	–	–	84	1	119
sourdough	1	134	–	–	–	–	99	1	75
wheat	1	127	–	–	–	–	101	2	106
whole wheat	1	134	4	0	–	0	175	2	139
Crystal Farms									
English Muffin	1	130	1	0	60	0	80	1	–

FOOD	PORTION	CALS	FIBER	VIT A	FOLIC	VIT C	CALCI	IRON	POTAS
Food For Life									
7 Sprouted Grains	1	160	6	–	–	–	–	–	150
Ezekiel 4:9 Cinnamon Raisin	1	160	4	–	–	–	–	–	–
Ezekiel 4:9 Sprouted Grain	1	160	6	–	–	–	–	–	150
Genesis 1:29 Original	1	180	6	–	–	–	–	–	220
Pepperidge Farm									
100% Whole Wheat	1	140	3	–	–	–	–	–	–
7 Grain	1	130	3	–	–	–	–	–	–
Sara Lee									
Heart Healthy Wheat w/ Honey	1	140	2	0	60	0	150	1	–
Original w/ Whole Grain	1	140	2	0	60	0	100	1	–
Thomas'									
100 Calories	1	100	5	0	–	0	80	1	–
Carb Consider	1	100	9	0	–	0	150	1	–
Corn	1	150	2	200	–	0	80	2	–
Hearty Grains 100% Whole Wheat	1	120	3	0	–	0	80	1	–
Hearty Grains Honey Wheat	1	130	2	0	–	0	60	1	–
Light Multi-Grain	1	100	8	0	–	0	100	1	–
Original	1	120	1	0	–	0	80	1	–
Raisin Cinnamon	1	140	1	0	–	0	20	1	–
Sandwich Size Original	1	190	2	0	–	0	100	3	–
Sourdough	1	120	1	0	–	0	80	2	–
Super Size Multi Grain	1	240	3	0	–	0	100	3	–
TAKE-OUT									
w/ butter	1 (2.2 oz)	189	–	136	57	1	103	2	69
w/ cheese & sausage	1 (4 oz)	393	–	380	67	1	168	2	215
w/ egg cheese & canadian bacon	1 (4.8 oz)	289	2	586	44	2	151	2	199
w/ egg cheese & sausage	1 (5.8 oz)	487	–	660	54	2	196	3	294
EPAZOTE									
fresh	1 tbsp (1 g)	tr	tr	tr	2	0	2	tr	5
fresh sprig	1 (2 g)	1	tr	1	4	tr	6	tr	13

FOOD	PORTION	CALS	FIBER	VIT A	FOLIC	VIT C	CALCI	IRON	POTAS
EPPAW									
raw	½ cup	75	–	0	–	7	55	1	170
FALAFEL									
Near East									
Falafel as prep	2½ patties	230	5	0	–	0	40	3	–
Sabra									
Burger	1 (1.8 oz)	90	3	200	–	5	20	1	–
VeggieLand									
FalafelBurger	1 (4 oz)	190	8	–	–	–	–	–	–
TAKE-OUT									
falafel	1 (1.2 oz)	57	–	2	13	tr	9	1	99
FAT									
bacon grease	1 tbsp	116	0	0	0	0	0	0	0
beef shortening	1 tbsp	115	0	0	0	0	0	0	0
beef suet	1 oz	242	0	0	0	0	1	tr	5
chicken	1 tbsp	115	0	–	–	–	–	–	–
chicken	1 cup	1846	0	–	–	–	–	–	–
cocoa butter	1 tbsp	120	0	–	–	–	–	–	–
duck	1 tbsp (13 g)	115	0	0	0	0	0	0	0
goose	1 tbsp	115	0	–	–	–	–	–	–
goose	1 oz	257	0	–	–	–	–	–	–
lamb new zealand	1 oz	182	0	–	–	–	6	tr	15
lard	1 cup (205 g)	1849	0	–	–	–	tr	–	tr
lard	1 tbsp (13 g)	115	0	–	–	–	tr	–	0
meat pan drippings	½ tbsp	124	0	0	0	0	0	0	0
nutmeg butter	1 tbsp	120	0	–	–	–	–	–	–
pork raw	1 oz	230	0	4	0	0	1	tr	18
salt pork	1 cube (1 oz)	215	0	0	0	0	2	tr	19
shortening	1 cup	1812	0	–	–	–	–	–	–
shortening	1 tbsp	113	0	–	–	–	–	–	–
turkey	1 tbsp	115	0	–	–	–	–	–	–
ucuhuba butter	1 tbsp	120	0	–	–	–	–	–	–
Crisco									
Shortening	1 tbsp	110	0	–	–	–	–	–	–

FOOD	PORTION	CALS	FIBER	VIT A	FOLIC	VIT C	CALCI	IRON	POTAS
Nebraska Land									
Pork Fatback	½ oz	110	0	0	–	0	0	0	–
Smart Balance									
Shortening	1 tbsp	110	0	–	–	–	–	–	–
Spectrum									
Organic Shortening	1 tbsp	110	0	0	–	0	0	0	0

FEIJOA

FOOD	PORTION	CALS	FIBER	VIT A	FOLIC	VIT C	CALCI	IRON	POTAS
fresh	1 (1.75 oz)	25	–	0	19	7	8	tr	78
puree	1 cup	119	–	0	93	32	41	tr	378

FENNEL

FOOD	PORTION	CALS	FIBER	VIT A	FOLIC	VIT C	CALCI	IRON	POTAS
fresh bulb	1 (8.2 oz)	72	–	–	62	28	116	–	969
fresh sliced	1 cup	27	–	–	23	11	43	–	360
leaves	1 oz	7	1	1119	29	27	31	1	–
seed	1 tsp	7	–	3	–	–	24	tr	34

FENUGREEK

FOOD	PORTION	CALS	FIBER	VIT A	FOLIC	VIT C	CALCI	IRON	POTAS
seed	1 tsp	12	–	–	2	tr	6	1	28

FIBER

FOOD	PORTION	CALS	FIBER	VIT A	FOLIC	VIT C	CALCI	IRON	POTAS
apple fiber	0.5 oz	40	7	–	–	–	–	–	–
Benefiber									
Supplement	1 pkg (4 g)	20	3	–	–	–	–	–	–
Choice									
Fiber Burst Lemon Lime	3 pieces	45	3	–	–	–	–	–	–
Fiber Burst Tropical Fruit	3 pieces	45	3	–	–	–	–	–	–
Metamucil									
Natural Fiber Regular Flavor	1 rounded tsp (7 g)	25	3	–	–	–	6	1	–
Wellements									
Fiber-Psyll	1 scoop (0.5 oz)	55	12	–	–	–	–	–	–

FIDDLEHEAD FERNS

FOOD	PORTION	CALS	FIBER	VIT A	FOLIC	VIT C	CALCI	IRON	POTAS
fresh	3.5 oz	34	–	3676	–	27	32	1	370

FIGS

FOOD	PORTION	CALS	FIBER	VIT A	FOLIC	VIT C	CALCI	IRON	POTAS
calimyrna	3 (5.4 oz)	120	4	200	–	4	60	tr	–
canned in heavy syrup	3	75	–	31	–	1	23	tr	85
canned in light syrup	3	58	–	32	–	1	23	tr	86

FOOD	PORTION	CALS	FIBER	VIT A	FOLIC	VIT C	CALCI	IRON	POTAS
canned water pack	3	42	–	31	–	1	22	tr	83
dried california	½ cup (3.5 oz)	200	17	100	24	2	150	3	710
dried cooked	½ cup	140	–	207	1	6	79	1	391
dried whole	10	477	17	248	14	2	269	4	1332
fresh	1 med	50	–	71	–	1	18	tr	116
Blue Ribbon									
California Figs	1 pkg (1.5 oz)	120	5	0	–	0	60	1	–
Figamajigs									
Chocolate Covered Bar	1 bar (1.4 oz)	130	5	–	–	–	40	1	–
Chocolate Covered Bar w/ Almonds	1 bar (1.4 oz)	150	4	–	–	–	60	tr	–
Jenny									
Sundried Kalamata	4	120	5	–	–	–	60	1	–
Trucco									
Kalamata	2	100	4	0	–	0	60	1	–

FIREWEED

FOOD	PORTION	CALS	FIBER	VIT A	FOLIC	VIT C	CALCI	IRON	POTAS
leaves chopped	1 cup (0.8 oz)	24	2	828	26	tr	99	1	114

FISH
CANNED
Beach Cliff

FOOD	PORTION	CALS	FIBER	VIT A	FOLIC	VIT C	CALCI	IRON	POTAS
Fish Steaks In Louisiana Hot Sauce	1 can (3.7 oz)	160	0	200	–	0	250	1	–
Fish Steaks In Mustard Sauce	1 can (3.7 oz)	160	0	200	–	0	250	1	–
Fish Steaks In Soybean Oil	1 can (3.7 oz)	200	0	200	–	0	200	2	–
Fish Steaks w/ Hot Green Chilies	1 can (3.7 oz)	160	0	200	–	0	400	2	–
Fish Steaks w/ Jalapeno Peppers	1 can (3.7 oz)	130	0	200	–	0	150	2	–
Brunswick									
Fish Steaks In Louisiana Hot Sauce	1 can (3.7 oz)	160	0	200	–	0	250	1	–
Fish Steaks In Mustard Sauce	1 can (3.7 oz)	160	0	200	–	0	250	1	–

FOOD	PORTION	CALS	FIBER	VIT A	FOLIC	VIT C	CALCI	IRON	POTAS
Fish Steaks In Soybean Oil	1 can (3.7 oz)	200	0	200	–	0	200	2	–
Fish Steaks In Spring Water	1 can (3.7 oz)	150	0	200	–	0	250	2	–
Fish Steaks w/ Hot Tabasco Peppers	1 can (3.7 oz)	220	0	200	–	0	150	2	–
Seafood Snacks Golden Smoked	1 can (3.2 oz)	170	0	0	–	0	70	2	–
Seafood Snacks In Lemon & Cracked Pepper	1 can (3.2 oz)	160	0	0	–	0	70	2	–
Seafood Snacks In Louisiana Hot Sauce	1 can (3.2 oz)	140	0	100	–	0	60	2	340
Seafood Snacks In Teriyaki Sauce	1 can (3.2 oz)	160	0	100	–	0	60	2	360
Seafood Snacks In Tomato & Basil Sauce	1 can (3.2 oz)	140	0	200	–	1	60	2	350
Seafood Snacks Kippered	1 can (3.2 oz)	160	0	100	–	0	130	2	–
Chicken Of The Sea									
Fish Steaks	½ can (2 oz)	70	1	200	–	1	200	1	–
FROZEN									
breaded fillet	1 (2 oz)	155	–	60	10	–	11	tr	149
sticks	1 stick (1 oz)	76	–	30	5	–	6	tr	73
Ian's									
Fillets	1 (3.4 oz)	260	2	100	–	1	100	3	–
Fish Stick Allergy Free	5 pieces	190	1	0	–	1	80	3	–
Fish Sticks	5 pieces	190	1	0	–	1	80	3	–
TAKE-OUT									
fish cake	1 (4.7 oz)	166	–	140	–	5	179	1	–
jamaican brown fish stew	1 serv	426	2	–	–	–	–	–	–
kedgeree	5.6 oz	242	1	640	–	0	58	1	–
mousse	1 serv (3.5 oz)	185	tr	170	–	tr	40	1	250

FOOD	PORTION	CALS	FIBER	VIT A	FOLIC	VIT C	CALCI	IRON	POTAS
stew	1 cup (7.9 oz)	157	–	160	–	11	32	1	–
taramasalata	2 tbsp	124	–	–	2	0	6	tr	16

FISH OIL
cod liver	1 tbsp	123	0	13600	0	0	0	0	0
herring	1 tbsp	123	0	0	0	0	0	0	0
menhaden	1 tbsp	123	0	0	0	0	0	0	0
salmon	1 tbsp	123	0	0	0	0	0	0	0
sardine	1 tbsp	123	0	0	0	0	0	0	0
shark	1 oz	270	0	–	–	–	–	–	–
whale	1 oz	270	0	–	–	–	–	–	–
Cormega									
Omega-E Orange	1 pkg	20	0	–	–	12	–	–	–
Spectrum									
Cod Liver Oil w/ Lemon	1 tsp	40	0	1250	–	–	–	–	–

FISH PASTE
fish paste	2 tsp	15	0	–	–	0	25	1	–

FLAXSEED
Arrowhead									
Organic Flax Seeds	¼ cup	140	6	–	–	–	–	–	–
Bob's Red Mill									
Flax Seed Meal	2 tbsp	60	4	–	–	–	–	–	–
Cracker Flax									
Organic Apple Raisin	1 oz	130	9	0	–	0	40	1	–
Hodgson Mill									
Milled	2 tbsp	60	4	0	–	0	20	1	–

FLOUNDER
FRESH
cooked	1 fillet (4.5 oz)	148	0	48	–	–	23	tr	436
cooked	3 oz	99	0	32	–	–	16	tr	292

TAKE-OUT
breaded & fried	3.2 oz	211	–	35	51	0	17	2	292
stuffed w/ crab	1 piece (7.6 oz)	332	1	495	59	6	124	2	792

FLOUR
arrowhead	1 cup	457	4	0	9	0	51	tr	14
buckwheat whole groat	1 cup	402	12	0	65	0	49	5	692

FOOD	PORTION	CALS	FIBER	VIT A	FOLIC	VIT C	CALCI	IRON	POTAS
corn masa	1 cup (4 oz)	416	11	552	213	0	161	8	340
cottonseed lowfat	1 oz	94	–	123	–	1	135	4	500
peanut defatted	1 cup	196	–	0	149	0	84	1	774
peanut lowfat	1 cup	257	–	–	–	–	78	3	815
potato	1 cup (6.3 oz)	628	–	0	–	34	59	31	2843
rice brown	1 cup (5.5 oz)	574	7	0	25	0	17	3	457
rice white	1 cup (5.5 oz)	578	4	0	6	0	16	1	120
rye dark	1 cup (4.5 oz)	415	29	0	77	0	72	8	934
rye light	1 cup (3.6 oz)	374	15	0	22	0	21	2	238
rye medium	1 cup (3.6 oz)	361	15	0	19	0	24	2	347
sesame lowfat	1 oz	95	–	18	8	–	42	4	113
triticale whole grain	1 cup (4.6 oz)	439	19	0	96	0	46	3	606
white all-purpose	1 cup (4.4 oz)	455	2	–	193	0	19	6	134
white bread	1 cup (4.8 oz)	495	3	0	211	0	21	6	137
white cake unsifted	1 cup (4.8 oz)	496	2	0	211	0	19	10	144
white self-rising	1 cup (4.4 oz)	443	3	0	193	0	423	6	155
white unbleached	1 cup (4.4 oz)	455	3	0	193	0	19	6	134
whole wheat	1 cup (4.2 oz)	407	15	0	53	0	41	5	486
Arrowhead									
Whole Grain Oat	⅓ cup	120	3	–	–	–	–	–	–
Bob's Red Mill									
Flour	⅓ cup	130	5	–	–	–	–	–	–
Gold Medal									
All Purpose	¼ cup (1 oz)	100	tr	0	40	0	0	1	40

FOOD	PORTION	CALS	FIBER	VIT A	FOLIC	VIT C	CALCI	IRON	POTAS
Better For Bread	¼ cup (1 oz)	100	tr	0	40	0	0	1	35
Organic All Purpose	¼ cup (1 oz)	100	tr	–	40	–	–	1	40
Self Rising	¼ cup (1 oz)	100	tr	0	40	0	60	1	35
Unbleached	¼ cup (1 oz)	100	tr	0	40	0	0	1	40
Wondra	¼ cup	100	tr	–	–	–	–	1	35
Heckers									
All Purpose Unbleached	¼ cup	100	tr	0	40	0	0	1	35
Whole Wheat	¼ cup	100	3	0	–	0	0	1	–
Hodgson Mill									
Best For Bread	¼ cup	100	1	0	–	0	0	1	–
Buckwheat	¼ cup	100	3	0	–	0	20	2	–
Oat Bran Flour	¼ cup	110	3	0	–	0	0	1	–
Kentucky Kernel									
Seasoned Flour	4 tsp	36	0	0	–	0	0	1	–
King Arthur									
All Purpose	¼ cup	110	tr	0	40	0	0	1	–
All Purpose Unbleached	¼ cup	110	1	0	40	0	0	1	–
Organic White Whole Wheat	¼ cup	100	3	0	–	0	20	1	–
Organic Whole Wheat	½ cup	110	4	0	–	0	20	1	–
Organic Artisan	¼ cup	110	tr	0	–	0	0	tr	–
Self-Rising	¼ cup	120	1	0	40	0	80	1	–
White Whole Wheat	¼ cup	100	3	0	–	0	20	1	–
Whole Wheat	¼ cup	110	4	0	–	0	0	tr	–
La Pina									
Flour	¼ cup (1 oz)	100	1	0	100	0	0	1	35
Lundberg									
Brown Rice	¼ cup	110	1	0	–	0	0	1	150
Manitoba Harvest									
Hemp Seed Flour	¼ cup	120	12	0	–	0	40	4	–
Red Band									
All Purpose	¼ cup (1 oz)	100	tr	0	–	0	0	1	40

FOOD	PORTION	CALS	FIBER	VIT A	FOLIC	VIT C	CALCI	IRON	POTAS
Self-Rising	¼ cup (1 oz)	100	tr	0	–	0	60	1	40

Robin Hood

Whole Wheat	¼ cup (1 oz)	90	3	0	–	0	0	1	110

FOOD COLORS

blue	1 tsp	0	0	–	–	–	–	–	–
orange	1 tsp	0	0	–	–	–	–	–	–
red	1 tsp	tr	0	–	–	tr	–	–	tr
yellow	1 tsp	tr	0	–	–	–	–	–	tr

FRENCH BEANS

dried cooked	1 cup	228	17	5	132	2	111	2	655

FRENCH TOAST
FROZEN

french toast	1 slice (2 oz)	126	2	110	14	–	63	1	79

Eggo

Toaster Sticks Original	2	220	1	1000	40	0	100	4	120

Ian's

Sticks	5 (3.2 oz)	250	6	0	–	0	60	1	–

TAKE-OUT

plain	1 slice	151	–	298	15	tr	64	1	86
sticks	5 (4.9 oz)	513	3	45	82	0	78	3	127
w/ butter	2 slices	356	–	473	73	tr	73	2	177

FROG LEGS
TAKE-OUT

as prep w/ seasoned flour & fried	1 (0.8)	70	–	0	tr	0	5	tr	–

FRUCTOSE
Estee

Fructose	1 tsp	15	0	–	–	–	–	–	–
Packet	1 pkg	10	0	–	–	–	–	–	–

FRUIT DRINKS
MIX
Bio Fruit

Mix	1 scoop (8 g)	42	1	–	–	106	20	1	–

FOOD	PORTION	CALS	FIBER	VIT A	FOLIC	VIT C	CALCI	IRON	POTAS
Luna									
Dragonfruit Kiwi	1 pkg	50	0	1000	200	30	150	2	–
Pomegranate Berry	1 pkg	50	0	1000	200	30	150	2	–
READY-TO-DRINK									
After The Fall									
Banana Casablanca	8 oz	150	–	–	–	60	150	–	300
Mango Montage	8 oz	150	–	500	–	60	150	–	190
Ceres									
Cranberry & Kiwi	8 oz	110	0	0	–	60	30	1	252
Medley	8 oz	130	2	200	–	60	20	1	248
Youngberry	8 oz	120	0	0	–	30	20	1	190
Champion Lyte									
All Flavors	1 bottle	0	0	0	–	0	0	0	25
Del Monte									
Peach Raspberry	5.5 fl oz	160	3	500	–	60	20	1	–
Pineapple Banana Orange	5.5 fl oz	170	1	100	–	60	20	2	–
Strawberry Peach Banana	5.5 fl oz	150	1	300	–	60	20	tr	–
Feel Good Drinks									
Spritz Cranberry & Lime No Sugar Added	1 bottle	159	–	–	–	60	–	–	–
Spritz Orange & Passionfruit No Sugar Added	1 bottle	151	–	–	–	60	–	–	–
Spritz Pink Citrus No Sugar Added	1 bottle	159	–	–	–	60	–	–	–
Frutzzo									
Organic 100% Juice Pomegranate Passionfruit	1 bottle (12 oz)	140	0	100	–	15	20	1	370
Organic 100% Juice Pomegranate Acai	1 bottle (12 oz)	140	0	200	–	2	0	1	410
Hansen's									
Fruit Punch 100% Juice	1 box (4.23 oz)	60	–	0	–	60	100	0	–
Juice Slam Wild Berry	1 box	120	–	1250	–	15	20	–	143

FOOD	PORTION	CALS	FIBER	VIT A	FOLIC	VIT C	CALCI	IRON	POTAS
Hog Wash									
All Flavors	1 bottle (10 oz)	37	0	1000	–	60	–	–	–
Hood									
Fruit Punch	1 cup	120	0	0	–	60	0	0	–
Kagome									
Burgundy Berry Blossom	8 oz	100	0	9000	–	15	20	1	170
Golden Peach Garden	8 oz	100	1	12000	–	18	20	1	200
Orange Carrot Blossom	8 oz	100	1	8500	–	27	20	0	230
Purple Roots & Fruits	8 oz	130	1	0	–	24	40	tr	280
L&A									
Pineapple Coconut	8 oz	140	1	–	–	30	40	1	–
Minute Maid									
Orange Passion	8 oz	130	–	–	40	72	350	–	300
Orange Tangerine	8 oz	110	–	–	40	72	350	–	450
Naked Juice									
Berry Blast	8 oz	120	1	5000	–	126	20	2	330
Blue Machine	8 oz	170	8	0	400	66	20	1	390
Green Machine	8 oz	130	1	4500	–	36	20	3	440
Mango Acai	8 oz	190	3	1000	–	72	40	1	110
Power C	8 oz	120	3	500	–	654	20	1	370
Protein Zone	8 oz	210	0	100	–	126	60	2	460
Red Machine	8 oz	160	4	200	400	6	40	3	290
Strawberry Banana C	8 oz	120	3	100	–	300	20	1	480
Very Berry	8 oz	130	1	100	–	300	20	1	370
Very Pro Berry	8 oz	190	1	100	–	300	80	2	420
Well Being	8 oz	140	0	300	–	150	20	1	460
Nantucket Nectars									
Peach Orange	8 oz	130	1	500	–	15	0	tr	–
Pomegranate Pear	8 oz	110	0	–	–	–	–	–	–
Noble									
Organic 100% Juice Orange Tangerine	8 oz	120	–	–	20	60	20	–	440
Northland									
Cranberry Blueberry	1 cup (8 oz)	140	–	–	–	78	–	–	180
Ocean Spray									
Cran*Grape	8 oz	170	0	0	–	60	–	–	–
Cran*Raspberry	8 oz	140	0	0	–	60	–	–	–

FOOD	PORTION	CALS	FIBER	VIT A	FOLIC	VIT C	CALCI	IRON	POTAS
Cran*Strawberry	8 oz	140	tr	0	–	60	–	–	–
Cranapple	8 oz	160	tr	0	–	60	–	–	–
Grape Cranberry	8 oz	170	–	0	–	60	–	–	0
Kiwi Strawberry	8 oz	120	0	0	–	60	–	–	0
Mandarin Magic	8 oz	120	0	1250	–	60	–	–	0
White Cranberry Apple Juice	8 oz	120	–	0	–	60	–	–	30
Odwalla									
Carrot Orange Apple	8 oz	100	1	14000	–	60	40	1	410
Rooty Fruity	8 oz	110	0	21000	–	48	20	1	–
Strawberry Banana	8 oz	120	3	200	–	66	20	1	510
Old Orchard									
100% Juice Pomegranate Black Currant	8 oz	130	–	0	–	0	0	tr	–
100% Juice Pomegranate Cherry	8 oz	140	–	0	–	0	0	0	–
Cocktail Apple Passion Mango	8 oz	120	–	0	–	78	0	0	95
Healthy Balance Apple Kiwi Strawberry	8 oz	30	–	0	–	78	0	0	78
Phat Phruit									
Peach Mango	8 oz	40	0	1000	–	60	200	–	–
Pineapple Orange	8 oz	40	0	2000	–	60	200	–	–
Purity Organic									
Citrus Punch	8 oz	123	tr	200	–	60	–	–	–
Tropicana									
Fruit Punch	1 cup	130	0	0	–	60	0	0	–
Light Fruit Punch	8 oz	10	0	0	–	60	0	0	–
Orange Tangerine Juice	8 oz	110	0	0	60	72	20	0	450
Orchard Berry	8 oz	110	0	0	–	60	0	0	230
Twister Berry Blast	8 oz	120	0	0	–	60	0	0	–
Twister Citrus Spark	8 oz	120	0	1500	–	60	0	0	–
Twister Fruit Fury	8 oz	120	0	0	–	60	0	0	–
Twister Light Strawberry Spiral	8 oz	40	0	0	–	60	0	0	–
V8									
Splash Fruit Medley	8 oz	80	–	5000	–	60	–	–	25

FOOD	PORTION	CALS	FIBER	VIT A	FOLIC	VIT C	CALCI	IRON	POTAS
Vruit									
Apple Carrot	1 box (8.45 oz)	120	–	5000	–	60	20	tr	334
Berry Veggie	1 box (8.45 oz)	110	–	5000	–	60	20	tr	370
Orange Veggie	1 box (8.45 oz)	110	–	5000	–	60	20	1	355
Tropical Blend	1 box (8.45 oz)	110	–	5000	–	60	20	tr	380
Wadda Juice									
All Flavors	8 oz	50	–	–	–	60	100	–	–
Welch's									
White Grape Peach 100% Juice	8 oz	160	–	–	–	60	–	–	–
FRUIT MIXED									
CANNED									
fruit cocktail in heavy syrup	½ cup	93	–	262	–	2	8	tr	112
fruit cocktail juice pack	½ cup	56	–	378	–	3	10	tr	118
fruit cocktail water pack	½ cup	40	–	305	–	3	6	tr	115
fruit salad in heavy syrup	½ cup	94	–	646	–	3	8	tr	103
fruit salad in light syrup	½ cup	73	–	541	–	3	8	tr	104
fruit salad juice pack	½ cup	62	–	744	–	4	14	tr	144
fruit salad water pack	½ cup	37	–	536	–	2	8	tr	95
mixed fruit in heavy syrup	½ cup	92	–	248	–	88	1	tr	108
tropical fruit salad in heavy syrup	½ cup	110	–	162	–	22	17	1	168
Del Monte									
Carb Clever Fruit Cocktail	½ cup	40	tr	300	–	48	0	tr	–
Fruit Cocktail In 100% Juice	½ cup	60	1	200	–	2	0	tr	–
Fruit Cocktail In Extra Light Syrup	½ cup	60	1	200	–	2	0	tr	–

FOOD	PORTION	CALS	FIBER	VIT A	FOLIC	VIT C	CALCI	IRON	POTAS
Fruit Cocktail In Heavy Syrup	½ cup	100	1	200	–	2	0	tr	–
Fruit Cup Mixed In Extra Light Syrup	1 pkg (4 oz)	50	1	100	–	12	0	tr	–
Fruit Naturals Tropical Medley	½ cup	70	tr	200	–	60	0	0	–
Orchard Select Premium Mixed	½ cup	80	tr	200	–	60	0	0	–
Snack Cups Strawberry Banana Peaches	1 pkg	70	tr	200	–	60	0	0	–
SunFresh Citrus Salad	½ cup	80	0	500	–	60	0	tr	–
Dole									
Tropical Fruit Salad	½ cup	80	1	2250	–	–	–	tr	90
Liberty Gold									
Fruit Cocktail In Heavy Syrup	½ cup	90	1	200	–	1	0	0	125
DRIED									
mixed	11 oz pkg	712	–	7155	–	11	110	8	2332
Goodniks									
Fruit Medley	¼ cup	110	2	500	–	0	0	1	–
Sun-Maid									
Mixed	¼ cup	100	3	300	–	2	20	1	310
Sunsweet									
Berry Blend	¼ cup (1.4 oz)	120	3	400	–	9	40	tr	115
Orchard Mix	¼ cup (1.4 oz)	100	3	200	–	2	20	1	160
Tropical Mix	⅓ cup	150	2	200	–	0	40	0	30
FROZEN									
mixed fruit sweetened	1 cup	245	–	806	–	188	18	1	327

FRUIT SNACKS

FOOD	PORTION	CALS	FIBER	VIT A	FOLIC	VIT C	CALCI	IRON	POTAS
fruit leather	1 bar (0.8 oz)	81	–	27	–	16	7	tr	32
fruit leather pieces	1 oz	97	–	33	–	16	5	tr	48
fruit leather pieces	1 pkg (0.9 oz)	92	–	31	–	15	5	tr	44
fruit leather rolls	1 lg (0.7 oz)	73	–	24	–	1	7	tr	62
fruit leather rolls	1 sm (0.5 oz)	49	–	16	–	1	4	tr	41

FOOD	PORTION	CALS	FIBER	VIT A	FOLIC	VIT C	CALCI	IRON	POTAS
CoolFruits									
Apple Grape	1 bar (0.5 oz)	51	1	100	–	0	20	tr	100
Apple Strawberry	1 bar (0.5 oz)	51	1	100	–	0	20	tr	–
Wild Blueberry	1 bar (0.5 oz)	51	1	100	–	0	20	tr	100
Sharkies									
Organic Energy Fruit Chews All Flavors	1 pkg (1.8 oz)	170	1	0	–	0	0	tr	45
Stretch Island									
Fruit Leather Bountiful Blueberry	1 pkg (0.5 oz)	45	1	0	–	2	0	0	95
Fruit Leather Harvest Grape	1 pkg (0.5 oz)	45	1	0	–	2	0	0	120
Fruit Leather Truly Tropical	1 pkg (0.5 oz)	45	1	0	–	1	0	0	100
Fruit Leathers Mango Sunrise	1 pkg (0.5 oz)	45	1	0	–	2	0	0	85
Organic Smooshed Fruit Apple	1 piece (0.4 oz)	40	1	0	–	0	0	0	80
Organic Smooshed Fruit Strawberry	1 piece (0.4 oz)	40	tr	0	–	0	0	0	85
Tropicana									
Fruit Wise Bars All Flavors	1 bar (1.4 oz)	140	2	0	–	60	20	tr	300
Fruit Wise Strips All Flavors	1 strip (0.7 oz)	70	1	0	–	60	0	tr	135
Welch's									
White Grape Peach	20 pieces	110	–	1250	–	60	–	tr	–
GARLIC									
clove	1	4	tr	0	tr	1	5	tr	12
fresh chopped	1 tbsp	18	tr	0	0	4	22	tr	48
powder	1 tsp	9	tr	0	0	1	2	tr	31
Dorot									
Crushed Cubes frzn	1 cube (4 g)	7	tr	–	–	–	–	–	–
Frieda's									
Elephant	1 tbsp	5	0	0	–	1	0	0	–
Vinegar Marinated	1 oz	30	0	0	–	6	40	tr	–

FOOD	PORTION	CALS	FIBER	VIT A	FOLIC	VIT C	CALCI	IRON	POTAS
McCormick									
Garlic Salt	¼ tsp	0	0	–	–	–	–	–	–
GEFILTE FISH									
sweet	1 piece (1.5 oz)	35	–	37	1	–	10	1	38
Mrs. Adler's									
Pike'n Whitefish	1 piece (1.8 oz)	50	0	–	–	–	20	1	–
GELATIN									
READY-TO-EAT									
Del Monte									
Mandarin Orange In Lite Orange Gel	1 pkg (4.5 oz)	60	0	0	–	18	20	tr	–
Mixed Fruit In Cherry Gel	1 pkg (4.5 oz)	90	0	0	–	18	20	0	–
Peaches In Peach Gel	1 pkg (4.5 oz)	90	0	0	–	18	20	tr	–
Peaches In Raspberry Gel	1 pkg (4.5 oz)	90	0	0	–	18	20	0	–
Peaches In Lite Strawberry Banana Gel	1 pkg (4.5 oz)	60	0	0	–	18	20	tr	–
Hunt's									
Snack Pack Juicy Gels Strawberry Orange	1 serv (3.5 oz)	100	0	0	–	–	–	–	–
Kozy Shack									
Gel Treats Cherry	1 pkg (4 oz)	85	1	0	–	0	11	0	67
Gel Treats Lemon Lime	1 pkg (4 oz)	85	1	0	–	0	11	0	67
Gel Treats Orange	1 pkg (4 oz)	85	1	0	–	0	17	0	67
Gel Treats Strawberry	1 pkg (4 oz)	85	1	0	–	0	11	0	67
Gel Treats Sugar Free Orange	1 pkg (4 oz)	11	1	0	–	0	20	0	81
Gel Treats Sugar Free Strawberry	1 pkg (4 oz)	11	1	0	–	0	20	0	81

FOOD	PORTION	CALS	FIBER	VIT A	FOLIC	VIT C	CALCI	IRON	POTAS
GIBLETS									
capon simmered	1 cup (5 oz)	238	0	19236	601	13	19	10	222
chicken floured & fried	1 cup (5 oz)	402	–	17298	550	13	26	15	478
chicken simmered	1 cup (5 oz)	228	–	10774	545	12	18	9	229
turkey simmered	1 cup (5 oz)	243	–	8753	501	3	18	10	291
GINGER									
ground	1 tsp	6	tr	3	1	tr	2	tr	24
pickled	0.5 oz	5	tr	–	–	–	3	tr	4
root fresh	5 slices	9	tr	0	1	1	2	tr	46
root fresh sliced	¼ cup	19	1	0	3	1	4	tr	100
Eden									
Pickled w/ Shiso Leaves	1 tbsp	20	tr	0	–	0	0	0	–
Frieda's									
Crystallized	9 pieces (1.1 oz)	100	0	500	–	0	40	1	–
Galanga Thai Ginger	⅔ cup	60	2	0	–	5	0	tr	–
GINKGO NUTS									
canned	1 oz	32	–	–	–	–	1	tr	51
dried	1 oz	99	–	310	–	8	6	tr	283
raw	1 oz	52	–	158	–	4	1	tr	145
GINSENG									
dried	1 oz	90	2	0	–	2	64	10	296
fresh	1 oz	28	tr	0	–	4	32	2	92
GIZZARDS									
chicken simmered	1 cup (5 oz)	222	–	273	77	2	14	6	259
turkey simmered	1 cup (5 oz)	236	–	268	75	2	22	8	306
GNOCCHI									
Bellino									
W/ Potato	1 cup	240	2	100	–	0	0	1	–
Vantia									
Gnocchi Whole Wheat	¾ cup	210	4	0	–	0	0	1	–

FOOD	PORTION	CALS	FIBER	VIT A	FOLIC	VIT C	CALCI	IRON	POTAS
GOAT									
roasted	3 oz	122	0	–	5	–	15	3	344
GOJI BERRIES									
dried	1 oz	106	2	–	–	25	32	3	323
Sunfood									
Organic	1 oz	90	3	100	–	2	20	2	–
GOOSE									
w/ skin roasted	½ goose (1.7 lbs)	2362	0	541	17	0	104	22	2546
w/ skin roasted	6.6 oz	574	0	131	4	0	25	5	618
w/o skin roasted	5 oz	340	0	–	–	–	20	4	554
w/o skin roasted	½ goose (1.3 lbs)	1406	0	–	–	–	84	17	2291
GOOSEBERRIES									
canned in light syrup	½ cup	93	–	174	4	13	20	tr	97
fresh	1 cup	67	–	435	–	42	38	tr	297
GRAPE JUICE									
bottled unsweetened	1 cup	154	tr	0	8	tr	23	1	334
Ceres									
Hanepoot White Grape	8 oz	130	0	0	–	27	40	1	190
Hansen's									
White Grape 100% Juice	1 box (4.23 oz)	90	–	0	–	60	0	0	–
Keto									
Kooler	½ tsp	0	0	–	–	–	–	–	–
Langers									
Plus 100% Juice	8 oz	160	–	–	–	60	100	–	–
White Grape Plus 100% Juice	8 oz	160	–	–	–	60	100	–	–
Old Orchard									
100% Juice White	8 oz	160	–	0	–	78	100	0	–
Tropicana									
Grape	1 bottle (14 oz)	270	0	0	–	72	0	0	–
Welch's									
100% Juice	8 oz	170	–	–	–	60	–	–	–
100% White	8 oz	160	–	–	–	60	–	–	–
Light White Grape	8 oz	70	–	–	–	60	100	–	–

FOOD	PORTION	CALS	FIBER	VIT A	FOLIC	VIT C	CALCI	IRON	POTAS
GRAPE LEAVES									
canned	1 (4 g)	3	–	210	3	1	12	tr	1
fresh raw	1 (3 g)	3	tr	826	2	tr	11	tr	8
Sabra									
Stuffed Meatless	1	45	1	300	–	9	20	1	–
TAKE-OUT									
dolmas w/ beef & rice	1 (0.7 oz)	50	1	345	7	2	21	tr	47
dolmas w/ lamb & rice	1 (0.7 oz)	56	1	375	5	2	22	tr	41
dolmas w/ rice	1 (2 oz)	92	2	680	21	3	50	1	86
GRAPEFRUIT									
CANNED									
juice pack	½ cup	46	–	0	–	42	19	tr	209
unsweetened	1 cup	93	–	18	26	72	18	1	378
water pack	½ cup	44	–	0	11	27	18	1	161
Del Monte									
Fruit Naturals Red	½ cup	60	tr	100	–	60	20	0	–
SunFresh Red	½ cup	80	2	100	–	60	20	0	–
SunFresh White In Real Fruit Juice	½ cup	45	2	0	–	60	20	2	–
FRESH									
pink	½	37	1	318	15	47	13	tr	158
pink sections	1 cup	69	1	595	28	88	25	tr	296
red	½	37	–	318	15	47	13	tr	158
red sections	1 cup	69	–	595	28	88	25	tr	296
white	½	39	1	12	12	39	17	tr	175
white sections	1 cup	76	1	23	23	77	28	tr	340
Ocean Spray									
Sweet Ruby	½ med	60	6	750	–	66	20	0	–
Sunkist									
Fresh	½ med	60	6	750	16	66	20	0	230
Oroblanco	½	100	4	0	60	66	40	tr	200
GRAPEFRUIT JUICE									
fresh	1 cup	96	–	–	–	94	22	tr	400
frzn as prep	1 cup	102	–	22	9	83	19	tr	337
frzn not prep	6 oz	302	–	65	26	248	18	1	1002
sweetened	1 cup	116	–	0	26	67	20	1	405

FOOD	PORTION	CALS	FIBER	VIT A	FOLIC	VIT C	CALCI	IRON	POTAS
Minute Maid									
Frozen + Calcium	8 oz	100	–	–	–	84	100	–	–
Ruby Red	8 oz	130	–	–	–	60	–	–	–
Ocean Spray									
100% Juice Pink	8 oz	110	0	0	–	60	–	–	280
100% White Juice	8 oz	100	tr	0	–	60	–	–	240
Ruby Drink	8 oz	120	–	0	–	60	–	–	10
Ruby Red Drink	8 oz	130	0	0	–	60	–	–	50
Odwalla									
Juice	8 oz	90	0	300	–	78	20	1	0
Tropicana									
Sweet	8 oz	130	0	0	40	60	20	0	300
GRAPES									
seedless red or green	20	69	1	66	2	11	10	tr	191
seedless red or green	1 cup	110	1	106	3	17	16	1	306
thompson seedless in heavy syrup	½ cup	93	1	82	4	1	13	1	132
thompson seedless water pack	½ cup	49	1	55	4	1	12	1	131
w/ seeds red or green	20	80	1	77	2	13	12	tr	222
w/ seeds red or green	1 cup	106	1	102	3	17	15	1	294
Chiquita									
Grapes	1½ cups (4.8 oz)	90	1	100	–	15	20	tr	–
Earthbound Farm									
Organic Black	½ cup	190	1	100	–	15	20	tr	–
Frieda's									
Champagne	½ cup (3 oz)	50	1	0	–	4	0	0	–
GRAVY									
CANNED									
au jus	1 cup	38	–	0	–	2	10	1	–
beef	1 cup	124	–	0	–	0	14	2	189
beef	1 can (10 oz)	155	–	0	–	0	17	2	236
chicken	1 cup	189	–	880	–	0	48	1	260
mushroom	1 cup	120	–	0	–	0	17	2	253
turkey	1 cup	122	–	0	–	0	10	2	–

FOOD	PORTION	CALS	FIBER	VIT A	FOLIC	VIT C	CALCI	IRON	POTAS
Heinz									
HomeStyle Chicken	¼ cup	25	0	200	–	0	0	tr	–
HomeStyle Roasted Turkey	¼ cup	25	0	0	–	0	0	0	–
Pacific Foods									
Natural Beef	1 cup	20	0	–	–	–	–	–	–
Natural Mushroom	¼ cup	20	1	–	–	–	–	–	–
Natural Turkey	¼ cup	25	0	–	–	–	–	–	–
FROZEN									
Tofurky									
Giblet & Mushroom	2 tbsp	30	1	–	–	–	–	–	–
MIX									
au jus as prep w/ water	1 cup	32	–	–	–	–	23	–	–
brown as prep w/ water	1 cup	75	–	–	–	–	66	tr	57
chicken as prep	1 cup	83	–	–	–	–	39	–	–
mushroom as prep	1 cup	70	–	–	–	–	49	–	–
onion as prep w/ water	1 cup	77	–	–	–	–	72	–	–
pork as prep	1 cup	76	–	–	–	–	32	–	–
turkey as prep	1 cup	87	–	–	–	–	50	–	–
Bournvita									
Extract	2 heaping tsp	34	–	tr	–	0	8	tr	–
Bovril									
Extract	1 heaping tsp	9	0	0	–	0	2	1	–
Marmite									
Extract	1 heaping tsp	9	–	0	–	0	5	tr	–
TAKE-OUT									
au jus	1 cup	62	tr	0	5	0	4	tr	34

GREAT NORTHERN BEANS

FOOD	PORTION	CALS	FIBER	VIT A	FOLIC	VIT C	CALCI	IRON	POTAS
canned	1 cup	299	13	3	213	3	139	4	919
dried cooked	1 cup	209	12	2	181	2	121	4	692
Eden									
Organic	½ cup	110	8	–	24	–	80	1	270

GREEN BEANS

FOOD	PORTION	CALS	FIBER	VIT A	FOLIC	VIT C	CALCI	IRON	POTAS
CANNED									
drained	1 cup	27	3	587	43	7	35	1	147
Del Monte									
Cut	½ cup	20	2	300	–	2	20	1	–
Cut Italian	½ cup	30	3	200	–	2	20	1	–
Cut w/ Potatoes & Ham Flavor	½ cup	30	tr	100	–	5	20	tr	–
French Style	½ cup	20	2	300	–	2	20	1	–
Whole	½ cup	20	2	300	–	2	20	1	–
Gertie's Finest									
Pickled	1 oz	15	1	100	–	0	20	0	–
S&W									
Blue Lake Cut	½ cup (4.2 oz)	20	2	300	–	4	20	1	–
French Style	½ cup (4.2 oz)	20	2	300	–	4	20	1	–
Whole Small	½ cup (4.2 oz)	20	2	300	–	4	20	1	–
Tillen Farms									
Crispy Dilly Beans Pickled	¼ cup	15	0	100	–	0	20	0	–
Veg-All									
French Style	½ cup	20	2	200	–	2	20	0	–
FRESH									
cooked w/o salt	1 cup	44	4	875	41	12	55	1	183
raw	1 cup	34	4	759	41	18	41	1	230
raw whole beans	10	17	2	380	20	9	20	1	115
Frieda's									
Purple Wax	⅔ cup	25	3	500	–	15	40	1	–
GreenLine									
Fresh Trimmed	3 oz	25	2	100	–	5	40	tr	–
FROZEN									
cooked	1 cup	38	4	752	31	6	66	1	170
Birds Eye									
Steamfresh Cut	½ cup	30	2	100	–	5	40	tr	–
C&W									
French Cut	1 cup	30	2	100	–	4	40	tr	–

FOOD	PORTION	CALS	FIBER	VIT A	FOLIC	VIT C	CALCI	IRON	POTAS
Fresh Like									
Cut	3.5 oz	29	1	534	–	11	41	1	149
French Cut	3.5 oz	29	1	459	–	9	46	1	174
Green Giant									
Green Bean Casserole	⅔ cup	110	1	200	–	4	20	tr	–
Pictsweet									
Cut	⅔ cup	30	2	100	–	4	40	tr	–
TAKE-OUT									
casserole w/ mushroom sauce	1 cup	108	3	180	21	4	79	1	176
pickled	½ cup	19	2	100	19	8	22	1	128

GREENS
Ready Pac

Microwave Leafy Greens as prep	½ cup	15	2	2500	–	0	80	4	–

GROUNDCHERRIES

fresh	½ cup	37	–	504	–	8	6	1	–

GROUPER

cooked	3 oz	100	0	–	–	–	18	1	403
cooked	1 fillet (7.1 oz)	238	0	–	–	–	42	2	959
raw	3 oz	78	0	–	–	–	23	1	410

GUAR GUM
Bob's Red Mill

Guar Gum	1 tbsp	20	6	–	–	–	–	–	–

GUAVA

fresh	1	45	–	713	–	165	18	tr	256
guava sauce	½ cup	43	–	337	–	174	8	tr	268
Frieda's									
Fresh	1 (3 oz)	45	5	750	–	156	0	0	–

GUAVA JUICE
Ceres

Guava	8 oz	120	0	250	–	60	20	tr	140
Nantucket Nectars									
Guava	8 oz	130	0	0	–	60	0	0	–

HADDOCK

fresh broiled	4 oz	127	0	71	15	0	48	2	452

FOOD	PORTION	CALS	FIBER	VIT A	FOLIC	VIT C	CALCI	IRON	POTAS
roe raw	1 oz	37	–	–	–	4	–	tr	–
smoked	1 oz	33	0	21	4	0	14	tr	118
TAKE-OUT									
breaded & fried	4 oz	229	1	550	24	0	66	2	380

HALIBUT

FOOD	PORTION	CALS	FIBER	VIT A	FOLIC	VIT C	CALCI	IRON	POTAS
atlantic & pacific cooked	3 oz	119	0	152	–	–	51	1	490
atlantic & pacific cooked	½ fillet (5.6 oz)	223	0	284	–	–	95	2	916
atlantic & pacific raw	3 oz	93	0	132	–	–	40	1	382
greenland baked	3 oz	203	0	51	1	–	3	1	292
greenland baked	5.6 oz	380	0	95	2	–	6	1	546

HAM

FOOD	PORTION	CALS	FIBER	VIT A	FOLIC	VIT C	CALCI	IRON	POTAS
boneless extra lean roasted	3 oz	123	0	0	3	0	7	1	244
boneless roasted	3 oz	151	0	0	3	0	7	1	348
canned extra lean roasted	3 oz	116	0	0	4	0	5	1	296
canned extra lean roasted	3 oz	142	0	0	4	0	6	1	298
center slice lean & fat roasted	3 oz	173	0	0	3	0	6	1	287
deviled	¼ cup	188	0	0	3	1	3	tr	121
ham salad spread	2 tbsp	65	0	0	0	0	2	tr	45
patty grilled	1 patty (2 oz)	205	0	0	2	0	5	1	146
prosciutto	4 slices (1.3 oz)	72	0	0	2	0	4	tr	188
sliced	3 slices (2.9 oz)	137	1	0	6	3	20	1	241
sliced extra lean	3 slices (2.2 oz)	69	0	0	3	0	6	1	221
westphalian smoked	1 oz	105	0	–	–	–	3	1	70
whole roasted	3 oz	207	0	0	3	0	6	1	243
Boar's Head									
Black Forest Smoked	2 oz	60	0	0	–	0	0	1	–
Deluxe	2 oz	60	0	0	–	0	0	1	–
Deluxe 42% Lowered Sodium	2 oz	60	0	0	–	0	0	tr	–

FOOD	PORTION	CALS	FIBER	VIT A	FOLIC	VIT C	CALCI	IRON	POTAS
Fresh Seasoned	2 oz	90	0	0	–	0	0	1	–
Maple Glazed Honey	2 oz	60	0	0	–	0	0	1	–
Pepper	2 oz	60	0	0	–	0	0	1	–
Rosemary & Sundried Tomato	2 oz	70	0	0	–	0	0	1	–
Virginia Smoked	2 oz	60	0	0	–	0	0	1	–
Hillshire									
Deli Select Honey Ham	6 slices (2 oz)	60	0	0	–	4	0	1	–
Oscar Mayer									
Brown Sugar	3 slices (1.8 oz)	60	0	0	–	0	0	1	–
Lunchables Ham Bagels	1 pkg	410	2	300	–	60	250	3	–
Lunchables Ham Wraps	1 pkg	430	2	300	–	60	300	3	–
Smoked	3 slices (2.2 oz)	60	0	0	–	0	0	1	–
Sara Lee									
Bavarian Oven Roasted Honey	2 oz	70	0	0	–	9	0	4	–
Brown Sugar	2 oz	70	0	0	–	0	0	tr	–
Homestyle Baked	2 oz	60	0	0	–	12	0	1	–
Maple Honey	2 oz	70	0	0	–	0	0	tr	–
TAKE-OUT									
thick slice fried	1 (2.2 oz)	140	0	0	2	0	4	1	202

HAM DISHES
TAKE-OUT

FOOD	PORTION	CALS	FIBER	VIT A	FOLIC	VIT C	CALCI	IRON	POTAS
croquette	1 (2.2 oz)	149	tr	245	11	tr	43	1	148
salad	½ cup	287	tr	253	22	1	33	2	232

HAMBURGER
Ian's

FOOD	PORTION	CALS	FIBER	VIT A	FOLIC	VIT C	CALCI	IRON	POTAS
Mini	2 (4.6 oz)	360	1	0	–	0	0	5	–
Mini Cheeseburger	2 (5 oz)	420	1	200	–	0	100	5	–
Kid Cuisine									
Cheeseburger Builder	1 meal	390	2	200	–	9	80	2	–
Lean Pockets									
Cheeseburger	1 (4.5 oz)	280	3	300	–	0	250	3	–
Oscar Mayer									
Lunchables All-Star Burgers	1 pkg	420	1	200	–	0	200	3	–

FOOD	PORTION	CALS	FIBER	VIT A	FOLIC	VIT C	CALCI	IRON	POTAS
Quaker Maid									
Pure Beef Patties	1 (4 oz)	240	0	0	–	0	0	1	–
Wellshire									
Beef	1 (4 oz)	260	0	0	–	0	0	2	–
Turkey Burgers	1 (4 oz)	200	0	0	–	0	0	1	–
TAKE-OUT									
cheeseburger + condiments	1 reg (4.5 oz)	347	1	170	26	1	164	3	221
double hamburger + condiments	1 reg (5.8 oz)	384	2	50	30	3	98	4	339
single patty + condiments	1 reg (4 oz)	299	2	30	67	5	104	3	277

HAMBURGER SUBSTITUTES

FOOD	PORTION	CALS	FIBER	VIT A	FOLIC	VIT C	CALCI	IRON	POTAS
Amy's									
All American Burger	1 (2.5 oz)	120	3	–	–	–	–	–	–
California Burger	1 (2.5 oz)	130	5	–	–	–	–	–	–
Chicago Burger	1 (2.5 oz)	160	3	–	–	–	–	–	–
Boca									
American Flame Grilled	1 (2.5 oz)	90	3	0	–	0	150	2	–
Cheeseburger	1 (2.5 oz)	100	3	100	–	5	0	2	–
Grilled Vegetable	1 (2.5 oz)	70	4	400	–	5	60	2	–
Ground Burger	1 serv (2 oz)	60	3	0	–	0	60	2	–
Original	1 (2.5 oz)	70	4	0	–	0	60	2	–
Original Vegan	1 patty (2.5 oz)	70	4	0	–	0	60	2	340
Dr. Praeger's									
California Burger	1 (2.7 oz)	100	4	2500	–	4	50	1	–
Fantastic									
Natures Burger Mix not prep	¼ cup	170	5	200	–	2	60	2	–
Tofu Burger Mix not prep	3 tbsp	80	1	0	–	0	40	1	–
Harmony Farms									
Soy Burger Onion	1 (2.5 oz)	90	3	0	–	0	40	1	–
Soy Burgers Garlic	1 (2.5 oz)	110	23	0	–	0	40	1	–
Soy Burgers Mushroom	1 (2.5 oz)	110	3	0	–	0	40	1	–
Soy Burgers Original	1 (2.5 oz)	110	4	0	–	0	40	1	–

FOOD	PORTION	CALS	FIBER	VIT A	FOLIC	VIT C	CALCI	IRON	POTAS
Lightlife									
Light Burgers	1 (3 oz)	120	3	–	–	–	–	–	520
Smart Menu Burger	1	80	2	–	–	–	–	–	200
Morningstar Farms									
Classic Burger	1 (2.2 oz)	150	3	0	–	0	0	2	350
Garden Veggie Patties	1 patty (2.4 oz)	100	4	200	–	0	40	1	180
Harvest Burger	1	140	5	0	–	0	80	3	380
Okara Pattie	1 (2.2 oz)	120	3	0	–	0	0	1	240
Vegan Burger	1 (2.5 oz)	100	5	0	–	0	20	3	260
Tofurky									
SuperBurgers Original	1 (3.5 oz)	120	2	500	–	0	80	tr	–
VeggieLand									
Veggie Burger Original	1 (3.5 oz)	132	7	0	–	0	40	3	–
Veggie Burger Peppadew	1 (5 oz)	210	4	1250	–	6	100	6	–
HAZELNUTS									
dried blanched	1 oz	191	–	20	–	–	55	1	131
dried unblanched	1 oz	179	–	19	20	tr	53	1	125
dry roasted unblanched	1 oz	188	–	–	–	–	55	1	131
oil roasted unblanched	1 oz	187	2	–	–	–	56	1	132
Kettle									
Butter Creamy Unsalted	2 tbsp	180	3	0	–	1	40	1	–
Love'n Bake									
Hazelnut Praline	2 tbsp	170	2	–	–	1	10	1	–
Low Carb Creations									
Soft Hazelnut Brittle	2 pieces (1 oz)	160	1	–	–	–	–	–	–
Torras									
Hazelnut Chocolate Spread	1 tsp	27	0	–	–	–	–	–	–
Twist									
Sugar Free Chocolate Hazelnut Spread	2 tbsp	180	0	–	–	–	–	–	–
HEART									
beef simmered	3 oz	140	0	0	4	0	4	5	186

FOOD	PORTION	CALS	FIBER	VIT A	FOLIC	VIT C	CALCI	IRON	POTAS
chicken cooked	1 (3 g)	5	0	0	0	0	0	tr	7
chicken diced simmered	½ cup	134	0	20	58	1	14	7	96
lamb braised	3 oz	157	0	0	2	6	12	5	160
pork braised	1 (4.5 oz)	191	0	28	5	3	9	8	266
turkey simmered	½ cup	94	0	46	6	2	5	4	211
veal braised	3 oz	158	0	0	2	9	7	4	169

HEARTS OF PALM

FOOD	PORTION	CALS	FIBER	VIT A	FOLIC	VIT C	CALCI	IRON	POTAS
canned	½ cup	20	2	0	28	6	42	2	129
canned	1 (1.2 oz)	9	1	0	13	3	19	1	58
Del Monte									
Hearts Of Palm	2–3 pieces	20	2	0	–	9	40	tr	–

HEMP

FOOD	PORTION	CALS	FIBER	VIT A	FOLIC	VIT C	CALCI	IRON	POTAS
Living Harvest									
Organic Hemp Nuts	2 tbsp (1 oz)	170	0	0	–	1	20	4	–
Organic Protein Powder	2 scoops (1 oz)	110	1	0	–	1	60	5	–
Manitoba Harvest									
Hemp Seed Butter	2 tbsp	160	1	0	–	0	0	4	–
Protein Powder	2 scoops (1 oz)	134	4	0	–	1	0	1	–
Shelled Seed	2 tbsp	160	1	0	–	0	0	4	–
Nutiva									
Organic Protein Powder	2 scoops (1 oz)	120	14	–	–	–	40	1	–
Shelled Hempseed	2 tbsp	110	1	–	–	–	–	2	210

HERBS/SPICES

FOOD	PORTION	CALS	FIBER	VIT A	FOLIC	VIT C	CALCI	IRON	POTAS
chinese five spice	1 tsp	7	tr	–	–	–	4	1	23
garam masala	1 tsp	8	–	2	0	0	15	1	29
poultry seasoning	1 tsp	5	–	39	–	tr	15	1	10
pumpkin pie spice	1 tsp	6	–	4	–	tr	12	tr	11
A Taste Of Thai									
Chicken & Rice Seasoning	¼ pkg (6 g)	15	0	0	–	–	20	–	–
Chef Paul Prudhomme's									
Magic Fajita	¼ tsp	0	0	–	–	–	–	–	–
Cut N Clean									
Greens Seasoning	1½ tsp	20	tr	400	–	2	20	tr	–

FOOD	PORTION	CALS	FIBER	VIT A	FOLIC	VIT C	CALCI	IRON	POTAS
Eden									
Shake Furikake	½ tsp	5	1	0	–	0	20	0	10
Nueva Cocina									
Picadillo	2 tsp	15	–	300	–	12	–	–	–
Taco Fresco	2 tsp	15	–	400	–	12	–	tr	–
Ortega									
Burrito Seasoning	1½ tsp	20	tr	1200	–	–	–	–	–
HERRING									
atlantic baked	4 oz	230	0	136	14	1	84	2	475
dried salted	1 fillet (1.4 oz)	161	0	125	9	1	62	1	331
pickled	1 oz	74	0	244	1	0	22	tr	20
pickled in cream sauce	1 oz	72	0	345	1	tr	24	tr	24
roe	1 tbsp	39	0	115	21	4	6	tr	62
smoked kippered	1 oz	620	0	38	4	tr	24	tr	127
Beach Cliff									
Kippered Snacks	1 can (4 oz)	220	0	300	–	0	60	1	–
TAKE-OUT									
breaded fried	1 serv (4 oz)	225	1	130	17	tr	68	1	264
HIBISCUS									
flowers dried sweetened	⅓ cup	100	2	0	–	0	40	0	–
HICKORY NUTS									
dried	1 oz	187	–	–	–	–	17	1	124
HOMINY									
CANNED									
white	1 cup (5.6 oz)	482	4	176	2	0	16	1	14
HONEY									
honey	1 tbsp (0.7 oz)	64	–	0	0	tr	1	tr	11
honey	1 cup (11.9 oz)	1031	–	0	5	2	20	2	176
orange blossom	1 tbsp	60	0	0	–	0	0	0	–

FOOD	PORTION	CALS	FIBER	VIT A	FOLIC	VIT C	CALCI	IRON	POTAS
Frieda's									
Honeycomb	½ cup (3 oz)	260	0	0	–	0	0	tr	–
Steel's									
Sugar Free	1 tbsp	24	0	–	–	–	–	–	–

HONEYDEW
FRESH

FOOD	PORTION	CALS	FIBER	VIT A	FOLIC	VIT C	CALCI	IRON	POTAS
cubed	1 cup	60	–	68	–	42	10	tr	461
wedge	¹⁄₁₀	46	–	52	–	32	8	tr	350
Chiquita									
Wedge	¹⁄₁₀ melon (4.7 oz)	50	1	100	–	27	0	tr	–

HORSE

FOOD	PORTION	CALS	FIBER	VIT A	FOLIC	VIT C	CALCI	IRON	POTAS
roasted	3 oz	149	0	–	–	2	7	4	322

HORSERADISH

FOOD	PORTION	CALS	FIBER	VIT A	FOLIC	VIT C	CALCI	IRON	POTAS
japanese wasabi	¼ tsp	1	0	tr	tr	1	2	tr	5
wasabi root raw	1 (5.9 oz)	184	12	78	30	71	216	2	960
wasabi root raw sliced	1 cup (4.6 oz)	142	10	60	23	71	166	1	738
Boar's Head									
Horseradish	1 tsp (5 g)	0	0	0	–	0	0	0	–
Horseradish & Beets	1 tsp	0	0	0	–	0	0	0	–
Eden									
Wasabi Powder	1 tsp	10	1	0	–	0	0	0	–

HOT CHOCOLATE

FOOD	PORTION	CALS	FIBER	VIT A	FOLIC	VIT C	CALCI	IRON	POTAS
mix as prep w/ water	7 oz	103	–	4	tr	1	96	tr	203
mix w/ equal as prep w/ water	7 oz	48	–	–	2	0	90	1	405
Carnation									
Hot Cocoa Rich Chocolate as prep w/ 2% milk	1 pkg	200	tr	400	–	0	300	1	–
Country Choice Naturals									
Irish Chocolate Mint Cocoa	1 pkg	100	tr	0	–	0	100	1	–
Royal Chocolate Cocoa	1 pkg	100	tr	0	–	0	100	1	–
Soy Cocoa Irish Chocolate Mint	1 pkg	100	1	0	–	0	60	1	–

FOOD	PORTION	CALS	FIBER	VIT A	FOLIC	VIT C	CALCI	IRON	POTAS
Soy Cocoa Royal Chocolate	1 pkg	100	1	0	–	0	60	1	–
Keto									
Hot Cocoa	1 tsp	12	1	–	–	–	–	–	–
Low Carb Creations									
Cocoa as prep	1 cup	30	0	0	–	0	0	tr	–
White Hot Chocolate	1 cup	25	0	0	–	0	0	tr	–
Sipper Sweets									
Sugar Free Low Carb Mix	1 serv	50	0	–	–	–	–	–	–
Swiss Miss									
Caramel Cream	1 serv	110	tr	0	–	0	40	0	–
Hot Cocoa Milk Chocolate Fat Free	1 pkg	50	tr	–	–	–	300	1	–
Milk Chocolate	1 pkg	120	1	0	–	0	40	1	–
Milk Chocolate w/ Marshmallows	1 pkg	120	tr	0	–	0	40	1	–
TAKE-OUT									
hot cocoa	1 cup	218	–	318	12	2	298	1	480
mexican hot chocolate	1 cup	173	1	503	13	2	306	tr	442

HOT DOG

FOOD	PORTION	CALS	FIBER	VIT A	FOLIC	VIT C	CALCI	IRON	POTAS
beef	1 (1.5 oz)	149	0	0	2	0	6	1	70
beef & pork	1 (1.5 oz)	137	1	26	2	0	5	1	75
beef low fat	1 (2 oz)	133	0	0	2	1	5	1	74
chicken	1 (1.5 oz)	116	0	59	2	0	43	1	38
fat free	1 (2 oz)	62	0	0	3	14	31	1	125
low fat	1 (2 oz)	88	0	0	2	0	6	1	86
low sodium	1 (2 oz)	180	0	0	2	0	11	1	95
pork and beef cheese smokie	1 (1.5 oz)	141	0	68	1	0	25	tr	89
turkey	1 (1.5 oz)	102	0	0	4	0	48	1	81
Ball Park									
Franks	1 (2 oz)	180	0	0	–	4	40	1	340
Franks Beef	1 (2 oz)	180	0	0	–	4	0	1	360
Franks Bun Size	1 (2 oz)	180	0	0	–	4	40	1	340
Franks Smoked White Turkey	1 (1.8 oz)	45	0	0	–	4	0	tr	450
Franks Fat Free	1 (1.8 oz)	40	0	0	–	4	0	tr	430
Franks Lite	1 (1.8 oz)	100	0	0	–	4	20	tr	340

FOOD	PORTION	CALS	FIBER	VIT A	FOLIC	VIT C	CALCI	IRON	POTAS
Franks Singles Cheese	1 (1.6 oz)	150	0	100	–	2	60	tr	280
Grillmaster Hearty Beef	1	250	0	0	–	8	0	1	520
Grillmaster Smokehouse	1	210	0	0	–	6	0	1	540
Boar's Head									
Beef	1 (2 oz)	160	0	300	–	0	0	1	–
Beef Lite	1 (1.6 oz)	90	0	100	–	0	0	1	–
Beef Cocktail	5 (2 oz)	170	0	100	–	–	0	1	–
Pork & Beef	1 (2 oz)	150	0	0	–	0	0	1	–
Dietz & Watson									
New York Style Beef	1 (2.3 oz)	130	0	0	–	0	0	tr	–
Healthy Choice									
Beef Low Fat	1 (1.8 oz)	70	0	0	–	2	0	tr	–
Hebrew National									
97% Fat Free Beef	1 (1.7 oz)	45	0	0	–	0	0	1	–
Beef	1 (1.7 oz)	150	0	0	–	0	0	1	–
Cocktail Franks	5 (2 oz)	180	0	0	–	0	0	1	–
Dinner Frank	1 (4 oz)	350	0	0	–	0	0	1	–
Franks In A Blanket	5 (2.8 oz)	290	1	0	–	0	0	1	–
Reduced Fat Beef	1 (1.7 oz)	120	0	0	–	0	0	1	–
Ian's									
Popcorn Turkey Corn Dog	5 pieces (3 oz)	237	0	0	–	0	0	2	–
Oscar Mayer									
Corn Dogs	1 (3.2 oz)	260	1	0	–	0	20	1	–
State Fair									
Corn Dogs	1 (2.67 oz)	180	1	–	–	–	–	1	–
Wellshire									
Beef Premium	1 (2 oz)	110	0	–	–	–	–	–	–
Cheese Franks	1 (2 oz)	110	0	–	–	–	–	1	–
Chicken Franks	1 (1.6 oz)	70	0	100	–	1	0	tr	–
Turkey Franks	1 (1.6 oz)	110	0	0	–	0	80	1	–
TAKE-OUT									
corndog	1	460	–	207	60	0	101	6	262
w/ bun chili	1	297	–	58	50	3	19	3	166
w/ bun plain	1	242	–	0	30	tr	24	2	143

FOOD	PORTION	CALS	FIBER	VIT A	FOLIC	VIT C	CALCI	IRON	POTAS
HOT DOG SUBSTITUTES									
Lightlife									
Smart Dogs	1	45	1	–	–	–	–	–	–
Smart Franks	1 (2 oz)	110	0	–	–	–	–	–	125
Tofu Pups	1 (1.5 oz)	60	1	–	–	–	–	–	180
Loma Linda									
Big Franks	1 (1.8 oz)	110	2	0	–	0	0	1	50
Big Franks Low Fat Vegan	1 (1.8 oz)	80	2	0	–	0	0	1	50
Morningstar Farms									
Corn Dog Veggie	1 (2.5 oz)	170	3	0	–	0	0	1	60
Quorn									
Meat-Free Dogs	1 (1.5 oz)	70	2	0	–	0	20	tr	–
HUMMUS									
Athenos									
Black Olive	2 tbsp	50	1	–	–	1	20	tr	–
Original	2 tbsp	50	1	0	–	0	20	tr	–
Travelers Hummus & Pita	1 pkg	325	3	0	–	3	100	7	–
Guiltless Gourmet									
Roasted Garlic	2 tbsp	35	1	0	–	0	0	tr	–
Sabra									
Homus	2 oz	110	3	0	–	2	20	1	–
Homus Spicy	½ cup	171	5	350	–	7	50	3	–
TAKE-OUT									
hummus	⅓ cup	140	–	20	49	6	41	1	142
HYACINTH BEANS									
dried cooked	1 cup	228	–	–	–	0	77	9	653
ICE CREAM AND FROZEN DESSERTS									
chocolate	½ cup (4 oz)	143	–	275	10	1	72	1	164
dixie cup chocolate	1 (3.5 oz)	125	–	241	9	tr	63	1	145
dixie cup strawberry	1 (3.5 oz)	112	–	185	7	5	70	tr	109
dixie cup vanilla	1 (3.5 oz)	116	–	237	3	tr	74	tr	115
freeze dried ice cream chocolate strawberry & vanilla	1 pkg (0.75 oz)	158	1	200	–	0	20	1	–
strawberry	½ cup (4 oz)	127	–	211	8	5	79	tr	124

FOOD	PORTION	CALS	FIBER	VIT A	FOLIC	VIT C	CALCI	IRON	POTAS
vanilla	½ cup (4 oz)	132	–	270	3	tr	85	tr	131
vanilla soft serve	½ cup	111	–	90	6	1	138	tr	194
Blue Bunny									
Blendz Peanut Butter Cup	1 (4.4 oz)	270	tr	200	–	–	150	tr	180
Caramel Sundae Bite Size	4 bars (3.1 oz)	340	1	200	–	–	100	–	180
Premium All Natural Vanilla	½ cup	160	0	300	–	–	100	–	150
Premium Bunny Tracks	½ cup	190	tr	200	–	–	80	–	130
Premium Butter Pecan	½ cup	150	0	200	–	–	80	–	135
Premium Cookies & Cream	½ cup	150	0	200	–	–	80	–	135
Premium Double Strawberry	½ cup	140	0	200	–	4	80	–	120
Premium Exquisite Mint	½ cup	170	0	200	–	–	80	–	120
Premium Rocky Road	½ cup	150	0	200	–	–	60	–	105
Premium Toasted Almond Fudge	½ cup	160	tr	200	–	–	80	–	115
Breyers									
Almond Joy	½ cup	140	tr	300	–	0	80	1	–
Bar Light Creamy Vanilla Chocolate Coated	1	160	3	200	–	0	100	0	–
Butter Almond	½ cup	160	tr	200	–	0	100	0	–
Butter Pecan	½ cup	170	0	200	–	0	100	0	–
Butter Pecan No Sugar Added	½ cup	120	tr	200	–	0	80	0	–
CarbSmart Chocolate	½ cup	130	3	300	–	0	60	tr	–
CarbSmart Strawberry	½ cup	130	3	300	–	0	60	0	–
CarbSmart Vanilla	½ cup	130	3	300	–	0	60	0	–
Chocolate	½ cup	150	tr	200	–	0	80	1	–
Chocolate 98% Fat Free	½ cup	90	4	200	–	0	80	1	–
Chocolate Caramel No Sugar Added	½ cup	110	tr	200	–	0	80	tr	–
Coffee	½ cup	140	0	200	–	0	100	0	–
Creamsicle	½ cup	130	0	200	–	0	60	0	–
Dulce De Leche	½ cup	150	0	200	–	0	100	0	–

FOOD	PORTION	CALS	FIBER	VIT A	FOLIC	VIT C	CALCI	IRON	POTAS
French Vanilla	½ cup	150	0	300	–	0	100	0	–
French Vanilla Light	½ cup	120	0	300	–	0	100	0	–
French Vanilla No Sugar Added	½ cup	110	0	200	–	0	100	0	–
Rocky Road	½ cup	160	tr	200	–	0	80	1	–
Strawberry	½ cup	120	0	200	–	6	80	0	–
Vanilla	½ cup	140	0	200	–	0	100	0	–
Vanilla Calcium Rich	½ cup	130	0	200	–	0	300	0	–
Vanilla Lactose Free	½ cup	130	0	200	–	0	80	0	–
Bubbies									
Mochi Mango	1 piece (1.3 oz)	110	0	200	–	2	20	0	–
Celestial Seasonings									
Tea Dreams Bars Chocolate Caramel Chai	1 (2.7 oz)	240	2	0	–	0	0	1	–
Tea Dreams Cinnamon Apple Spice	½ cup	140	1	0	–	0	20	0	–
Tea Dreams Vanilla Ginger Spice Chai	½ cup	140	1	0	–	0	20	0	–
Edy's									
Slow Churned Light Vanilla	½ cup	100	–	–	–	–	60	–	–
Good Humor									
Bar Toasted Almond	1 (3 oz)	180	tr	0	–	0	40	0	–
Bar Vanilla Dark Chocolate	1 (3 oz)	190	tr	100	–	0	60	tr	–
Bar Vanilla Milk Chocolate	1 (3 oz)	180	0	100	–	0	80	0	–
Bar Strawberry Shortcake	1 (4 oz)	230	tr	0	–	0	40	1	–
Chocolate Eclair Bar	1 (4 oz)	220	tr	0	–	0	40	1	–
Cone Premium Sundae	1 (4.3 oz)	270	tr	200	–	0	60	1	–
Cone Strawberry Shortcake	1 (4.3 oz)	230	tr	0	–	0	20	1	–
Giant Sandwich Neapolitan	1 (6 oz)	250	tr	200	–	0	100	1	–
Giant Sandwich Vanilla	1 (6 oz)	250	0	200	–	0	100	1	–

FOOD	PORTION	CALS	FIBER	VIT A	FOLIC	VIT C	CALCI	IRON	POTAS
King Cone	1 (4.6 fl oz)	250	tr	200	–	0	80	1	–
Sandwich Chocolate Chip Cookie	1 (4.5 oz)	290	1	100	–	0	60	1	–
Sandwich Vanilla	1 (3.5 oz)	160	0	100	–	0	40	1	–
Sundae Twist Cup	1 (6 oz)	160	0	100	–	0	150	0	–
GoodBody									
Chocolate Banana	1 bar (3.5 oz)	120	4	1250	80	66	300	1	510
Chocolate Double Dutch	1 bar (3.5 oz)	130	4	1250	80	60	300	1	430
Chocolate Peanut Butter	1 bar (3.5 oz)	180	5	1250	80	60	300	1	460
Vanilla & Raspberry Sorbet	1 bar (3.5 oz)	120	4	1250	80	60	300	0	180
Vanilla & Strawberry Sorbet	1 bar (3.5 oz)	120	4	1250	80	60	300	0	180
Vanilla & Tropical Sorbet	1 bar (3.5 oz)	120	4	1250	80	60	300	0	180
Haagen-Dazs									
Bars Chocolate & Almonds	1 (3.7 oz)	380	2	500	–	0	150	1	–
Bars Chocolate & Dark Chocolate	1 (3.6 oz)	350	2	500	–	0	100	2	–
Bars Vanilla & Almonds	1 (3.7 oz)	380	1	500	–	0	150	1	–
Bars Vanilla & Dark Chocolate	1 (3.6 oz)	350	1	500	–	0	100	2	–
Bars Vanilla & Milk Chocolate	1 (3.5 oz)	340	tr	500	–	0	150	1	–
Butter Pecan	½ cup	310	tr	500	–	0	100	tr	–
Chocolate	½ cup	270	1	500	–	0	150	1	–
Coffee	½ cup	270	0	750	–	0	150	0	–
Rum Raisin	½ cup	270	0	500	–	0	100	0	–
Strawberry	½ cup	250	tr	500	–	6	150	0	–
Vanilla	½ cup	270	0	750	–	0	150	0	–
Vanilla Fudge	½ cup	290	0	500	–	0	150	tr	–
Healthy Choice									
Bar Sorbet & Cream	1	100	tr	0	–	0	100	0	–
Brownie Bliss	½ cup	130	1	200	–	0	100	2	–

FOOD	PORTION	CALS	FIBER	VIT A	FOLIC	VIT C	CALCI	IRON	POTAS
Butter Pecan Crunch	½ cup	100	2	100	–	0	100	0	150
Cappuccino Chocolate Chunk	½ cup	120	tr	200	–	0	100	0	–
Caramel Fudge Brownie	½ cup	120	1	200	–	0	100	tr	–
Cherry Chocolate Mambo	½ cup	130	1	200	–	0	100	0	–
Chocolate Chocolate Chunk	½ cup	120	1	200	–	0	100	1	–
Cookies 'N Cream	½ cup	120	tr	200	–	0	100	0	–
Crazy Caramel	½ cup	120	tr	100	–	0	100	0	–
Double Karma	½ cup	140	tr	200	–	0	100	0	–
French Silk	½ cup	120	2	0	–	0	100	tr	190
Happy Together	½ cup	150	1	200	–	0	100	1	–
Jumpin' Java	½ cup	130	tr	100	–	0	100	tr	170
Low Fat Bar Fudge	1	90	0	500	–	0	80	tr	–
Low Fat Bar Mocha Fudge	1	90	2	0	–	0	100	tr	160
Low Fat Bar Strawberry & Cream	1	90	tr	500	–	0	60	0	–
Mint Chocolate Chip	½ cup	120	tr	200	–	0	100	0	–
No Sugar Added Chocolate Fudge Brownie	½ cup	120	1	200	–	0	100	0	–
No Sugar Added Coffee Almond Fudge	½ cup	110	1	200	–	0	100	tr	–
No Sugar Added Mint Chocolate Chip	½ cup	110	1	200	–	0	100	0	–
No Sugar Added Vanilla	½ cup	100	1	200	–	0	100	0	–
Peanut Butter Cup	½ cup	120	tr	200	–	0	100	tr	–
Praline & Caramel	½ cup	120	tr	200	–	0	100	0	–
Rocky Road	½ cup	130	tr	200	–	0	100	1	–
Sandwich Caramel	1	140	tr	100	–	0	20	2	–
Sandwich Fudge Swirl	1	140	tr	100	–	0	20	2	–
Sandwich Vanilla	1	130	tr	100	–	0	20	2	–
Turtle Fudge Cake	½ cup	130	tr	100	–	0	100	1	190
Vanilla	½ cup	110	tr	200	–	0	100	0	–
Vanilla Bean	½ cup	120	tr	200	–	0	100	0	–
Vanilla Caramel Fudge	½ cup	140	tr	200	–	0	100	0	–

FOOD	PORTION	CALS	FIBER	VIT A	FOLIC	VIT C	CALCI	IRON	POTAS
Hood									
Butterscotch Blast	½ cup	160	0	200	–	0	80	0	–
Chocolate	½ cup	140	0	300	–	0	80	1	–
Chocolate Eclair	1 bar (2.2 oz)	150	0	0	–	0	20	0	–
Creamy Coffee	½ cup	140	0	300	–	0	80	0	–
Fat Free Chocolate Passion	½ cup	100	0	300	–	0	80	1	–
Fat Free Very Vanilla	½ cup	100	0	300	–	0	80	0	–
Grasshopper Pie	½ cup	160	0	200	–	0	80	1	–
Hoodsie Cups	1 (1.7 oz)	100	0	200	–	0	40	0	–
Light Butter Pecan	½ cup	140	0	300	–	0	80	0	–
Light Creamy Vanilla	½ cup	110	0	300	–	0	100	0	–
Low Fat No Sugar Added Vanilla Dream	½ cup	90	3	300	–	0	100	0	–
Maple Walnut	½ cup	160	0	300	–	0	80	0	–
No Sugar Added Chocolate Chip	½ cup	100	3	300	–	0	100	0	–
Orange Cream	1 bar (2.2 oz)	90	0	0	–	0	40	0	–
Sandwich Vanilla	1	180	tr	200	–	0	60	0	–
Sandwich Vanilla Light	1 (2.2 oz)	160	tr	200	–	0	60	1	–
Sandwich Vanilla Lowfat	1 (2.8 oz)	80	2	0	–	0	40	0	–
Spumoni	½ cup	140	0	300	–	0	80	0	–
Klondike									
Slim-A-Bear 98% Fat Free Sandwich Vanilla	1	130	3	200	–	0	100	tr	–
Slim-A-Bear No Sugar Added Cone Vanilla	1	270	4	200	–	0	250	tr	–
Slim-A-Bear No Sugar Added Fudge Bar	1	90	4	0	–	0	100	tr	–
Slim-A-Bear No Sugar Added Reduced Fat Bar Vanilla	1	160	4	200	–	0	250	0	–
Slim-A-Bear No Sugar Added Sandwich Vanilla	1	120	2	200	–	0	150	0	–

FOOD	PORTION	CALS	FIBER	VIT A	FOLIC	VIT C	CALCI	IRON	POTAS
Natural Choice									
Organic Double Chocolate	½ cup	230	0	400	–	2	150	0	–
Organic Strawberry	½ cup	210	0	400	–	5	150	0	–
Organic Vanilla	½ cup	220	0	400	–	2	150	0	–
No Pudge!									
Giant Chocolate Eclair Low Fat	1 bar	110	4	300	–	0	100	0	–
Giant Cone Chocolate No Sugar Added	1	110	6	300	–	0	100	tr	–
Giant Cone Cookies & Cream Low Fat	1	140	3	200	–	0	100	tr	–
Giant Cone Fudgy Brownie Low Fat	1	140	4	200	–	0	100	3	–
Giant Cone Vanilla No Sugar Added	1	110	5	300	–	0	100	tr	–
Giant Cookie & Cream Low Fat No Sugar Added	1 bar	100	6	300	–	0	100	1	–
Giant Fudgy Fat Free No Sugar Added	1 bar	60	6	400	–	0	100	0	–
Giant Sandwich Brownie Batter Low Fat	1	140	3	300	–	0	100	1	–
Giant Sandwich Brownie Chunk Low Fat	1	140	4	200	–	0	80	2	–
Giant Sandwich Vanilla & Chocolate No Sugar Added	1	130	6	300	–	0	100	1	–
Giant Strawberry Shortcake 98% Fat Free	1 bar	90	4	300	–	0	100	0	–
Rice Dream									
Bar Vanilla w/ Chocolate Coating	1 (3 oz)	230	tr	0	–	1	0	tr	–
Carob Almond	½ cup	180	2	0	–	0	40	tr	–
Frozen Pie Chocolate	1 (3.4 oz)	330	2	0	–	1	0	1	–
Mint Carob Chip	½ cup	170	0	0	–	0	0	0	–
Strawberry	½ cup	160	2	0	–	0	20	tr	–

FOOD	PORTION	CALS	FIBER	VIT A	FOLIC	VIT C	CALCI	IRON	POTAS
Silhouette									
The Skinny Cow Low Fat Ice Cream Sandwich Vanilla	1	130	2	0	–	0	80	0	–
Skinny Cow									
Sandwich Low Fat	1 (2.5 oz)	140	3	300	–	0	80	0	–
Slim-Fast									
Chocolate Fudge Bar	1 bar	110	tr	750	–	9	250	1	–
Ice Cream Sandwich Chocolate	1	130	tr	750	–	9	250	1	–
Ice Cream Sandwich Vanilla	1	130	tr	750	–	9	250	tr	–
Soy Dream									
Butter Pecan	½ cup	140	tr	0	–	0	20	tr	–
Sandwich Lil' Dreamers Chocolate	1 (1.4 oz)	100	tr	0	–	0	0	0	–
Vanilla	½ cup	140	tr	0	–	0	20	tr	–
Starbucks									
Caramel Cappuccino Swirl	½ cup	240	0	750	–	0	100	0	–
Classic Coffee	½ cup	230	0	750	–	0	100	0	–
Coffee Almond Fudge	½ cup	250	1	500	–	0	100	1	–
Frappuccino Bar Java Fudge	1 bar	130	4	200	–	0	100	0	–
Frappuccino Bar Mocha	1 bar	120	3	200	–	0	100	0	–
Java Chip	½ cup	250	0	500	–	0	100	tr	–
Low Fat Latte	½ cup	170	0	400	–	0	100	0	–
Mud Pie	½ cup	240	1	500	–	0	100	tr	–
White Chocolate Latte	½ cup	280	0	500	–	0	100	0	–
Turkey Hill									
Butter Pecan	½ cup	170	0	300	–	0	80	0	–
Carb IQ Vanilla Bean	½ cup	110	5	300	–	0	60	0	–
Light Butter Pecan	½ cup	130	0	300	–	0	100	0	–
Light Vanilla Bean	½ cup	110	0	300	–	0	100	0	–
Neapolitan	½ cup	150	0	300	–	0	80	0	–
Rocky Road	½ cup	170	0	200	–	0	80	0	–
Vanilla Bean	½ cup	140	0	300	–	0	80	0	–
Weight Watchers									
English Toffee Crunch	1 bar	110	2	100	–	0	40	1	–

FOOD	PORTION	CALS	FIBER	VIT A	FOLIC	VIT C	CALCI	IRON	POTAS
Smart Ones Giant Sundae	1 serv (8 oz)	150	7	500	–	0	200	tr	–
TAKE-OUT									
cone vanilla light soft serve	1 (4.6 oz)	164	–	211	5	1	153	tr	169
gelato chocolate hazelnut	½ cup (5.3 oz)	370	2	76	35	1	179	2	352
gelato vanilla	½ cup (3 oz)	211	0	191	15	tr	67	tr	77
sundae caramel	1 (5.4 oz)	303	–	263	12	3	189	tr	318
sundae hot fudge	1 (5.4 oz)	284	–	221	9	2	207	tr	395
sundae strawberry	1 (5.4 oz)	269	–	222	18	2	161	tr	270

ICE CREAM CONES AND CUPS

FOOD	PORTION	CALS	FIBER	VIT A	FOLIC	VIT C	CALCI	IRON	POTAS
wafer cone	1	17	tr	0	7	0	1	tr	4
waffle cone	1 lg	121	1	0	50	0	7	1	32

ICE CREAM TOPPINGS

FOOD	PORTION	CALS	FIBER	VIT A	FOLIC	VIT C	CALCI	IRON	POTAS
marshmallow cream	1 oz	88	–	0	0	–	1	tr	1
nuts in syrup	2 tbsp	184	1	3	11	tr	14	tr	62
pineapple	2 tbsp (1.5 oz)	106	–	9	1	25	9	tr	133
strawberry	2 tbsp (1.5 oz)	107	–	9	1	11	10	tr	31
Lollipop Tree									
Hot Fudge Sauce	1 tbsp	80	tr	100	–	0	0	1	–
Maple Walnut Cream	2 tbsp	190	0	400	–	0	40	0	–
Sanders									
Butterscotch Caramel	2 tbsp	90	0	100	–	–	20	–	–
Smucker's									
Butterscotch Caramel	2 tbsp	130	tr	0	–	0	40	0	–
Dove Dark Chocolate	2 tbsp	140	1	0	–	0	0	1	105
Dove Milk Chocolate	2 tbsp	130	1	0	–	0	60	1	115
Hot Fudge	2 tbsp	140	tr	0	–	0	60	1	–
Hot Fudge Sugar Free Fat Free	2 tbsp	90	1	0	–	0	20	1	–

ICED TEA
MIX
A La Source

FOOD	PORTION	CALS	FIBER	VIT A	FOLIC	VIT C	CALCI	IRON	POTAS
Organic as prep	8 oz	90	–	–	–	6	–	–	–

FOOD	PORTION	CALS	FIBER	VIT A	FOLIC	VIT C	CALCI	IRON	POTAS
Organic Green Tea as prep	8 oz	90	–	–	–	6	–	–	–
Organic Herbal Tea Red Rooibos	8 oz	80	–	–	–	6	20	–	–
Lipton									
Chailatta Chocolate as prep	8 oz	120	–	–	–	–	80	–	–
Chailatta Original as prep	8 oz	120	–	–	–	–	80	–	–
READY-TO-DRINK									
Anteadote									
All Flavors	8 oz	0	0	–	–	60	–	–	–
Arizona									
Green Tea w/ Ginseng & Honey	8 oz	70	0	0	–	21	0	0	–
Lemon	8 oz	90	0	0	–	21	0	0	–
Bolthouse Farms									
Perfectly Protein Vanilla Chai Tea w/ Soy	8 oz	160	0	0	–	108	300	3	530
Brazil Gourmet									
Nectar Tea All Flavors	8 oz	90	0	500	–	6	–	–	–
Nectar Tea Light Mango Passion	8 oz	60	0	500	–	6	–	–	–
Delta Blues									
Spearmint Tea Punch	8 oz	90	0	0	–	5	–	–	–
Fuze									
LemonAID	8 oz	70	–	1250	–	60	–	–	–
Vitamin Tea Diet Peach	8 oz	5	0	1250	–	30	–	–	–
Vitamin Tea Green Tea w/ Ginseng	8 oz	60	–	2500	–	30	–	–	–
Vitamin Tea Lemon	8 oz	70	–	1250	–	30	–	–	–
White Tea	8 oz	60	–	–	100	60	–	–	–
White Tea No Carb Diet Pomegranate	8 oz	0	0	–	100	60	–	–	–
Glaceau Vitamin Water									
Vital-T	8 oz	50	–	–	–	36	–	–	–
Hansen's									
Chai	8 oz	150	–	–	–	60	–	–	–
China Black	8 oz	90	–	–	–	60	–	–	–

FOOD	PORTION	CALS	FIBER	VIT A	FOLIC	VIT C	CALCI	IRON	POTAS
Green	8 oz	70	–	–	–	60	–	–	–
Green Diet Lemon	8 oz	0	0	–	–	60	–	–	–
Green Diet Peach	8 oz	0	0	–	–	60	–	–	–
Green Lemon	8 oz	70	–	–	–	60	–	–	–
Green Peach	8 oz	70	–	–	–	60	–	–	–
Oolong	8 oz	70	–	–	–	60	–	–	–
Spice	8 oz	90	–	–	–	60	–	–	–
Hawaiian									
Iced Tea	1 can	120	0	0	–	60	0	0	–
Honest Tea									
Assam	8 oz	17	–	–	–	12	–	–	–
Hood									
Iced Tea	1 cup	100	0	0	–	72	0	0	–
Old Orchard									
Green Tea w/ Lemon & Honey	8 oz	45	0	0	–	0	0	0	–
Green Tea w/ Pomegranate	8 oz	45	0	0	–	0	0	0	–
Pacific Foods									
Organic Lemon	8 oz	70	0	0	–	60	0	0	–
Organic Peach	8 oz	70	0	0	–	60	0	0	–
Organic Raspberry	8 oz	70	0	0	–	60	0	0	–
Organic Sweetened Black Tea	8 oz	60	0	0	–	60	0	0	–
Organic Unsweetened Green Tea	8 oz	0	0	0	–	60	0	0	–
Solebury Home									
Organic All Flavors	8 oz	33	–	–	–	60	–	–	–
Sri Lankan									
Apple	8 oz	70	0	0	–	24	0	0	–
Lemon	8 oz	60	0	0	–	24	0	0	–
Sweet Leaf Tea									
Hibiscus Herbal	8 oz	25	–	–	–	72	–	–	–
XS Energy									
Energy Tea Berry Typhoon	1 can (8.4 oz)	12	–	0	–	0	0	0	25

ICES AND ICE POPS
Blue Bunny
Bar Big Fudge	1 (2.7 oz)	110	0	–	–	–	100	–	170

FOOD	PORTION	CALS	FIBER	VIT A	FOLIC	VIT C	CALCI	IRON	POTAS
Chill Cups Double Lemon	1 (4 oz)	100	0	–	–	60	–	–	–
FrozFruit Creamy Coconut	1 bar (3 oz)	150	tr	300	–	–	40	0	45
Frozfruit Strawberries & Cream	1 bar (4 oz)	190	tr	200	–	18	20	tr	35
The Original Bomb	1 (1.8 oz)	50	0	–	–	–	–	–	–
Breyers									
Fruit Bars No Sugar Added	1 (1.75 oz)	25	0	0	–	2	0	0	–
CoolFruits									
Fruite Juice Freezer Pops Grape & Cherry	3 pops (3 oz)	70	0	–	–	–	–	–	100
Haagen-Dazs									
Sorbet Bars Chocolate	1 (2.7 oz)	80	1	0	–	0	0	1	–
Sorbet Bars Orange	1 (2.5 oz)	120	0	200	–	6	40	0	–
Sorbet Bars Raspberry & Vanilla Yogurt	1 (2.5 oz)	90	tr	0	–	1	60	0	–
Sorbet Bars Strawberry & Vanilla Ice Cream	1 (2.5 oz)	110	0	200	–	5	40	0	–
Sorbet Chocolate	½ cup	120	2	0	–	0	0	1	–
Sorbet Mango	½ cup	120	tr	750	–	2	0	0	–
Sorbet Orange	½ cup	120	tr	100	–	15	0	0	–
Sorbet Orchard Peach	½ cup	130	tr	200	–	4	0	0	–
Sorbet Raspberry	½ cup	120	2	0	–	2	0	0	–
Sorbet Strawberry	½ cup	120	1	0	–	12	0	0	–
Sorbet Zesty Lemon	½ cup	120	tr	0	–	4	0	0	–
Hendrie's									
Citrus N' Berry Stix	1 (1.9 oz)	15	0	0	–	27	0	0	–
Fudge Stix Fat Free	1 bar (1.8 oz)	70	0	0	–	0	60	0	–
Hood									
Hoodsie Pop	1 (3.3 oz)	60	0	0	–	0	0	0	–
Minute Maid									
Fruit Bars	1 bar	60	–	–	–	60	–	–	–
Natural Choice									
Organic Vegan Fruit Bars Coconut	1 (2.75 oz)	90	1	0	–	0	20	1	–

FOOD	PORTION	CALS	FIBER	VIT A	FOLIC	VIT C	CALCI	IRON	POTAS
Organic Vegan Fruit Bars Pink Lemonade	1 (2.75 oz)	50	0	0	–	18	20	tr	–
Organic Vegan Grape	1 (2.75 oz)	50	0	0	–	18	20	tr	–
Organic Vegan Sorbet Blueberry	½ cup	110	tr	0	–	5	20	1	–
Organic Vegan Sorbet Lemon	½ cup	110	0	0	–	15	20	1	–
Organic Vegan Sorbet Mango	½ cup	110	1	1250	–	12	20	tr	–
Popsicle									
All Natural Ice Pops	1 (1.75 oz)	50	–	–	–	–	100	–	–
Bar Fruti Holanda Strawberry	1 (3 oz)	90	–	–	–	2	–	–	–
Bar Mega Warheads	1 (4 oz)	110	0	0	–	4	20	0	–
Big Stick Pops Cherry Pineapple	1 (3.5 oz)	50	0	–	–	–	–	–	–
Creamsicle Bar	1 (2.5 oz)	100	0	0	–	0	40	0	–
Creamsicle Sugar Free	2 (3.3 oz)	40	6	–	–	–	20	0	–
Creamsicle Pop No Sugar Added	1 (1.75 oz)	25	0	0	–	0	60	0	–
Cup Frostee Fudge	1 (10 oz)	280	2	400	–	2	200	1	–
Fruti Holanda Coconut Bar	1 (3 oz)	120	tr	–	–	–	–	–	–
Fudgsicle Bar	1 (2.5 oz)	90	tr	0	–	0	80	tr	–
Fudgsicle Bar Fat Free	1 (1.75 oz)	60	tr	0	–	0	80	tr	–
Fudgsicle Pop	1 (1.75 oz)	60	tr	0	–	0	60	0	–
Fudgsicle Pops No Sugar Added	2 (1.75 oz)	90	1	–	–	–	80	1	–
Minis Fudge Bar	2 (2.4 oz)	80	tr	0	–	0	80	1	–
Pop Sherbet Cyclone	1 (1.8 oz)	50	0	0	–	30	20	0	–
Pop Ups Orange Burst	1 (2.75 oz)	80	0	0	–	27	20	0	–
Pop Ups Reckless Rainbow	1 (2.75 oz)	90	0	0	–	27	20	0	–
Pop Ups SpongeBob	1 (2.75 oz)	90	0	0	–	0	20	0	–
Rainbow Floats	1 (1.75 oz)	60	0	0	–	0	20	0	–

FOOD	PORTION	CALS	FIBER	VIT A	FOLIC	VIT C	CALCI	IRON	POTAS
Sugar Free Pops Orange Cherry Grape	1 (1.75 oz)	15	–	–	–	6	–	–	–
Silhouette									
Fat Free Fudge Bars	1	90	–	–	–	–	100	–	–
Tropicana									
Fruit Juice Bar Orange	1	45	0	400	–	6	0	0	–
Fruit Juice Bar Raspberry	1	45	0	0	–	0	0	0	–
Strawberry	1	45	0	0	–	1	0	0	–
Wawona									
Peach	1 pop	78	1	172	0	63	9	tr	140
Strawberry	1 pop	77	1	19	0	27	17	tr	89

JACKFRUIT

FOOD	PORTION	CALS	FIBER	VIT A	FOLIC	VIT C	CALCI	IRON	POTAS
fresh	3.5 oz	70	–	tr	–	9	27	1	407

JAM/JELLY/PRESERVES

FOOD	PORTION	CALS	FIBER	VIT A	FOLIC	VIT C	CALCI	IRON	POTAS
apple butter	1 tbsp (0.6 oz)	33	–	0	–	tr	1	tr	16
orange marmalade	1 tbsp (0.7 oz)	49	–	9	7	1	8	tr	7
strawberry jam	1 tbsp (0.7 oz)	48	tr	2	7	2	4	tr	15
Eden									
Organic Apple Butter	1 tbsp	20	1	–	–	–	–	–	50
Organic Butter Apple Cherry	1 tbsp	25	tr	–	–	–	–	–	40
Organic Cherry Butter	1 tbsp	35	1	200	–	0	–	–	110
El Angel									
Strawberry Marmalade	1 tbsp	25	0	–	–	6	18	0	–
Lollipop Tree									
Butter Cranberry Pear	1 tbsp	25	–	0	–	0	0	0	–
Butter Pumpkin Maple Pecan	1 tbsp	30	tr	1250	–	0	0	0	–
Jam Raspberry Peach	1 tbsp	50	–	0	–	0	0	0	–
Jam Triple Cherry	1 tbsp	50	–	0	–	0	0	0	–
Jelly Hot Pepper	1 tbsp	60	–	100	–	1	0	0	–
Jelly Wasabi Lime Pepper	1 tbsp	60	0	–	–	0	0	0	–
Polaner									
All Fruit Apricot	1 tbsp	40	–	–	–	4	–	–	–

FOOD	PORTION	CALS	FIBER	VIT A	FOLIC	VIT C	CALCI	IRON	POTAS
Sarabeth's									
Spreadable Fruit Orange Apricot	1 tbsp	30	–	–	–	2	–	–	–
Spreadable Fruit Peach Apricot	1 tbsp	40	1	–	–	1	–	–	–
Spreadable Fruit Strawberry Raspberry	1 tbsp	40	tr	–	–	1	–	–	–
JICAMA									
fresh	1 sm (12.8 oz)	139	18	77	44	74	44	2	548
raw sliced	1 cup	46	6	25	14	24	14	1	180
Frieda's									
Jicama	¾ cup	35	1	0	–	18	0	tr	–
JUJUBE									
dried	1 oz	82	–	–	–	4	23	1	151
JUTE									
cooked	1 cup	32	2	4511	90	29	184	3	479
KALE									
chopped cooked w/o salt	1 cup	36	3	17707	17	53	94	1	296
fresh cooked w/ fat	1 cup	69	2	4605	18	53	93	1	297
scotch chopped cooked w/o salt	1 cup	36	2	2592	17	69	172	3	356
Glory									
Fresh Greens	1 serv (2.8 oz)	40	2	7000	–	96	100	1	–
Seasoned canned	½ cup	35	1	8500	–	24	40	1	–
KEFIR									
kefir	8 oz	98	0	17	12	2	284	tr	370
KETCHUP									
ketchup	1 tbsp	15	0	140	2	2	3	tr	57
ketchup	1 pkg (0.2 oz)	6	tr	61	1	1	1	tr	29
low sodium	1 tbsp	15	0	140	2	2	3	tr	57
Del Monte									
Ketchup	1 tbsp	15	0	100	–	1	0	0	–

FOOD	PORTION	CALS	FIBER	VIT A	FOLIC	VIT C	CALCI	IRON	POTAS
Heinz									
Ketchup	1 tbsp	15	0	300	–	0	0	0	–
No Salt	1 tbsp	20	0	0	–	0	0	0	–
One Carb	1 tbsp	5	0	0	–	0	0	0	–
Organic	1 tbsp	20	0	200	–	0	0	0	–
Hunt's									
Ketchup	1 tbsp	15	0	0	–	0	0	0	–
No Salt Added	1 tbsp	20	0	0	–	0	0	0	40
Muir Glen									
Organic	1 tbsp (0.6 oz)	15	0	100	–	1	0	0	–
KIDNEY									
beef simmered	3 oz	134	0	0	71	0	16	5	115
lamb braised	3 oz	116	0	387	69	10	15	11	151
pork braised	3 oz	128	0	221	35	9	11	5	122
veal braised	3 oz	139	0	569	18	7	25	3	135
KIDNEY BEANS									
canned	½ cup	108	6	0	46	2	44	2	303
dried cooked w/o salt	½ cup	112	6	0	115	1	31	2	358
Bush's									
Light Red	½ cup	110	7	100	–	1	80	2	–
Eden									
Chili Beans	½ cup	130	7	200	–	–	60	3	400
Organic	½ cup	100	10	–	–	–	60	1	440
Organic Cannellini	½ cup	100	5	–	–	–	40	2	250
Organic Refried	½ cup	80	6	–	–	–	40	2	410
Goya									
Dark	½ cup	90	7	0	–	0	40	2	–
Rienzi									
Cannellini	½ cup	80	7	0	–	0	40	2	–
Red	½ cup	90	7	0	–	0	40	2	–
KIWI									
fresh	1 lg (3.2 oz)	56	3	79	23	84	31	tr	284
Zespri									
Gold	2 med	80	2	0	–	186	20	tr	420
Green	2 med	100	4	100	–	144	60	1	480

FOOD	PORTION	CALS	FIBER	VIT A	FOLIC	VIT C	CALCI	IRON	POTAS
KIWI JUICE									
Auna									
Kiwifruit Juice	1 bottle (12 oz)	120	4	–	8	336	20	–	–
KIWIS									
fresh	1 med (2.6 oz)	46	2	66	19	71	26	tr	237
Chiquita									
Fresh	2 med (5.2 oz)	100	4	100	–	144	60	1	–
KNISH									
TAKE-OUT									
cheese	1 (2.1 oz)	205	1	610	36	0	22	1	60
meat	1 (1.8 oz)	174	1	430	26	tr	13	1	84
potato	1 (2.1 oz)	212	1	620	35	1	13	1	94
potato	1 lg (7 oz)	332	1	225	35	8	54	2	358
KOHLRABI									
sliced cooked w/o salt	1 cup	48	2	58	20	89	41	1	561
Frieda's									
Kohlrabi	⅔ cup	25	3	0	–	54	20	0	–
TAKE-OUT									
creamed	1 cup	150	1	375	19	58	122	1	485
KRILL									
fresh	1 oz	22	0	210	–	1	114	1	81
KUMQUATS									
canned in syrup	1	13	1	5	1	3	5	tr	15
fresh	1	13	1	55	3	8	12	tr	35
LAMB									
cubed lean & fat braised	4 oz	253	0	0	24	0	17	3	295
cubed lean broiled	4 oz	211	0	0	26	0	15	3	380
ground broiled	4 oz	321	0	0	22	0	25	2	384
leg roasted	4 oz	213	0	0	16	0	13	2	225
loin chop lean & fat broiled	1 chop (4 oz)	222	0	0	10	0	15	1	201
rib chop lean & fat broiled	1 chop (1.6 oz)	165	0	0	6	0	9	1	124

FOOD	PORTION	CALS	FIBER	VIT A	FOLIC	VIT C	CALCI	IRON	POTAS
rib roast baked	4 oz	386	0	0	18	0	25	2	314
shank lean & fat braised	4 oz	360	0	0	25	0	30	3	380
shoulder chop lean & fat cooked	1 chop (5.5 oz)	274	0	0	21	0	20	2	249
shoulder w/ bone braised	4 oz	231	0	0	18	0	17	2	210

LAMB DISHES
TAKE-OUT

FOOD	PORTION	CALS	FIBER	VIT A	FOLIC	VIT C	CALCI	IRON	POTAS
lamb curry	1 cup	257	1	0	28	1	38	3	493
moussaka	4 in sq (16 oz)	659	8	146	82	27	210	5	1089
stew w/ potatoes & vegetables	1 cup	260	4	590	30	9	33	3	592

LAMBSQUARTERS

FOOD	PORTION	CALS	FIBER	VIT A	FOLIC	VIT C	CALCI	IRON	POTAS
chopped cooked w/ salt	1 cup	58	4	17460	25	67	464	1	518

LEEKS

FOOD	PORTION	CALS	FIBER	VIT A	FOLIC	VIT C	CALCI	IRON	POTAS
chopped cooked w/o salt	¼ cup	8	tr	12	6	1	8	tr	23
cooked	1 (4.4 oz)	38	1	57	30	5	37	1	108
freeze dried	1 tbsp	1	0	1	1	tr	1	tr	5
Frieda's									
Fresh	1 cup	50	2	0	–	9	60	2	–

LEMON

FOOD	PORTION	CALS	FIBER	VIT A	FOLIC	VIT C	CALCI	IRON	POTAS
fresh	1 med (4 oz)	22	5	32	–	83	66	1	157
peel	1 tsp	1	tr	1	0	3	3	tr	3
peel	1 tbsp	3	1	3	1	8	8	tr	10
wedge	1 (7 g)	2	tr	0	1	4	2	tr	10
Sunkist									
Fresh	1 (2 oz)	15	tr	0	8	24	20	0	90

LEMON CURD

FOOD	PORTION	CALS	FIBER	VIT A	FOLIC	VIT C	CALCI	IRON	POTAS
lemon curd made w/ egg	2 tsp	29	0	70	–	1	2	tr	–
Lollipop Tree									
Lemon Curd	1 tbsp	50	–	0	–	0	0	0	–

LEMON GRASS

FOOD	PORTION	CALS	FIBER	VIT A	FOLIC	VIT C	CALCI	IRON	POTAS
fresh	1 tbsp	5	–	0	4	tr	3	tr	35

FOOD	PORTION	CALS	FIBER	VIT A	FOLIC	VIT C	CALCI	IRON	POTAS
LEMON JUICE									
bottled	1 tbsp	3	tr	2	2	4	2	tr	15
fresh	1 oz	8	tr	6	4	14	2	tr	38
from 1 lemon	1.6 oz	12	tr	9	6	22	3	tr	58
LEMONADE									
MIX									
Low Carb Creations									
Lemonade as prep	1 serv	10	0	0	–	0	0	tr	–
Raspberry as prep	1 serv	10	0	0	–	0	0	tr	–
READY-TO-DRINK									
Adina									
Hibiscus Lemon Bissap	8 oz	80	–	–	–	2	40	tr	–
Hood									
Lemonade	1 cup	110	0	0	–	72	0	0	–
Naked Juice									
Just Made	8 oz	110	0	–	–	6	20	–	65
Odwalla									
Pure Squeezed	8 oz	96	0	0	–	15	0	0	–
Purity Organic									
Lemonade	8 oz	123	tr	200	–	60	–	–	–
Santa Cruz									
Organic	1 can	160	–	–	–	60	–	1	–
Tropicana									
Light	1 cup	10	0	–	–	60	0	0	–
Orchard Style	8 oz	120	0	0	–	60	0	0	–
Uncle Matt's									
Organic	8 oz	120	0	0	–	0	0	0	310
Zeigler's									
Old Fashioned	8 oz	120	0	0	–	9	0	0	–
LENTILS									
dried cooked	1 cup	230	16	16	358	3	38	7	731
Eden									
Organic Green w/ Onion & Bay Leaf	½ cup	90	4	–	–	–	40	2	230
Near East									
Lentil Pilaf as prep	1 cup	200	8	750	–	1	20	3	–
Sabra									
Dardara	2 oz	40	1	0	–	1	0	0	–

FOOD	PORTION	CALS	FIBER	VIT A	FOLIC	VIT C	CALCI	IRON	POTAS
Shiloh Farms									
Organic Green not prep	¼ cup (1.6 oz)	150	7	0	–	0	40	3	–
TastyBite									
Bengal Lentils	½ pkg (5 oz)	190	1	0	–	0	80	2	–
Jodhpur Lentils	½ pkg (5 oz)	190	2	0	–	0	50	2	–
Madras Lentils	½ pkg (5 oz)	130	5	0	–	0	50	3	–
TAKE-OUT									
lentil loaf	1 slice (1.6 oz)	83	3	0	63	1	17	1	155
yemiser selatta ethiopian lentil salad	1 serv (3 oz)	115	2	89	73	56	19	2	234

LETTUCE

FOOD	PORTION	CALS	FIBER	VIT A	FOLIC	VIT C	CALCI	IRON	POTAS
arugula	6 leaves (0.4 oz)	3	tr	70	12	2	19	tr	44
arugula shredded	1 cup	5	tr	120	19	3	32	tr	74
boston	1 head (5.7 oz)	21	2	5399	119	6	57	2	388
boston chopped	6 leaves	7	1	1822	40	2	19	1	131
cornsalad field salad	1 cup (1.9 oz)	7	1	1790	80	19	19	1	232
iceberg	1 lg head (26.5 oz)	106	9	3790	219	21	136	3	1065
iceberg	6 med leaves	7	1	241	14	1	9	tr	68
iceberg shredded	1 cup	10	1	361	21	2	13	tr	102
looseleaf outer leaves	6 (5 oz)	22	2	10663	55	26	52	1	279
looseleaf shredded	1 cup	5	1	2666	14	7	13	tr	70
red leaf	6 leaves (3.6 oz)	16	1	7642	37	4	34	1	191
red leaf shredded	1 cup	4	tr	2098	10	1	9	tr	52
romaine	3 leaves (3 oz)	14	2	4878	114	20	28	1	207
romaine heart	6 leaves (1.3 oz)	6	1	520	49	9	12	tr	89
romaine shredded	1 cup	8	1	2729	64	11	16	tr	116

FOOD	PORTION	CALS	FIBER	VIT A	FOLIC	VIT C	CALCI	IRON	POTAS
Andy Boy									
Romaine Hearts	6 leaves (3 oz)	20	1	1000	–	2	40	tr	140
Dole									
Classic Romaine	1½ cups (3 oz)	15	1	3500	–	21	40	1	–
Shredded	1½ cups (3 oz)	15	1	200	–	4	0	0	–
Earthbound Farm									
Organic Baby Romaine Salad	2 cups	15	1	5000	–	54	40	4	–
Frieda's									
Limestone	⅔ cup	10	1	300	–	4	0	tr	–
Green Giant									
Hearts Of Romaine	6 leaves (3 oz)	14	2	5000	–	21	20	1	210
Mann's									
Romaine Jumbo Hearts	3 oz	15	1	2250	–	21	40	1	–
Ocean Mist									
Romaine Hearts	6 leaves	20	1	1000	–	2	20	tr	140
Ready Pac									
Baby Arugula	4 cups	20	2	2000	–	12	150	1	–
Bella Romaine	1½ cups	15	1	1000	–	5	20	1	–
River Ranch									
Hearts Of Romaine	1½ cups	12	1	1100	208	20	–	1	247
Romaine Chopped	1½ cups	10	1	2250	120	21	40	1	–
Romaine Hearts	1½ cups	10	1	2250	120	21	40	1	–
LILY ROOT									
dried	1 oz	89	tr	25	–	5	9	1	195
fresh	1 oz	32	tr	3	–	6	1	tr	–
LIMA BEANS									
CANNED									
lima beans	½ cup	95	6	0	60	0	25	2	265
Del Monte									
Green	½ cup	80	4	100	–	5	20	1	–
Hanover									
Butter Beans In Sauce	½ cup	100	5	0	–	0	0	2	–

FOOD	PORTION	CALS	FIBER	VIT A	FOLIC	VIT C	CALCI	IRON	POTAS
S&W									
Small Green	½ cup (4.4 oz)	80	4	100	–	5	20	1	–
Veg-All									
Baby Green	½ cup	90	3	0	–	0	20	1	–
DRIED									
cooked	½ cup	150	5	314	22	9	27	2	484
FROZEN									
C&W									
Baby	½ cup	110	5	0	–	9	40	1	–
Fresh Like									
Baby	3.5 oz	138	2	231	–	19	34	2	494
LIME									
fresh	1 (2.4 oz)	20	1	5	5	20	22	tr	68
wedge	1 (8 g)	2	tr	0	1	2	3	tr	8
Sunkist									
Fresh	1 (2 oz)	20	2	100	–	19	20	tr	–
LIME JUICE									
bottled	1 oz	6	tr	5	2	2	4	tr	23
fresh	1 oz	8	tr	15	3	9	4	tr	36
from 1 lime	1.1 oz	11	tr	22	4	13	6	tr	51
Odwalla									
Summertime Lime	8 fl oz	90	0	0	–	5	0	0	–
LING									
fresh baked	3 oz	95	0	98	–	–	37	1	413
LIQUOR/LIQUEUR									
7&7	1 serv	178	0	–	–	–	4	tr	3
alabama slammer	1 serv	103	tr	13	2	3	1	tr	13
amaretto sour	1 serv	295	4	388	55	98	75	tr	362
angel's kiss	1 serv	85	0	47	tr	tr	7	tr	12
antifreeze	1 serv	177	tr	372	56	93	20	tr	372
apricot sour	1 serv	164	tr	6	4	14	3	tr	49
bahama breeze	1 serv	70	tr	17	5	6	3	tr	34
bahama mama	1 serv	153	tr	12	33	27	23	tr	207
banana colada	1 serv	376	3	94	77	36	49	1	736
bay breeze	1 serv	173	tr	815	19	73	17	tr	302
bend me over	1 serv	242	tr	316	47	78	18	tr	319
betsy ross	1 serv	206	0	–	1	–	2	tr	44

FOOD	PORTION	CALS	FIBER	VIT A	FOLIC	VIT C	CALCI	IRON	POTAS
black devil	1 serv	220	tr	18	–	2	5	tr	6
bloody mary	1 serv	150	1	1068	21	32	11	tr	195
blue whale	1 serv	222	0	13	–	2	1	tr	18
bourbon & soda	1 serv (4 oz)	105	0	0	0	0	4	–	2
bourbon sour	1 serv	166	tr	6	4	14	3	tr	49
brandy alexander	1 serv	266	0	190	–	tr	29	tr	48
brandy sour	1 serv	164	tr	6	4	14	4	tr	49
bushwacker	1 serv	286	tr	–	3	tr	tr	tr	18
coffee liqueur	1 serv (1.5 oz)	175	0	0	0	0	1	tr	16
cosmopolitan martini	1 serv	126	tr	2	1	7	2	tr	18
creme de menthe	1 serv (1.5 oz)	186	0	0	0	0	0	tr	0
daiquiri	1 serv (2 oz)	112	tr	2	1	1	2	tr	13
daiquiri banana	1 serv	277	1	48	11	5	4	tr	235
frozen daiquiri pineapple	1 serv	186	2	59	37	123	21	tr	365
frozen tequila screwdriver	1 serv	159	1	202	39	84	16	tr	287
fuzzy navel	1 serv	247	tr	186	28	47	10	tr	188
gimlet vodka	1 serv	150	1	2	2	6	7	tr	21
gin	1 serv (1.5 oz)	110	0	0	0	0	0	0	0
gin & tonic	1 serv (7.5 oz)	171	–	2	1	1	4	–	12
gin ricky	1 serv	114	tr	2	1	5	10	tr	20
grasshopper	1 serv	275	0	142	1	tr	22	tr	38
happy hawaiian	1 serv	434	tr	9	43	20	32	1	266
harvey wallbanger	1 serv	198	tr	310	47	78	17	tr	311
hot buttered rum	1 serv	219	4	170	4	101	101	3	49
hot toddy	1 serv	188	5	33	5	4	102	3	33
hurricane	1 serv	205	tr	31	7	9	3	tr	43
long island iced tea	1 serv	292	0	6	–	1	1	tr	10
lynchburg lemonade	1 serv	465	1	145	15	27	11	1	107
mai tai	1 serv	165	tr	10	–	1	2	tr	24
margarita strawberry	1 serv	106	1	18	13	41	11	tr	128
martini	1 serv (3 oz)	206	0	0	0	0	1	tr	14
martini apple	1 serv	147	tr	tr	tr	tr	2	tr	38
martini rum	1 serv	131	tr	tr	–	1	1	tr	3

FOOD	PORTION	CALS	FIBER	VIT A	FOLIC	VIT C	CALCI	IRON	POTAS
mexican grasshopper	1 serv	638	0	673	2	tr	42	tr	79
mint julep	1 serv	136	tr	162	4	1	8	tr	19
mississippi mud	1 serv	496	0	476	4	1	87	tr	132
orange crush	1 serv	461	tr	10	1	90	8	tr	46
painkiller	1 serv	277	tr	68	38	29	26	1	231
pina colada	1 serv (4.5 oz)	245	tr	3	17	7	11	tr	100
planter's cocktail	1 serv	105	tr	3	2	7	1	tr	19
planter's punch	1 serv	233	4	573	67	124	79	tr	447
presbyterian	1 serv	170	tr	tr	tr	1	8	tr	5
purple passion	1 serv	215	0	272	6	23	11	tr	102
rob roy	1 serv	171	tr	tr	tr	1	3	tr	15
rum	1 serv (1.5 oz)	97	0	0	0	0	0	tr	1
rum boogie	1 serv	134	tr	1	1	3	5	tr	12
rum cola	1 serv	209	tr	2	1	4	7	tr	19
rum punch	1 serv	448	1	147	34	217	33	1	300
sake	1 serv (1 oz)	39	0	0	0	0	1	tr	7
salty dog	1 serv	210	tr	815	19	71	18	tr	304
scotch & soda	1 serv	104	tr	tr	tr	1	10	tr	5
screwdriver rum	1 serv	166	tr	310	47	78	17	tr	311
sea breeze	1 serv	207	tr	275	6	57	8	tr	118
sex on the beach	1 serv	190	tr	49	–	34	4	tr	58
sloe gin fizz	1 serv (2.5 oz)	132	0	5	tr	11	2	0	35
sour rum	1 serv	156	tr	6	4	14	4	tr	49
tequila gimlet	1 serv	150	1	2	2	6	7	tr	21
tequila sour	1 serv	156	tr	6	4	14	3	tr	48
tequila sunrise	1 serv (6.8 oz)	232	0	205	23	41	0	tr	21
tom collins	1 serv (7.5 oz)	121	–	2	2	4	10	–	18
vermouth cassis	1 serv	97	tr	2	1	4	14	tr	31
vodka	1 serv (1.5 oz)	97	0	0	0	0	0	0	0
vodka sour	1 serv	138	tr	2	1	4	1	tr	17
whiskey	1 serv (1.5 oz)	105	0	0	0	0	0	tr	0

FOOD	PORTION	CALS	FIBER	VIT A	FOLIC	VIT C	CALCI	IRON	POTAS
whiskey sour	1 serv (3.5 oz)	162	0	0	0	2	1	tr	19
white russian	1 serv	290	0	328	1	tr	14	tr	27
zombie	1 serv	235	tr	124	19	31	8	tr	129

LITCHI JUICE
Ceres
Litchi	8 oz	120	0	0	–	60	0	tr	190

LIVER
beef braised	1 slice (2.4 oz)	130	0	21566	172	1	4	4	239
beef pan-fried	1 slice (2.8 oz)	142	0	21131	211	1	5	5	284
chicken fried	3 oz	146	0	12221	476	2	8	11	268
chicken simmered	3 oz	142	0	11329	491	24	9	10	224
lamb braised	3 oz	187	0	21203	62	3	7	7	188
lamb fried	3 oz	202	0	22098	340	11	8	9	299
moose braised	3 oz	132	–	81600	–	19	6	6	200
pork braised	3 oz	140	0	15297	139	20	8	15	128
turkey simmered	1 liver (2.9 oz)	227	0	62526	574	19	4	9	175
veal braised	1 slice (2.8 oz)	154	0	56451	265	1	5	4	263
veal pan fried	1 slice (2.4 oz)	129	0	44883	234	1	5	4	237

TAKE-OUT
calves liver w/ onions	1 serv (5 oz)	177	1	34035	236	3	17	6	399

LOBSTER
northern cooked	1 cup	142	–	126	16	–	88	1	510
northern cooked	3 oz	83	–	74	9	–	52	tr	299

LOGANBERRIES
frzn	1 cup	80	–	52	38	23	38	1	213

LOTUS
root sliced cooked	10 slices	59	–	0	–	24	23	1	323
seeds dried	1 oz	94	–	14	–	0	46	1	389

Eden
Dried Sliced	5 slices (0.3 oz)	35	2	0	–	0	20	tr	160

FOOD	PORTION	CALS	FIBER	VIT A	FOLIC	VIT C	CALCI	IRON	POTAS
Frieda's									
Lotus Root Fresh	1 cup	50	4	0	–	36	40	1	–

LYCHEES
fresh	1	6	–	0	–	7	0	tr	16
Frieda's									
Fresh	6 to 8 (3.5 oz)	60	1	0	–	60	0	0	–

MACADAMIA NUTS
dry roasted w/ salt	11 nuts (1 oz)	200	1	0	–	–	20	1	100
oil roasted	1 oz	204	–	3	–	0	13	1	94
Hawaiian Host									
White Choco	3 pieces (1.4 oz)	230	0	0	–	0	40	0	–
Keto									
Chocolately Covered	1 oz	171	4	0	–	0	60	3	–
Mauna Loa									
Milk Chocolate Coated	3 pieces	230	1	0	–	0	60	tr	–
Milk Chocolate Toffee	7 pieces	210	1	0	–	0	40	1	–

MACE
ground	1 tsp	8	–	14	–	–	4	tr	8

MACKEREL
CANNED
jack	1 cup	296	0	825	10	2	458	4	369
Brunswick									
Jack In Water	2 oz	100	0	0	–	0	200	1	–
Chicken Of The Sea									
Jack In Tomato Sauce	¼ cup	70	0	0	–	0	150	1	–
Jack In Water	⅓ cup	90	0	100	–	0	250	1	–
Orleans									
Jack	¼ cup	90	0	100	–	0	260	1	–
DRIED									
Eden									
Bonito Flakes	2 tbsp	5	0	0	–	0	0	0	13
FRESH									
atlantic cooked	3 oz	223	0	153	–	tr	13	1	341
jack baked	3 oz	171	0	40	2	–	25	1	442
jack fillet baked	6.2 oz	354	0	82	4	–	52	3	916

FOOD	PORTION	CALS	FIBER	VIT A	FOLIC	VIT C	CALCI	IRON	POTAS
king baked	3 oz	114	0	713	7	–	34	2	474
pacific baked	3 oz	171	0	40	2	–	25	1	442
spanish cooked	3 oz	134	0	–	–	–	11	1	471
SMOKED									
atlantic	3.5 oz	296	0	350	1	0	20	1	310
MAHI MAHI									
fresh baked	4 oz	192	0	320	14	2	22	1	377
MALANGA									
dasheen mashed	1 cup	226	8	40	29	6	84	1	1075
dasheen pieces boiled	1 cup	212	8	35	27	6	78	1	1004
pieces fried	1 cup	304	8	30	21	6	27	1	721
root raw	1 (10.7 oz)	299	5	24	52	16	27	3	1824
Frieda's									
Malanga	⅔ cup	90	2	0	–	4	60	tr	–
MALT									
malt liquor	1 bottle (12 oz)	148	tr	0	22	0	18	tr	90
nonalcoholic	1 bottle (12 oz)	133	0	0	50	2	25	tr	29
MALTED MILK									
chocolate as prep w/ milk	1 cup	179	1	505	21	1	266	tr	437
chocolate flavor powder	3 heaping tsp (0.7 oz)	79	1	5	11	tr	13	tr	130
natural flavor as prep w/ milk	1 cup	186	tr	575	19	1	308	tr	463
natural flavor powder	3 heaping tsp (0.7 oz)	87	tr	85	10	1	63	tr	159
MAMMY-APPLE									
fresh	1	431	–	1946	–	118	93	6	398
MANGO									
fresh	1	135	–	8060	–	57	21	tr	322
C&W									
Chunks	¾ cup	90	3	1000	–	36	0	0	–
Sunsweet									
Philippine dried	6 pieces (1.5 oz)	130	2	1000	–	18	0	tr	190

FOOD	PORTION	CALS	FIBER	VIT A	FOLIC	VIT C	CALCI	IRON	POTAS
Thailand dried	⅓ cup (1.4 oz)	140	1	500	–	1	80	tr	10
Tomorrow's Tropicals									
Fresh	½ (3.6 oz)	70	1	2000	–	9	0	0	–

MANGO JUICE
Ceres
Mango	8 oz	120	1	500	–	60	20	1	190
Naked Juice									
Mighty Mango	8 oz	120	0	5000	–	162	20	2	280
Old Orchard									
Nectar Cocktail	8 oz	120	–	0	–	78	0	0	93

MANGOSTEEN
canned in syrup	1 cup	143	4	69	61	6	24	1	94

MARGARINE
squeeze	1 tsp	34	0	155	tr	tr	3	–	4
stick corn	1 tsp	34	0	155	tr	tr	1	–	2
tub corn	1 tsp	34	0	155	tr	tr	1	–	2
tub diet	1 tsp	17	0	159	tr	tr	1	–	1
Benecol									
Spread Light	1 tbsp	50	0	500	–	–	–	–	–
Spread Regular	1 tbsp	70	0	500	–	–	–	–	–
Blue Bonnet									
Light Stick	1 tbsp	50	0	500	–	–	–	–	–
Soft Spread	1 tbsp	60	0	500	–	–	–	–	–
Soft Spread Light	1 tbsp	40	0	500	–	–	–	–	–
Stick	1 tbsp	80	0	500	–	–	–	–	–
Brummel & Brown									
Made With Natural Yogurt	1 tbsp	45	0	500	–	–	–	–	–
Crystal Farms									
60/40 Margarine Butter	1 tbsp	100	0	400	–	0	0	0	–
Margarine	1 tbsp	100	0	500	–	0	0	0	–
I Can't Believe Its Not Butter									
Regular Stick	1 tbsp	90	0	500	–	–	–	–	–
Soft Fat Free	1 tbsp	5	0	500	–	–	–	–	–
Soft Light	1 tbsp	50	0	500	–	–	–	–	–
Soft Regular	1 tbsp	80	0	500	–	–	–	–	–
Soft w/ Calcium	1 tbsp	50	0	500	–	–	100	–	–

FOOD	PORTION	CALS	FIBER	VIT A	FOLIC	VIT C	CALCI	IRON	POTAS
Squeeze	1 tbsp	60	0	500	–	–	–	–	–
Stick Light	1 tbsp	50	0	500	–	–	–	–	–
Parkay									
Light Spread	1 tbsp	50	0	500	–	0	–	–	–
Promise									
Buttery Spread	1 tbsp	80	0	500	–	–	–	–	–
Smart Balance									
37% Light	1 tbsp	45	0	500	–	–	–	–	–
Omega Plus w/ Flax Oil	1 tbsp	80	0	500	–	–	–	–	–
Spectrum									
Essential Omega	1 tbsp	80	0	0	–	0	0	0	0
Spread	1 tbsp	88	0	0	–	0	0	0	0
Take Control									
Spread	1 tbsp (0.5 oz)	80	0	500	–	–	–	–	–
MARJORAM									
dried	1 tsp	2	–	48	–	–	12	1	9
MARLIN									
raw	3 oz	110	0	20	–	1	8	1	–
MARSHMALLOW									
marshmallow	1 reg (0.3 oz)	23	–	0	0	0	0	tr	0
MATZO									
brie	1 piece (0.5 oz)	54	tr	35	2	0	4	tr	10
egg	1 (1 oz)	109	1	12	7	0	11	1	42
matzo ball	1 med (1.2 oz)	48	tr	60	4	0	6	tr	20
plain	1 (1 oz)	111	1	0	5	0	4	1	31
whole wheat	1 (1 oz)	98	3	0	10	0	6	1	88
Horowitz Margareten									
Egg	1 (1.2 oz)	130	1	0	–	0	0	tr	–
Manischewitz									
Dark Chocolate Coated Egg	½ (1.5 oz)	90	2	0	–	0	20	1	–
Egg	1 (1.2 oz)	120	1	0	–	0	0	tr	–
Egg & Onion	1 (1 oz)	100	2	0	60	0	10	1	50

FOOD	PORTION	CALS	FIBER	VIT A	FOLIC	VIT C	CALCI	IRON	POTAS
Matzo Meal	¼ cup (1 oz)	130	1	0	–	0	0	0	–
Thin Unsalted	1 (0.8 oz)	90	0	0	64	0	0	1	35
Streit's									
Egg	1 (1.1 oz)	120	1	0	–	0	0	tr	–
Egg & Onion	1 (1 oz)	100	1	0	–	0	0	1	–
Passover	1 (1 oz)	110	1	0	–	0	0	tr	–

MAYONNAISE

FOOD	PORTION	CALS	FIBER	VIT A	FOLIC	VIT C	CALCI	IRON	POTAS
diet	1 tbsp	36	0	0	0	0	0	tr	2
mayonnaise	1 tbsp	99	0	55	1	0	2	tr	5
Blue Plate									
Squeeze	1 tbsp	100	0	0	–	0	0	0	–
Miracle Whip									
Light	1 tbsp	25	0	0	–	0	0	0	–
Original	1 tbsp	40	0	0	–	0	0	0	–
Nasoya									
Fat Free Nayonaise	1 tbsp	10	0	0	–	0	0	0	–
Nayonaise	1 tbsp	35	0	0	–	0	0	0	–
Spectrum									
Canola Squeeze	1 tbsp	100	0	0	–	0	0	0	0
Canola Squeeze Light Eggless Vegan	1 tbsp	35	0	0	–	0	0	0	0
Organic Dijon	1 tbsp	90	0	0	–	0	0	0	–
Organic Olive Oil	1 tbsp	100	0	0	–	0	0	0	0
Organic Roasted Garlic	1 tbsp	100	0	0	–	0	0	0	0
Organic Squeeze	1 tbsp	100	0	0	–	0	0	0	0
Organic Wasabi	1 tbsp	100	0	0	–	0	0	0	0

MEAT STICKS

FOOD	PORTION	CALS	FIBER	VIT A	FOLIC	VIT C	CALCI	IRON	POTAS
jerky beef	1 piece (0.7 oz)	82	tr	0	27	0	4	1	119
pork jerky	1 strip (0.5 oz)	62	tr	0	20	0	3	1	90
venison jerky	1 strip (0.5 oz)	55	0	0	1	0	2	1	55
Jack Link's									
Beef Jerky Teriyaki	1 oz	80	0	0	–	0	0	0	–
Pemmican									
Homestyle Tender All Flavors	1 oz	80	1	0	–	0	0	2	–

FOOD	PORTION	CALS	FIBER	VIT A	FOLIC	VIT C	CALCI	IRON	POTAS
Kippered Beef Original	1 pkg (1 oz)	60	0	0	–	0	0	1	–
Kippered Beef Peppered	1 pkg (1 oz)	60	0	0	–	0	0	1	–
Kippered Beef Sweet & Hot	1 pkg (1 oz)	70	0	0	–	0	0	tr	–
Kippered Beef Teriyaki	1 pkg (1 oz)	60	0	0	–	0	0	2	–
Long Lasting Hot & Spicy	1 oz	60	0	0	–	0	0	1	–
Long Lasting Original	1 oz	60	0	0	–	0	0	1	–
Long Lasting Peppered	1 oz	60	0	0	–	0	0	1	–
Long Lasting Teriyaki	1 oz	70	0	0	–	0	0	1	–
Premium Cut Beef Jerky	1 oz	80	1	0	–	0	0	2	–
Premium Cut Turkey Peppered	1 oz	70	0	0	–	0	0	tr	–
Premium Cut Turkey Sweet Smoked	1 oz	70	0	0	–	0	0	tr	–
Shredded Beef Jerky All Flavors	¼ cup	80	1	0	–	0	0	2	–
Steak Tips All Flavors	1 oz	70	0	0	–	0	0	1	–

MEAT SUBSTITUTES
Fantastic
FOOD	PORTION	CALS	FIBER	VIT A	FOLIC	VIT C	CALCI	IRON	POTAS
Sloppy Joe Mix not prep	¼ cup	70	3	100	–	9	60	1	–
Taco Filling not prep	¼ cup	80	4	300	–	2	80	2	–

Lightlife
FOOD	PORTION	CALS	FIBER	VIT A	FOLIC	VIT C	CALCI	IRON	POTAS
Balogna	4 slices (2 oz)	60	2	–	–	–	–	–	30
Smart Deli Country Ham	4 slices (2 oz)	90	1	–	–	–	–	–	160
Smart Ground Original	⅓ cup (1.9 oz)	80	3	–	–	–	–	–	330
Smart Menu Meatless Meatballs	5	160	2	–	–	–	–	–	150
Smart Menu Steak Strips	1 serv (3 oz)	80	5	–	–	–	–	–	520

Loma Linda
FOOD	PORTION	CALS	FIBER	VIT A	FOLIC	VIT C	CALCI	IRON	POTAS
Dinner Cuts	2 slices (3.2 oz)	90	2	0	–	0	0	tr	20

FOOD	PORTION	CALS	FIBER	VIT A	FOLIC	VIT C	CALCI	IRON	POTAS
Swiss Stake	1 piece (3.2 oz)	130	3	0	–	0	0	1	200
Morningstar Farms									
Meal Starters Steak Strips	12 pieces (3 oz)	140	1	0	–	0	40	5	460
Quorn									
Grounds	⅔ cup (3 oz)	80	4	0	–	0	20	1	–
VeggieLand									
Veg-T-Balls	3 (3 oz)	113	5	0	–	0	30	2	–
Viana									
Cowgirl Veggie Steaks	1 (3.7 oz)	260	4	0	–	0	60	4	–
Veggie Cevapcici	4 pieces (2.8 oz)	240	3	0	–	0	40	3	–
Veggie Gyros	24 strips (3 oz)	220	2	0	–	0	40	3	–
Veggie Kebab	½ cup	210	2	0	–	0	10	2	–
Worthington									
Bolono	3 slices (2 oz)	80	2	0	–	0	20	2	100
Choplets	2 slices (3.2 oz)	90	2	0	–	0	0	tr	40
Corned Beef Vegetarian	3 slices (2 oz)	140	0	0	–	0	0	2	130
Dinner Roast	1 slice (3 oz)	180	3	0	–	0	20	2	120
Multigrain Cutlets	2 slices (3.2 oz)	100	3	0	–	0	0	1	30
Prime Stakes	1 piece (3.2 oz)	120	1	0	–	0	0	2	90
Vegetable Skallops	½ cup (3 oz)	90	3	0	–	0	0	tr	10
Wham	2 slices (2 oz)	110	0	0	–	0	60	2	110

MEATBALL SUBSTITUTES

FOOD	PORTION	CALS	FIBER	VIT A	FOLIC	VIT C	CALCI	IRON	POTAS
meatless	2 (1.3 oz)	71	2	0	28	0	9	1	65
Loma Linda									
Tender Rounds	6 (2.8 oz)	120	1	0	–	0	20	1	80

FOOD	PORTION	CALS	FIBER	VIT A	FOLIC	VIT C	CALCI	IRON	POTAS
Quorn									
Meatballs	4 (2.4 oz)	110	1	0	–	0	80	tr	–
MEATBALLS									
beef	1 med (1 oz)	74	0	0	3	0	7	1	84
beef	1 lg (1.5 oz)	111	0	0	4	0	10	1	126
beef cocktail	1 (0.2 oz)	18	0	0	1	0	2	tr	21
Mama Lucia									
Homestyle	4	207	1	0	–	0	40	2	–
Italian Style	4	280	0	0	–	0	40	1	–
Sausage Beef	8	220	1	0	–	0	40	2	–
Shady Brook									
Turkey Meatballs Italian Style	3 (3 oz)	190	tr	100	–	1	60	2	–
TastyBite									
Meatballs Vindaloo	1 pkg (9.5 oz)	270	4	1000	–	12	60	4	–
TAKE-OUT									
albondigas w/ sauce	3 + sauce (5.3 oz)	372	1	90	22	4	38	3	480
porcupine + tomato sauce	3 + sauce	160	1	30	21	5	19	2	213
swedish w/ cream sauce	3 + sauce (4.7 oz)	215	tr	225	16	2	73	2	317
sweet & sour	3 + sauce (4.5 oz)	188	1	65	14	tr	46	2	268
MELON									
melon balls frzn	1 cup	55	–	3096	45	11	17	1	484
Frieda's									
Camouflage	1 cup (5 oz)	50	1	0	–	36	0	0	–
SpriteMelon	1 (10.5 oz)	115	2	0	–	90	0	1	–
Temptation	1/10 melon (4.7 oz)	55	1	0	–	24	0	tr	–
MILK									
CANNED									
condensed sweetened	1 cup	982	–	1004	34	8	868	1	1136

FOOD	PORTION	CALS	FIBER	VIT A	FOLIC	VIT C	CALCI	IRON	POTAS
evaporated	½ cup	169	–	306	10	2	329	tr	382
evaporated skim	½ cup	99	–	500	11	2	369	tr	423
Meyenberg									
Evaporated Goat Milk	8 oz	145	–	343	80	–	298	–	–
DRIED									
buttermilk	1 tbsp	25	–	14	3	tr	77	tr	103
nonfat instantized	1 pkg (3.2 oz)	244	–	2157	45	5	837	tr	1552
Carnation									
Instant Nonfat as prep	1 cup	80	0	500	–	1	300	–	390
Meyenberg									
Instant Goat Milk as prep	1 cup	142	–	316	80	–	307	–	–
REFRIGERATED									
1%	1 cup	102	–	500	12	2	300	tr	381
2%	1 cup	121	–	500	12	2	297	tr	377
buffalo	7 oz	224	–	–	–	6	390	tr	200
buttermilk	1 cup	99	–	81	–	2	285	tr	371
goat	1 cup	168	–	451	1	3	326	tr	499
human	1 cup	171	–	593	13	12	79	tr	126
indian buffalo	1 cup	236	–	434	14	5	412	tr	434
nonfat	1 cup	86	–	500	13	2	302	tr	406
sheep	1 cup	264	–	360	–	10	474	tr	334
whole	1 cup	150	–	307	12	2	291	tr	370
Borden									
Fat Free Skim	1 cup	80	0	500	–	2	300	0	–
Farmland									
Buttermilk	8 oz	160	0	100	–	4	450	0	–
Fat Free	8 oz	80	0	500	–	1	300	0	–
Special Request 1% Plus Omega-3	8 oz	130	0	500	–	1	400	0	–
Special Request Skim Plus	8 oz	110	0	500	–	1	400	0	–
Special Request Skim Plus 100% Lactose Free	8 oz	110	0	500	–	1	400	0	–
Whole	8 oz	160	0	100	–	4	450	0	–
Hood									
1%	1 cup	110	0	500	–	6	300	0	–
2%	1 cup	130	0	500	–	6	300	0	–

FOOD	PORTION	CALS	FIBER	VIT A	FOLIC	VIT C	CALCI	IRON	POTAS
Buttermilk Fat Free	1 cup	90	0	0	–	2	300	0	–
Calorie Countdown 2%	8 oz	90	0	500	–	0	300	0	–
Calorie Countdown Fat Free	8 oz	45	0	500	–	0	300	0	–
Fat Free	1 cup	80	0	500	–	6	300	0	–
Simply Smart 0% Fat	1 cup	90	0	500	–	0	350	0	–
Simply Smart 1% Fat	1 cup	120	0	500	–	0	350	0	–
Whole	1 cup	150	0	300	–	6	300	0	–
Horizon Organic									
Fat Free	8 oz	90	0	500	–	1	300	0	–
Lactaid									
1% Lowfat	1 cup	110	0	500	–	0	300	0	–
2% Reduced Fat	1 cup	130	0	500	–	0	300	0	–
Calcium Fortified	1 cup	80	0	500	–	0	500	0	–
Fat Free	1 cup	90	0	500	–	0	300	0	–
Whole	1 cup	150	0	300	–	0	300	0	–
Meyenberg									
Goat Milk	8 oz	142	–	316	–	–	307	–	–
Goat Milk Low Fat	8 oz	89	–	500	–	–	268	–	–
Skinny Cow									
Fat Free	8 oz	110	0	500	–	0	400	0	–
Stonyfield Farm									
Organic Whole Milk	1 cup (8 oz)	180	0	400	–	2	540	0	447
Organic Whole Milk Vanilla	1 cup (8 oz)	230	0	300	–	2	450	0	439
Tuscan									
Whole	8 oz	150	0	300	–	2	300	0	–
Welsh Farms									
Fat Free	8 oz	80	0	500	–	1	300	0	–
SHELF-STABLE									
Parmalat									
2% Reduced Fat	8 oz	130	0	500	–	1	300	0	–
Fat Free	8 oz	80	0	500	–	1	300	0	–
Lactose Free 2% Reduced Fat	8 oz	130	0	500	–	1	300	0	–

MILK DRINKS

FOOD	PORTION	CALS	FIBER	VIT A	FOLIC	VIT C	CALCI	IRON	POTAS
chocolate milk	1 cup	208	–	302	12	2	280	1	417
chocolate milk 1%	1 cup	158	–	500	12	2	287	1	426
chocolate milk 2%	1 cup	179	–	500	12	2	284	1	422

FOOD	PORTION	CALS	FIBER	VIT A	FOLIC	VIT C	CALCI	IRON	POTAS
Bravo!									
Blenders Creamy Double Chocolate	1 bottle (11 oz)	180	2	2250	100	30	500	5	800
Blenders Creamy French Vanilla	1 bottle (11 oz)	160	2	2250	100	30	500	5	970
Cocio									
Chocolate Milk	1 bottle	225	tr	150	–	5	390	2	–
Farmland									
Really Really Good! Chocolate Milk	8 oz	160	0	500	–	2	300	0	–
Garelick									
Colossal Coffee	1 cup	145	0	500	–	2	300	0	–
Ultimate Chocolate	1 cup	150	1	500	–	2	300	0	–
Hershey's									
Chocolate Milk Fat Free	1 bottle	160	tr	500	–	–	500	–	–
Chocolate Milk Reduced Fat	1 bottle	200	1	500	–	–	500	–	–
Hood									
Calorie Countdown Chocolate 2%	8 oz	90	1	500	–	0	300	1	–
Chocolate Lowfat	1 cup	170	tr	500	–	0	500	1	–
Chocolate Milk	1 cup	230	tr	300	–	0	500	1	–
Coffee Lowfat Milk	1 cup	170	0	500	–	15	300	0	–
Horizon Organic									
Lowfat Chocolate Milk	8 oz	170	tr	500	–	18	200	tr	–
Strawberry	8 oz	200	0	500	–	0	250	0	–
Parmalat									
Chocolate Milk 2% Reduced Fat	1 cup	190	1	500	–	1	300	tr	–
Quaker									
Chocolate	8 oz	140	3	500	–	6	200	0	–
Strawberry	8 oz	130	tr	500	–	6	200	0	–
Vanilla	8 oz	130	tr	500	–	6	200	0	–

MILK SUBSTITUTES

8th Continent

FOOD	PORTION	CALS	FIBER	VIT A	FOLIC	VIT C	CALCI	IRON	POTAS
Soymilk Chocolate	8 oz	140	1	500	–	0	300	2	–
Soymilk Fat Free Original	8 oz	60	0	500	–	0	300	1	–

FOOD	PORTION	CALS	FIBER	VIT A	FOLIC	VIT C	CALCI	IRON	POTAS
Soymilk Fat Free Vanilla	8 oz	70	0	500	–	0	300	1	–
Soymilk Light Chocolate	8 oz	90	tr	500	–	0	300	1	–
Soymilk Light Original	8 oz	50	0	500	–	0	300	1	–
Soymilk Light Vanilla	8 oz	60	0	500	–	0	300	1	–
Soymilk Original	8 oz	80	0	500	–	0	300	1	–
Soymilk Vanilla	8 oz	100	0	500	–	0	300	1	–
Almond Breeze									
Chocolate	8 oz	115	1	500	–	0	205	1	209
Original	8 oz	57	1	500	–	0	198	tr	179
Original Unsweetened	8 oz	40	1	500	–	0	200	tr	190
Vanilla	8 oz	91	1	500	–	0	200	tr	182
DariFree									
Fat Free as prep	8 oz	70	0	500	–	6	300	1	50
Fat Free Chocolate as prep	8 oz	110	tr	750	–	9	300	1	360
EdenBlend									
Organic	8 oz	120	tr	–	24	–	40	1	250
Edensoy									
Organic Carob	8 oz	170	tr	–	80	–	80	1	350
Organic Chocolate	8 oz	180	tr	–	40	–	100	2	410
Organic Original	8 oz	140	tr	–	40	–	100	2	440
Organic Original Unsweetened	8 oz	120	tr	–	60	–	40	2	460
Organic Original Light	8 oz	100	0	0	60	–	100	1	220
Organic Vanilla	8 oz	150	tr	–	40	–	80	1	320
Organic Vanilla Light	8 oz	110	0	–	16	–	100	1	200
Hansen's									
Soy Smoothie Lemon Chiffon	8 oz	150	tr	5000	–	60	300	4	73
Soy Smoothie Orange Dream	8 oz	150	tr	5000	–	60	300	1	73
Living Harvest									
Hempmilk Original	1 cup	130	1	900	25	0	460	3	113
Hempmilk Vanilla	1 cup	130	1	900	25	0	460	3	113
Lundberg									
Organic Drink Rice Original	8 oz	120	tr	500	–	0	300	1	85

FOOD	PORTION	CALS	FIBER	VIT A	FOLIC	VIT C	CALCI	IRON	POTAS
Manitoba Harvest									
Hemp Bliss Chocolate	8 oz	160	1	0	–	0	40	4	–
Hemp Bliss Original	1 cup	110	1	0	–	0	20	4	–
Hemp Bliss Vanilla	8 oz	150	1	0	–	0	20	4	–
Pacific Foods									
Almond Low Fat Original	1 cup	70	1	500	–	0	300	tr	–
Almond Low Fat Vanilla	1 cup	100	1	500	–	0	300	tr	–
Multi Grain Low Fat Original	1 cup	160	1	500	–	0	–	1	–
Oat Organic Low Fat Original	1 cup	130	2	500	–	0	–	tr	–
Soy Organic Unsweetened Original	1 cup	90	2	100	–	0	20	4	–
Soy Select Low Fat Plain	1 cup	70	tr	0	–	0	20	1	–
Soy Ultra	1 cup	130	1	500	–	0	500	2	–
Soy Ultra Plain	1 cup	120	1	500	–	0	500	2	–
Rice Dream									
Carob	8 oz	150	tr	0	–	0	0	0	–
Heartwise Vanilla	8 oz	140	3	500	–	0	300	tr	30
Horchata	8 oz	130	2	0	–	0	40	2	140
Original	8 oz	120	0	0	–	0	20	tr	–
Original Enriched	8 oz	120	0	500	–	0	300	1	–
Vanilla Enriched	8 oz	130	0	500	–	0	300	tr	–
Silk									
Chocolate	1 cup	140	0	500	24	0	300	1	100
Organic Plain	1 cup	100	0	500	24	0	300	1	80
Vanilla	1 bottle (11 oz)	140	0	750	32	0	400	1	110
Sno*e									
Tofu as prep	8 oz	80	0	500	–	6	300	tr	95
Tofu Low Fat as prep	8 oz	70	0	500	–	6	300	tr	86
Soy Dream									
Classic Vanilla	8 oz	140	2	0	–	0	40	7	140
Original Enriched	8 oz	100	2	500	–	0	350	7	250
Vitamite									
Non-Dairy	1 cup (8 oz)	110	0	500	–	0	300	tr	170
Vitasoy									
Classic Original	8 oz	120	1	0	–	0	40	1	380

FOOD	PORTION	CALS	FIBER	VIT A	FOLIC	VIT C	CALCI	IRON	POTAS
Complete Original	8 oz	70	4	300	–	0	300	1	240
Complete Vanilla	8 oz	50	4	300	–	0	300	1	180
Creamy Original	8 oz	110	1	300	60	0	300	1	320
Green Tea Soymilk	8 oz	120	1	0	–	0	40	1	300
Light Original	8 oz	60	0	500	24	0	300	1	190
Light Chocolate	8 oz	100	0	300	24	0	300	1	200
Lite Vanilla	8 oz	70	0	300	24	0	300	1	200
Original Unsweetened	8 oz	80	tr	300	60	0	300	1	340
Rich Chocolate	8 oz	160	1	300	60	0	300	1	320
Smooth Vanilla	8 oz	120	1	300	60	0	300	1	320
Vanilla Delight	8 oz	120	1	0	–	0	40	1	320
White Wave									
Mocha	1 cup	140	1	300	–	0	200	3	–
MILKSHAKE									
chocolate	1 serv (10 oz)	393	2	665	20	1	269	2	524
malted milk shake	1 serv (10 oz)	402	1	710	20	1	311	tr	487
vanilla	1 serv (10 oz)	379	1	665	14	8	275	tr	396
Ben & Jerry's									
Cherry Garcia	1 bottle (8 oz)	320	–	500	–	0	200	2	–
Chocolate Fudge Brownie	1 bottle (8 oz)	340	–	500	–	0	150	2	–
Chunky Monkey	1 bottle (8 oz)	330	–	400	–	0	150	0	–
Breyers									
Quick Vanilla	1 serv (10 oz)	320	0	500	–	1	200	0	–
Carb Options									
Chocolate Delite	1 can (11 oz)	190	4	1750	120	60	350	3	480
Creamy Vanilla	1 can (11 oz)	190	4	1750	120	60	350	3	350
MILLET									
cooked	1 cup (6.1 oz)	207	2	0	33	0	5	1	108

FOOD	PORTION	CALS	FIBER	VIT A	FOLIC	VIT C	CALCI	IRON	POTAS
MISO									
dried	1 oz	86	1	0	–	0	51	2	219
miso	½ cup	284	7	120	46	0	92	4	226
Eden									
Hacho	1 tbsp	40	tr	0	–	2	20	1	180
Organic Genmai	1 tbsp	25	2	0	–	2	20	tr	80
Organic Mugi	1 tbsp	25	tr	0	–	0	0	tr	60
Organic Shiro	1 tbsp	30	tr	0	–	0	0	0	15
Tekka	1 tsp	5	0	0	–	0	0	tr	16
MOLASSES									
blackstrap	1 tbsp (0.7 oz)	47	–	0	0	–	172	4	498
molasses	1 tbsp (0.7 oz)	53	–	0	0	–	41	1	293
Brer Rabbit									
Dark	1 tbsp	60	–	–	–	–	20	1	231
Grandma's									
Robust	1 tbsp	60	–	0	–	0	100	4	–
MOOSE									
roasted	3 oz	114	0	–	–	4	5	4	284
MOTH BEANS									
dried cooked	1 cup	207	–	17	–	2	6	6	538
MOUSSE									
TAKE-OUT									
chocolate	½ cup (7.1 oz)	447	–	1134	–	–	202	1	296
MUFFIN									
MIX									
Glory									
Golden Sweet Corn as prep	1	170	1	100	–	0	40	1	–
Jiffy									
Apple Cinnamon as prep	1	190	1	0	–	0	60	1	–
Banana Nut as prep	1	180	2	0	–	0	60	1	–
Blueberry as prep	1	190	1	0	–	0	60	1	–
Bran w/ Dates as prep	1	170	3	0	–	0	60	1	–

FOOD	PORTION	CALS	FIBER	VIT A	FOLIC	VIT C	CALCI	IRON	POTAS
Corn as prep	1	180	1	0	–	0	80	1	–
Raspberry as prep	1	180	1	0	–	0	60	1	–
King Arthur									
Cranberry Orange Whole Grain not prep	¼ cup	180	3	0	–	2	100	1	–
Miracle Maize									
Country Style as prep	1	155	1	0	–	0	30	tr	–
Sweet as prep	1	180	1	0	–	0	60	tr	–
READY-TO-EAT									
Fred's Incredible Muffins									
All Flavors	1 (2.5 oz)	100	–	4500	–	1	100	1	–
Natural Ovens									
Blueberry	1 (2.5 oz)	180	2	0	60	24	80	1	–
Carrot Nut	1 (2.5 oz)	170	2	4000	100	42	100	1	–
Raisin Bran	1 (2.5 oz)	170	5	0	80	30	100	1	–
Otis Spunkmeyer									
Apple Cinnamon	1 (4 oz)	420	tr	0	–	2	40	2	–
Cheese Streusel	½ muffin (2 oz)	220	tr	100	32	0	20	1	–
Low Fat Wild Blueberry	1 (2.25 oz)	200	tr	0	–	0	20	1	–
Uncle Wally's									
Chocolate Passion	1 (2 oz)	130	1	0	–	0	0	1	–
Cranberry Orange Supreme	1 (2 oz)	130	1	0	–	1	20	1	–
Fat Free Apple Cinnamon Delight	1 (2 oz)	110	1	0	–	0	20	1	–
Fat Free Wild Blueberry Bliss	1 (2 oz)	120	1	0	–	0	0	1	–
Golden Waves Of Corn	1 (2 oz)	120	1	0	–	0	0	1	–
Honey Raisin Bran	1 (2 oz)	130	1	0	–	0	20	1	–
No Nut Banana	1 (2 oz)	130	1	0	–	0	0	1	–
VitaMuffin									
Apple Berry Bran	1 (2 oz)	100	5	2500	200	30	20	9	170
Blue Bran	1 (2 oz)	100	4	2500	200	30	20	9	–
Cran Bran	1 (2 oz)	100	4	2500	200	30	20	9	–
Deep Chocolate	1 (4 oz)	200	12	5000	400	60	40	18	340
Multi Bran	1 (2 oz)	100	4	2500	200	30	20	9	–
VitaTops Apple Berry Bran	1 (2 oz)	100	5	2500	200	30	20	9	170

FOOD	PORTION	CALS	FIBER	VIT A	FOLIC	VIT C	CALCI	IRON	POTAS
VitaTops Blue Bran	1 (2 oz)	100	4	2500	200	30	20	9	–
VitaTops Cran Bran	1 (2 oz)	100	4	2500	200	30	20	9	–
VitaTops Deep Chocolate	1 (2 oz)	100	6	2500	200	30	20	9	170
VitaTops MultiBran	1 (2 oz)	100	4	2500	200	30	20	9	–
TAKE-OUT									
corn	1 lg (2.5 oz)	214	2	130	55	0	152	2	104
raisin bran lowfat	1 (4 oz)	270	5	0	–	0	60	4	–

MULBERRIES

fresh	1 cup	61	–	35	–	51	55	3	271

MULLET

striped cooked	3 oz	127	0	120	–	–	26	1	389

MUNG BEANS

dried cooked	1 cup	213	–	48	321	2	55	3	536

MUNGO BEANS

dried cooked	1 cup	190	–	56	170	2	95	3	416

MUSHROOMS
CANNED

caps	8 (1.6 oz)	12	1	0	6	0	5	tr	61
caps pickled	6 (0.8 oz)	5	tr	0	2	tr	1	tr	59
chanterelle	3.5 oz	12	6	1	–	3	5	1	155
pickled	1 cup	33	1	0	14	2	5	1	395
pieces	½ cup	20	1	0	9	0	9	1	101
straw	1 cup	58	5	0	69	0	18	3	142
Green Giant									
Pieces & Stems	½ cup	30	2	0		0	0	tr	–
Sunny Dell									
Portabella Sliced	½ cup	20	2	0		2	0	1	–
DRIED									
chanterelle	1 oz	25	17	–	–	tr	24	5	1
shiitake	1 (3.6 g)	11	tr	0	6	tr	0	tr	55
tree ear	½ cup (0.4 oz)	36	–	8	19	0	14	1	85
wood ear mok yee	½ cup (0.4 oz)	25	4	10	–	–	30	12	91

FOOD	PORTION	CALS	FIBER	VIT A	FOLIC	VIT C	CALCI	IRON	POTAS
Eden									
Maitake Sliced	10 pieces (0.3 oz)	35	4	0	–	0	0	tr	230
Shitake	3 (0.4 oz)	35	5	0	–	0	0	1	200
Shitake Sliced	3 pieces (0.3 oz)	35	5	0	–	0	0	1	200
Frieda's									
Chanterelle	2 pieces (4 g)	15	1	0	–	0	0	tr	–
Wood Ear	3 pieces (4 g)	15	1	0	–	0	0	1	–
FRESH									
brown italian or crimini sliced	1 cup	19	tr	0	10	0	13	tr	323
brown italian or crimini whole	1 (0.7 oz)	5	tr	0	3	0	4	tr	90
chanterelle	3.5 oz	11	6	–	–	6	8	7	507
enoki raw	1 lg (5 g)	2	tr	0	3	0	0	tr	18
enoki sliced	1 cup	29	2	0	34	0	1	1	239
enoki whole	1 cup	28	2	0	33	0	1	1	236
maitake diced	1 cup	26	2	0	20	0	1	tr	143
maitake whole	1 (6.6 g)	2	tr	0	2	0	0	tr	13
morel	3.5 oz	9	7	–	–	5	11	1	390
oyster	1 sm (0.5 oz)	5	tr	7	4	0	0	tr	63
oyster sliced	1 cup	30	2	41	23	0	3	1	361
portobello raw	1 cap (3 oz)	22	1	0	18	0	7	1	407
portobello sliced grilled	1 cup (4.2 oz)	42	3	0	23	0	5	1	630
raw sliced	½ cup	8	tr	0	6	1	1	tr	111
shiitake pieces cooked	1 cup	81	3	0	30	tr	4	1	170
shiitake cooked	4 (2.5 oz)	40	2	0	15	tr	2	tr	84
white	1 (0.6 oz)	4	tr	0	3	tr	1	tr	57
white sliced cooked	1 cup	28	2	0	22	0	4	tr	428
Frieda's									
Enoki	¼ pkg (1 oz)	10	1	0	–	4	0	0	–

FOOD	PORTION	CALS	FIBER	VIT A	FOLIC	VIT C	CALCI	IRON	POTAS
FROZEN									
Alexia									
Mushroom Bites	1 serv (2 oz)	110	1	0	–	0	0	tr	120
TAKE-OUT									
battered fried	1 lg (0.6 oz)	39	tr	20	5	tr	4	tr	37
creamed	1 cup	171	3	435	22	1	128	1	306
stuffed	1 (0.8 oz)	67	1	120	8	1	39	1	90
MUSSELS									
fresh blue cooked	3 oz	147	–	–	–	–	28	6	228
MUSTARD									
dry mustard	1 tsp	15	–	2	–	–	17	tr	23
yellow ready-to-use	1 tsp	5	–	0	–	0	4	tr	7
Boar's Head									
Delicatessen Style	1 tsp (5 g)	0	0	0	–	0	0	0	–
Bone Suckin'									
Fat Free Gluten Free	1 tbsp	25	0	0	–	0	0	0	–
French's									
Honey	1 tsp	10	–	200	–	–	–	–	–
Luzianne									
Creole Mustard	1 tbsp	10	0	0	–	0	0	0	–
Sara Lee									
Country Honey	1 tbsp	10	0	0	–	0	0	0	–
Cranberry Honey	1 tbsp	10	0	0	–	0	0	0	–
MUSTARD GREENS									
fresh chopped cooked	½ cup	11	–	2122	–	18	52	tr	141
frozen chopped cooked	½ cup	14	–	3352	–	10	75	1	104
Allen's									
Seasoned Southern Style	½ cup	30	2	2750	–	6	100	1	115
Glory									
Seasoned canned	½ cup	35	1	4000	–	15	40	tr	–
NATTO									
natto	½ cup	187	–	0	–	11	191	8	642

FOOD	PORTION	CALS	FIBER	VIT A	FOLIC	VIT C	CALCI	IRON	POTAS
NAVY BEANS									
CANNED									
navy	1 cup	296	–	4	163	2	123	5	755
Eden									
Organic	½ cup	110	7	–	–	–	80	2	300
DRIED									
cooked	1 cup	259	–	3	255	2	128	5	669
NECTARINE									
fresh	1	67	2	1001	5	7	6	tr	288
Chiquita									
Fresh	1 med (4.9 oz)	70	2	200	–	9	0	tr	–
Sunsweet									
Dried	3 pieces (1.4 oz)	100	3	200	–	2	20	1	160
NEUFCHATEL									
neufchatel	1 oz	74	–	321	3	0	21	tr	32
Back To Nature									
Organic	⅛ pkg (1 oz)	70	0	300	–	0	20	0	–
NOODLES									
cellophane	1 cup	492	–	0	–	0	35	3	14
chow mein	1 cup (1.6 oz)	237	2	39	39	0	9	2	52
egg cooked	1 cup (5.6 oz)	213	2	32	102	0	19	3	45
japanese soba cooked	1 cup (4 oz)	113	–	0	8	0	5	1	40
japanese somen cooked	1 cup (6.2 oz)	231	–	0	4	0	14	1	51
korean acorn noodles not prep	2 oz	195	tr	0	–	0	–	1	–
rice cooked	1 cup (6.2 oz)	192	2	0	5	0	7	tr	7
spinach/egg cooked	1 cup (5.6 oz)	211	4	165	102	0	30	2	59
Annie Chun's									
Chow Mein	2 oz	200	3	0	–	0	0	2	–
Noodle Bowl Teriyaki	1 pkg	310	2	400	–	2	20	1	–

FOOD	PORTION	CALS	FIBER	VIT A	FOLIC	VIT C	CALCI	IRON	POTAS
Noodle Express Chinese Chow Mein	½ pkg	160	1	0	–	0	0	0	–
Noodle Express Singapore Curry	½ pkg	160	2	0	–	0	20	tr	–
Noodle Express Spicy Szechuan	½ pkg	170	1	100	–	2	0	tr	–
Noodle Express Teriyaki	½ pkg	160	1	0	–	0	20	tr	–
Noodle Express Thai Peanut	½ pkg	200	1	0	–	1	40	1	–
Rice	2 oz	210	0	0	–	0	0	2	–
Rice Pad Thai	2 oz	210	0	0	–	0	0	2	–
Azumaya									
Asian Style Thin Cut	1 cup	210	2	0	–	0	20	3	–
Hodgson Mill									
Egg Whole Wheat not prep	2 oz	190	4	100	28	0	20	2	–
Manischewitz									
Egg Medium	1¼ cups	220	2	0	120	0	20	2	–
Fine Egg	1½ cups	220	2	0	120	0	20	2	–
Fine Yolk Free	1½ cups	210	2	0	120	0	0	2	–
Wide Yolk Free	1¾ cups	210	2	0	120	0	0	2	–
Nasoya									
Chinese	1 cup	210	2	0	–	0	20	3	–
Japanese	1 cup	210	2	0	–	0	20	3	–
Spinach	1 cup	210	2	0	–	0	20	3	–
No Yolks									
Extra Broad	2 oz	210	3	0	120	0	0	2	–
Pennsylvania Dutch									
Yolk Free Ribbons as prep	1½ cups	210	2	0	100	0	0	2	–

NUTMEG

ground	1 tsp	12	–	2	–	–	4	tr	8

NUTRITION SUPPLEMENTS

Boost									
Breeze	8 oz	160	–	70	80	60	150	0	230
Diabetic	8 oz	250	3	1200	80	100	276	4	270
DiabetiTrim									
Shake French Vanilla	1 pkg	90	4	1000	80	18	300	5	390

FOOD	PORTION	CALS	FIBER	VIT A	FOLIC	VIT C	CALCI	IRON	POTAS
Enlive!									
Drink All Flavors	1 box (8.1 oz)	300	0	1250	–	24	60	3	40
Ensure									
Creamy Milk Chocolate Shake	1 can (8 oz)	350	tr	1250	100	30	200	5	500
Plus Vanilla Shake	1 bottle (8 oz)	350	0	1250	100	30	200	5	440
GeniSoy									
Soy Natural Protein Powder	1 scoop (1 oz)	100	0	1250	100	15	250	5	90
Glucerna									
Shakes All Flavors	1 can (8 oz)	220	3	1750	–	60	250	5	60
Jelly Belly									
Sport Beans Berry Blue	1 pkg (1 oz)	100	0	0	–	6	0	0	40
Nutribar									
Shake Chocolate Supreme as prep w/ 2% milk	1 serv (10 oz)	262	2	1750	140	13	370	5	790
Pria									
Complete Shake Creamy Milk Chocolate	1 pkg (11.6 oz)	170	7	2250	100	30	500	5	570
Complete Shake French Vanilla	1 pkg (11.6 oz)	170	7	2250	100	30	300	5	440
Resource									
Optisource High Protein Drink	1 box (4 oz)	100	0	0	–	0	150	0	70
Slim-Fast									
Optima Ready-To-Drink Creamy Milk Chocolate	1 can (11 oz)	190	5	1750	120	60	500	3	605
Optima Shake Mix Chocolate Royale as prep w/ fat free milk	1 serv	190	4	1250	100	27	500	5	580

FOOD	PORTION	CALS	FIBER	VIT A	FOLIC	VIT C	CALCI	IRON	POTAS
Optima Shake Mix French Vanilla as prep w/ fat free milk	1 serv	200	4	1250	100	27	500	6	540
Vitasoy									
Weight Management Meal All Flavors	1 bottle (10 oz)	200	8	1250	140	21	500	6	100

NUTS MIXED

FOOD	PORTION	CALS	FIBER	VIT A	FOLIC	VIT C	CALCI	IRON	POTAS
dry roasted w/ peanuts salted	¼ cup	203	3	10	17	tr	24	1	204
dry roasted w/ peanuts w/o salt	¼ cup	203	3	5	17	tr	24	1	204
oil roasted w/o peanuts salted	¼ cup	221	2	3	20	tr	38	1	196
oil roasted w/o peanuts w/o salt	¼ cup	221	2	7	20	tr	38	1	196
Good Sense									
Deluxe Mix	¼ cup	180	2	0	–	0	40	1	–
Here's Howe									
Royal Mixed Nuts	1 oz	180	2	0	–	0	40	1	–
Kind									
Nut Delight	1 bar (1.4 oz)	203	3	0	–	0	45	1	–
MaraNatha									
Cashew Macadamia Butter	2 tbsp	210	2	0	–	0	20	1	–
Tamari Organic	¼ cup	160	2	0	–	0	20	1	–
Tamari Roasted	¼ cup	160	2	0	–	0	20	1	–
Organic Trails									
Tamari Roasted Nuts & Seeds	¼ cup	190	5	0	–	0	40	1	–
Peanut Better									
Mixed Nut Butter Creamy & Crunchy	2 tbsp	190	3	0	–	0	60	1	–
Planters									
NUT-rition Energy Mix	¼ cup	180	3	0	–	0	40	1	135
NUT-rition Heart Healthy Mix	1 (0.9 oz)	170	3	0	–	0	40	1	–

FOOD	PORTION	CALS	FIBER	VIT A	FOLIC	VIT C	CALCI	IRON	POTAS
OCA									
Frieda's									
Oca	½ cup	70	1	0	–	18	0	1	–
OCTOPUS									
fresh steamed	3 oz	140	–	–	–	–	90	8	–
OHELOBERRIES									
fresh	1 cup	39	–	1162	–	8	10	tr	54
OIL									
butter oil	1 tbsp	112	0	480	–	–	–	–	–
canola	1 tbsp	124	0	–	–	–	–	–	–
coconut	1 tbsp	117	0	–	–	–	–	tr	–
corn	1 tbsp	120	0	–	–	–	–	–	–
grapeseed	1 tbsp	120	0	0	0	0	0	0	0
olive	1 tbsp	119	0	–	–	–	tr	tr	–
palm	1 tbsp	120	0	–	–	–	–	0	–
peanut	1 tbsp	119	0	–	–	–	tr	0	0
rice bran	1 tbsp	120	0	–	–	–	–	tr	–
safflower	1 tbsp	120	0	–	–	–	–	–	–
soybean	1 tbsp	120	0	–	–	–	tr	0	–
Alpha									
Hazelnut	1 oz	257	0	–	–	–	tr	–	–
Carapelli									
Grapeseed	1 tbsp	120	0	0	–	0	0	0	–
Olive Extra Virgin	1 tbsp	120	0	0	–	0	0	0	–
Enova									
Oil	1 tbsp	120	0	–	–	–	–	–	–
House Of Tsang									
Mongolian Fire	1 tsp	45	0	0	–	0	0	0	0
Wok Oil	1 tbsp	130	0	0	–	0	0	0	0
Kinloch Plantation									
100% Virgin Pecan	1 tbsp	130	0	0	–	0	0	0	–
Living Harvest									
Organic Hemp Oil	2 tbsp	250	0	0	–	0	0	0	–
Manitoba Harvest									
Hemp Seed Oil	1 tbsp	126	0	0	–	0	0	0	–
Orville Redenbacher's									
Popping & Topping	1 tbsp	120	0	0	–	0	0	0	–
Spectrum									
Almond	1 tbsp	120	0	0	–	0	0	0	–

FOOD	PORTION	CALS	FIBER	VIT A	FOLIC	VIT C	CALCI	IRON	POTAS
Apricot Kernel	1 tbsp	120	0	0	–	0	0	0	–
Avocado	1 tbsp	120	0	0	–	0	0	0	–
Canola Organic	1 tbsp	120	0	0	–	0	0	0	–
Coconut Organic	1 tbsp	120	0	0	–	0	0	0	–
Corn	1 tbsp	120	0	0	–	0	0	0	–
Grapeseed	1 tbsp	120	0	0	–	0	0	0	–
Grapeseed Oil Spray	⅓ sec spray	0	0	0	–	0	0	0	0
Hazelnut Toasted Organic	1 tbsp	120	0	0	–	0	0	0	0
Mediterranean Olive Organic	1 tbsp	120	0	0	–	0	0	0	0
Organic Extra Virgin Oil Spray	⅓ sec spray	0	0	0	–	0	0	0	0
Peanut	1 tbsp	120	0	0	–	0	0	0	–
Pumpkin Seed Organic	1 tbsp	120	0	0	–	0	0	0	–
Sesame Organic	1 tbsp	120	0	0	–	0	0	0	–
Sesame Toasted Organic	1 tbsp	120	0	0	–	0	0	0	0
Soy Organic	1 tbsp	120	0	0	–	0	0	0	0
Sunflower Organic	1 tbsp	120	0	0	–	0	0	0	0
Walnut Organic	1 tbsp	120	0	0	–	0	0	0	0

OKRA
CANNED
pickled	6 pods (2.3 oz)	18	2	40	32	9	44	tr	161

Glory
Cut	½ cup	25	2	500	–	12	60	tr	–

FRESH
cooked w/ salt	8 pods	19	2	241	39	14	65	tr	115
luffa chinese okra cooked	1 cup	39	4	100	82	29	137	1	239
sliced cooked w/ salt	½ cup	18	2	226	37	13	62	tr	108

TAKE-OUT
batter dipped fried	10 pieces (2.6 oz)	142	2	65	36	8	50	1	155

OLIVES
green	3 extra lg	15	tr	40	–	0	8	tr	7

FOOD	PORTION	CALS	FIBER	VIT A	FOLIC	VIT C	CALCI	IRON	POTAS
green	4 med	15	tr	40	–	0	8	tr	7
green olive tapenade	1 tbsp	25	0	200	–	2	20	tr	–
ripe	1 sm	4	tr	13	0	0	3	tr	0
ripe	1 lg	5	tr	18	0	0	4	tr	0
ripe	1 jumbo	7	–	29	–	tr	8	tr	1
ripe	1 colossal	12	–	53	–	tr	14	1	1
spanish stuffed	5 (0.5 oz)	15	0	200	–	0	20	0	–
Peloponnese									
Amfissa	3	45	0	0	–	0	0	0	–
Ionian Green	3	25	0	0	–	0	0	0	–
Kalamata Pitted	5	45	0	0	–	0	0	0	–
Kalamata Spread	1 tsp	15	0	0	–	0	0	0	–

ONION
CANNED
cocktail	½ cup	41	2	0	14	5	20	tr	153

Boar's Head
Sweet Vidalia In Sauce	1 tbsp	10	0	0	–	0	0	0	–

DRIED
flakes	1 tbsp	17	1	1	8	4	13	tr	81
powder	1 tsp	7	tr	0	4	tr	9	tr	23
shallots	1 tbsp	3	–	505	1	tr	2	tr	15

FRESH
cooked w/o salt	1 lg (4.5 oz)	56	2	3	19	7	28	tr	212
cooked w/o salt	1 med (3.3 oz)	41	1	2	14	5	21	tr	156
cooked w/o salt	1 sm (2 oz)	26	1	1	9	3	13	tr	100
cooked w/o salt chopped	1 tbsp	7	tr	0	2	1	3	tr	25
raw chopped	1 tbsp	4	tr	0	2	1	2	tr	15
raw chopped	½ cup	32	1	2	15	6	18	tr	117
raw slice	1 (0.5 oz)	6	tr	0	3	1	3	tr	20
raw sliced	½ cup	23	1	1	11	4	13	tr	84
scallions raw	1 med (0.5 oz)	5	tr	150	10	3	11	tr	41
scallions raw chopped	¼ cup	8	1	249	16	5	18	tr	69
shallots raw chopped	¼ cup	29	–	476	14	3	15	tr	134
sweet whole raw	1 (11.6 oz)	106	3	3	76	16	66	1	394

FOOD	PORTION	CALS	FIBER	VIT A	FOLIC	VIT C	CALCI	IRON	POTAS
whole raw	1 lg (5.3 oz)	60	3	3	28	11	34	tr	219
whole raw	1 med (4 oz)	44	2	2	21	8	25	tr	161
whole raw	1 sm (2.5 oz)	28	1	1	13	5	16	tr	102
Antioch Farms									
Vidalia	1 med	60	3	tr	tr	12	40	tr	200
Arrowfarms									
Cipoline	2 (1.1 oz)	20	5	0	–	0	0	0	–
Blue Ribbon									
Yellow	1 med (5.2 oz)	60	3	0	–	12	40	tr	–
Christopher Ranch									
Shallots	1 (1 oz)	20	1	0	–	0	0	0	–
Earthbound Farm									
Organic Green Onions	¼ cup	10	1	100	–	5	0	0	–
Organic Red	1 med (5.2 oz)	60	3	0	–	12	40	tr	–
Frieda's									
Cipolline	3 (3 oz)	30	2	0	–	6	0	0	–
Maui	⅓ cup (1.1 oz)	10	1	0	–	2	0	0	–
Pearl	⅔ cup (3 oz)	30	2	0	–	6	0	0	–
Shallots	1 tbsp (1 oz)	20	0	350	–	2	0	tr	–
Nature's Harvest									
Onion	1 med (5.2 oz)	60	3	0	–	12	40	tr	–
OsoSweet									
Onion	1 med (5 oz)	60	3	0	–	12	40	tr	–
FROZEN									
Alexia									
Onion Rings	6 (3 oz)	230	4	0	–	2	20	1	–
C&W									
Petite Whole	⅔ cup (3 oz)	30	tr	0	–	0	0	0	–

FOOD	PORTION	CALS	FIBER	VIT A	FOLIC	VIT C	CALCI	IRON	POTAS
Ian's									
Rings & Strings	5–9 pieces (2.5 oz)	152	1	0	–	0	20	tr	–
TAKE-OUT									
creamed	1 cup	187	2	390	27	8	132	1	369
fried	½ cup	57	1	–	–	1	9	tr	58
rings breaded & fried	8–9 (3 oz)	276	–	8	55	1	73	1	129

ORANGE
CANNED
Del Monte

FOOD	PORTION	CALS	FIBER	VIT A	FOLIC	VIT C	CALCI	IRON	POTAS
SunFresh Mandarin	½ cup	80	tr	0	–	60	0	1	–
FRESH									
california navel	1	65	3	256	47	80	56	tr	250
california valencia	1	59	3	278	47	59	48	tr	217
florida	1	69	4	302	26	68	65	tr	254
peel	1 tbsp	6	–	25	–	8	10	tr	13
sections	1 cup	85	4	369	55	96	52	tr	326
Frieda's									
Cara Cara	1 med (5 oz)	70	3	300	–	72	60	0	–
Mandarin Delite	1 cup (5 oz)	60	3	1250	–	42	0	0	–
Mandarin Page	1 cup (5 oz)	60	3	1250	–	42	0	0	–
Mandarin Pixie	1 cup (5 oz)	60	3	1250	–	42	0	0	–
Mandarin Satsuma	1 (5 oz)	60	3	1250	–	42	0	0	–
Melogold	½ (6 oz)	50	2	200	–	60	0	0	–
Seville	1 (3 oz)	40	2	200	–	48	40	0	–
Sunkist									
Cara Cara Navel	1 med	80	7	1500	60	90	20	0	260
Minneola Tangelo	1 (3.8 oz)	70	2	200	320	60	40	0	220
Moro	1 (5.4 oz)	70	3	400	60	66	40	tr	260
Orange	1 med	80	7	100	60	78	60	tr	260
Satsuma Mandarin	1 (3.8 oz)	50	2	100	32	66	40	tr	200

ORANGE JUICE

FOOD	PORTION	CALS	FIBER	VIT A	FOLIC	VIT C	CALCI	IRON	POTAS
canned	1 cup	104	–	432	–	86	21	1	436
chilled	1 cup	110	–	194	45	82	24	tr	473

FOOD	PORTION	CALS	FIBER	VIT A	FOLIC	VIT C	CALCI	IRON	POTAS
fresh	1 cup	111	–	496	–	124	27	1	496
mandarin orange	7 oz	94	–	tr	–	64	38	tr	–
After The Fall									
24 Karrot Orange	8 oz	120	–	10000	–	90	150	–	390
Dole									
100% Juice	8 oz	110	–	–	40	60	20	–	430
Florida's Natural									
Calcium & Vitamin D	8 oz	110	0	–	60	72	350	–	450
Hood									
100% Juice	1 cup	120	0	0	–	72	0	0	–
Italian Volcano									
Blood Orange Organic	1 serv (6.75 oz)	84	1	–	–	100	–	5	–
Minute Maid									
Country Style	8 oz	110	–	–	60	72	20	–	450
Heart Wise	8 oz	110	–	–	60	72	20	–	450
Kids+	8 oz	110	–	1000	60	72	350	–	450
Light	8 oz	50	–	–	24	72	350	–	450
Original	8 oz	110	–	–	60	72	20	–	450
Plus Calcium	8 oz	110	–	–	60	72	350	–	450
W/ Extra Vitamin C & E Plus Zinc	8 oz	110	–	–	60	144	20	–	450
Naked Juice									
Just OJ	8 oz	110	0	400	–	108	20	tr	470
Odwalla									
Organic	8 fl oz	110	–	0	–	144	20	0	450
Simply Orange									
Calcium Pulp Free	8 oz	110	–	–	60	84	350	–	450
Tropicana									
Antioxidant Advantage	8 oz	110	0	0	60	144	20	0	450
Calcium + Vitamin D	8 oz	110	0	0	60	72	350	0	450
Fiber	8 oz	120	3	0	60	72	20	0	450
Healthy Heart	8 oz	120	0	0	60	60	20	0	450
Healthy Kids	8 oz	110	0	1000	60	72	350	0	450
Light 'n Healthy w/ Calcium	8 oz	50	0	500	24	72	200	0	450
Light 'n Healthy w/ Pulp	8 oz	50	0	1000	28	72	0	0	450

FOOD	PORTION	CALS	FIBER	VIT A	FOLIC	VIT C	CALCI	IRON	POTAS
No Pulp	8 oz	110	0	0	60	72	20	0	450
Orangeade	8 oz	1113	0	0	–	60	0	0	–
Uncle Matt's									
Organic 100% Juice Pulp Free	8 oz	110	0	0	60	72	0	0	450
Organic 100% Juice w/ Pulp	8 oz	110	0	0	60	72	0	0	450
TAKE-OUT									
orange julius	1 serv (24 oz)	443	1	427	92	219	40	tr	713

OREGANO

FOOD	PORTION	CALS	FIBER	VIT A	FOLIC	VIT C	CALCI	IRON	POTAS
ground	1 tsp	5	–	104	–	–	24	1	25

OYSTERS

FOOD	PORTION	CALS	FIBER	VIT A	FOLIC	VIT C	CALCI	IRON	POTAS
canned eastern	1 cup	112	0	486	15	8	73	11	371
eastern baked	6 med	47	0	37	14	4	33	5	90
eastern raw	6 med	50	0	21	15	4	37	5	104
eastern sauteed	6 med	76	0	255	6	2	30	4	106
smoked	6	33	0	70	5	2	22	3	75
Brunswick									
Smoked	1 can (3 oz)	140	1	500	–	0	40	8	–
Bumble Bee									
Smoked	¼ cup	120	0	300	–	0	10	13	–
Whole	¼ cup	70	0	200	–	0	20	6	–
Chicken Of The Sea									
Smoked In Oil	1 can (3.75 oz)	140	–	200	–	0	20	5	–
Smoked In Water	1 can (3.75 oz)	120	0	300	–	0	20	7	–
Smoked Teriyaki	1 can (3.75 oz)	120	1	300	–	4	20	7	–
Whole	½ can (2 oz)	80	0	200	–	0	20	5	–
TAKE-OUT									
breaded & fried	6	368	–	363	31	4	28	4	182
fritter	1 (1.4 oz)	121	tr	105	21	1	62	2	58
oysters rockefeller	1 cup	302	4	3125	143	27	226	10	627
stew	1 cup	208	0	820	15	3	235	6	380

PANCAKE/WAFFLE SYRUP

FOOD	PORTION	CALS	FIBER	VIT A	FOLIC	VIT C	CALCI	IRON	POTAS
lite	¼ cup	98	0	0	0	0	1	tr	2
pancake syrup	¼ cup	209	0	0	0	0	4	tr	5

PANCAKES

FROZEN

Eggo

Buttermilk	3	280	1	1000	60	0	40	4	70
Minis	11	260	1	1000	60	0	40	4	75

Golden

Potato	1 (1.3 oz)	70	1	0	–	0	0	0	–

Ian's

Blueberry	1 (1.3 oz)	100	1	0	–	0	60	1	–
Pancake	1 (1.3 oz)	100	1	0	–	0	60	1	–

McCain

Homestyle BabyCakes	4 pieces (2.6 oz)	150	2	0	–	5	0	tr	220

MIX

Aunt Jemima

Buttermilk Pancake & Waffle Mix not prep	⅓ cup	160	1	0	40	0	150	2	–
Pancake & Waffle Mix Whole Wheat as prep	3 pancakes	200	3	200	40	0	150	3	170

Big Train

Low Carb Pancake & Waffle Mix as prep	3	190	5	200	–	0	50	1	–

Don's Chuck Wagon

Buckwheat Mix	⅓ cup	160	1	0	–	0	20	3	–

Hodgson Mill

Buckwheat not prep	⅓ cup	140	3	0	–	0	0	1	–
Whole Wheat Buttermilk not prep	⅓ cup	120	4	0	–	0	150	1	–

King Arthur

Multi-Grain Buttermilk not prep	6 tbsp	160	5	0	–	0	150	2	–

TAKE-OUT

buckwheat	1 (7 in)	142	2	188	14	0	175	1	160
plain	1 (7 in)	183	1	115	33	tr	50	3	58
potato	1 (1.3 oz)	70	1	45	9	6	9	tr	165

FOOD	PORTION	CALS	FIBER	VIT A	FOLIC	VIT C	CALCI	IRON	POTAS
w/ butter & syrup	2 (8.1 oz)	520	–	281	30	4	128	3	251
whole wheat	1 (7 in)	183	3	190	14	0	155	1	188

PAPAYA
fresh	1	117	–	6122	–	188	72	tr	780
fresh cubed	1 cup	54	–	2819	–	87	33	tr	359

Del Monte
In Extra Light Syrup w/ Passion Fruit Puree	½ cup	70	1	300	–	6	0	0	–

Frieda's
Mexican	1 cup (5 oz)	50	3	400	–	84	40	0	–

PAPAYA JUICE
nectar	1 cup	142	–	277	5	8	24	1	78

Ceres
Papaya	8 oz	120	0	0	–	30	20	tr	190

Langers
Papaya Delight 100% Juice	8 oz	130	1	–	–	48	–	–	–

Old Orchard
Nectar Cocktail	8 oz	120	–	0	–	78	0	0	93

PAPRIKA
paprika	1 tsp	6	–	1273	–	1	4	1	49

PARSLEY
dry	1 tbsp	1	–	253	6	1	1	tr	25
dry	1 tsp	1	–	70	–	tr	4	tr	11
fresh chopped	½ cup	11	–	1560	46	40	41	2	166

Dorot
Chopped Cubes frzn	1 cube (4 g)	5	tr	–	–	–	–	–	–

Frieda's
Parsley Root	⅔ cup	10	1	0	–	0	0	0	–

PARSNIPS
fresh cooked	1 (5.6 oz)	130	–	0	93	21	59	1	588
fresh sliced cooked	½ cup	63	–	0	45	10	29	tr	287
raw sliced	½ cup	50	–	0	45	11	24	tr	251

Frieda's
Sliced	1 cup	100	7	0	–	21	–	1	–

FOOD	PORTION	CALS	FIBER	VIT A	FOLIC	VIT C	CALCI	IRON	POTAS
PASSION FRUIT									
purple fresh	1	18	–	126	–	5	2	tr	63
PASSION FRUIT JUICE									
purple	1 cup	126	–	1771	–	74	9	1	–
yellow	1 cup	149	–	5953	–	45	9	1	687
Ceres									
Passion Fruit	8 oz	120	0	0	–	30	20	1	190
PASTA									
DRY									
corn cooked	1 cup (4.9 oz)	176	7	80	8	0	1	tr	43
elbows	1 cup	389	–	0	19	0	19	4	170
elbows cooked	1 cup (4.9 oz)	197	2	0	98	0	10	2	43
shells small cooked	1 cup (4 oz)	162	2	0	81	0	8	2	36
spaghetti cooked	1 cup (4.9 oz)	197	2	0	98	0	10	2	43
spinach spaghetti cooked	1 cup (4.9 oz)	182	–	213	17	0	42	1	81
spirals cooked	1 cup (4.7 oz)	189	2	0	94	0	9	2	42
vegetable cooked	1 cup (4.7 oz)	172	6	71	87	0	15	1	42
whole wheat all shapes cooked	1 cup	174	4	0	7	0	21	1	62
Annie Chun's									
Soba Noodles	2 oz	200	3	0	–	0	0	2	–
Barilla									
Pastina	2 oz	210	2	0	120	0	0	2	–
Penne	1 cup (2 oz)	200	2	0	120	0	0	2	–
Plus Penne	2 oz	200	4	0	120	0	20	2	–
Plus Rotini not prep	2 oz	210	4	0	160	0	20	3	–
Tortelloni Porcini Mushroom	¾ cup	240	5	0	–	0	60	1	–
Tortelloni Ricotta & Asparagus	¾ cup	240	5	100	–	0	60	1	–

FOOD	PORTION	CALS	FIBER	VIT A	FOLIC	VIT C	CALCI	IRON	POTAS
Tortelloni Ricotta & Spinach	¾ cup	240	4	300	–	0	100	1	–
Bella Vita									
Low Carb Penne Rigate	2 oz	190	8	0	–	0	150	8	–
Catelli									
Bistro Cracked Black Pepper Fettucine	¼ pkg	320	2	0	320	0	20	4	–
Bistro Italian Herb Fettuccine	¼ pkg	310	3	0	320	0	60	4	–
Bistro Lemon Pepper Linguine	¼ pkg	320	3	0	320	0	20	4	–
Bistro Rainbows	3 oz	320	2	0	320	0	40	4	–
Bistro Spinach Lasagne	3 oz	320	3	100	320	0	80	4	–
Bistro Sun Dried Tomato & Basil Spaghettini	¼ pkg	320	3	100	320	0	40	4	–
Bistro Vegetable Fusilli	3 oz	320	2	0	320	0	40	4	–
Healthy Harvest Flax Omega-3	3 oz	290	6	0	320	0	40	5	–
Healthy Harvest Multigrain	3 oz	310	6	0	320	0	20	5	–
Healthy Harvest Organic Whole Wheat	3 oz	320	3	0	–	0	0	1	–
Healthy Harvest Whole Wheat All Shapes	3 oz	310	5	100	320	0	20	5	–
Darielle									
All Shapes not prep	2 oz	160	8	–	–	–	–	–	–
DaVinci									
Rotini	1 cup	210	2	0	140	0	20	2	–
Spaghetti	2 oz	210	2	0	140	0	20	2	–
DeCecco									
Spaghetti w/ Spinach (2 oz)	⅛ pkg	200	2	0	120	0	20	2	–
Dreamfields									
Lasagna not prep	2 pieces (2 oz)	190	5	0	160	0	0	2	–
Rotini not prep	⅔ cup (2 oz)	190	5	0	120	0	0	2	–

FOOD	PORTION	CALS	FIBER	VIT A	FOLIC	VIT C	CALCI	IRON	POTAS
Due Amici									
Pasta Lite Low Carb Fusilli	2 oz	160	7	0	–	0	150	6	–
Eden									
Bifun Pasta not prep	2 oz	200	0	0	–	0	0	1	10
Harusame Pasta not prep	2 oz	190	0	0	–	0	0	2	10
Kudzu	2 oz	200	2	0	–	0	0	1	0
Organic Gemelli Spelt & Buckwheat not prep	½ cup (2 oz)	210	4	–	24	–	–	2	240
Organic Ribbons Artichoke not prep	½ cup (2 oz)	210	2	0	16	0	20	1	260
Organic Rigatoni Kamut & Buckwheat not prep	½ cup (2 oz)	200	5	–	16	–	20	3	220
Organic Spaghetti 100% Whole Wheat not prep	2 oz	210	6	100	–	0	20	3	260
Organic Spirals Flax Rice not prep	½ cup (2 oz)	200	4	–	24	–	20	2	240
Organic Spirals Kamut Vegetable not prep	½ cup (2 oz)	210	6	200	24	0	20	4	210
Organic Spirals Rye not prep	½ cup (2 oz)	200	8	0	80	1	20	2	300
Organic Spirals Spinach not prep	½ cup (2 oz)	210	5	0	24	0	20	2	320
Organic Udon not prep	¼ pkg	200	3	0	–	0	20	2	115
Organic Udon Spelt not prep	¼ pkg	200	2	–	24	–	–	1	45
Organic Vegetable Alphabets not prep	½ cup (2 oz)	210	4	0	24	0	20	2	280
Organic Vegetable Shells not prep	½ cup (2 oz)	210	4	0	24	0	0	2	280
Organic Ziti Rigati Spelt not prep	½ cup (2 oz)	210	5	0	24	0	0	2	260
Soba Japanese 100% Buckwheat not prep	2 oz	200	3	0	–	0	20	1	200
Soba Japanese Lotus Root not prep	2 oz	190	4	0	–	0	20	2	170
Soba Japanese Mugwort not prep	2 oz	190	2	0	–	0	20	2	140

FOOD	PORTION	CALS	FIBER	VIT A	FOLIC	VIT C	CALCI	IRON	POTAS
Soba Japanese Wild Yam not prep	2 oz	190	2	0	–	0	20	1	150
Udon Japanese Brown Rice not prep	2 oz	190	2	0	–	0	0	1	125
Udon Japanese not prep	2 oz	190	3	0	–	0	0	2	170
Food For Life									
Ezekiel 4:9 Sprouted Grain	2 oz	210	7	0	–	0	20	2	–
Hodgson Mill									
Lasagne Whole Wheat not prep	2 oz	190	6	0	28	0	20	3	–
Organic Fettuccine Whole Wheat w/ Milled Flax Seed not prep	2 oz	200	6	0	32	0	20	3	–
Pasta Ribbons Whole Wheat not prep	2 oz	190	5	0	28	0	20	2	–
Spaghetti Whole Wheat not prep	2 oz	190	6	0	28	0	20	3	–
Veggie Bows not prep	2 oz	200	1	0	–	0	0	3	–
Wagon Wheels Veggie not prep	2 oz	200	1	0	120	0	0	3	–
Keto									
Elbows not prep	1.6 oz	108	1	–	–	–	–	–	–
Spaghetti not prep	1.3 oz	130	2	–	–	–	–	–	–
LifeStream									
Organic All Shapes	2 oz	208	8	100	–	0	30	3	–
Lundberg									
Organic Spaghetti Brown Rice	2 oz	210	3	0	–	0	0	1	190
Mueller's									
Elbow Macaroni not prep	½ cup	210	2	0	100	0	0	2	–
Multi Grain Rotini not prep	1 cup (2 oz)	190	5	0	–	0	20	3	–
Notta Pasta									
Rice Pasta All Shapes	2 oz	200	2	0	–	0	20	1	–
Pastalia									
Heart Health Low Carb not prep	2 oz	176	3	–	–	–	–	–	–

FOOD	PORTION	CALS	FIBER	VIT A	FOLIC	VIT C	CALCI	IRON	POTAS
Real Torino									
Tirali not prep	1 cup (2 oz)	210	2	0	140	0	20	2	–
Revival									
Soy Penne	⅙ box	200	1	–	–	–	25	3	88
Soy Thin Spaghetti	⅙ box	200	1	–	–	–	25	3	88
Ronzoni									
Elbows not prep	½ cup (2 oz)	210	2	–	100	–	–	2	–
Healthy Harvest Multigrain Spaghetti	⅐ pkg (2 oz)	190	5	–	140	–	–	3	–
Healthy Harvest Whole Wheat Blend Spaghetti	⅐ pkg (2 oz)	180	6	–	120	–	–	2	–
Healthy Harvest Whole Wheat Rotini not prep	¾ cup (2 oz)	180	6	–	120	–	–	2	–
Lasagne	2½ pieces (2 oz)	210	2	–	100	–	–	2	–
San Giorgio									
Elbows not prep	½ cup	210	2	–	100	–	–	2	–
Soy7									
Pasta All Shapes	2 oz	200	2	–	–	–	–	–	–
Whey Cool									
High Protein Xtreme Rotini	1 serv (2 oz)	210	1	–	–	–	–	–	–
FRESH									
cooked	2 oz	75	–	11	36	0	3	1	14
spinach cooked	2 oz	74	–	59	36	0	10	1	21
REFRIGERATED									
Buitoni									
Angel Hair	1¼ cups	230	2	0	–	0	20	2	–
Fettuccine	1¼ cups	240	2	0	–	0	20	2	–
Fettuccine Spinach	1¼ cups	260	2	300	–	1	60	3	–
Linguine	1¼ cups	240	2	0	–	0	20	2	–
Ravioletti Three Cheese	1 cup	270	2	100	–	0	100	1	–
Ravioli Chicken & Roasted Garlic	1¼ cups	340	2	0	–	0	40	2	–
Ravioli Chicken Parmesan	1¼ cups	310	2	200	–	0	40	1	–

FOOD	PORTION	CALS	FIBER	VIT A	FOLIC	VIT C	CALCI	IRON	POTAS
Ravioli Classic Beef	1¼ cups	340	2	100	–	0	60	2	–
Ravioli Doublestuffed Mozzarella & Herb	1½ cups	340	3	200	–	0	250	2	–
Ravioli Four Cheese	1¼ cups	330	3	0	–	0	150	2	–
Ravioli Garden Vegetable	1 cup	250	2	300	–	2	100	2	–
Ravioli Light Four Cheese	1¼ cups	230	2	0	–	0	100	1	0
Tortellini Herb Chicken	1 cup	340	2	200	–	0	20	2	–
Tortellini Mixed Cheese	1 cup	320	3	200	–	0	150	2	–
Tortellini Spinach Cheese	1 cup	320	3	200	–	0	200	2	–
Tortellini Three Cheese	1 cup	320	3	100	–	0	150	1	–
Tortelloni Cheese & Roasted Garlic	1 cup	270	2	100	–	0	150	1	–
Tortelloni Chicken & Prosciutto	1 cup	320	2	0	–	0	40	2	–
Tortelloni Mozzarella & Herb	1 cup	330	2	200	–	0	150	2	–
Tortelloni Mozzarella & Pepperoni	1 cup	330	2	100	–	0	150	1	–
Tortelloni Portabello Mushroom & Cheese	1 cup	290	3	0	–	0	40	2	–
Tortelloni Sun Dried Tomato	1 cup	310	3	300	–	0	80	1	–
Tortelloni Sweet Italian Sausage	1 cup	330	3	0	–	0	40	2	–
Pasta Prima									
Ravioli Spinach & Mozzarella	1 cup	200	4	8000	–	9	100	1	–
Ravioli Sun Dried Tomato & Mozzarella	1 cup	200	3	1500	–	9	30	1	–

PASTA DINNERS
CANNED
Annie's Homegrown

FOOD	PORTION	CALS	FIBER	VIT A	FOLIC	VIT C	CALCI	IRON	POTAS
Organic All Stars	1 cup	150	tr	200	–	2	40	1	–
Organic BernieOs	1 cup	150	tr	200	–	2	40	1	–

FOOD	PORTION	CALS	FIBER	VIT A	FOLIC	VIT C	CALCI	IRON	POTAS
Organic Cheesy Ravioli	1 cup	180	3	500	–	2	80	2	–
Organic P'sghetti Loops	1 cup	190	2	400	–	4	60	2	–
FROZEN									
Amy's									
Bowl Stuffed Pasta Shells	1 pkg (10 oz)	300	5	–	–	–	–	–	–
Cannelloni w/ Vegetables	1 pkg (9 oz)	330	6	–	–	–	–	–	–
Lasagna Cheese	1 pkg (10.25 oz)	330	5	–	–	–	–	–	–
Lasagna Garden Vegetable	1 pkg (10.25 oz)	290	5	–	–	–	–	–	–
Macaroni & Cheese	1 pkg (9 oz)	410	3	–	–	–	–	–	–
Macaroni & Soy Cheese	1 pkg (9 oz)	370	4	–	–	–	–	–	–
Pasta & Vegetable Alfredo	1 cup	220	4	–	–	–	–	–	–
Pasta Primavera	1 pkg (9 oz)	300	3	–	–	–	–	–	–
Ravioli w/ Sauce	1 pkg (8 oz)	340	3	–	–	–	–	–	–
Rice Mac & Cheese	1 pkg (9 oz)	140	3	–	–	–	–	–	–
Skillet Meals	1 cup	250	3	–	–	–	–	–	–
Tofu Vegetable Lasagna	1 pkg (9.5 oz)	300	6	–	–	–	–	–	–
Vegetable Lasagna	1 pkg (9.5 oz)	280	3	–	–	–	–	–	–
Bertolli									
Meatballs Pomodoro & Penne	1 serv (12 oz)	600	6	1250	–	12	150	4	–
Boca									
Lasagna Meatless	1 pkg (9.4 oz)	290	5	1500	–	4	300	4	–
Celentano									
Cheese Ravioli	4 (4.3 oz)	230	2	200	–	0	100	2	–
Contessa									
Ravioli Portobello	6 (6.7 oz)	360	2	300	–	0	100	tr	–

FOOD	PORTION	CALS	FIBER	VIT A	FOLIC	VIT C	CALCI	IRON	POTAS
Glory									
Macaroni & Cheese	1 pkg	480	1	750	–	0	450	2	–
Glutino									
Gluten Free Duo Mushroom Penne	1 pkg (10.5 oz)	380	5	0	–	1	60	1	–
Gluten Free Macaroni & Cheese	1 pkg (8.8 oz)	430	2	700	–	0	500	11	–
Gluten Free Penne Alfredo	1 pkg (10.5 oz)	400	4	200	–	1	400	1	–
Golden Cuisine									
Cheese Manicotti	1 pkg	360	6	3559	233	20	629	3	546
Spaghetti & Meatballs	1 pkg	490	12	4828	237	14	104	4	365
Tuna Casserole	1 pkg	386	8	625	219	31	187	4	347
Healthy Choice									
Beef Macaroni	1 meal (8.5 oz)	220	5	500	–	54	40	3	–
Breaded Chicken Breast w/ Mac & Cheese	1 pkg	290	3	0	–	0	150	1	–
Breaded Chicken Breast Strips w/ Macaroni & Cheese	1 meal (8 oz)	270	1	0	–	1	150	1	–
Cheese Ravioli Parmigiana	1 meal (9 oz)	260	6	750	–	0	150	2	–
Fettuccine Alfredo	1 pkg	280	3	200	–	0	200	1	390
Fettuccini Alfredo Chicken	1 pkg	290	3	0	–	0	100	1	–
Lasagna Bake	1 pkg	270	4	400	–	0	100	2	–
Macaroni & Cheese	1 meal (9 oz)	240	3	0	–	0	200	1	–
Macaroni & Cheese	1 pkg	290	5	0	–	0	150	1	–
Manicotti	1 pkg	280	4	750	–	0	400	2	–
Manicotti w/ Three Cheeses	1 meal (11 oz)	300	5	750	–	0	250	2	–
Rigatoni w/ Broccoli & Chicken	1 pkg	270	5	400	–	12	80	1	450
Spaghetti w/ Meat Sauce	1 pkg	310	7	100	–	0	60	3	600

FOOD	PORTION	CALS	FIBER	VIT A	FOLIC	VIT C	CALCI	IRON	POTAS
Spaghetti & Sauce w/ Seasoned Beef	1 meal (10 oz)	260	5	500	–	15	40	4	–
Stuffed Pasta Shells	1 pkg	290	5	500	–	6	300	3	–
Joseph's Pasta									
Grilled Chicken Ravioli w/ Roasted Red Pepper Sauce	1 pkg (14 oz)	540	6	1500	–	7	180	3	–
Kashi									
Chicken Pasta Promodoro	1 pkg (10 oz)	280	6	500	–	18	100	2	510
Kid Cuisine									
Cheese Blaster Mac & Cheese	1 meal	380	5	1250	–	18	150	0	–
Twist & Twirl Spaghetti w/ Mini Meatballs	1 meal	460	6	100	–	2	80	5	–
Lean Cuisine									
Cafe Classics Bow Tie Pasta & Chicken	1 pkg (9.5 oz)	240	3	1500	–	5	60	1	590
Cafe Classics Bowl Three Cheese Stuffed Rigatoni	1 pkg (10 oz)	260	4	4500	–	9	200	1	600
Cafe Classics Cheese Lasagna w/ Chicken Breast Scallopini	1 pkg (10 oz)	290	3	500	–	6	150	1	760
Cafe Classics Four Cheese Cannelloni	1 pkg (9.1 oz)	260	3	500	–	6	450	1	630
Cafe Classics Grilled Chicken & Penne Pasta	1 pkg (12 oz)	320	4	1250	–	54	100	1	630
Cafe Classics Jumbo Rigatoni w/ Meatballs	1 pkg (15.4 oz)	400	6	1250	–	12	200	2	1100
Cafe Classics Lasagna w/ Meat Sauce	1 pkg (10.5 oz)	310	4	300	–	5	200	1	610
Cafe Classics Macaroni & Beef	1 pkg (9.5 oz)	270	3	200	–	2	60	2	750
Cafe Classics Macaroni & Cheese	1 pkg (10 oz)	300	1	0	–	0	300	1	500

FOOD	PORTION	CALS	FIBER	VIT A	FOLIC	VIT C	CALCI	IRON	POTAS
Cafe Classics Penne Pasta w/ Tomato Basil Sauce	1 pkg (10 oz)	270	5	750	–	6	60	1	520
Cafe Classics Roasted Chicken w/ Lemon Pepper Fettuccini	1 pkg (8.1 oz)	250	2	750	–	4	80	1	420
Cafe Classics Shrimp & Angel Hair Pasta	1 pkg (10 oz)	240	2	2000	–	24	100	1	460
Cafe Classics Spaghetti w/ Meat Sauce	1 pkg (11.5 oz)	280	3	500	–	2	100	2	570
Cafe Classics Spaghetti w/ Meatballs	1 pkg (9.5 oz)	270	3	200	–	4	80	2	490
Dinnertime Selects Chicken Fettuccini	1 pkg (12 oz)	360	4	200	–	54	200	1	550
One Dish Favorites Alfredo Pasta w/ Chicken & Broccoli	1 pkg (10 oz)	270	3	500	–	6	150	1	460
One Dish Favorites Angel Hair Pasta Marinara	1 pkg (10 oz)	260	4	500	–	4	100	2	600
One Dish Favorites Cheese Ravioli	1 pkg (8.5 oz)	250	3	400	–	1	150	1	510
One Dish Favorites Chicken Fettuccini	1 pkg (9.25 oz)	280	2	0	–	0	150	1	490
One Dish Favorites Lasagna Cheese Florentine Bake	1 pkg (10 oz)	270	3	1000	–	0	250	1	620
One Dish Favorites Lasagna Chicken Florentine	1 pkg (10 oz)	270	3	1000	–	0	250	1	620
One Dish Favorites Lasagna Classic Five Cheese	1 pkg (11.5 oz)	330	4	500	–	6	300	2	640
Skillet Chicken Alfredo	1 serv	180	3	2000	–	18	100	1	510
Marie Callender's									
Cheese Ravioli In Marinara Sauce w/ Spirals & Garlic Bread	1 meal (16 oz)	750	11	1000	–	0	500	5	–

FOOD	PORTION	CALS	FIBER	VIT A	FOLIC	VIT C	CALCI	IRON	POTAS
Extra Cheese Lasagna	1 meal (15 oz)	590	7	2250	–	0	800	3	–
Fettuccine Alfredo & Garlic Bread	1 meal (14 oz)	920	3	200	–	0	250	3	–
Fettuccine Alfredo Supreme	1 meal (13 oz)	450	4	200	–	1	150	2	–
Fettuccine Primavera w/ Tortellini	1 meal (14 oz)	750	6	2250	–	6	200	2	–
Fettuccine w/ Broccoli & Chicken	1 meal (13 oz)	710	6	500	–	9	150	3	–
Macaroni & Cheese	1 meal (12 oz)	540	5	100	–	0	400	1	–
Meat Lasagna	1 cup	240	2	400	–	0	150	2	–
Skillet Meal Chicken Alfredo	½ pkg	490	7	2500	–	30	150	2	–
Skillet Meal Penne Pasta & Meatballs	½ pkg	600	4	1000	–	0	150	5	–
Skillet Meal Rigatoni Vegetables In Cheese Sauce	1 cup	290	4	0	–	4	200	1	–
Spaghetti w/ Meat Sauce & Garlic Bread	1 meal (17 oz)	670	9	750	–	0	150	2	–
Stuffed Pasta Trio	1 meal (10.5 oz)	380	5	750	–	1	500	2	–
Michelina's									
Lasagna w/ Meat Sauce	1 pkg (9 oz)	340	3	1000	–	12	150	3	–
Morton									
Macaroni & Cheese	1 serv (8 oz)	240	3	200	–	0	100	1	–
Spaghetti w/ Meat Sauce	1 meal (8.5 oz)	200	4	500	–	0	20	1	–
Savvy Faire									
Lasagna Florentine	1 pkg (9.2 oz)	300	5	3500	–	21	250	4	–
Seeds Of Change									
Chicken Fettuccine Alfredo	1 pkg (10 oz)	340	3	300	–	15	200	2	–
Lasagna Creamy Spinach	1 pkg (11 oz)	370	7	2500	–	0	300	2	–

FOOD	PORTION	CALS	FIBER	VIT A	FOLIC	VIT C	CALCI	IRON	POTAS
Lasagna Vegetable	1 pkg (11 oz)	310	5	1250	–	15	400	4	–
Penne Marinara	1 pkg (11 oz)	290	5	1000	–	12	250	4	–
Slim-Fast									
Fettuccine Alfredo	1 pkg	240	5	1500	120	60	400	3	400
Rotini w/ Tomato & Italian Herb	1 pkg	240	4	1500	120	60	250	3	400
Shells & Creamy Cheese Sauce	1 pkg	240	5	1500	120	60	400	3	400
South Beach Diet									
Penne & Chicken In Roasted Red Pepper Sauce w/ Broccoli	1 pkg	290	8	500	–	12	150	2	–
Stouffer's									
Lasagna w/ Meat Sauce	1 cup	260	3	200	–	2	150	1	–
Weight Watchers									
Smart Ones Lasagna w/ Meat Sauce	1 pkg (10.5 oz)	300	5	750	–	5	300	2	–
MIX									
A Taste Of Thai									
Coconut Ginger	1 cup	280	1	0	–	–	20	–	–
Pad Thai For Two	½ pkg	345	4	0	–	–	30	–	–
Peanut Noodles as prep	1 cup	330	1	0	–	–	60	–	–
Red Curry Noodles as prep	1 cup	280	2	200	–	–	40	–	–
Annie's Homegrown									
Gluten Free Rice Pasta & Cheddar as prep	1 cup	330	0	100	–	0	150	0	–
Organic Shells & Real Aged Wisconsin Cheddar as prep	1 cup	370	2	1000	–	0	150	1	–
Organic Skillet Meals Beef Stroganoff as prep	1 cup	320	1	400	–	1	100	3	–
Organic Skillet Meals Cheddar & Herb Chicken as prep	1 cup	310	1	400	–	2	100	1	–

FOOD	PORTION	CALS	FIBER	VIT A	FOLIC	VIT C	CALCI	IRON	POTAS
Organic Skillet Meals Cheese Lasagna as prep	1 cup	280	1	400	–	2	40	3	–
Organic Skillet Meals Cheeseburger Macaroni as prep	1 cup	350	1	500	–	1	150	3	–
Organic Skillet Meals Chicken Fettucine as prep	1 cup	330	1	200	–	0	100	1	–
Organic Skillet Meals Creamy Tuna Spirals as prep	1 cup	260	1	300	–	1	150	1	–
Organic Whole Wheat Shells & Cheddar as prep	1 cup	360	5	500	–	0	150	3	–
Shells & Real Aged Wisconsin Cheddar as prep	1 cup	290	1	200	–	0	150	1	–
Shells & White Cheddar as prep	1 cup	290	1	100	–	0	100	1	–
Back To Nature									
Alfredo & Gemelli as prep	1 cup	340	1	300	–	0	150	2	–
Macaroni & Cheese as prep	1 cup	320	1	300	–	0	150	2	–
White Cheddar & Spirals as prep	1 cup	330	1	400	–	0	150	2	–
Carapelli									
Penne Alfredo as prep	1 cup	240	4	0	–	0	60	1	–
Spirals Creamy Tomato as prep	1 cup	240	4	200	–	1	40	1	–
Keto									
Macaroni & Cheese not prep	1 serv	112	1	–	–	–	–	–	–
Near East									
Angel Hair w/ Spicy Tomato as prep	1 cup	240	3	750	–	12	20	2	–
Radiatore Basil & Herb as prep	1 cup	240	3	300	–	9	20	1	–

FOOD	PORTION	CALS	FIBER	VIT A	FOLIC	VIT C	CALCI	IRON	POTAS
Vermicelli Garlic & Oil as prep	1 cup	310	3	100	–	4	20	2	–
Whey Cool									
High Protein Macaroni & Cheese as prep	1 serv	260	1	–	–	–	–	–	–
REFRIGERATED									
Country Crock									
Elbow Macaroni & Cheese	1 cup	380	1	750	–	0	300	2	–
SHELF-STABLE									
It's Pasta Anytime									
Penne With Tomato Italian Sausage Sauce	1 pkg (15.25 oz)	540	12	750	–	9	80	5	–
TAKE-OUT									
bami goreng indonesian noodle dish	1 cup	170	4	400	–	2	40	1	–
lasagna meatless	1 piece (9 oz)	356	3	510	79	10	335	3	425
lasagna w/ meat	1 piece (8 oz)	362	3	336	67	8	278	3	427
lasagna w/ vegetables	1 serv (9 oz)	315	4	1025	95	20	302	3	512
macaroni & cheese w/ ham	1 cup	542	3	925	66	0	311	3	343
manicotti cheese filled marinara sauce	1 (5 oz)	229	1	450	40	3	214	2	233
manicotti cheese filled w/ meat sauce	1 (5 oz)	239	3	420	39	3	203	2	246
pasta w/ pesto sauce	1 cup	370	2	115	78	2	179	3	189
ravioli cheese & spinach filled w/ cream sauce	1 cup	362	2	1740	115	3	238	4	356
ravioli meat filled w/ marinara sauce	1 cup	372	3	460	70	7	72	5	535
ravioli cheese w/ tomato sauce	1 cup	335	2	760	72	5	162	3	375
rigatoni w/ sausage sauce	¾ cup	260	3	999	8	16	44	3	286

FOOD	PORTION	CALS	FIBER	VIT A	FOLIC	VIT C	CALCI	IRON	POTAS
spaghetti w/ red clam sauce	1 cup	285	3	260	109	14	64	10	379
spaghetti w/ sauce & meatballs	2 cups	670	12	595	60	21	188	6	1052
spaghetti w/ white clam sauce	1 cup	456	3	670	37	16	82	23	513
tortellini cheese w/ tomato sauce	1 cup	332	2	760	72	5	150	3	375
tortellini meat filled w/ marinara sauce	1 cup	281	2	355	82	3	92	3	258
tortellini spinach filled w/ marinara sauce	1 cup	238	2	530	104	5	110	3	278

PASTA SALAD
MIX
Dole

FOOD	PORTION	CALS	FIBER	VIT A	FOLIC	VIT C	CALCI	IRON	POTAS
Veggie Pasta Salads Broccoli Ranch	1½ cups	230	2	2000	–	24	40	1	–
Veggie Pasta Salads Cheddar Bacon Ranch	1½ cups	370	3	1500	–	30	100	3	–
Veggie Pasta Salads Garden Vegetable	1½ cups	240	2	2250	–	21	40	1	–
Veggie Pasta Salads Italian Herb	1½ cups	270	2	3000	–	30	60	2	–

TAKE-OUT

FOOD	PORTION	CALS	FIBER	VIT A	FOLIC	VIT C	CALCI	IRON	POTAS
pasta salad w/ crab vegetables mayonnaise	1 cup	317	2	115	92	2	46	2	179
tortellini salad cheese filled w/ vinaigrette dressing	1 cup	333	1	475	61	tr	137	2	122

PATE

FOOD	PORTION	CALS	FIBER	VIT A	FOLIC	VIT C	CALCI	IRON	POTAS
chicken liver canned	1 tbsp	26	0	94	42	1	1	1	12
fish pate	1 oz	76	–	–	–	–	52	1	45
liver w/ truffle	1 serv (2 oz)	183	–	8400	34	1	39	2	77
mushroom anchovy pate	1 can (2.25 oz)	130	1	300	–	1	20	1	–
pate de foie gras smoked canned	1 tbsp	60	0	433	8	tr	9	1	18

FOOD	PORTION	CALS	FIBER	VIT A	FOLIC	VIT C	CALCI	IRON	POTAS
pork pate	1 oz	107	0	6000	29	tr	11	1	27
pork pate en croute	1 oz	91	tr	–	–	–	–	–	–
rabbit pate	1 oz	66	–	–	–	tr	3	1	89
shrimp	1 can (2.25 oz)	140	0	1500	–	1	20	1	–

PEACH
CANNED
FOOD	PORTION	CALS	FIBER	VIT A	FOLIC	VIT C	CALCI	IRON	POTAS
halves in heavy syrup	1 half	60	–	269	3	2	8	tr	74
halves in light syrup	1 half	44	–	286	3	2	3	tr	79
halves juice pack	1 half	34	–	294	–	3	15	tr	98
halves water pack	1 half	18	–	410	3	2	2	tr	76
peach sauce	½ cup	120	1	500	–	6	0	0	–
spiced in heavy syrup	1 fruit	66	–	279	–	5	5	tr	75
spiced in heavy syrup	1 cup	180	–	768	–	13	15	1	206
Del Monte									
Carb Clever Sliced	½ cup	30	1	300	–	54	0	tr	–
Freestone Lite Slices	½ cup	60	1	100	–	1	0	tr	–
Freestone Sliced	½ cup	100	1	100	–	1	0	0	–
Fruit Cup Diced Extra Light Syrup	1 pkg (4 oz)	50	1	200	–	12	0	tr	–
Fruit Cup Diced In Heavy Syrup	1 serv (4 oz)	80	1	200	–	12	0	tr	–
Fruit Naturals Chunks	½ cup	70	tr	200	–	60	0	0	–
Fruit To Go Banana Berry Peaches	1 pkg (4 oz)	70	1	200	–	60	0	0	–
Fruit To Go Peachy Peaches	1 pkg (4 oz)	70	1	200	–	60	0	0	–
Halves In Heavy Syrup	½ cup	100	1	0	–	2	0	0	–
Orchard Select Sliced Cling	½ cup	80	tr	100	–	60	0	0	–
Sliced In 100% Juice	½ cup	60	1	300	–	5	0	tr	–
Sliced Light Syrup Raspberry Flavor	½ cup	80	tr	300	–	4	0	0	–
Dole									
All Natural Yellow Cling Sliced	½ cup	80	tr	300	–	24	–	–	–
Liberty Gold									
Sliced Cling In Heavy Syrup	½ cup	100	1	300	–	1	0	0	110

FOOD	PORTION	CALS	FIBER	VIT A	FOLIC	VIT C	CALCI	IRON	POTAS
S&W									
Slices Lightly Sweetened Juice	½ cup	80	1	400	–	1	0	0	–
Yellow Cling In Heavy Syrup	½ cup	100	1	300	–	5	0	tr	110
DRIED									
halves	1 cup	383	13	3461	–	8	45	7	1594
halves	10	311	11	2812	–	6	37	5	1295
halves cooked w/ sugar	½ cup	139	–	243	tr	5	11	2	395
halves cooked w/o sugar	½ cup	99	–	254	tr	5	12	2	413
Crispy Green									
Crispy Peaches	1 pkg (0.36 oz)	38	tr	100	–	1	0	0	–
FRESH									
peach	1	37	1	465	3	6	5	tr	171
sliced	1 cup	73	–	910	6	11	9	tr	334
Chiquita									
Peach	1 med (3.4 oz)	40	2	100	–	6	0	0	–
FROZEN									
slices sweetened	1 cup	235	–	709	–	235	6	1	325
C&W									
Ultimate Sliced	¾ cup	50	2	500	–	168	0	tr	–
PEACH JUICE									
nectar	1 cup	134	–	643	–	13	13	tr	101
After The Fall									
Georgia Peach	8 oz	130	–	–	–	60	150	–	250
Ceres									
Peach	8 oz	120	0	0	–	60	0	1	240
PEANUT BUTTER									
chunky	1 cup	1520	17	0	237	0	105	5	1928
chunky	2 tbsp	188	2	0	29	0	13	1	239
chunky w/o salt	2 tbsp	188	2	0	29	0	13	1	239
chunky w/o salt	1 cup	1520	17	0	237	0	105	5	1928
smooth	2 tbsp	188	2	0	25	0	11	1	231
smooth	1 cup	1517	15	0	202	0	88	4	1861

FOOD	PORTION	CALS	FIBER	VIT A	FOLIC	VIT C	CALCI	IRON	POTAS
smooth w/o salt	2 tbsp	188	2	0	25	0	11	1	231
smooth w/o salt	1 cup	1517	15	0	201	0	88	4	1861
Carb Options									
Creamy	2 tbsp	190	2	0	40	0	0	1	–
Cream-Nut									
Natural	2 tbsp	190	2	0	–	0	0	tr	–
Estee									
Creamy Low Sodium	2 tbsp	180	2	–	–	–	–	–	–
Jif									
Creamy	2 tbsp	190	2	–	–	–	–	1	–
Creamy To Go	1 pkg (2.25 oz)	270	4	0	–	0	20	1	–
Extra Crunchy	2 tbsp	190	2	–	–	–	–	1	–
Peanut Butter & Honey	2 tbsp	190	2	–	–	–	–	1	–
Reduced Fat Creamy	2 tbsp	190	2	–	24	–	–	1	–
Reduced Fat Crunchy	2 tbsp	190	2	–	24	–	–	1	–
Simply	2 tbsp	190	2	–	–	–	–	1	–
Kettle									
Organic Unsalted	2 tbsp	170	2	0	–	0	20	tr	–
MaraNatha									
Crunchy	2 tbsp	190	2	–	–	–	–	–	–
Salted	2 tbsp	190	2	0	–	0	20	1	–
P.B.									
Slices	1 slice (1 oz)	170	1	–	–	–	–	–	–
Peanut Better									
Cinnamon Currant	2 tbsp	180	3	0	–	0	0	tr	–
Deep Chocolate	2 tbsp	170	2	0	–	0	0	1	–
Hickory Smoked	2 tbsp	190	3	0	–	0	0	tr	–
Onion Parsley	2 tbsp	180	3	0	–	0	20	1	–
Peanut Praline	2 tbsp	180	3	0	–	0	0	tr	–
Rosemary Garlic	2 tbsp	180	3	0	–	0	20	1	–
Spicy Southwestern	2 tbsp	190	3	200	–	0	0	1	–
Sweet Molasses	2 tbsp	180	2	0	–	0	40	1	–
Thai Ginger & Red Pepper	2 tbsp	180	3	0	–	0	0	1	–
Vanilla Cranberry	2 tbsp	170	2	0	–	0	1	tr	–
Peanut Butter & Co.									
Cinnamon Raisin Swirl	2 tbsp	143	2	0	–	0	10	1	–
Crunch Time	2 tbsp	200	2	0	–	0	0	1	–

FOOD	PORTION	CALS	FIBER	VIT A	FOLIC	VIT C	CALCI	IRON	POTAS
Dark Chocolate Dreams	2 tbsp	175	2	0	–	0	10	1	–
Smooth Operator	2 tbsp	200	2	0	–	0	0	1	–
The Heat Is On	2 tbsp	164	2	0	–	0	10	1	–
White Chocolate Wonderful	1 tbsp	165	2	0	–	0	10	1	–
Peanut Wonder									
Low Sodium	2 tbsp	100	0	0	–	5	40	tr	–
Regular	2 tbsp	100	0	0	–	5	40	tr	–
Reese's									
Creamy	2 tbsp	200	2	0	–	0	200	tr	–
Skippy									
Creamy	2 tbsp	190	2	0	–	0	0	tr	–
Creamy w/ 2 slices white bread	1 sandwich	340	–	–	–	–	40	2	–
Reduced Fat Creamy	2 tbsp	190	2	0	24	0	0	1	–
Roasted Honey Nut	2 tbsp	190	2	0	–	0	0	tr	–
Roasted Honey Nut Super Chunk	2 tbsp	190	2	0	–	0	0	tr	–
Squeeze Stix	1 pkg	140	2	0	–	21	0	tr	–
Squeeze Stix Chocolate	1 pkg	140	2	0	–	0	0	tr	–
Squeez'It	2 tbsp	190	2	0	–	0	0	1	–
Super Chunk	2 tbsp	190	2	0	–	0	0	tr	–
Super Chunk Reduced Fat	2 tbsp	190	2	0	24	0	0	1	–
Smucker's									
Goober All Flavors	3 tbsp	240	2	0	–	0	20	1	–
Natural Chunky	2 tbsp	210	2	0	–	0	0	tr	–
Natural Creamy	2 tbsp	210	2	0	–	0	0	tr	–
Natural Honey	2 tbsp	200	2	0	–	0	0	tr	–
Natural No Salt Added Creamy	2 tbsp	210	2	0	–	0	0	tr	–
Natural Reduced Fat Creamy	2 tbsp	200	2	0	24	0	0	tr	–
Teddies									
Old Fashioned	2 tbsp	190	3	0	–	0	20	1	–
Tropical Source									
Chips Dairy Free	13 pieces (1.5 oz)	80	0	0	–	0	0	tr	–

FOOD	PORTION	CALS	FIBER	VIT A	FOLIC	VIT C	CALCI	IRON	POTAS
PEANUTS									
chocolate coated	¼ cup	193	2	46	3	0	39	tr	187
cooked w/ salt	½ cup	286	8	0	68	0	50	1	162
dry roasted w/ salt	28 nuts (1 oz)	164	1	0	41	0	15	1	187
dry roasted w/o salt	¼ cup	214	3	0	53	0	20	1	240
dry roasted w/o salt	28 (1 oz)	164	2	0	41	0	15	1	184
honey roasted	¼ cup	191	3	0	36	tr	18	tr	218
milk chocolate coated	1	21	tr	5	0	0	4	tr	20
sugar coated	¼ cup	203	2	0	29	0	30	tr	158
yogurt coated	¼ cup	230	2	0	48	tr	65	1	203
A Taste Of Thai									
Spicy Peanut Bake	¼ pkg	45	1	0	–	–	20	–	–
Brach's									
Double Dippers Chocolate Covered	15 pieces	210	2	–	–	–	20	1	–
Low Carb Creations									
Soft Peanut Brittle	2 pieces (1 oz)	140	2	–	–	–	–	–	–
Planters									
Cocktail	1 oz	170	2	0	–	0	0	tr	–
Dry Roasted	1 oz	170	2	0	–	0	20	tr	–
PEAR									
CANNED									
halves in heavy syrup	1 cup	188	–	0	3	3	12	1	165
halves in heavy syrup	1 half	68	–	0	1	1	4	tr	51
halves in light syrup	1 half	45	–	0	1	1	4	tr	52
halves juice pack	1 cup	123	–	14	–	4	21	1	238
halves water pack	1 half	22	–	0	1	1	–	3	5
Del Monte									
Carb Clever Sliced	½ cup	40	1	0	–	48	0	0	–
Fruit Cup Diced In Heavy Syrup	1 pkg (4 oz)	80	1	0	–	12	0	0	–
Fruit Cup Diced Extra Light Syrup	1 pkg (4 oz)	50	1	0	–	12	0	0	–
Halves In 100% Juice	½ cup	60	1	0	–	2	0	0	–
Halves In Light Syrup	½ cup	60	1	0	–	2	0	0	–
Orchard Select Sliced Bartlett	½ cup	80	2	300	–	60	0	0	–

FOOD	PORTION	CALS	FIBER	VIT A	FOLIC	VIT C	CALCI	IRON	POTAS
S&W									
Halves In Lightly Sweetened Juice	½ cup	80	2	0	–	1	0	tr	–
DRIED									
halves	10	459	–	6	–	12	59	4	932
halves	1 cup	472	–	6	–	13	60	4	959
halves cooked w/ sugar	½ cup	196	–	56	0	5	22	1	344
halves cooked w/o sugar	½ cup	163	–	54	0	5	21	1	331
FRESH									
asian	1 (4.3 oz)	51	–	0	10	2	5	–	148
pear	1	98	4	33	12	7	19	tr	208
sliced w/ skin	1 cup	97	4	33	12	7	19	tr	207
Chiquita									
Pear	1 med (5.8 oz)	100	4	0	–	6	20	0	–

PEAR JUICE

FOOD	PORTION	CALS	FIBER	VIT A	FOLIC	VIT C	CALCI	IRON	POTAS
nectar	1 cup	149	–	1	–	3	11	1	33
Ceres									
Pear	8 oz	120	0	0	–	30	20	tr	190
Langers									
Kid's 100% Juice	4 oz	60	–	0	–	60	0	0	–

PEAS

FOOD	PORTION	CALS	FIBER	VIT A	FOLIC	VIT C	CALCI	IRON	POTAS
CANNED									
green	½ cup	59	–	653	38	8	17	1	147
green low sodium	½ cup	59	–	653	38	8	17	1	147
Del Monte									
Sweet	½ cup	60	4	300	–	9	20	1	–
Sweet No Salt Added	½ cup	60	4	300	–	9	20	1	–
Sweet Very Young Small	½ cup	60	4	300	–	9	0	1	–
Green Giant									
Sweet	½ cup	60	3	300	–	6	20	1	–
Libby's									
No Salt No Sugar Added	½ cup	70	3	300	–	12	20	1	105

FOOD	PORTION	CALS	FIBER	VIT A	FOLIC	VIT C	CALCI	IRON	POTAS
S&W									
Petite	½ cup (4.4 oz)	70	4	500	–	9	20	1	–
Small	½ cup (4.4 oz)	70	4	500	–	9	20	1	–
Tillen Farms									
Crispy Snapper Pickled	¼ cup	15	1	300	–	0	0	3	–
Veg-All									
Tender Sweet	½ cup	60	3	300	–	9	20	1	–
DRIED									
split cooked	1 cup	231	–	14	127	1	26	3	710
Snapea Crisps									
Baked Original	22 (1 oz)	70	2	0	–	4	60	1	–
FRESH									
green cooked	½ cup	67	–	478	51	11	22	1	217
green raw	½ cup	58	–	461	47	29	18	1	176
snap peas cooked	½ cup	34	2	104	–	38	33	2	192
snap peas raw	½ cup	30	2	105	–	43	36	2	144
Frieda's									
Snow Peas	1 cup	35	2	100	–	54	40	2	–
Sugar Snap	⅔ cup (3 oz)	35	2	100	–	54	40	1	–
River Ranch									
Sugar Snap	1½ cups	35	2	100	32	54	40	2	–
FROZEN									
green cooked	½ cup	63	–	534	47	8	19	1	134
snap peas cooked	½ cup	42	–	133	–	18	48	2	173
Birds Eye									
Steamfresh Garlic Baby Peas & Mushrooms	¾ cup	80	3	300	–	6	20	1	–
Steamfresh Sweet Peas	⅓ cup	70	4	400	–	6	0	1	–
C&W									
Alfredo	½ cup	110	4	0	–	9	40	1	–
Early Harvest Petite No Salt Added	⅔ cup	70	4	400	–	6	0	1	–
Sugar Snap	⅔ cup	40	2	200	–	9	40	1	–
Fresh Like									
Garden	3.5 oz	85	2	698	–	20	23	2	149

FOOD	PORTION	CALS	FIBER	VIT A	FOLIC	VIT C	CALCI	IRON	POTAS
Green Giant									
Sweet	⅔ cup	70	4	300	–	9	0	1	–
La Choy									
Snow Pea Pods	½ pkg (3 oz)	35	2	200	–	15	20	1	–
Pictsweet									
Green Peas	⅔ cup	70	4	400	–	6	0	1	–
SHELF-STABLE									
TastyBite									
Agra Peas & Greens	½ pkg (5 oz)	260	1	0	–	0	50	1	–
TAKE-OUT									
pea & potato curry	1 serv (7 oz)	284	6	550	–	12	56	2	–
pea curry	1 serv (4.4 oz)	438	4	2600	–	14	41	3	–

PECANS

FOOD	PORTION	CALS	FIBER	VIT A	FOLIC	VIT C	CALCI	IRON	POTAS
candied	1 oz	190	5	0	–	0	0	1	–
dry roasted	1 oz	187	–	–	12	–	10	1	105
dry roasted salted	1 oz	187	–	–	12	–	10	1	105
halves dry roasted w/ salt	20 (1 oz)	200	3	–	8	–	20	1	120
halves dried	1 cup	721	7	138	42	2	39	2	423
oil roasted	1 oz	195	–	–	–	–	10	1	102
oil roasted salted	1 oz	195	–	–	–	–	10	1	102
Emerald									
Glazed Pecan Pie	¼ cup	150	1	0	–	0	20	tr	65
Keto									
Chocolately Covered	1 oz	207	5	0	–	0	40	2	–
Sweet Delights									
Pecan Roasters	⅓ pkg (1 oz)	210	2	–	–	–	–	–	–

PECTIN

FOOD	PORTION	CALS	FIBER	VIT A	FOLIC	VIT C	CALCI	IRON	POTAS
liquid	1 oz	3	1	0	0	0	0	0	0
powder	1 pkg (1.75 oz)	162	4	2	0	0	4	1	4

FOOD	PORTION	CALS	FIBER	VIT A	FOLIC	VIT C	CALCI	IRON	POTAS
PEPEAO									
dried	¼ cup	18	–	0	10	tr	7	tr	42
raw sliced	1 cup	25	–	0	19	1	16	1	43
PEPPER									
black	1 tsp	5	–	4	–	–	9	1	26
cayenne	1 tsp	6	–	749	–	1	3	tr	36
red	1 tsp	6	–	749	–	1	3	tr	36
white	1 tsp	7	–	–	–	–	6	tr	2
PEPPERS									
CANNED									
chili pepper paste	1 tbsp	6	1	120	–	–	21	1	40
chili green	1 cup (5.5 oz)	29	2	175	75	0	50	2	157
chili green hot chopped	½ cup	17	–	415	–	46	5	tr	–
chili red hot	1 (2.6 oz)	18	–	8681	–	50	5	tr	–
chili red hot chopped	½ cup	17	–	8087	–	46	5	tr	–
green halves	½ cup	13	–	109	–	33	28	1	102
jalapeno chopped	½ cup	17	–	1156	–	9	18	2	92
red halves	½ cup	13	–	364	–	33	28	1	102
B&G									
Sweet Fried	1 oz	25	1	300	–	42	–	–	–
Gertie's Finest									
Piquillo	1 oz	10	tr	500	–	25	10	3	–
Las Palmas									
Diced Green Chiles	2 tbsp	5	1	0	–	6	40	0	–
Jalapenos Sliced	3 tbsp	10	0	100	–	6	20	0	–
Old El Paso									
Green Chiles Chopped	2 tbsp (1 oz)	5	1	0	–	6	40	0	–
Tillen Farms									
Bell Peppers Pickled Sweet	¼ cup	25	0	100	–	15	0	0	–
DRIED									
ancho	1 (0.6 oz)	48	4	3474	12	0	10	2	410
ancho	1 tsp	3	tr	204	1	0	1	tr	24
casabel	1 tsp	3	tr	90	–	1	1	tr	–
chipotle smoked	1 tsp	3	tr	25	–	0	3	tr	–
green	1 tbsp	1	–	25	1	8	1	tr	13

FOOD	PORTION	CALS	FIBER	VIT A	FOLIC	VIT C	CALCI	IRON	POTAS
guajillo	1 tsp	3	tr	165	–	1	1	tr	–
mulato	1 tsp	3	tr	140	–	1	1	tr	–
pasilla	1 (7 g)	24	2	2503	12	0	7	1	156
pasilla	1 tsp	3	tr	358	2	0	1	tr	22
red	1 tbsp	1	–	309	1	8	1	tr	13
Frieda's									
California Chili	2 tbsp	15	0	3000	–	0	0	0	–
FRESH									
banana	1 (4 in) (1.2 oz)	9	1	112	10	27	5	tr	84
banana	1 cup (4.4 oz)	33	4	422	36	27	17	1	317
chili green hot	1	18	–	346	11	109	8	1	153
chili green hot chopped	½ cup	30	–	578	18	182	13	1	255
chili red chopped	½ cup	30	–	8063	18	182	13	1	255
chili red hot	1 (1.6 oz)	18	–	4838	11	109	8	1	153
green	1 (2.6 oz)	20	1	468	16	95	7	tr	131
green chopped	½ cup	13	1	316	11	45	5	tr	89
green chopped cooked	½ cup	19	–	403	11	51	6	tr	113
green cooked	1 (2.6 oz)	20	–	432	11	54	7	tr	121
habanero	1 tsp	9	1	85	7	27	5	1	99
hungarian	1 (0.9 oz)	8	0	38	14	0	3	tr	55
jalapeno	1 (0.5 oz)	4	tr	30	7	6	1	tr	30
jalapeno sliced	1 cup (3.2 oz)	27	3	194	42	6	9	1	197
red	1 (2.6 oz)	20	1	4218	16	141	7	tr	131
red chopped	½ cup	13	1	2850	11	95	5	tr	69
red chopped cooked	½ cup	19	–	2745	11	125	6	tr	113
red cooked	1 (2.6 oz)	20	–	2745	11	125	7	tr	121
serrano	1 (6 g)	2	tr	57	1	3	1	tr	19
serrano chopped	1 cup (3.7 oz)	34	4	984	24	3	12	1	320
yellow	10 strips	14	–	124	14	95	6	–	110
yellow	1 (6.5 oz)	50	–	442	48	341	20	–	393
Chiquita									
Pepper	1 med (5.2 oz)	30	2	400	–	114	20	tr	–

FOOD	PORTION	CALS	FIBER	VIT A	FOLIC	VIT C	CALCI	IRON	POTAS
Frieda's									
Peppadew	⅓ cup	40	3	300	–	60	0	1	–
FROZEN									
green chopped	1 oz	6	–	103	4	16	3	tr	26
red chopped	1 oz	6	–	1333	4	16	3	tr	26
C&W									
Strips	¾ cup	25	1	300	–	21	0	tr	–
Roast Works									
Flame Roasted Red	1 serv (3 oz)	45	3	1000	–	27	40	1	–
PERCH									
FRESH									
cooked	3 oz	99	0	–	–	–	87	1	293
cooked	1 fillet (1.6 oz)	54	0	–	–	–	47	1	158
ocean perch atlantic cooked	3 oz	103	0	39	–	–	117	1	298
ocean perch atlantic cooked	1 fillet (1.8 oz)	60	0	23	–	–	69	1	175
ocean perch atlantic raw	3 oz	80	0	34	–	–	91	1	232
raw	3 oz	77	0	–	–	–	68	1	228
red raw	3.5 oz	114	0	tr	–	1	22	1	308
PERSIMMONS									
dried japanese	1 (1.2 oz)	93	5	261	–	0	8	tr	273
fresh	1 (6 oz)	118	6	2733	13	13	13	tr	271
Frieda's									
Dried Fuyu	⅓ cup (1.4 oz)	140	3	400	–	72	20	tr	–
PHEASANT									
breast cooked	½ breast (4.5 oz)	312	0	360	6	3	20	2	343
leg cooked	1 (2.6 oz)	184	0	215	4	2	12	1	202
PHYLLO									
sheet	1 (0.7 oz)	57	tr	0	17	0	2	1	14
Ekizian									
Sheets	¼ lb	433	–	260	31	0	24	5	117

FOOD	PORTION	CALS	FIBER	VIT A	FOLIC	VIT C	CALCI	IRON	POTAS
Fillo Factory									
Fillo Dough Whole Wheat Vegan	3 sheets (2 oz)	190	3	–	–	–	–	–	–
PICKLES									
bread & butter	6 slices	39	1	67	2	4	15	tr	96
dill	1 lg (4.7 oz)	24	2	247	1	3	12	1	157
dill low sodium	1 med (2.3 oz)	12	1	214	1	1	6	tr	75
dill sliced	6 slices	7	1	71	0	1	3	tr	45
sweet gherkin	1 (1.2 oz)	41	tr	267	0	tr	1	tr	11
tsukemono japanese pickles sliced	¼ cup	10	1	10	9	tr	13	tr	200
Claussen									
Kosher Dills Whole	½ (1 oz)	5	0	0	–	0	20	0	–
Del Monte									
Dill Halves	1 piece (1 oz)	5	1	0	–	0	40	0	–
Hamburger Dill Chips	1 serv (1 oz)	0	0	0	–	0	20	tr	–
Sweet	1 serv (1 oz)	40	tr	0	–	0	0	0	–
Sweet Gerkins	1 serv (1 oz)	40	tr	0	–	0	0	0	–
Tiny Kosher Dill	1 serv (1 oz)	5	tr	0	–	0	20	0	–
PIE									
TAKE-OUT									
apple	⅛ of 9 in pie (5.4 oz)	411	3	90	7	3	11	2	123
banana cream	⅛ of 9 in pie (5.2 oz)	398	–	386	17	2	110	2	245
blueberry	⅛ of 9 in pie (5.2 oz)	360	–	61	7	1	10	2	74
butterscotch	⅛ of 9 in pie (4.5 oz)	355	–	383	14	1	128	2	221
cherry	⅛ of 9 in pie (6.3 oz)	486	–	737	12	2	18	3	138

FOOD	PORTION	CALS	FIBER	VIT A	FOLIC	VIT C	CALCI	IRON	POTAS
chocolate creme	1 slice (4 oz)	344	–	–	8	–	41	1	144
coconut creme	⅛ of 9 in pie (4.7 oz)	396	–	379	14	1	113	1	183
coconut custard	⅙ of 8 in pie (3.6 oz)	271	–	114	–	–	84	1	182
custard	⅛ of 9 in pie (4.5 oz)	262	2	281	13	1	107	1	159
key lime	1 slice (5 oz)	420	tr	500	–	0	60	1	–
lemon meringue	1 slice (4.5 oz)	303	1	198	10	4	63	1	100
mince	⅛ of 9 in pie (5.8 oz)	477	–	36	9	10	37	2	335
pecan	1 slice (4 oz)	452	4	198	7	1	19	1	84
pumpkin	1 slice (3.8 oz)	229	3	–	17	–	66	1	168
vanilla cream	⅛ of 9 in pie (4.4 oz)	350	–	385	14	1	113	1	158
PIE CRUST									
FROZEN									
baked	⅛ of 9 in pie	113	tr	0	12	0	5	1	24
baked	9 in crust	884	2	0	95	0	36	4	189
puff pastry shell	1 (1.4 oz)	223	1	0	22	0	4	1	25
tart shell	1 (1 oz)	149	tr	0	16	0	6	1	32
READY-TO-EAT									
chocolate crumb	⅛ of 9 in pie	132	tr	275	14	0	8	1	44
chocolate crumb	1 (9 in crust)	1063	3	2215	111	0	63	6	353
graham cracker	⅛ of 9 in pie	109	tr	182	5	0	5	tr	19
graham cracker	1 (9 in crust)	1037	3	1735	50	0	44	5	185
graham cracker dessert shell	1 (1.1 oz)	148	tr	248	7	0	6	1	26

FOOD	PORTION	CALS	FIBER	VIT A	FOLIC	VIT C	CALCI	IRON	POTAS
PIE FILLING									
apple	⅛ can (2.6 oz)	74	1	–	0	–	3	tr	33
apple	1 can (21 oz)	599	6	–	0	–	27	2	268
cherry	⅛ can (2.6 oz)	85	–	152	3	–	8	tr	78
cherry	1 can (21 oz)	683	–	1220	24	–	65	1	625
pumpkin pie mix	1 cup	282	–	22405	–	10	99	3	372
Colac									
All Flavors	1 tbsp	19	0	–	–	–	–	–	–
Comstock									
Blueberry	⅓ cup	100	1	0	–	0	0	0	–
Country Cherry	⅓ cup	90	1	100	–	0	0	tr	–
Light Cherry	⅓ cup	60	1	300	–	0	0	0	–
Farmer's Market									
Organic Pumpkin Pie Mix	½ cup	120	2	2250	–	0	20	0	–
PIEROGI									
potato	¾ cup (4.4 oz)	307	–	246	8	1	156	2	101
Mrs. T's									
Broccoli & Cheddar	3 (4.2 oz)	200	2	300	–	12	40	2	–
Jalapeno & Cheddar	3 (4.2 oz)	190	2	100	–	9	40	2	–
Potato & American Cheese	3 (4.2 oz)	220	2	100	–	6	40	2	–
Potato & Roasted Garlic	3 (4.2 oz)	190	2	200	–	9	20	2	–
Potato & 4 Cheese Blend	3 (4.2 oz)	230	1	0	–	9	40	1	–
Potato & Cheddar	3 (4.2 oz)	180	1	100	–	6	40	1	–
Potato & Onion	3 (4.2 oz)	180	2	0	–	9	20	1	–
Rogies Cheddar & Bacon	7 (3 oz)	140	1	100	–	4	10	1	–
Rogies Jalapeno & Cheddar	7 (3 oz)	120	1	0	–	5	20	1	–

FOOD	PORTION	CALS	FIBER	VIT A	FOLIC	VIT C	CALCI	IRON	POTAS
PIGEON PEAS									
dried cooked	½ cup	102	–	2	93	0	36	1	322
dried cooked	1 cup	204	–	4	186	0	72	2	644
PIG'S FEET									
cooked	1	201	0	0	2	0	0	1	29
pickled	1	177	0	0	3	0	28	1	204
PIKE									
northern cooked	3 oz	96	0	69	3	–	62	1	282
northern cooked	½ fillet (5.4 oz)	176	0	125	–	6	113	1	514
northern raw	3 oz	75	0	60	–	3	48	tr	220
roe raw	1 oz	37	–	–	–	4	–	tr	–
walleye baked	3 oz	101	0	–	–	–	120	1	424
walleye fillet baked	4.4 oz	147	0	–	–	–	175	2	618
PILLNUTS									
canarytree dried	1 oz	204	–	12	–	–	41	1	144
PIMIENTOS									
canned	1 tbsp	3	–	319	1	10	1	tr	19
canned	1 slice	0	–	27	0	1	0	tr	2
PINE NUTS									
pignolia dried	1 oz	146	–	–	–	–	7	3	170
pignolia dried	1 tbsp	51	–	–	–	–	3	1	60
pinyon dried	1 oz	161	–	8	–	1	2	1	178
Frieda's									
Pine Nuts	¼ cup	150	1	750	–	–	–	–	–
Good Sense									
Pignolias	¼ cup	190	4	0	–	1	0	1	–
PINEAPPLE									
CANNED									
chunks in heavy syrup	1 cup	199	–	37	12	19	35	1	264
chunks juice pack	1 cup	150	–	95	–	24	34	1	304
crushed in heavy syrup	1 cup	199	–	37	12	19	35	1	264
slices in heavy syrup	1 slice	45	–	8	3	4	8	tr	60
slices in light syrup	1 slice	30	–	9	3	4	8	tr	61
slices juice pack	1 slice	35	–	22	–	6	8	tr	70
slices water pack	1 slice	19	–	9	3	5	9	tr	74
tidbits in heavy syrup	1 cup	199	–	37	12	19	35	1	264

FOOD	PORTION	CALS	FIBER	VIT A	FOLIC	VIT C	CALCI	IRON	POTAS
tidbits in juice	1 cup	150	–	95	–	24	34	1	304
tidbits in water	1 cup	79	–	37	12	19	37	1	313
Del Monte									
Chunks In Heavy Syrup	½ cup	90	1	0	–	12	0	tr	–
Chunks In Its Own Juice	½ cup	70	1	0	–	12	0	tr	–
Crushed In Heavy Syrup	½ cup	90	1	0	–	12	0	tr	–
Crushed In Its Own Juice	½ cup	70	1	0	–	12	0	tr	–
Fruit Cup Tidbits	1 pkg (4 oz)	50	1	0	–	12	0	tr	–
Fruit Naturals Chunks	½ cup	70	tr	0	–	60	0	0	–
Dole									
All Natural Chunks	½ cup	60	tr	–	–	24	–	tr	–
Chunks Juice Pack	½ cup	60	1	–	–	15	–	tr	–
Liberty Gold									
Crushed No Sugar Added	½ cup	80	2	200	–	12	20	1	–
Slices Natural Juice	½ cup	80	2	200	–	12	20	1	–
DRIED									
Sunsweet									
Pineapples	⅓ cup (1.4 oz)	130	1	0	–	0	20	0	135
FRESH									
diced	1 cup	77	2	35	16	24	11	1	175
slice	1 slice	42	1	19	9	13	6	tr	95
Cala Fruit									
Golden Sliced	1 serv (3.5 oz)	50	1	0	–	15	0	tr	–
Frieda's									
Zululand Queen	1 cup (5 oz)	70	2	0	–	21	0	tr	–
Frosty Fresh									
Peeled & Cored	½ cup	60	1	–	–	18	–	tr	–
FROZEN									
chunks sweetened	½ cup	104	–	37	–	10	11	tr	122
Europe's Best									
Aloha Gold	1 cup	70	2	100	–	54	20	tr	–

FOOD	PORTION	CALS	FIBER	VIT A	FOLIC	VIT C	CALCI	IRON	POTAS
Roast Works									
Flame Roasted	1 serv (3 oz)	80	1	0	–	15	20	tr	–
PINEAPPLE JUICE									
canned	1 cup	139	–	12	58	27	42	1	334
frzn as prep	1 cup	129	–	25	–	30	28	1	340
frzn not prep	6 oz	387	–	108	–	91	84	2	1020
Adina									
Pineapple Ginger Gin-Jah	8 oz	80	–	–	–	8	–	–	–
Ceres									
Pineapple	8 oz	120	2	0	–	60	40	1	300
Del Monte									
Juice	6 fl oz	80	0	0	–	60	20	tr	–
Langers									
100% Juice	8 oz	130	–	–	–	72	–	–	–
PINK BEANS									
dried cooked	1 cup	252	–	0	284	0	88	4	858
PINTO BEANS									
CANNED									
Eden									
Organic Spicy	½ cup	120	7	200	–	–	80	3	380
Organic Spicy Refried	½ cup	90	7	–	–	–	40	1	420
DRIED									
cooked	1 cup	245	15	0	294	1	79	4	746
TAKE-OUT									
stewed w/ viandas	1 cup	222	6	5	97	8	51	2	546
PISTACHIOS									
dry roasted w/ salt	49 nuts (1 oz)	161	3	74	14	1	31	1	295
dry roasted w/o salt	49 nuts (1 oz)	162	3	74	14	1	31	1	295
in shells	½ cup	165	3	20	14	1	32	1	302
Love'n Bake									
Pistachio Paste	2 tbsp	160	2	100	–	1	20	1	–
Sweet Delights									
Pistachio Roasters	⅓ pkg (1 oz)	190	3	–	–	–	–	–	300

FOOD	PORTION	CALS	FIBER	VIT A	FOLIC	VIT C	CALCI	IRON	POTAS
PITANGA									
fresh	1	2	–	105	–	2	1	tr	7
fresh	1 cup	57	–	2595	–	46	16	tr	178
PIZZA									
Alexia									
Pizza Snack Sweet Italian Sausage Roasted Peppers & Parmesan	6 pieces (3 oz)	210	1	200	–	6	60	3	–
Pizza Snacks Pesto Chicken w/ Fresh Mozzarella	6 pieces (3 oz)	220	1	300	–	4	100	5	–
Amy's									
Cheese	⅓ pie	300	2	–	–	–	–	–	–
Mushroom & Olive	⅓ pie	250	2	–	–	–	–	–	–
Pesto	⅓ pie	310	2	–	–	–	–	–	–
Pocket Sandwich Cheese Pizza	1 (4.5 oz)	300	4	–	–	–	–	–	–
Pocket Sandwich Vegetarian Pizza	1 (4.5 oz)	250	4	–	–	–	–	–	–
Roasted Vegetable	⅓ pie	260	2	–	–	–	–	–	–
Snacks Cheese	5–6 pieces	180	2	–	–	–	–	–	–
Soy Cheese	⅓ pie	290	2	–	–	–	–	–	–
Spinach	⅓ pie	300	2	–	–	–	–	–	–
Veggie Combo	⅓ pie	280	2	–	–	–	–	–	–
Boca									
Supreme w/ Rising Crust Sausage & Pepperoni	⅓ pkg (4.3 oz)	280	3	500	–	9	150	1	–
Celeste									
4 Cheese	1 (5.7 oz)	360	2	500	–	6	350	3	–
Ellio's									
All Cheesy	1 slice	160	1	200	–	1	100	1	–
Cheese	1 slice	150	1	200	–	1	80	1	–
Microwave Single Slice	1 slice	360	4	400	–	2	200	2	–
Pepperoni	1 slice	160	1	300	–	0	80	1	–
Freschetta									
Pepperoni	½ pie (5.8 oz)	470	2	400	–	0	200	4	–

FOOD	PORTION	CALS	FIBER	VIT A	FOLIC	VIT C	CALCI	IRON	POTAS
Glutino									
Gluten Free Duo Cheese	1 (6.1 oz)	420	2	400	–	0	250	1	–
Gluten Free Spinach & Feta	1 (6.1 oz)	430	4	1250	–	0	250	3	–
Healthy Choice									
French Bread Cheese	1 pie	340	5	500	–	0	350	4	–
French Bread Cheese	1 piece (6 oz)	340	5	100	–	0	250	5	–
French Bread Pepperoni	1 pie	340	5	500	–	0	250	4	–
French Bread Pepperoni	1 piece (6 oz)	340	6	300	–	0	300	4	–
French Bread Sausage	1 piece (6 oz)	320	5	200	–	0	150	3	–
French Bread Supreme	1 pie	340	5	400	–	0	200	5	–
French Bread Supreme	1 piece (6.35 oz)	330	6	200	–	0	150	4	–
French Bread Vegetable	1 pie	320	6	400	–	0	300	4	–
Ian's									
Cheese	1 slice (1.5 oz)	100	1	250	–	1	20	tr	–
Jeno's									
Crisp 'n Tasty Cheese	1 pie (6.8 oz)	460	2	0	–	0	350	1	–
Jiffy									
Crust Mix as prep	⅕ crust	180	2	0	–	0	0	2	–
Lean Cuisine									
Casual Eating Deluxe	1 pkg (6 oz)	370	3	200	–	2	150	2	300
Casual Eating Four Cheese	1 pkg (6 oz)	400	3	200	–	0	250	2	260
Casual Eating French Bread Cheese	1 serv (6 oz)	320	3	200	–	1	300	1	390
Casual Eating French Bread Deluxe	1 pkg (6.1 oz)	310	3	500	–	15	150	3	300
Casual Eating French Bread Pepperoni	1 pkg (5.25 oz)	300	2	300	–	2	100	2	360
Casual Eating Margherita	1 pkg (6 oz)	320	4	1000	–	1	150	3	120

FOOD	PORTION	CALS	FIBER	VIT A	FOLIC	VIT C	CALCI	IRON	POTAS
Casual Eating Pepperoni	1 pkg (6 oz)	380	3	200	–	0	200	2	280
Casual Eating Roasted Vegetable	1 pkg (6 oz)	330	3	300	–	6	150	1	280
Casual Eating Spinach & Mushroom	1 pkg (6.1 oz)	310	4	500	–	0	200	3	90
Casual Eating Three Meat	1 pkg (6.4 oz)	350	4	500	–	6	200	4	280
Mr. P's									
Cheese	1 pie (6.5 oz)	410	5	1000	–	0	350	3	–
Red Baron									
Deep Dish Single Pepperoni	1 pizza	460	2	400	–	1	200	3	–
French Bread Supreme	1 pie (5.8 oz)	370	2	500	–	12	200	5	–
South Beach Diet									
Deluxe w/ Wheat Crust	1 pie	340	10	750	–	12	300	3	–
Four Cheese w/ Wheat Crust	1 pie	340	10	500	–	0	500	2	–
Grilled Chicken & Vegetable w/ Wheat Crust	1 pie	330	10	1000	–	6	350	3	–
Pepperoni w/ Wheat Crust	1 pie	350	9	500	–	1	400	2	–
Tony's									
Pizza For One Cheese	1 (6.5 oz)	500	3	400	–	0	250	4	–
Totino's									
Crisp Crust Cheese	½ pie	320	2	0	–	0	300	2	–
TAKE-OUT									
cheese	16 in pie	3384	23	4845	1067	4	2575	23	1974
cheese	⅛ of 16 in pie	423	3	605	133	1	322	3	247
cheese deep dish individual	1 (5.5 oz)	460	2	400	–	1	250	3	–
cheese & vegetables	⅛ of 16 in pie	428	3	270	97	18	292	4	361
ground beef	16 in pie	3753	20	1935	698	41	2145	30	2569
ham & pineapple	⅛ of 16 in pie	439	3	240	92	19	269	4	374

FOOD	PORTION	CALS	FIBER	VIT A	FOLIC	VIT C	CALCI	IRON	POTAS
no cheese	⅛ of 16 in pie	262	2	45	78	5	22	3	218
pepperoni	⅛ of 16 in pie	469	3	240	87	5	268	4	321
white pizza	⅛ of 16 in pie	484	2	375	114	tr	366	4	133

PIZZA CRUST

FOOD	PORTION	CALS	FIBER	VIT A	FOLIC	VIT C	CALCI	IRON	POTAS
crust	1 slice (1.7 oz)	130	1	0	40	0	0	1	–
whole wheat	⅛ crust	140	1	0	–	0	0	tr	–
Alvarado Street Bakery									
Sprouted Wheat California Style	⅛ pie	190	1	0	–	0	40	1	–
Boboli									
Thin Crust	⅕ crust (2 oz)	160	1	0	40	0	20	1	–
Carbsense									
Garlic & Herb as prep	1 slice	100	4	–	–	–	–	–	–
Keto									
Dough Mix as prep	1 slice	79	3	–	–	–	–	–	–
MiniCarb									
Parmesan Herb Mix as prep	1 slice	130	3	–	–	–	–	–	–

PIZZA SAUCE

FOOD	PORTION	CALS	FIBER	VIT A	FOLIC	VIT C	CALCI	IRON	POTAS
Hunt's									
Family Favorites	¼ cup	25	1	100	–	4	0	1	240
Muir Glen									
Organic	¼ cup (2.2 oz)	40	2	100	–	1	0	tr	–

PLANTAINS

FOOD	PORTION	CALS	FIBER	VIT A	FOLIC	VIT C	CALCI	IRON	POTAS
cooked mashed	1 cup	232	5	1818	52	22	4	1	930
sliced cooked	1 cup	179	4	1400	40	17	3	1	716
Chester's									
Chips	1 oz	150	2	0	–	5	0	0	–
Grab Em Snacks									
Chips Black Pepper	1 oz	150	2	1250	–	9	0	0	200
TAKE-OUT									
mofongo	1 serv	320	5	501	63	25	21	2	1303

FOOD	PORTION	CALS	FIBER	VIT A	FOLIC	VIT C	CALCI	IRON	POTAS
ripe fried	2.8 oz	214	4	80	–	10	5	1	–
sweet baked w/ ice cream	1 serv	285	3	621	35	14	37	1	678

PLUMS

canned in heavy syrup	1 cup	163	3	730	5	1	18	2	170
canned purple juice pack	1 cup	146	2	2543	8	7	25	1	388
canned purple water pack	1 cup	102	2	2276	7	7	17	tr	314
dried japanese	1	9	tr	5	0	0	2	tr	28
fresh	1	30	1	228	3	6	4	tr	104
pickled	1	34	tr	15	1	2	1	tr	35

Chiquita

Fresh	2 med (4.6 oz)	80	2	300	–	12	0	0	–

Eden

Umeboshi Plum Paste	1 tsp	5	0	–	–	–	–	–	10
Umeboshi Plums	1 (8 g)	5	0	–	–	–	–	–	20

POI

poi	½ cup	134	–	24	–	5	19	1	220

POKEBERRY SHOOTS

cooked	½ cup	16	–	7134	–	67	43	1	–
fresh	½ cup	18	–	6960	–	109	42	1	–

POLENTA

Frieda's

Organic	2 slices (3.5 oz)	70	1	300	–	7	0	tr	–

POLLACK

atlantic fillet baked	5.3 oz	178	0	61	–	–	116	1	689
atlantic baked	3 oz	100	0	34	–	–	65	1	388

POMEGRANATE

fresh	1 (5.4 oz)	105	1	166	9	9	5	tr	399

POMEGRANATE JUICE

Frutzzo

Organic 100% Juice	1 bottle (12 oz)	130	0	100	–	6	0	1	320

FOOD	PORTION	CALS	FIBER	VIT A	FOLIC	VIT C	CALCI	IRON	POTAS
Langers									
100% Juice	8 oz	150	–	–	–	27	–	1	590
Naked Juice									
Pomegranate Passion	8 oz	150	0	0	–	48	0	tr	340
Odwalla									
PomaGrand Berry	8 oz	140	0	0	–	0	40	tr	540
PomaGrand Mango	8 oz	160	0	0	–	0	40	tr	420
Old Orchard									
100% Pure	8 oz	140	–	0	–	0	0	0	–
POM									
100% Juice	8 oz	140	0	0	–	0	40	tr	430
Pomegranate Blueberry	8 oz	140	0	0	–	0	40	1	280
Pomegranate Cherry	8 oz	140	0	0	–	0	60	tr	390
Pomegranate Mango	8 oz	140	0	0	–	0	40	1	330
Pomegranate Tangerine	8 oz	150	0	0	–	0	20	1	390
POMPANO									
broiled	4 oz	192	0	320	14	2	22	1	377
smoked	2 oz	109	0	95	9	0	15	tr	252
steamed	4 oz	232	0	185	17	0	32	1	459
TAKE-OUT									
battered & fried	4 oz	304	tr	155	26	0	46	1	398
breaded & fried	4 oz	361	1	225	40	0	69	2	476
POPCORN									
air popped	1 cup (0.3 oz)	31	2	16	2	0	1	tr	24
caramel coated	1 cup (1.2 oz)	152	2	18	–	0	15	1	38
caramel coated w/ peanuts	⅔ cup (1 oz)	114	1	18	–	0	19	1	101
cheese	1 cup (0.4 oz)	58	1	27	–	tr	12	tr	29
oil popped	1 cup (0.4 oz)	55	1	17	2	0	1	tr	25
Cape Cod									
White Cheddar	2⅓ cups	170	2	100	–	4	0	tr	–
Chester's									
Microwave Butter	3 cups	170	3	2250	–	0	0	1	–
Microwave Cheddar Cheese	3 cups	200	2	750	–	0	0	1	–

FOOD	PORTION	CALS	FIBER	VIT A	FOLIC	VIT C	CALCI	IRON	POTAS
Cracker Jack									
Butter Toffee	¾ cup	140	1	0	–	0	0	0	–
Original	½ cup	120	1	0	–	0	0	1	–
Dale & Thomas									
Caramel	½ cup	75	0	0	–	0	0	tr	–
Hall Of Fame Kettlecorn	½ cup	34	1	0	–	0	0	tr	–
North Country Cheddar	½ cup	73	1	0	–	0	0	tr	–
Peanut Butter & White Chocolate Drizzlecorn	½ cup	115	1	0	–	0	0	tr	–
Purepopped Natural	½ cup	26	1	0	–	0	0	tr	–
Sweet Georgia Pecan	½ cup	96	1	0	–	0	0	tr	–
Toffee Crunch Drizzlecorn	½ cup	107	1	0	–	0	0	0	–
Husman's									
Cheese Corn	2¼ cups (1 oz)	160	1	0	–	0	10	1	–
Jay's									
Caramel	¾ cup	110	1	0	–	0	0	0	–
Ok-Ke-Doke Cheese	1 oz	160	2	0	–	0	20	tr	–
LesserEvil									
Black&White	1 cup	120	1	0	–	0	0	1	–
KettleCorn	1 cup	120	2	100	–	0	0	tr	–
MaplePecan	1 cup	120	3	0	–	0	0	tr	–
PeanutButter & Choco	1 cup	120	1	0	–	0	0	tr	–
SinNamon	1 cup	120	2	100	–	0	40	1	–
Newman's Own									
Microwave 94% Fat Free	3½ cups	110	4	0	–	0	0	1	–
Microwave Butter	3½ cups	130	3	0	–	0	0	1	–
Microwave Butter Boom	3½ cups	130	3	0	–	0	0	1	–
Microwave Light Butter	3½ cups	120	4	0	–	0	0	1	–
Microwave Low Sodium Butter	3½ cups	130	3	0	–	0	0	1	–
Microwave Natural	3½ cups	130	3	0	–	0	0	1	–

FOOD	PORTION	CALS	FIBER	VIT A	FOLIC	VIT C	CALCI	IRON	POTAS
Organic Pop's Corn Butter	3½ cups	160	1	–	–	–	–	–	–
Organic Pop's Corn No Butter No Salt 94% Fat Free	3½ cups	120	1	–	–	–	–	–	–
Oogie's									
Romano & Pesto	1 oz	138	3	150	–	1	30	1	–
Smoked Gouda	1 oz	132	3	50	–	0	20	1	–
Spicy Chipotle & Lime	1 oz	143	3	50	–	0	0	1	–
White Cheddar	1 oz	142	3	50	–	0	20	1	–
Orville Redenbacher's									
Microwave Natural Light	1 cup	20	1	0	–	0	0	0	–
Microwave Regular Natural	1 cup	15	1	0	–	0	0	0	–
Microwave Regular Old Fashioned Butter	1 cup	35	1	0	–	0	0	0	–
Microwave Smart Pop Kettle Korn	1 cup	20	1	0	–	0	0	0	–
Poppycock									
The Original	½ cup	160	1	100	–	0	0	0	–
Smart Balance									
Light as prep	4 cups	120	4	0	–	0	0	1	–
Low Fat as prep	5 cups	120	5	0	–	0	0	1	–
Movie Style as prep	3.5 cups	170	3	0	–	0	0	1	–
Smartfood									
Reduced Fat White Cheddar	3 cups	140	3	0	–	0	20	1	–
White Cheddar	1 pkg	160	2	0	–	0	40	tr	–
Snyder's Of Hanover									
Butter	⅝ oz	100	1	0	–	0	0	0	–
Wise									
Butter	1 pkg (0.5 oz)	80	1	750	–	0	0	0	–
Hot Cheese	1 oz	150	2	0	–	0	20	tr	–

POPCORN CAKES
Orville Redenbacher's

FOOD	PORTION	CALS	FIBER	VIT A	FOLIC	VIT C	CALCI	IRON	POTAS
Butter	2	60	2	0	–	0	0	0	–
Caramel	1	40	tr	0	–	0	0	0	–

FOOD	PORTION	CALS	FIBER	VIT A	FOLIC	VIT C	CALCI	IRON	POTAS
Chocolate	1	45	tr	0	–	0	0	0	–
Mini Butter	8	60	1	0	–	0	0	0	–
Mini Caramel	7	50	1	0	–	0	0	0	–
Mini Peanut Caramel Crunch	6	60	1	0	–	0	0	0	–
Mini Peanut Crunch	6	60	2	0	–	0	0	0	–
Mini Sour Cream & Onion	8	60	2	0	–	0	0	0	–
White Cheddar	2	60	2	0	–	0	0	0	–

POPOVER
home recipe as prep w/ 2% milk	1 (1.4 oz)	87	–	117	7	tr	38	1	65
home recipe as prep w/ whole milk	1 (1.4 oz)	90	–	97	7	tr	37	1	64
mix as prep	1 (1.2 oz)	67	–	–	–	–	9	1	25

POPPY SEEDS
poppy seeds	1 tsp	15	–	0	–	–	41	0	20
Love'n Bake									
Poppy Seed Filling	2 tbsp	120	tr	0	–	0	150	1	–

PORGY
fresh	3 oz	77	0	–	–	–	41	tr	415

PORK
FRESH
boneless loin lean & fat roasted	3.5 oz	195	0	0	–	0	7	1	348
center loin chop bone in broiled	1 (3 oz)	178	0	0	–	0	20	1	293
center rib chop lean & fat bone in broiled	1 (3 oz)	189	0	0	–	0	24	1	279
country style ribs bone in lean & fat braised	3.5 oz	288	0	0	–	0	36	1	299
dehydrated oriental style	1 cup (0.8 oz)	135	0	0	0	0	2	tr	31
fresh ham rump half lean & fat roasted	4 oz	278	0	10	3	tr	13	1	413
fresh ham shank half lean & fat roasted	4 oz	319	0	10	6	tr	17	1	373

FOOD	PORTION	CALS	FIBER	VIT A	FOLIC	VIT C	CALCI	IRON	POTAS
fresh ham whole lean & fat roasted	4 oz	302	0	11	11	tr	15	1	389
ground cooked	4 oz	328	0	8	7	1	24	1	400
ham hock cooked	1	167	0	10	2	tr	9	1	187
shoulder chop bone in braised	1 (3 oz)	229	0	0	–	0	22	1	259
sirloin roast lean & fat bone in roasted	4 oz	231	0	0	–	0	15	1	340
spareribs bone in roasted	3 oz	304	0	0	–	0	16	1	225
tail simmered	3 oz	336	0	0	3	0	11	1	–
tenderloin roast boneless lean & fat roasted	4 oz	145	0	0	–	0	6	1	419
top loin chop boneless lean & fat broiled	1 (3.5 oz)	195	0	0	–	0	7	1	358
Boar's Head									
Smoked Shoulder Butt Roast	3 oz	170	–	300	–	–	–	1	–
Freirich									
Porkette	4 oz	220	0	0	–	0	40	1	–
Smithfield									
Smoked Pork Chop	3 oz	100	0	0	–	0	20	1	–
READY-TO-EAT									
Sara Lee									
Oven Roasted	2 oz	70	0	0	–	1	0	5	–
TAKE-OUT									
chicharrones pork cracklings fried	1 cup	492	0	50	2	0	10	1	514
chop breaded & fried	1 lg (5 oz)	441	1	95	28	tr	76	2	453
chop breaded & fried	1 med (3.4 oz)	304	1	65	19	tr	53	2	313
chop stewed	1 lg (4.6 oz)	315	0	18	4	1	28	1	494

PORK DISHES

Hormel

Center Cut Loin Lemon Garlic	1 serv (4 oz)	130	0	0	–	1	0	tr	–

FOOD	PORTION	CALS	FIBER	VIT A	FOLIC	VIT C	CALCI	IRON	POTAS
Extra Lean Apple Bourbon	1 serv (4 oz)	140	0	0	–	0	0	1	–
Extra Lean Teriyaki	4 oz	140	0	0	–	0	0	1	–
Pork Roast Au Jus	1 serv (5 oz)	180	0	–	–	–	–	1	–

Morton's Of Omaha

Tender Pork Roast w/ Gravy & Vegetables	1 serv (5 oz)	210	1	750	–	4	20	1	–

Smithfield

Pulled Pork w/ Barbecue Sauce	2 oz	90	–	0	–	2	20	1	–
Tenderloin Garlic & Herb	3 oz	100	tr	200	–	2	0	2	–
Tenderloin Hickory Sweet	4 oz	110	0	100	–	1	0	1	–

Tyson

Lemon Pepper Pork Roast	1 serv (3 oz)	110	0	0	–	1	20	1	–

Wellshire

Baby Back Ribs w/ Sauce	2 ribs (5 oz)	260	0	500	–	3	0	1	–
Shredded Pork In BBQ Sauce	¼ cup	90	0	200	–	0	0	tr	–

TAKE-OUT

spareribs barbecued w/ sauce	2 med (2.8 oz)	248	tr	10	3	2	32	1	230
tourtiere	1 piece (4.9 oz)	451	–	10	–	–	18	3	–

POT PIE
Amy's

Broccoli	1 (7.5 oz)	430	4	–	–	–	–	–	–
Country Vegetable	1 (7.5 oz)	370	4	–	–	–	–	–	–
Shepherd's	1 (8 oz)	160	5	–	–	–	–	–	–
Vegetable	1 (7.5 oz)	420	4	–	–	–	–	–	–
Vegetable Non-Dairy	1 (7.5 oz)	320	4	–	–	–	–	–	–

Ian's

Chicken	1 pkg (9.4 oz)	510	2	2500	–	1	40	4	–

FOOD	PORTION	CALS	FIBER	VIT A	FOLIC	VIT C	CALCI	IRON	POTAS
TAKE-OUT									
beef	1 8 in pie (14.6 oz)	938	5	1795	129	14	42	6	709
chicken	1 8 in pie (14.6 oz)	897	6	2625	133	17	108	6	646
ham	1 serv (11 oz)	752	4	535	104	12	38	4	588
oyster	1 serv (11.5 oz)	817	3	246	115	4	220	10	515
POTATO									
CANNED									
potatoes	½ cup	54	–	–	6	5	5	1	206
Del Monte									
New Whole	2 med (5.5 oz)	60	2	0	–	9	20	tr	–
Savory Sides Au Gratin	½ cup	80	1	100	–	6	40	tr	–
S&W									
Whole Small	2 (5.5 oz)	60	2	0	–	9	20	tr	–
FRESH									
baked skin only	1 skin (2 oz)	115	2	0	–	8	20	4	332
baked w/ skin	1 (6.5 oz)	220	–	0	22	26	20	3	844
baked w/o skin	1 (5 oz)	145	2	0	14	20	8	1	610
baked w/o skin	½ cup	57	1	–	6	8	3	tr	238
boiled	½ cup	68	1	0	8	10	4	tr	295
microwaved	1 (7 oz)	212	–	–	24	31	22	3	903
microwaved w/o skin	½ cup	78	–	–	10	12	4	tr	321
raw w/o skin	1 (3.9 oz)	88	–	0	14	22	8	1	608
Arrowfarms									
Yukon Gold	1 med (5 oz)	100	3	0	–	27	20	1	–
Dole									
Idaho	1 (5.3 oz)	100	3	0	24	27	20	1	720
Frieda's									
Fingerling	4 (5 oz)	100	3	0	–	27	20	1	–
Green Giant									
Red Potatoes	1 med (5 oz)	100	3	0	–	27	20	1	720

FOOD	PORTION	CALS	FIBER	VIT A	FOLIC	VIT C	CALCI	IRON	POTAS
Lucinda's									
Red "C"	1 med (5.2 oz)	100	3	0	–	27	20	1	–
SunLite									
SunLite	1 (5 oz)	87	4	0	24	24	40	1	680
FROZEN									
french fries	10 strips	111	2	–	8	6	4	1	229
french fries thick cut	10 strips	109	–	–	9	5	5	1	240
hashed brown	½ cup	170	–	–	–	5	12	1	340
potato puffs	½ cup	138	–	10	10	4	19	1	236
potato puffs as prep	1	16	–	1	1	1	2	tr	27
Alexia									
Hashed Brown	1 serv (3 oz)	80	2	0	–	1	0	0	250
Mashed Red w/ Garlic & Parmesan	½ cup	150	2	200	–	2	40	1	–
Mashed Yukon Gold & Sea Salt	½ cup	150	2	300	–	0	20	1	–
Oven Crinkles Classic	1 serv (3 oz)	120	3	0	–	1	0	1	–
Oven Crinkles Salt & Pepper	1 serv (3 oz)	120	3	0	–	1	0	tr	–
Oven Fries Garlic	12 pieces	140	2	0	–	4	0	1	–
Oven Reds	1 serv (3 oz)	120	2	0	–	9	30	1	250
Waffle Fries	8 pieces	150	3	0	–	0	0	1	–
Yukon Gold Fries w/ Sea Salt	1 serv (3 oz)	130	2	300	–	9	0	3	–
Funster									
BBQ Lite	14 pieces (3 oz)	140	<2	100	–	2	20	1	–
Cheddar	14 pieces (3 oz)	135	<2	50	–	2	30	1	–
Original	14 pieces (3 oz)	135	2	0	–	2	20	1	–
Healthy Choice									
Cheddar Broccoli Potatoes	1 pkg	270	7	300	–	12	150	1	–

FOOD	PORTION	CALS	FIBER	VIT A	FOLIC	VIT C	CALCI	IRON	POTAS
Ian's									
Alphatots	1 serv (3.5 oz)	156	1	–	–	5	–	1	–
Fries Sweet Potato	7 pieces (2.5 oz)	70	1	12500	–	9	20	tr	–
Inland Valley									
Crinkle Cuts	15 pieces (3 oz)	150	2	–	–	6	–	tr	350
Crisscut Fries	13 pieces (3 oz)	160	2	–	–	–	60	1	480
Curly QQQ's	1⅓ cups (3 oz)	180	2	–	–	5	–	1	330
Fajita Fries	17 pieces (3 oz)	170	2	–	–	–	40	1	300
French Fries	15 pieces (3 oz)	130	2	–	–	4	–	tr	360
Hash Browns	⅔ cup	70	2	–	–	6	–	tr	280
Home Browns	1 patty (2.2 oz)	130	2	–	–	2	–	tr	280
Mashed Homestyle	⅔ cup	160	3	–	–	1	40	tr	270
Simply Shreds	1 cup	70	2	–	–	9	–	tr	350
Stix	5 pieces (3 oz)	170	2	–	–	2	–	tr	330
Stuffed Spudz w/ Cheese	5 pieces	210	2	200	–	–	150	1	150
Tater Babies	8 pieces (3 oz)	130	2	–	–	–	80	1	330
Tater Puffs	10 pieces	160	2	–	–	1	–	1	310
Twice Baked	1 (5.2 oz)	230	2	400	–	12	150	5	–
Twice Baked Sour Cream Bacon & Chives	1 (5.2 oz)	240	3	300	–	6	40	4	–
Twice Baked Triple Cheese	1 (5.2 oz)	250	3	400	–	6	80	4	–
Larry's									
Mashed Broccoli & Cheddar Cheese	1 serv (5 oz)	180	2	0	–	4	80	0	–
Mashed Cheddar Cheese	1 serv (5 oz)	190	2	0	–	2	100	tr	–

FOOD	PORTION	CALS	FIBER	VIT A	FOLIC	VIT C	CALCI	IRON	POTAS
Mashed Old Fashioned Butter	1 serv (5 oz)	190	2	200	–	2	80	tr	–
Mashed Sour Cream & Chives	1 serv (5 oz)	180	2	0	–	2	80	tr	–
Mashed Sweet Potatoes	1 serv (4 oz)	140	2	4000	–	4	200	1	–
Lean Cuisine									
One Dish Favorites Deluxe Cheddar	1 pkg (10.4 oz)	260	5	300	–	18	250	1	1040
McCain									
French Fries Crinkle Cut	18 pieces (3 oz)	130	2	0	–	4	0	tr	260
Mash-Bites	1 serv (3 oz)	50	1	0	–	0	0	1	280
Roasters All American	1 serv (3 oz)	120	tr	0	–	4	0	1	340
Roasters Grilled Garlic & Onion	1 serv (3 oz)	120	2	0	–	4	0	1	370
Seasoned Wedges Skin On	1 serv (3 oz)	120	2	0	–	2	0	tr	320
Shoestring French Fries	45 pieces (3 oz)	140	2	0	–	4	0	tr	280
Smiles	6 pieces (3 oz)	160	2	0	–	4	0	0	380
Steak Fries	8 pieces (3 oz)	120	2	0	–	4	0	tr	250
Tasti Tater	1 serv (3 oz)	160	3	0	–	2	0	tr	220
Oh Boy!									
Stuffed w/ Onion Sour Cream & Chives	1 (5 oz)	110	2	0	–	0	40	1	–
Roast Works									
Roasted Seasoned Wedge	1 serv (3 oz)	100	1	0	–	5	0	tr	–
Roasted Wedges Rosemary Redskin	1 serv (3 oz)	110	2	0	–	0	20	1	–
Roasted Wedges Yukon Gold	1 serv (3 oz)	110	1	0	–	2	0	0	–
MIX									
au gratin as prep	½ cup	160	–	322	10	12	146	1	483

FOOD	PORTION	CALS	FIBER	VIT A	FOLIC	VIT C	CALCI	IRON	POTAS
instant mashed flakes as prep w/ whole milk & butter	½ cup	118	–	189	8	10	52	tr	245
instant mashed flakes not prep	½ cup	78	–	–	9	18	5	tr	239
instant mashed granules as prep w/ whole milk & butter	½ cup	114	–	195	8	6	37	tr	152
instant mashed granules not prep	½ cup	372	–	9	40	37	41	1	703
scalloped	½ cup	105	–	165	10	13	70	1	461
Idahoan									
AuGratin as prep	½ cup	150	2	300	–	6	80	tr	–
Hash Browns as prep	½ cup	160	1	300	–	1	40	tr	–
Hash Browns Cheesy not prep	½ cup	120	2	0	–	6	20	tr	–
Mashed Baked as prep	½ cup	110	2	0	–	9	40	tr	–
Mashed Butter & Herb as prep	½ cup	110	1	0	–	9	20	tr	–
Mashed Buttery Homestyle as prep	½ cup	110	1	0	–	6	20	tr	–
Mashed Four Cheese as prep	½ cup	100	1	0	–	9	40	tr	–
Mashed Southwest as prep	½ cup	110	2	0	–	5	20	tr	–
Roasted Garlic as prep	½ cup	600	1	0	–	6	40	tr	–
Scalloped as prep	½ cup	150	1	300	–	6	80	tr	–
REFRIGERATED									
Country Crock									
Garlic Mashed	⅔ cup	170	3	300	–	0	0	1	–
Homestyle Mashed	⅔ cup	190	3	400	–	0	20	1	–
PurelyIdaho									
Cheddar Crusted	¾ cup	120	2	50	–	15	30	tr	–
Simply Potatoes									
Diced w/ Onion	⅔ cup	60	1	0	–	0	0	tr	–
Homestyle Slices	⅔ cup	70	1	0	–	0	0	tr	–
Mashed	⅔ cup	170	1	400	–	0	40	tr	–
Mashed Sweet Potatoes	⅔ cup	160	2	19500	–	21	60	1	–

FOOD	PORTION	CALS	FIBER	VIT A	FOLIC	VIT C	CALCI	IRON	POTAS
Red Potato Wedges	½ cup	50	2	0	–	2	0	tr	–
Shredded Hash Browns	½ cup	50	tr	0	–	0	0	0	–
SHELF-STABLE									
TastyBite									
Bombay Potatoes	½ pkg (5 oz)	190	6	0	–	0	50	3	–
Mumbai Pav Bhaji	½ pkg (5 oz)	229	7	50	–	1	40	3	–
Simla Potatoes	½ pkg (5 oz)	180	1	0	–	0	20	2	–
TAKE-OUT									
au gratin w/ cheese	½ cup	178	–	392	–	12	156	1	375
baked topped w/ cheese sauce	1	475	–	834	28	26	310	3	1167
baked topped w/ cheese sauce & bacon	1	451	–	627	28	29	309	3	1179
baked topped w/ cheese sauce & broccoli	1	402	–	1695	61	49	334	3	1440
baked topped w/ cheese sauce & chili	1	481	–	768	50	32	409	6	1570
baked topped w/ sour cream & chives	1	394	–	1346	32	34	105	3	1383
curry	1 serv (6 oz)	292	4	1000	–	14	47	2	–
french fries	1 reg	235	–	22	25	4	12	1	541
hash brown	½ cup (2.5 oz)	151	–	18	8	6	7	tr	267
indian yogurt potatoes	1 serv	315	0	–	–	–	–	–	–
mashed	½ cup	111	–	177	0	6	27	tr	303
o'brien	1 cup	157	–	934	16	32	70	1	516
potato dumpling	3.5 oz	334	3	–	–	–	–	–	–
potato pancakes	1 (1.3 oz)	101	–	53	9	8	9	1	291
potato salad	½ cup	179	2	196	9	13	24	1	318
red new boiled	5 sm (5 oz)	120	2	0	–	24	20	1	680
scalloped	½ cup	127	–	196	–	13	66	1	401
twice baked w/ cheese	1 half (10 oz)	392	4	0	–	29	400	1	–

FOOD	PORTION	CALS	FIBER	VIT A	FOLIC	VIT C	CALCI	IRON	POTAS
POTATO STARCH									
potato starch	1 oz	96	–	–	–	0	10	tr	4
POUT									
ocean baked	3 oz	86	0	–	–	–	11	tr	–
ocean fillet baked	4.8 oz	139	0	–	–	–	18	tr	–
PRETZELS									
chocolate covered	1 (0.4 oz)	47	tr	10	15	0	7	tr	23
soft	1 lg (5 oz)	483	2	0	34	0	33	6	126
twists salted	10 (2.1 oz)	229	2	0	50	0	22	1	88
twists w/o salt	10 (2.1 oz)	229	2	0	103	0	22	3	88
whole wheat	2 sm (1 oz)	103	2	0	15	tr	8	1	122
yogurt covered	1 cup (3 oz)	391	1	5	79	tr	101	2	191
yogurt covered	1 (4 g)	19	tr	0	4	0	5	tr	9
Aramana									
Soy Pretzels	15 (1 oz)	100	4	–	–	–	–	–	–
Cape Cod									
Pretzels	25	130	tr	0	–	0	0	tr	–
Combos									
Cheddar Cheese Cracker	1 pkg (1.7 oz)	240	1	–	–	–	40	tr	–
Nacho Cheese	1 pkg (1.7 oz)	230	1	–	–	–	80	tr	–
Pizzeria Pretzel	1 pkg (1.7 oz)	230	1	–	–	–	60	tr	–
Glenny's									
Organic Original Salted	8 (1 oz)	110	1	–	–	–	–	–	–
Organic Sourdough	6 (1 oz)	110	1	–	–	–	–	–	–
Glutino									
Gluten Free All Shapes	44 (1.4 oz)	190	0	0	–	0	0	0	–
Goodniks									
Yogurt Pretzels	15	180	0	0	–	0	80	1	–

FOOD	PORTION	CALS	FIBER	VIT A	FOLIC	VIT C	CALCI	IRON	POTAS
Handi-Snacks									
Mister Salty Pretzels 'n Cheez	1 pkg	90	0	100	–	0	40	tr	–
Healthy Handfuls									
Python Pretzels	1 box (1.5 oz)	170	1	0	–	0	0	0	–
Landies Candies									
Sugar Free Chocolate	4 (1.5 oz)	220	tr	0	–	0	20	tr	–
Newman's Own									
Organic Bavarian Sour Dough	1	90	1	–	–	–	–	–	–
Organic Hi Protein	22	120	4	–	–	–	–	–	–
Organic Salt & Pepper Rounds	8	100	1	–	–	–	–	–	–
Organic Salt & Pepper Thins	10	120	tr	–	–	–	–	–	–
Organic Salted Nuggets	20	120	2	–	–	–	–	–	–
Organic Salted Rods	4	120	2	–	–	–	–	–	–
Organic Salted Rounds	8	110	tr	–	–	–	–	–	–
Organic Salted Sticks	13	110	1	–	–	–	–	–	–
Organic Salted Thins	10	110	1	–	–	–	–	–	–
Organic Spelt	20	120	4	–	–	–	–	–	–
Organic Unsalted Rounds	8	110	tr	–	–	–	–	–	–
Quinlan									
Low Fat Mini	1 oz	110	tr	0	–	0	0	0	–
Rold Gold									
Braided Twists	8	110	1	0	–	0	0	1	–
Braided Twists Honey Wheat	8	110	1	0	–	0	0	1	–
Checkers	20	110	1	0	–	0	0	1	–
Rods	3	110	1	0	–	0	0	1	–
Sourdough Hard	1	100	1	0	–	0	0	tr	–
Sourdough Specials	5	110	1	0	–	0	0	0	–
Sticks	48	100	1	0	–	0	0	1	–
Thins	9 pieces	110	1	0	–	0	0	2	–
Tiny Twists	18 pieces	110	1	0	–	0	0	1	–
Tiny Twists Cheddar	20	110	1	0	–	0	0	1	–
Tiny Twists Honey Mustard	13	110	1	0	–	0	0	1	–

FOOD	PORTION	CALS	FIBER	VIT A	FOLIC	VIT C	CALCI	IRON	POTAS
Snyder's Of Hanover									
100 Calorie Pack Snaps	1 pkg (0.9 oz)	100	tr	0	–	0	0	0	–
100 Calorie Pack Stick	1 pkg (0.9 oz)	100	tr	0	–	0	0	tr	–
Dips Milk Chocolate	1 oz	140	tr	0	–	0	40	tr	–
Dips Special Dark Chocolate	1 oz	140	2	0	–	0	0	tr	–
Mini Unsalted	1 oz	110	tr	0	–	0	0	tr	–
MultiGrain Sticks Lightly Salted	1 oz	120	3	0	–	0	0	0	–
MultiGrain Twists	1 oz	120	2	0	–	0	0	0	–
Nibblers Sourdough	1 oz	120	tr	0	–	0	0	1	–
Old Tyme	1 oz	120	1	0	–	0	0	0	–
Organic Honey Wheat	1 oz	130	1	0	–	0	0	1	–
Organic Oat Bran	1 oz	120	2	0	–	0	0	1	–
Pieces Garlic Bread	1 oz	140	1	0	–	0	0	0	–
Pieces Honey Mustard & Onions	1 oz	140	tr	0	–	0	0	0	–
Pieces Hot Buffalo Wing	1 oz	140	tr	0	–	0	0	1	–
Pretzel Sandwich Peanut Butter	1 oz	140	tr	0	–	0	0	tr	–
Rods	1 oz	120	1	0	–	0	0	tr	–
Snaps	1 oz	120	1	0	–	9	0	0	–
Sourdough Unsalted	1 oz	100	1	0	–	0	0	tr	–
Sticks 12 Multi Grain	1 oz	130	3	0	–	1	20	1	–
Spinzels									
Braided	1 pkg (0.5 oz)	55	tr	0	–	0	0	tr	–
Utz									
Rods	3 (1 oz)	120	1	0	–	0	0	tr	–
Wege									
Honey Wheat	1 (0.8 oz)	120	1	0	–	0	0	0	–
PRUNE JUICE									
jarred	1 cup	182	3	0	0	11	31	3	707
L&A									
100% Juice	8 oz	180	3	200	–	9	–	3	540
Langers									
Plus 100% Juice	8 oz	180	1	500	–	60	100	–	480

FOOD	PORTION	CALS	FIBER	VIT A	FOLIC	VIT C	CALCI	IRON	POTAS
Ocean Spray									
100% Juice	8 oz	180	0	0	–	5	–	–	480
Old Orchard									
Healthy Balance	8 oz	70	5	0	–	60	150	1	135
Sunsweet									
100% Juice	8 oz	180	3	100	–	0	20	1	540
PlumSmart	8 oz	160	3	0	8	72	20	tr	290
PRUNES									
cooked w/o sugar	½ cup	133	4	424	0	4	24	1	398
dried	1	20	1	66	0	tr	4	tr	61
Love'n Bake									
Prune Lekvar	2 tbsp	90	1	100	–	1	0	tr	–
Newman's Own									
Organic	½ cup	110	2	–	–	–	–	–	–
St Dalfour									
French Prunes	3	100	3	500	–	0	20	tr	–
Sunsweet									
Pitted Dried	5	100	3	400	–	0	20	tr	290
PUDDING									
MIX									
Keto									
Banana not prep	½ scoop	62	2	–	–	–	–	–	–
Chocolate not prep	½ scoop	66	3	–	–	–	–	–	–
French Vanilla not prep	½ scoop	62	2	–	–	–	–	–	–
Uncle Ben's									
Rice Pudding Cinnamon & Raisins as prep	½ cup	160	1	0	40	0	20	1	–
Rice Pudding French Vanilla as prep	½ cup	120	1	0	60	0	20	tr	–
READY-TO-EAT									
Boost									
Vanilla	1 pkg (5 oz)	240	0	750	84	36	250	3	250
Hunt's									
Dessert Favorites Banana Cream Pie	1 serv (3.5 oz)	140	0	–	–	–	40	–	–

FOOD	PORTION	CALS	FIBER	VIT A	FOLIC	VIT C	CALCI	IRON	POTAS
Dessert Favorites Chocolate Brownie	1 serv (3.5 oz)	190	0	–	–	–	40	1	–
Dessert Favorites Chocolate Mud Pie	1 serv (3.5 oz)	170	0	–	–	–	60	1	–
Dessert Favorites Chocolate Peanut Butter Pie	1 serv (3.5 oz)	190	0	–	–	–	40	1	–
Dessert Favorites Dulce De Leche Caramel Cream	1 serv (3.5 oz)	140	0	–	–	–	40	–	–
Dessert Favorites Lemon Merinque Pie	1 serv (3.5 oz)	130	0	–	–	–	–	–	–
Snack Pack Butterscotch	1 serv (3.5 oz)	130	0	0	–	0	40	–	–
Snack Pack Chocolate	1 serv (3.5 oz)	104	0	0	–	0	60	1	–
Snack Pack Chocolate Fudge	1 serv (3.5 oz)	150	0	0	–	0	60	1	–
Snack Pack Chocolate Marshmallow	1 serv (3.5 oz)	130	0	0	–	0	40	–	–
Snack Pack Fat Free Chocolate	1 serv (3.5 oz)	90	0	0	–	0	40	1	–
Snack Pack Fat Free Tapioca	1 serv (3.5 oz)	80	0	–	–	–	40	–	–
Snack Pack Fat Free Vanilla	1 serv (3.5 oz)	80	0	0	–	0	40	–	–
Snack Pack Lemon	1 serv (3.5 oz)	120	0	0	–	–	–	–	–
Snack Pack Swirl Chocolate Caramel	1 serv (3.5 oz)	140	0	0	–	0	60	tr	–
Snack Pack Swirl S'mores	1 serv (3.5 oz)	140	0	0	–	0	40	–	–
Snack Pack Tapioca	1 serv (3.5 oz)	130	0	0	–	0	60	–	–
Snack Pack Vanilla	1 serv (3.5 oz)	130	0	0	–	0	60	–	–

FOOD	PORTION	CALS	FIBER	VIT A	FOLIC	VIT C	CALCI	IRON	POTAS
Jell-O									
100 Calorie Pack Fat Free Chocolate Vanilla Swirl	1 serv (4 oz)	100	tr	0	–	0	100	tr	–
100 Calorie Pack Fat Free Tapioca	1 serv (4 oz)	100	0	0	–	0	100	0	–
Fat Free Chocolate Fudge & Caramel	1 serv (4 oz)	100	0	100	–	0	60	0	–
Fat Free Vanilla Caramel	1 serv (4 oz)	100	0	0	–	0	40	0	–
Tapioca	1 serv (4 oz)	110	0	0	–	0	40	0	–
Kozy Shack									
Black Forest	1 pkg (4 oz)	120	1	100	–	0	100	0	–
Chocolate	1 pkg (4 oz)	139	1	121	–	0	119	tr	224
Chocolate No Sugar Added	1 pkg (4 oz)	93	1	100	–	0	131	tr	244
Rice	1 pkg (4 oz)	135	0	138	–	0	116	1	155
Tapioca	1 pkg (4 oz)	130	0	100	–	1	100	0	–
Tapioca No Sugar Added	1 pkg	90	4	100	–	1	100	0	–
Vanilla	1 pkg (4 oz)	130	0	133	–	0	119	tr	151
Vanilla No Sugar Added	1 pkg (4 oz)	90	0	100	–	0	128	tr	162
Swiss Miss									
Low Fat Tapioca	1 pkg (4 oz)	130	0	–	–	–	200	tr	–
Low Fat Vanilla	1 serv (4 oz)	120	–	–	–	–	200	tr	–
TAKE-OUT									
blancmange	1 serv (4.7 oz)	154	tr	350	–	tr	149	tr	–
bread w/ raisins	1 cup	306	2	650	40	1	238	2	432
coconut	1 cup	291	2	510	13	tr	258	tr	370
corn	1 cup	328	4	750	83	9	100	1	440

FOOD	PORTION	CALS	FIBER	VIT A	FOLIC	VIT C	CALCI	IRON	POTAS
indian pudding	½ cup	156	1	200	23	0	146	1	345
noodle pudding kugel	1 cup	297	2	510	56	2	39	3	194
plum pudding	1 slice (1.5 oz)	125	1	215	6	tr	43	1	197
queen of puddings	1 serv (4.4 oz)	266	tr	625	–	1	99	1	–
rice pudding	1 cup	302	1	415	9	tr	225	1	403
sweet potato	1 cup	215	5	8200	15	25	101	1	519
tapioca	1 cup	236	0	615	18	0	211	1	291
yorkshire	1 serv (3 oz)	177	tr	270	3	0	37	tr	45

PUFFERFISH

FOOD	PORTION	CALS	FIBER	VIT A	FOLIC	VIT C	CALCI	IRON	POTAS
raw	3 oz	72	0	0	–	0	12	1	246

PUMMELO

FOOD	PORTION	CALS	FIBER	VIT A	FOLIC	VIT C	CALCI	IRON	POTAS
fresh	1	228	–	0	–	372	23	1	1317
sections	1 cup	71	–	0	–	116	7	tr	411
Sunkist									
Fresh	¼	90	4	0	60	72	40	tr	270

PUMPKIN

FOOD	PORTION	CALS	FIBER	VIT A	FOLIC	VIT C	CALCI	IRON	POTAS
butter	1 tbsp	32	–	1000	–	–	–	–	–
canned	½ cup	41	–	26908	15	5	32	2	251
cooked mashed	½ cup	24	–	1320	–	6	18	1	281
flowers cooked	½ cup	10	–	1162	–	3	25	1	71
flowers raw	1	0	–	39	–	1	1	tr	3
leaves cooked	½ cup	7	–	866	–	tr	15	1	153
leaves raw	½ cup	4	–	388	–	2	8	tr	87
raw cubed	½ cup	15	–	928	–	5	12	tr	197
Farmer's Market									
Organic Puree	½ cup	50	4	14000	–	2	20	1	–
Libby's									
Puree	½ cup	40	5	15000	–	0	20	1	–

PUMPKIN SEEDS

FOOD	PORTION	CALS	FIBER	VIT A	FOLIC	VIT C	CALCI	IRON	POTAS
dried	1 oz	154	–	108	–	–	12	4	229
roasted	¼ cup	296	–	–	–	–	24	9	457
salted & roasted	¼ cup	296	–	–	–	–	24	9	457
whole roasted	1 oz	127	–	–	–	–	16	1	261
whole roasted	¼ cup	71	–	–	–	–	9	1	147
whole salted roasted	¼ cup	71	–	–	–	–	9	1	147

FOOD	PORTION	CALS	FIBER	VIT A	FOLIC	VIT C	CALCI	IRON	POTAS
David									
All Natural	¼ cup	160	1	–	–	–	–	3	–
Eden									
Dry Roasted & Salted	¼ cup	200	5	–	–	–	0	2	270
Good Sense									
Roasted & Salted	½ cup	160	1	0	–	0	0	4	–
PURSLANE									
cooked	1 cup	21	–	2130	–	12	90	1	561
fresh	1 cup	7	–	568	–	9	28	1	213
QUAIL									
cooked bone removed	1 (2.7 oz)	177	0	265	5	2	11	3	163
QUICHE									
TAKE-OUT									
cheese	⅛ (9 in) pie	566	1	1535	52	1	317	2	232
lorraine	⅛ (9 in) pie	568	1	1400	52	1	230	2	267
mushroom	1 slice (3 oz)	256	1	745	–	tr	180	1	–
spinach	⅛ (9 in) pie	342	1	1595	80	5	223	2	275
QUINCE									
fresh	1	53	–	37	–	14	10	1	181
QUINOA									
quinoa not prep	1 cup (6 oz)	636	10	0	83	0	102	16	1258
Eden									
Quinoa not prep	¼ cup	180	11	200	32	0	20	3	260
Seeds Of Change									
French Herb Quinoa Blend as prep	1 cup	290	3	1000	16	0	40	3	–
RABBIT									
domestic w/o bone roasted	3 oz	167	0	–	9	0	16	2	325
wild w/o bone stewed	3 oz	147	0	–	–	–	15	4	292

FOOD	PORTION	CALS	FIBER	VIT A	FOLIC	VIT C	CALCI	IRON	POTAS
RACCOON									
roasted	3 oz	217	0	–	–	–	–	–	–
RADICCHIO									
raw shredded	½ cup	5	–	5	12	2	4	–	60
RADISHES									
chinese dried	½ cup	157	–	0	–	0	165	4	2027
chinese raw	1 (12 oz)	62	–	0	–	74	91	1	767
chinese raw sliced	½ cup	8	–	0	–	10	12	tr	100
chinese sliced cooked	½ cup	13	–	0	–	11	12	tr	211
daikon dried	½ cup	157	–	0	–	0	365	4	2027
daikon raw	1 (12 oz)	62	–	0	–	74	91	1	767
daikon raw sliced	½ cup	8	–	0	–	10	12	tr	100
daikon sliced cooked	½ cup	13	–	0	–	11	12	tr	211
red raw	10	7	–	3	12	10	9	tr	104
red sliced	½ cup	10	–	4	16	13	12	tr	134
white icicle raw	1 (0.5 oz)	2	–	0	2	5	5	tr	48
white icicle raw sliced	½ cup	7	–	0	7	15	14	tr	140
Eden									
Daikon Dried Shredded	2 tbsp	45	3	0	–	0	60	1	420
Frieda's									
Black	¾ cup	15	1	0	–	18	0	0	–
Chinese Lo Bok	⅔ cup	25	2	0	–	18	20	0	–
Daikon	½ cup	15	0	100	–	9	0	0	–
Korean Moo	⅔ cup	15	1	0	–	18	20	0	–
TAKE-OUT									
korean kimchee	½ cup	31	–	–	–	7	3	–	–
moo namul saengche korean salad	1 serv (3.7 oz)	34	2	81	15	13	19	tr	247
RAISINS									
cinnamon coated	¼ cup	108	1	0	2	1	18	1	271
cooked	¼ cup	162	1	0	1	1	18	1	232
golden seedless	¼ cup	109	1	0	1	1	19	1	270
jumbo golden	¼ cup	130	2	0	–	0	20	1	–
milk chocolate coated	28 (1 oz)	109	1	24	2	tr	24	tr	144
milk chocolate coated	¼ cup	176	2	38	3	tr	39	1	231
seedless	55 (1 oz)	86	1	0	1	1	14	1	214
sultanas	1 oz	88	2	20	–	0	18	1	–

FOOD	PORTION	CALS	FIBER	VIT A	FOLIC	VIT C	CALCI	IRON	POTAS
Amazin'									
Raisin All Flavors	1 oz	84	2	0	–	0	20	1	–
Brach's									
California Chocolate Covered	35 pieces	170	1	0	–	0	0	1	–
Earthbound Farm									
Organic Jumbo Flame Seedless	¼ cup	120	2	0	–	1	20	1	–
Estee									
Chocolate Covered Fructose Sweetened	¼ cup	180	1	–	–	–	–	–	–
Goodniks									
Yogurt Raisins	3 tbsp	145	1	0	–	0	60	tr	–
Newman's Own									
Organic	¼ cup	130	2	–	–	–	–	–	310
Sun-Maid									
California Golden	¼ cup	130	2	0	–	0	20	1	310
California Seedless	¼ cup	130	2	0	–	0	20	1	310
Sunsweet									
Red Flame	¼ cup	130	2	0	–	0	20	1	310

RASPBERRIES

FOOD	PORTION	CALS	FIBER	VIT A	FOLIC	VIT C	CALCI	IRON	POTAS
canned in heavy syrup	½ cup	117	–	43	13	11	14	1	120
fresh	1 cup	61	–	160	–	31	27	1	187
fresh	1 pint	154	–	406	–	78	69	2	474
frozen sweetened	1 cup	256	–	149	65	41	38	2	285
frozen sweetened	1 pkg (10 oz)	291	–	169	74	47	43	2	324
frzn unsweetened	¾ cup	130	2	500	–	36	40	2	–
C&W									
Ultimate Red	¾ cup	70	7	0	–	24	20	1	
Europe's Best									
Raspberries frzn	¾ cup	60	2	100	–	24	20	tr	–
Frieda's									
Dried	⅓ cup (1.4 oz)	145	6	50	–	5	30	1	–

RASPBERRY JUICE
Naked Juice
FOOD	PORTION	CALS	FIBER	VIT A	FOLIC	VIT C	CALCI	IRON	POTAS
Raspberry Ade	8 oz	90	0	0	–	6	20	0	60

FOOD	PORTION	CALS	FIBER	VIT A	FOLIC	VIT C	CALCI	IRON	POTAS
Old Orchard									
Organic 100% Juice	8 oz	120	–	0	–	78	0	tr	280
RED BEANS									
Bean Cuisine									
Pasta & Beans Barcelona Red With Radiatore	1 serv	210	4	1000	–	42	60	3	–
RELISH									
cranberry orange	½ cup	246	–	97	–	25	15	tr	53
hamburger	1 tbsp	19	–	40	–	tr	1	tr	11
hamburger	½ cup	158	–	325	–	3	5	1	93
hot dog	½ cup	111	–	203	–	1	7	2	95
hot dog	1 tbsp	14	–	25	–	tr	1	tr	12
piccalilli	1.4 oz	13	1	–	–	0	10	tr	–
sweet	½ cup	159	–	189	–	1	4	1	30
sweet	1 tbsp	19	–	23	–	tr	0	tr	4
Del Monte									
Hamburger	1 tbsp	20	tr	200	–	0	0	0	–
Hot Dog	1 tbsp	15	tr	0	–	0	0	0	–
Sweet Pickle	1 tbsp	20	0	0	–	0	0	0	–
Frieda's									
Kim Chee	¼ cup	15	1	500	–	6	0	tr	–
Matouk's									
Hot Chow	2 tbsp	20	0	–	–	–	–	–	–
Kuchela	1 tsp	9	0	–	–	–	–	–	–
Patak's									
Brinjal Eggplant Sweet Spicy	1 tbsp	70	1	0	–	0	0	0	–
Garlic	1 tbsp	45	0	0	–	0	0	1	–
Lime Mild	1 tbsp	30	0	0	–	4	0	0	–
Mango Mild	1 tbsp	40	0	0	–	2	0	0	–
Peloponnese									
Sun Dried Tomato	1 tbsp	25	0	0	–	0	0	0	–
RENNIN									
tablet	1 (0.9 g)	1	–	0	–	0	34	tr	3
RHUBARB									
fresh	½ cup	13	–	61	4	5	52	tr	175

FOOD	PORTION	CALS	FIBER	VIT A	FOLIC	VIT C	CALCI	IRON	POTAS
frozen	½ cup	60	–	73	6	3	132	tr	73
frzn as prep w/ sugar	½ cup	139	–	83	6	4	174	tr	115

RICE

FOOD	PORTION	CALS	FIBER	VIT A	FOLIC	VIT C	CALCI	IRON	POTAS
brown long grain cooked	1 cup (6.8 oz)	216	4	0	8	0	20	1	84
brown medium grain cooked	1 cup (6.8 oz)	218	4	0	8	0	20	1	154
glutinous cooked	1 cup (6.1 oz)	169	2	0	2	0	3	tr	17
starch	1 oz	98	–	–	–	–	6	–	2
white long grain cooked	1 cup (5.5 oz)	205	1	0	92	0	16	2	55
white long grain instant cooked	1 cup (5.8 oz)	162	1	0	68	0	13	1	7
white medium grain cooked	1 cup (6.5 oz)	242	1	0	108	0	6	3	54
white short grain cooked	1 cup (6.5 oz)	242	–	0	110	0	2	3	48

A Taste Of Thai

FOOD	PORTION	CALS	FIBER	VIT A	FOLIC	VIT C	CALCI	IRON	POTAS
Coconut Garlic Basil as prep	¾ cup	160	0	0	–	–	0	–	–
Coconut Ginger as prep	¾ cup	190	2	0	–	–	0	–	–
Jasmine not prep	¼ cup	160	0	0	–	–	0	–	–
Yellow Curry as prep	¾ cup	180	0	0	–	–	0	–	–

Amy's

FOOD	PORTION	CALS	FIBER	VIT A	FOLIC	VIT C	CALCI	IRON	POTAS
Bowls Brown Rice & Vegetables	1 pkg (10 oz)	240	5	–	–	–	–	–	–

Buitoni

FOOD	PORTION	CALS	FIBER	VIT A	FOLIC	VIT C	CALCI	IRON	POTAS
Risotto Garden Vegetable	1 serv	210	0	750	–	0	20	tr	–
Risotto Portobello Mushrooms	1 serv	210	0	0	–	0	0	0	–
Risotto Rosemary & Potatoes	1 serv	210	2	100	–	0	20	tr	–
Risotto Tomato Basil	1 serv	210	0	0	–	0	0	0	–

Carolina

FOOD	PORTION	CALS	FIBER	VIT A	FOLIC	VIT C	CALCI	IRON	POTAS
Black Beans & Rice Mix as prep	1 serv	200	5	0	40	0	60	3	–

FOOD	PORTION	CALS	FIBER	VIT A	FOLIC	VIT C	CALCI	IRON	POTAS
Gold as prep	1 cup	160	tr	0	80	0	0	1	–
Spanish Rice Mix as prep	1 serv	180	2	0	80	4	20	2	–
Country Crock									
Chicken Rice w/ Herbs	1 cup	210	1	1000	–	0	0	0	–
Fantastic									
Arborio not prep	¼ cup	160	tr	0	–	0	0	tr	–
Basmati not prep	¼ cup	160	tr	0	–	0	0	tr	–
Jasmine not prep	¼ cup	160	tr	0	–	0	0	tr	–
Gourmet House									
Brown & White not prep	¼ cup	160	1	100	–	0	0	1	113
Lundberg									
Eco-Farmed Black Japonica not prep	¼ cup	170	3	0	–	0	0	1	–
Eco-Farmed Brown California Basmati not prep	¼ cup	160	2	0	–	0	0	tr	–
Eco-Farmed White California Arborio not prep	¼ cup	10	1	0	–	0	0	0	–
Organic Brown Golden Rose not prep	¼ cup	160	1	0	–	0	20	1	–
Organic Rice Sensations Ginger Miso not prep	½ cup	116	1	350	–	0	0	tr	59
Organic Risotto Porcini Mushroom not prep	½ cup	143	1	0	–	0	0	0	–
Organic White Sushi Rice not prep	¼ cup	150	1	0	–	0	0	0	–
Organic Wild Blend not prep	¼ cup	150	3	0	–	0	0	tr	–
RiceXpress Chicken Herb	½ pkg (4.4 oz)	250	6	500	–	1	0	tr	76
RiceXpress Santa Fe Grill	½ pkg (4.4 oz)	260	3	200	–	2	20	1	110
Risotto Butternut Squash not prep	½ cup	143	1	1000	–	1	20	1	35
Mahatma									
Jambalaya as prep	1 cup	190	1	1500	–	1	20	tr	–

FOOD	PORTION	CALS	FIBER	VIT A	FOLIC	VIT C	CALCI	IRON	POTAS
Nacho Cheese Mix as prep	1 serv	250	tr	300	80	0	60	2	–
Thai Jasmine as prep	¾ cup	160	2	0	60	0	0	1	–
Marrakesh Express									
Pilaf Tomato & Basil as prep	1 cup	190	0	100	–	0	40	2	–
Risotto Parmesan as prep	1 cup	200	1	0	–	0	20	0	–
Near East									
Creative Grains Chicken & Herb as prep	1 cup	270	6	300	–	0	20	1	–
Creative Grains Creamy Parmesan as prep	1 cup	280	3	200	–	0	80	1	–
Creative Grains Roasted Garlic as prep	1 cup	220	5	0	–	0	20	1	–
Creative Grains Roasted Pecan as prep	1 cup	240	4	0	–	0	20	1	–
Long Grain & Wild Rice Garlic & Herb as prep	1 cup	220	2	100	–	0	20	1	–
Long Grain & Wild Rice Roasted Vegetable & Chicken as prep	1 cup	220	2	400	–	6	20	1	–
Pilaf Brown Rice as prep	1 cup	210	3	400	–	0	20	1	–
Pilaf Chicken as prep	1 cup	220	2	100	–	9	20	1	–
Pilaf Mix Curry as prep	1 cup	220	2	500	–	4	20	1	–
Pilaf Mix Garlic & Herb as prep	1 cup	220	1	0	–	0	0	tr	–
Pilaf Mix Long Grain & Wild as prep	1 cup	220	2	300	–	2	20	1	–
Pilaf Mix Rice as prep	1 cup	220	1	100	–	0	0	tr	–
Pilaf Mix Roasted Chicken & Garlic as prep	1 cup	220	2	100	–	0	20	tr	–
Pilaf Mix Spanish Rice as prep	1 cup	310	2	500	–	18	20	1	–
Pilaf Mix Toasted Almond as prep	1 cup	230	2	100	–	0	20	1	–

FOOD	PORTION	CALS	FIBER	VIT A	FOLIC	VIT C	CALCI	IRON	POTAS
Pilaf Mix Wild Mushroom & Herb as prep	1 cup	220	2	100	–	0	20	1	–
Nueva Cocina									
Arroz A La Mexicana	1 cup	190	2	1250	–	6	40	2	–
Arroz Con Pollo	1 cup	150	1	500	–	18	–	2	–
Gallo Pinto	⅓ pkg	220	3	200	–	2	–	2	–
Moros Y Cristianos	⅓ pkg	220	3	200	–	–	40	2	–
Paella	⅓ pkg	160	1	500	–	18	–	2	–
Pacific Foods									
Ready-To-Serve Lemon & Herb	½ pkg	240	1	0	–	0	20	1	–
Ready-To-Serve Roasted Chicken	½ pkg	240	1	100	–	0	20	1	–
Ready-To-Serve Spanish Style	½ pkg	230	1	100	–	0	20	1	–
Ready-To-Serve Wild Rice & Mushroom	½ pkg	230	1	100	–	0	20	1	–
Patak's									
Basmati	1 pkg	430	2	0	–	0	20	1	0
Coconut	1 pkg	500	4	0	–	0	40	1	0
Yellow	1 pkg	440	2	0	–	0	40	1	0
Rice Expressions									
Indian Basmati	1 cup	180	tr	0	–	0	0	0	–
Organic Brown	1 cup	160	3	0	–	0	0	0	–
Organic Long Grain	1 cup	180	tr	0	–	0	0	0	–
Organic Rice Pilaf	1 cup	170	2	3000	–	5	20	1	–
Organic Tex Mex	1 cup	190	tr	0	–	0	0	0	–
Rice Select									
Royal Blend w/ Lentils	1 serv	130	1	–	–	–	–	–	–
Royal Blend w/ Red Beans	1 serv	130	2	–	–	–	–	–	–
Texmati Brown	1 serv	170	2	–	–	–	–	–	–
Texmati Light Brown	1 serv	170	1	–	–	–	–	–	–
River Rice									
Brown Long Grain not prep	¼ cup	150	tr	0	–	0	0	1	–
S&W									
Arborio as prep	¾ cup	150	tr	0	60	0	0	1	–
Basmati Mix as prep	¾ cup	160	0	0	60	0	0	1	–

FOOD	PORTION	CALS	FIBER	VIT A	FOLIC	VIT C	CALCI	IRON	POTAS
Brown Long Grain not prep	¼ cup	150	1	0	–	0	0	1	–
Long Grain Organic not prep	¼ cup	150	0	0	–	0	0	1	–
Seeds Of Change									
Moroccan Lentil Rice Pilaf as prep	1 cup	180	3	750	16	1	20	1	–
Tuscan Rice & Beans as prep	1 cup	180	2	750	16	0	20	1	–
Success									
Boil-In-Bag Brown as prep	1 cup	150	2	0	–	0	0	tr	–
Boil-In-Bag Jasmine as prep	¾ cup	150	0	0	60	0	0	1	–
Boil-In-Bag White as prep	1 cup	190	1	0	80	0	20	1	–
Ready To Serve Brown	1 cup	170	2	0	8	0	20	tr	–
Ready To Serve White	1 pkg	190	0	0	80	0	20	1	–
Ready To Serve Yellow Rice Mix	1 pkg	190	1	0	60	0	40	1	–
Whole Grain Herb Roasted Chicken as prep	1 cup	290	3	0	–	21	20	1	–
Whole Grain Multigrain Pilaf as prep	1 cup	230	3	1000	–	2	40	1	–
Whole Grain Portobello Mushroom as prep	1 cup	220	3	0	–	4	40	1	–
TastyBite									
Pilaf Curried Vegetable	½ pkg (4.5 oz)	180	9	0	–	1	50	4	–
Pilaf Green Peas	½ pkg (4.5 oz)	208	4	0	–	1	20	1	–
Pilaf Vegetable Kofta	½ pkg (4.5 oz)	229	7	0	–	8	30	1	–
Uncle Ben's									
Boil-In-Bag	1 cup	190	1	0	80	0	0	2	–
Country Inn Chicken & Broccoli as prep	1 cup	190	1	750	120	12	20	4	–
Country Inn Chicken & Vegetables as prep	1 cup	200	1	750	120	2	20	4	–

FOOD	PORTION	CALS	FIBER	VIT A	FOLIC	VIT C	CALCI	IRON	POTAS
Country Inn Mexican Fiesta as prep	1 cup	200	1	500	120	9	40	4	–
Country Inn Oriental Fried as prep	1 cup	200	1	1000	120	2	20	4	–
Country Inn Three Cheese as prep	1 cup	200	1	0	100	0	60	3	–
Country Inn Wheat	1 cup	200	1	0	100	0	20	4	–
Fast & Natural	1 cup	190	2	0	–	0	0	tr	–
Flavorful Four Cheese as prep	1 cup	190	1	0	100	0	60	2	–
Flavorful Garlic & Butter as prep	1 cup	200	tr	0	–	0	40	tr	–
Flavorful Lemon & Herb as prep	1 cup	200	tr	0	–	1	40	tr	–
Flavorful Spanish as prep	1 cup	200	tr	200	–	2	40	tr	–
Instant	1 cup	190	1	0	80	0	20	2	–
Long Grain & Wild Butter Herb as prep	1 cup	190	1	100	100	2	40	4	–
Long Grain & Wild Fast Cook as prep	1 cup	200	1	200	80	4	2	2	–
Long Grain & Wild Original as prep	1 cup	200	1	300	100	5	60	3	–
Long Grain & Wild Roasted Garlic as prep	1 cup	200	1	200	80	4	40	3	–
Ready Rice Long Grain & Wild as prep	1 cup	240	1	100	–	1	40	1	80
Ready Rice Original as prep	1 cup	230	1	0	–	0	40	1	65
Ready Rice Roasted Chicken as prep	1 cup	230	1	0	–	0	40	1	60
Ready Rice Teriyaki as prep	1 cup	190	1	0	–	0	40	1	–
Ready Rice Whole Grain Brown	1 cup	220	1	0	–	0	0	1	115
White Original as prep	1 cup	170	0	–	80	0	20	2	–
Water Maid									
White Medium Grain not prep	¼ cup	160	tr	0	80	0	0	1	–

FOOD	PORTION	CALS	FIBER	VIT A	FOLIC	VIT C	CALCI	IRON	POTAS
TAKE-OUT									
coconut rice	1 serv	500	2	–	–	–	–	–	–
congee	½ cup (4.1 oz)	44	–	–	–	–	4	tr	13
nasi goreng (fried rice)	1 serv	206	5	–	–	–	–	–	–
nasi goreng indonesian rice & vegetables	1 cup (4.9 oz)	130	1	2250	–	5	20	1	–
paella	1 serv (7 oz)	308	3	0	–	10	52	3	386
pilaf	½ cup	84	3	726	24	15	21	1	206
risotto	1 serv (6.6 oz)	426	3	730	–	tr	46	1	–
spanish	¾ cup	363	–	763	14	26	22	2	369

RICE CAKES

Lundberg

FOOD	PORTION	CALS	FIBER	VIT A	FOLIC	VIT C	CALCI	IRON	POTAS
Eco-Farmed Apple Cinnamon	1 (0.7 oz)	80	tr	100	–	0	0	0	75
Eco-Farmed Brown Rice Salt Free	1 (0.7 oz)	70	tr	0	–	0	0	0	63
Eco-Farmed Toasted Sesame	1 (0.7 oz)	70	1	0	–	0	20	0	65
Organic Caramel Corn	1 (0.7 oz)	80	1	0	–	1	0	0	40
Organic Green Tea w/ Lemon	1 (0.7 oz)	80	1	0	–	0	0	0	–
Organic Mochi Sweet	1 (0.7 oz)	70	tr	0	–	0	0	0	65

Mr. Krispers

FOOD	PORTION	CALS	FIBER	VIT A	FOLIC	VIT C	CALCI	IRON	POTAS
Baked Rice Krisps Barbecue	37	110	1	0	–	0	20	tr	–
Baked Rice Krisps Nacho	37	120	1	100	–	1	20	tr	–
Baked Rice Krisps Sea Salt & Pepper	37	110	1	0	–	0	0	tr	–
Baked Rice Krisps Sour Cream & Onion	37	110	1	0	–	0	20	tr	–

Tastemorr

FOOD	PORTION	CALS	FIBER	VIT A	FOLIC	VIT C	CALCI	IRON	POTAS
Rice Crisps Caramel	7	55	0	–	–	–	–	–	–

FOOD	PORTION	CALS	FIBER	VIT A	FOLIC	VIT C	CALCI	IRON	POTAS
ROCKFISH									
pacific cooked	1 fillet (5.2 oz)	180	0	327	–	–	18	1	774
pacific cooked	3 oz	103	0	186	–	–	10	tr	442
pacific raw	3 oz	80	0	162	–	–	8	tr	344
ROE									
fresh baked	1 oz	58	0	86	26	5	8	tr	80
ROLL									
FROZEN									
Alexia									
Ciabatta	1 (1.5 oz)	100	1	0	–	2	40	tr	–
French	1 (1.5 oz)	100	1	0	–	4	20	tr	–
Three Cheese Focaccia	1 (1.5 oz)	110	tr	100	–	2	40	tr	–
Whole Grain	1 (1.5 oz)	90	3	0	–	4	20	1	–
Eggo									
Toaster Swirlz Cinnamon Roll Minis	4 (1.6 oz)	120	tr	500	16	0	40	2	25
Pepperidge Farm									
Hearth Fired Hearty Wheat Dinner Roll	1	120	2	0	–	0	0	1	–
Pillsbury									
Dinner Rolls Crusty French	1	110	0	0	–	0	0	2	–
Sara Lee									
Deluxe Cinnamon Rolls w/ Icing	1 (2.7 oz)	320	1	300	–	0	20	1	–
READY-TO-EAT									
bialy	1 (2.2 oz)	138	1	–	–	–	–	–	–
brioche sweet roll	1 (3.5 oz)	410	3	950	–	tr	43	2	201
brown & serve	1 (1 oz)	85	–	–	8	–	34	1	38
cheese	1 (2.3 oz)	238	–	–	–	–	78	1	–
cinnamon raisin	1 (2¾ in)	223	1	129	14	1	43	1	67
dinner	1 (1 oz)	85	–	–	8	–	34	1	38
egg	1 (2½ in)	107	1	–	–	0	21	1	–
french	1 (1.3 oz)	105	–	–	–	0	35	1	43
hamburger	1 (1.5 oz)	123	–	–	–	–	60	1	60
hamburger multi-grain	1 (1.5 oz)	113	2	–	–	0	41	2	–

FOOD	PORTION	CALS	FIBER	VIT A	FOLIC	VIT C	CALCI	IRON	POTAS
hamburger reduced calorie	1 (1.5 oz)	84	3	–	–	–	26	1	34
hard	1 (3½ in)	167	–	0	8	0	54	2	61
hot cross bun	1	202	1	220	–	0	72	1	–
hot dog	1 (1.5 oz)	123	–	–	–	–	60	1	60
hot dog reduced calorie	1 (1.5 oz)	84	3	–	–	–	26	1	34
hot dog whole wheat	1 (1.5 oz)	110	2	0	–	0	20	1	–
kaiser	1 (3½ in)	167	–	0	8	0	54	2	61
oat bran	1 (1.2 oz)	78	1	–	–	0	28	1	–
rye	1 (1 oz)	81	–	–	–	0	9	1	51
submarine	1 (4.7 oz)	155	–	0	–	0	24	1	49
wheat	1 (1 oz)	77	–	0	–	0	50	1	–
whole wheat	1 (1 oz)	75	–	0	8	0	30	1	77
Alvarado Street Bakery									
Sprouted Wheat Burger Bun	1 (2.2 oz)	140	3	0	–	0	0	1	–
Country Kitchen									
Wheat Light	1	80	4	0	32	0	60	1	–
Natural Ovens									
Best Burger Bun	1	178	3	500	40	12	50	2	–
Better Wheat Buns	1	140	5	0	80	0	150	2	–
Gourmet Dinner	1	70	4	0	0	0	100	1	0
Nature's Own									
100% Whole Grain Sugar Free	1 (1.9 oz)	110	4	0	16	0	40	1	–
Butter Buns	1 (1.7 oz)	120	1	0	40	0	40	1	–
Pepperidge Farm									
Kaiser Soft 100% Whole Wheat	1	200	3	–	–	–	–	–	–
Sara Lee									
Hamburger Bun Classic	1 (2.6 oz)	200	1	0	60	0	100	2	–
Hamburger Bun Classic Wheat	1 (2.6 oz)	200	3	0	60	0	60	3	–
Heart Healthy Hamburger Bun Wheat	1 (2.6 oz)	190	3	0	80	0	60	2	–
Hot Dog Gourmet	1 (1.5 oz)	120	tr	0	40	0	40	1	–

FOOD	PORTION	CALS	FIBER	VIT A	FOLIC	VIT C	CALCI	IRON	POTAS
Super Bakery									
Daily Donut Reduced Fat	1 (2.2 oz)	200	1	1500	140	30	150	7	–
Organic Sandwich Bun	1 (3.6 oz)	250	10	0	–	0	0	2	–
Sub Roll	1 (3.6 oz)	250	10	0	–	0	0	1	–
REFRIGERATED									
cinnamon w/ frosting	1	109	–	–	–	–	10	1	19
crescent	1 (1 oz)	98	–	0	–	0	6	1	45
Pillsbury									
Crecents Reduced Fat	1 (1 oz)	100	0	0	–	0	0	1	–
Crescent	1 (1.7 oz)	170	tr	0	–	0	0	1	–
ROSE APPLE									
fresh	3.5 oz	32	–	tr	–	22	20	1	–
ROSE HIP									
fresh	1 oz	26	–	–	–	tr	73	tr	83
ROSELLE									
fresh	1 cup	28	–	163	–	7	123	1	118
ROSEMARY									
dried	1 tsp	4	–	38	–	1	15	tr	11
ROUGHY									
orange baked	3 oz	75	0	–	–	–	–	tr	–
RUTABAGA									
cooked mashed	½ cup	41	–	0	19	26	50	1	344
raw cubed	½ cup	25	–	0	14	18	33	tr	236
Glory									
Cut Fresh	1 cup	50	4	750	–	36	60	1	–
SABLEFISH									
baked	3 oz	213	0	–	–	–	–	1	390
fillet baked	5.3 oz	378	0	–	–	–	–	2	693
smoked	1 oz	72	0	–	–	–	–	–	132
smoked	3 oz	218	0	–	–	–	–	–	401
SAFFLOWER									
seeds dried	1 oz	147	–	–	–	–	22	–	–

FOOD	PORTION	CALS	FIBER	VIT A	FOLIC	VIT C	CALCI	IRON	POTAS
SAFFRON									
saffron	1 tsp	2	–	–	–	–	1	tr	12
SAGE									
ground	1 tsp	2	–	41	–	tr	12	tr	7
SALAD									
Dole									
American Blend	1½ cups	15	1	1250	–	12	20	tr	–
Baby Spinach Salad	1½ cups (3 oz)	20	2	5500	–	24	80	3	–
Butter & Red Leaf	1½ cups (3 oz)	10	1	1250	–	6	40	0	–
Classic Iceberg	1½ cups (3 oz)	15	1	1750	–	6	20	0	–
Classic Romaine	1½ cups (3 oz)	15	1	3500	–	21	40	1	–
European Blend	1½ cups (3 oz)	15	1	1000	–	9	20	tr	–
Field Greens	1½ cups (3 oz)	15	2	3000	–	5	40	0	–
French Blend	1½ cups (3 oz)	15	2	4450	–	6	20	0	–
Greener Selection	1½ cups (3 oz)	15	1	2000	–	12	20	1	–
Hearts Delight	1½ cups (3 oz)	15	1	2000	–	15	40	1	–
Italian Blend	1½ cups (3 oz)	15	1	2000	–	18	20	1	–
Kits Asian Crunch	1½ cups (3.5 oz)	120	2	2000	–	21	20	1	–
Kits Bacon Lettuce Toss	1½ cups (3.5 oz)	130	1	1750	–	4	20	tr	–
Kits Caesar	1½ cups (3 oz)	170	2	1750	–	15	60	1	–
Kits Caesar Light	1½ cups (3 oz)	100	1	1750	–	18	60	1	–
Kits Fall Harvest	1½ cups (3.5 oz)	150	–	2500	–	9	40	1	–
Kits Romano	1½ cups (3 oz)	150	2	1500	–	15	40	1	–

FOOD	PORTION	CALS	FIBER	VIT A	FOLIC	VIT C	CALCI	IRON	POTAS
Kits Spring Garden	1½ cups (3.5 oz)	140	2	8000	–	12	20	3	–
Kits Sunflower Ranch	1½ cups (3 oz)	160	2	2000	–	6	100	tr	–
Mediterranean Blend	1½ cups	15	2	1250	–	5	40	tr	–
Very Veggie Blend	1½ cups (3 oz)	20	1	3500	–	15	20	1	–
Earthbound Farm									
Organic Baby Arugula Salad	2 cups	20	1	2000	–	12	150	1	–
Organic Baby Lettuce Salad	2 cups	15	1	7000	–	18	60	4	–
Organic Baby Spinach Salad	2 cups	10	7	4500	–	21	60	5	–
Organic Fresh Herb Salad	2 cups	15	2	6000	–	36	80	4	–
Organic Mixed Baby Greens	2 cups	15	2	5500	–	30	60	4	–
Fresh Express									
Baby Spinach Trio	4 cups (3 oz)	20	1	7000	–	21	80	2	–
Krakus									
Bordeaux	1 pkg (5 oz)	35	2	2000	–	6	80	1	–
Mann's									
Rainbow	3 oz	25	2	2500	48	54	40	1	260
Ready Pac									
All American	2.5 cups	15	1	2250	–	4	20	1	–
Bowl Salad Chef	1 pkg	350	2	750	–	6	350	1	–
Bowl Salad Chicken Caesar	1 pkg	380	2	2500	–	24	350	2	–
Bowl Salad Greek	1 pkg	400	3	2000	–	21	150	1	–
Bowl Salad Spinach Bacon	1 pkg	300	1	2000	–	4	150	1	–
Bowl Salad Spring Mix Veggie	1 pkg	330	3	2500	–	48	300	2	–
Caesar Romaine	1½ cups	15	1	1000	–	5	20	1	–
Classic Crisp Salad	2¼ cups	10	tr	750	–	9	20	2	–
Continental	3 cups	20	2	2000	–	15	40	tr	–
Costa Brava	3 cups	15	2	3000	–	15	40	tr	–

FOOD	PORTION	CALS	FIBER	VIT A	FOLIC	VIT C	CALCI	IRON	POTAS
Hearty Green Salad	2½ cups	10	tr	750	–	9	20	2	–
Lafayette	3 cups	10	1	750	–	5	20	tr	–
Milano	3 cups	15	2	1000	–	9	40	1	–
Organic Caesar Romaine	2¼ cups	15	tr	400	–	9	20	2	–
Organic Mesclun Blend	1 pkg (4.5 oz)	35	3	2000	–	6	40	1	–
Organic Monterey	3 cups	15	2	3000	–	18	40	1	–
Parisian	2 cups	20	1	2250	–	12	40	1	–
Portofino	1 pkg (5 oz)	25	2	3000	–	0	150	1	–
Santa Barbara	3½ cups	15	tr	750	–	0	20	tr	–
Spring Mix	1 pkg (5 oz)	35	3	2000	–	6	40	1	–
River Ranch									
American Blend	1½ cups	15	1	2750	60	9	20	tr	–
Caesar Kit	1½ cups	110	2	2000	100	18	60	1	–
European Blend	1¾ cups	10	1	750	60	6	20	1	–
Garden	1½ cups	15	1	2500	40	6	<20	tr	–
Garden Supreme	1½ cups	15	1	3000	60	12	20	1	–
Italian Blend	1¾ cups	15	1	2000	100	18	40	1	–
Raspberry Vinaigrette Kit	1¾ cups	130	2	1250	100	15	20	1	–
Riviera Blend	1½ cups	10	tr	780	60	6	20	tr	–
TAKE-OUT									
7-layer salad	2 cups	557	3	820	81	18	150	2	324
caesar	4 cups	734	7	4170	415	73	372	5	873
chef salad w/o dressing	3 cups	535	–	2106	202	33	469	4	802
chef w/o dressing	1½ cups	386	–	1197	56	15	317	3	330
cobb w/ dressing	4 cups	645	11	2065	258	44	243	3	1383
greek w/ dressing	4 cups	424	4	2165	160	20	491	4	714
mixed salad greens shredded	1 cup	9	1	695	59	9	26	1	160
somen w/ lettuce egg fish pork	2 cups	550	4	865	93	7	109	4	669
spinach no dressing	4 cups	429	6	2650	275	26	181	5	926
tossed w/ avocado w/o dressing	2 cups	90	5	1115	64	13	31	1	473

FOOD	PORTION	CALS	FIBER	VIT A	FOLIC	VIT C	CALCI	IRON	POTAS
tossed w/ chicken w/o dressing	3 cups	194	2	230	51	16	49	2	535
tossed w/ egg w/o dressing	2 cups	93	2	1495	51	10	49	1	347
tossed w/ seafood w/o dressing	3 cups	120	3	885	68	21	142	2	559
tossed w/ shrimp & egg w/o dressing	3 cups	185	2	370	57	11	219	3	351
tossed w/o dressing	2 cups	22	2	110	36	5	31	tr	240
waldorf	1 cup	242	3	110	21	5	26	1	196
wilted lettuce w/ bacon dressing	1 cup	99	1	1860	36	16	38	1	236

SALAD DRESSING
MIX
A Taste Of Thai
FOOD	PORTION	CALS	FIBER	VIT A	FOLIC	VIT C	CALCI	IRON	POTAS
Peanut Dressing as prep	2 tbsp	40	1	0	–	–	40	–	–

READY-TO-EAT
FOOD	PORTION	CALS	FIBER	VIT A	FOLIC	VIT C	CALCI	IRON	POTAS
blue cheese	1 tbsp	77	–	32	–	tr	12	0	–
french	1 tbsp	67	–	–	–	–	2	tr	12
french reduced calorie	1 tbsp	22	–	–	–	–	2	tr	13
italian	1 tbsp	69	–	–	–	–	1	0	2
italian reduced calorie	1 tbsp	16	–	–	–	–	0	0	2
russian	1 tbsp	76	–	106	–	1	3	tr	24
russian reduced calorie	1 tbsp	23	–	–	–	–	3	tr	26
thousand island	1 tbsp	59	–	50	–	–	2	tr	18
thousand island reduced calorie	1 tbsp	24	–	49	–	–	2	tr	17

Annie's Naturals
FOOD	PORTION	CALS	FIBER	VIT A	FOLIC	VIT C	CALCI	IRON	POTAS
Organic Buttermilk	2 tbsp	70	–	–	–	–	20	–	–
Organic Papaya Poppy Seed	2 tbsp	120	–	–	–	2	–	–	–

Bernstein's
FOOD	PORTION	CALS	FIBER	VIT A	FOLIC	VIT C	CALCI	IRON	POTAS
Chunky Blue Cheese	2 tbsp	120	0	0	–	0	20	0	–
Creamy Caesar	2 tbsp	120	0	0	–	0	20	0	–
Italian Restaurant Recipe	2 tbsp	120	0	0	–	0	20	0	–
Light Fantastic Roasted Garlic Balsamic	2 tbsp	45	0	0	–	0	0	0	–

FOOD	PORTION	CALS	FIBER	VIT A	FOLIC	VIT C	CALCI	IRON	POTAS
Red Wine & Garlic Italian	2 tbsp	110	0	0	–	0	0	tr	–
Carb Options									
Italian	2 tbsp	70	0	0	–	0	0	0	–
Ranch	2 tbsp	150	0	0	–	0	0	1	–
Ken's									
Bacon Ranch	2 tbsp	140	0	0	–	0	0	0	–
Caesar	2 tbsp	170	0	0	–	0	0	0	–
Country French w/ Vermont Honey	2 tbsp	150	0	200	–	0	0	0	–
Fat Free Italian	2 tbsp	25	0	0	–	0	0	0	–
Fat Free Raspberry Pecan	2 tbsp	50	0	0	–	0	0	0	–
Honey Mustard	2 tbsp	130	0	0	–	0	0	0	–
Italian w/ Aged Romano	2 tbsp	110	0	0	–	0	0	0	–
Lite Chunky Blue Cheese	2 tbsp	80	0	0	–	0	20	0	–
Lite Italian	2 tbsp	50	0	0	–	0	0	0	–
Lite Ranch	2 tbsp	80	0	0	–	0	20	0	–
Lite Red Wine Vinegar & Olive Oil	2 tbsp	50	0	0	–	2	0	0	–
Lite Vinaigrette Balsamic & Basil	2 tbsp	50	0	0	–	0	0	0	–
Red Wine Vinegar & Olive Oil	2 tbsp	120	0	0	–	2	0	0	–
Russian	2 tbsp	140	0	0	–	0	0	0	–
Thousand Island	2 tbsp	140	0	0	–	0	0	0	–
Kraft									
Free French	2 tbsp	50	0	0	–	0	0	0	–
Free Ranch	2 tbsp	50	1	0	–	0	0	0	–
Free Thousand Island	2 tbsp	45	0	0	–	0	0	0	–
LaMartinique									
Blue Cheese Vinaigrette	2 tbsp	160	0	0	–	0	40	0	–
Poppy Seed	2 tbsp	170	0	0	–	0	0	0	–
Milo's									
Gorgonzola Pear Riesling	2 tbsp	70	0	0	–	0	20	0	–
Pomegranate Port	2 tbsp	90	0	0	–	5	20	0	–

FOOD	PORTION	CALS	FIBER	VIT A	FOLIC	VIT C	CALCI	IRON	POTAS
Nasoya									
Creamy Dill	1 tbsp	30	0	0	–	0	0	0	–
Creamy Italian	2 tbsp	70	0	0	–	0	0	0	–
Garden Herb	2 tbsp	60	0	0	–	0	0	0	–
Sesame Garlic	2 tbsp	60	0	0	–	0	0	0	–
Newman's Own									
Caesar	2 tbsp	150	0	0	–	0	20	0	–
Lighten Up Balsamic Vinaigrette	2 tbsp	45	0	–	–	–	–	–	–
Lighten Up Caesar	2 tbsp	70	0	0	–	0	40	0	–
Lighten Up Honey Mustard	2 tbsp	70	0	0	–	0	40	0	–
Lighten Up Low Fat Sesame Ginger	2 tbsp	35	0	0	–	0	0	tr	–
Lighten Up Raspberry & Walnut	2 tbsp	70	0	0	–	0	0	0	–
Old Dutch									
Sweet & Sour	2 tbsp	50	0	0	–	0	0	0	–
Seeds Of Change									
Vinaigrette Balsamic	2 tbsp	60	0	0	–	0	0	0	–
Vinaigrette Greek Feta	2 tbsp	60	0	0	–	0	0	0	–
Vinaigrette Roasted Garlic	2 tbsp	60	0	0	–	0	0	0	–
Vinaigrette Sweet Basil	2 tbsp	60	0	0	–	0	0	0	–
Sonoma									
Creamy Tomato Bacon	2 tbsp	150	0	0	–	0	0	0	–
South Beach Diet									
Balsamic Vinaigrette	2 tbsp	50	0	0	–	0	0	0	–
Italian	2 tbsp	60	0	200	–	0	0	0	–
Ranch	2 tbsp	70	0	–	–	–	–	–	–
Spectrum									
Honey Dijon	2 tbsp	35	0	0	–	0	0	0	0
Organic Creamy Dill	2 tbsp	25	0	0	–	0	0	0	0
Organic Creamy Garlic	2 tbsp	20	0	0	–	0	0	0	0
Organic Greek Goddess	2 tbsp	110	0	0	–	0	20	tr	0
Organic Porcini Mushroom Vinaigrette	2 tbsp	70	0	0	–	0	0	0	0
Organic Rocky Mountain Ranch	2 tbsp	130	0	0	–	0	0	0	0

FOOD	PORTION	CALS	FIBER	VIT A	FOLIC	VIT C	CALCI	IRON	POTAS
Organic Sweet Onion & Garlic	2 tbsp	15	0	0	–	0	0	0	0
Organic Toasted Sesame	2 tbsp	15	0	0	–	0	0	0	0
Organic Omega 3 Balsamic Vinaigrette	2 tbsp	80	0	0	–	6	0	0	0
Organic Omega 3 Ginger Garlic Vinaigrette	2 tbsp	80	0	0	–	6	0	0	0
Organic Omega 3 Raspberry Vinaigrette	2 tbsp	80	0	0	–	6	0	0	0
Provencal Garlic Lover's	2 tbsp	50	0	0	–	0	0	0	0
Zesty Italian	2 tbsp	30	0	0	–	0	0	0	0
Steel's									
Honey Mustard	1 tbsp	90	0	–	–	–	–	–	–
Sweet Ginger Lime	1 tbsp	68	1	–	–	–	–	–	–
Wishbone									
Blue Cheese w/ Gorgonzola	2 tbsp	140	0	0	–	0	0	0	–
Caesar w/ Aged Romano	2 tbsp	80	0	0	–	2	0	0	–
Classic Ranch Extra Thick	2 tbsp	140	0	0	–	0	0	0	–
Creamy Caesar	2 tbsp	170	0	0	–	0	0	0	–
Creamy Italian	2 tbsp	110	0	0	–	1	20	0	–
Deluxe French	2 tbsp	50	tr	400	–	0	0	0	–
Fat Free Chunky Blue Cheese	2 tbsp	35	tr	0	–	0	20	0	–
Fat Free Italian	2 tbsp	20	0	0	–	2	0	0	–
Fat Free Ranch	2 tbsp	30	tr	0	–	0	0	0	–
Five Cheese Italian	2 tbsp	120	0	0	–	1	0	0	–
Italian	2 tbsp	90	0	0	–	2	0	0	–
Just 2 Good Blue Cheese	2 tbsp	45	0	0	–	0	0	0	–
Just 2 Good Creamy Caesar	2 tbsp	50	0	0	–	0	0	0	–
Just 2 Good Deluxe French	2 tbsp	50	tr	400	–	0	0	0	–
Just 2 Good Italian	2 tbsp	35	0	0	–	0	0	0	–
Just 2 Good Ranch	2 tbsp	40	0	0	–	0	0	0	–

FOOD	PORTION	CALS	FIBER	VIT A	FOLIC	VIT C	CALCI	IRON	POTAS
Just 2 Good Thousand Island	2 tbsp	50	0	0	–	0	0	0	–
Just 2 Good Western	2 tbsp	70	0	100	–	0	0	1	–
Light Vinaigrette Asian Sesame	2 tbsp	70	0	0	–	0	0	0	–
Light Vinaigrette Raspberry Walnut	2 tbsp	80	0	0	–	0	0	0	–
Light Ranch Extra Thick	2 tbsp	70	0	0	–	0	0	0	–
Ranch	2 tbsp	160	0	0	–	0	0	0	–
Russian	2 tbsp	110	0	0	–	1	0	0	–
Salad Spritzers Balsamic Breeze	10 sprays	10	0	0	–	0	0	0	–
Salad Spritzers Italian	10 sprays	10	0	0	–	0	0	0	–
Salad Spritzers Red Wine Mist	10 sprays	10	0	0	–	0	0	0	–
Thousand Island	2 tbsp	130	0	0	–	0	20	0	–
Vinaigrette Berry	2 tbsp	50	0	0	–	0	0	0	–
Vinaigrette Lemon Garlic & Herb	2 tbsp	70	0	0	–	4	0	0	–
Vinaigrette Olive Oil	2 tbsp	60	0	0	–	0	0	0	–
Western	2 tbsp	160	0	100	–	0	0	1	–

SALAD TOPPINGS
Salad Pizazz!

FOOD	PORTION	CALS	FIBER	VIT A	FOLIC	VIT C	CALCI	IRON	POTAS
Asian Medley	1 tbsp	40	tr	0	–	0	20	tr	–
Cherry Cranberry Pecano	1 tbsp	35	tr	0	–	0	0	0	–
Honey Toasted Delites	1 tbsp	40	1	0	–	0	0	0	–
Orange Cranberry Almondine	1 tbsp	35	tr	0	–	0	0	0	–
Raspberry Cranberry Walnut Frisco	1 tbsp	30	0	0	–	0	0	0	–
Tomato 'N Bacon Parmesano	1 tbsp	30	tr	100	–	0	20	tr	–
Tomato Pinenut Tuscano	1 tbsp	130	tr	100	–	0	0	tr	–

SALMON
CANNED

FOOD	PORTION	CALS	FIBER	VIT A	FOLIC	VIT C	CALCI	IRON	POTAS
w/ bone	½ cup	106	0	90	10	0	165	1	251

FOOD	PORTION	CALS	FIBER	VIT A	FOLIC	VIT C	CALCI	IRON	POTAS
Bumble Bee									
Blueback	¼ cup	110	0	100	–	0	100	tr	–
Keta	¼ cup	90	0	0	–	0	100	tr	–
Pink	¼ cup	90	0	0	–	0	100	tr	–
Red	¼ cup	110	0	100	–	0	100	tr	–
Skinless & Boneless	¼ cup	50	0	0	–	0	0	0	–
Smoked Fillets In Oil	⅓ cup	150	0	200	–	0	150	1	–
Chicken Of The Sea									
Pink	1 pkg (3 oz)	90	0	0	–	0	0	1	–
Pink Skinless Boneless	¼ cup	60	0	0	–	0	0	tr	–
Red	¼ cup	110	0	100	–	0	100	tr	–
Smoked Pacific	1 pkg (3 oz)	120	0	0	–	1	20	1	–
Libby's									
Alaskan Sockeye Red	¼ cup	110	0	100	–	–	100	tr	–
Pink Skinless Boneless	¼ cup	50	0	0	–	0	0	0	–
Red	¼ cup	110	0	100	–	0	100	tr	–
FRESH									
atlantic farmed baked	4 oz	233	0	57	39	4	17	tr	435
cloudberry native alaska	3.5 oz	51	–	210	–	–	18	1	–
coho wild poached	4 oz	209	0	122	10	1	52	1	516
pink baked	4 oz	169	0	154	6	0	19	1	469
roe raw	1 oz	59	–	–	–	5	–	–	–
sockeye baked	4 oz	245	0	237	6	0	8	1	425
SMOKED									
lox	1 oz	33	0	25	1	0	3	tr	50
TAKE-OUT									
guisado stew salmon	1 serv (7.4 oz)	320	3	125	34	15	276	2	825
roulette w/ spinach stuffing	1 serv (4 oz)	160	tr	1000	–	6	40	1	–
salmon cake	1 (4.2 oz)	264	1	115	24	4	179	1	385
salmon loaf	1 slice (3.7 oz)	206	tr	495	29	2	192	1	287
SALSA									
black bean & corn	2 tbsp	15	tr	0	–	5	20	tr	–
citrus	2 tbsp (1 oz)	10	0	0	–	1	0	0	–

FOOD	PORTION	CALS	FIBER	VIT A	FOLIC	VIT C	CALCI	IRON	POTAS
peach	2 tbsp	15	0	0	–	5	0	tr	–
tomato-less corn & chile	2 tbsp	45	tr	100	–	2	0	0	–
Bone Suckin'									
Fat Free Gluten Free	2 tbsp	40	0	0	–	0	0	0	–
Cape Cod									
Medium & Mild	2 tbsp	15	1	0	–	5	0	0	–
Del Salsa									
Fire Roasted All Flavors	2 tbsp	8	0	–	–	–	–	–	–
Emeril's									
Original Recipe	2 tbsp	10	0	200	–	0	20	tr	–
Gringo Billy's									
Salsa Mix	1 tsp	5	1	–	–	–	–	–	–
Muir Glen									
Black Bean & Corn Medium	2 tbsp (1.1 oz)	15	tr	200	–	4	0	tr	–
Chipotle Medium	2 tbsp (1.1 oz)	10	0	300	–	5	0	tr	–
Fire Roasted Tomato Medium	2 tbsp (1.1 oz)	10	0	300	–	4	0	tr	–
Garlic Cilantro Medium	2 tbsp (1.1 oz)	10	0	200	–	5	0	tr	–
Habanero Hot	2 tbsp (1.1 oz)	10	0	200	–	4	0	tr	–
Organic Medium	2 tbsp (1.1 oz)	10	0	200	–	5	0	tr	–
Organic Mild	2 tbsp (1.1 oz)	10	0	200	–	1	0	tr	–
Roasted Garlic Medium	2 tbsp (1.1 oz)	10	0	200	–	4	0	tr	–
Newman's Own									
Bandito Mild	2 tbsp	10	1	–	–	–	–	–	–
Bandito Peach	2 tbsp	25	tr	750	–	0	0	0	–
Bandito Pineapple	2 tbsp	15	1	–	–	–	–	–	–
Bandito Roasted Garlic	2 tbsp	10	1	–	–	–	–	–	–
Bandito Tequila Lime	2 tbsp	15	–	200	–	0	20	tr	–
Ortega									
Garden Style Mild	2 tbsp	10	tr	400	–	4	–	–	–
Picante Mild	2 tbsp	10	–	–	–	1	–	–	–

FOOD	PORTION	CALS	FIBER	VIT A	FOLIC	VIT C	CALCI	IRON	POTAS
Seeds Of Change									
Black Bean & Tomato Mild	2 tbsp	15	tr	200	–	0	0	tr	–
Garlic & Cilantro Mild	2 tbsp	15	tr	200	–	0	0	tr	–
Snyder's Of Hanover									
Sweet	2 tbsp	20	0	200	–	4	20	0	–
Tostitos									
All Natural	2 tbsp	15	1	100	–	0	0	0	–
Con Queso	2 tbsp	40	tr	100	–	0	40	0	–
Monterey Jack Queso	2 tbsp	40	0	0	–	0	20	0	–
Restaurant Style	2 tbsp	15	tr	200	–	1	0	tr	–
SALSIFY									
fresh sliced cooked	½ cup	46	–	0	–	3	32	tr	192
Frieda's									
Salsify	¾ cup	70	3	0	–	6	60	1	–
SALT SUBSTITUTES									
gomasio sesame salt	2 tsp	34	1	–	–	–	60	1	29
AlsoSalt									
Butter Flavored	¼ tsp	1	0	–	–	–	–	–	320
Garlic Flavored	¼ tsp	1	0	–	–	–	–	–	300
Salt Substitute	¼ tsp	tr	0	–	–	–	–	–	356
Eden									
Organic Seaweed Gomasio Sesame Salt	1 tsp	15	0	0	–	0	20	tr	15
Organic Gomasio Sesame Salt	1 tsp	15	0	0	–	0	20	tr	10
French's									
No Salt	¼ cup	0	0	–	–	–	–	–	650
SALT/SEASONED SALT									
salt	1 tbsp (18 g)	0	0	–	–	–	4	tr	1
salt	1 tsp (6 g)	0	0	–	–	–	1	tr	0
SANDWICHES									
Amy's									
Pocket Sandwich Broccoli & Cheese	1 (4.5 oz)	270	3	–	–	–	–	–	–
Pocket Sandwich Roasted Vegetables	1 (4.5 oz)	220	4	–	–	–	–	–	–

FOOD	PORTION	CALS	FIBER	VIT A	FOLIC	VIT C	CALCI	IRON	POTAS
Pocket Sandwich Spinach Feta	1 (4.5 oz)	250	3	–	–	–	–	–	–
Pocket Sandwich Tofu Scramble	1 (4 oz)	160	tr	–	–	–	–	–	–
Pocket Sandwich Vegetable Pie	1 (5 oz)	300	3	–	–	–	–	–	–
Toaster Pops Grilled Cheese	1	180	0	–	–	–	–	–	–
Guiltless Gourmet									
Wrap California Veggie	1 (5.7 oz)	270	4	500	–	0	100	2	–
Wrap Mediterranean Spinach	1 (5.7 oz)	270	4	3500	–	0	150	2	–
Ian's									
Mini Chicken Patty	2 (5.3 oz)	368	1	0	–	4	0	4	–
Lean Pockets									
Chicken Fajita	1 (4.5 oz)	260	3	400	–	1	200	2	–
Meatballs & Mozzarella	1 (4.5 oz)	290	3	500	–	0	300	3	–
Sausage Egg & Cheese	1 (4.5 oz)	140	2	100	–	1	80	2	–
Turkey & Ham w/ Cheddar	1 (4.5 oz)	280	3	750	–	0	200	2	–
Madalena's Masterpiece									
Calzone Artichoke Parmesan	1 (10 oz)	570	2	500	–	–	500	–	–
Calzone Grilled Chicken	1 (10 oz)	520	1	750	–	–	500	–	–
Calzone Sausage Pepperoni	1 (10 oz)	640	tr	750	–	–	450	–	–
Panini Garlic Chicken	1 (8 oz)	450	2	1500	–	9	400	4	–
Panini Honey Ham	1 (8 oz)	520	tr	300	–	0	350	3	–
Panini Turkey Pesto	1 (8 oz)	500	0	500	–	1	350	–	–
Panini Veggie	1 (8 oz)	480	1	1000	–	27	450	4	–
Quesabake Mexican Sausage	1 (7 oz)	510	2	6500	–	–	900	–	–
Quesabake Roasted Veggie	1 (7 oz)	460	1	1250	–	18	900	3	–

FOOD	PORTION	CALS	FIBER	VIT A	FOLIC	VIT C	CALCI	IRON	POTAS
Smucker's									
Uncrustables Grilled Cheese	1 (1.8 oz)	150	tr	300	–	0	150	1	–
Uncrustables Peanut Butter & Grape Jelly	1 (2 oz)	210	2	0	–	1	20	1	–
Uncrustables Peanut Butter & Strawberry Jam	1 (2 oz)	210	2	0	–	0	20	1	–
South Beach Diet									
Breakfast Wraps All American	1 serv (4.6 oz)	200	15	300	–	1	300	1	–
Breakfast Wraps Denver	1 serv (4.6 oz)	180	15	400	–	15	250	1	–
Breakfast Wraps Southwestern	1 serv (4.6 oz)	160	15	500	–	15	250	1	–
Breakfast Wraps Vegetable Medley	1 serv (4.6 oz)	160	15	400	–	2	250	1	–
Wrap Kit Deli Ham & Turkey	1 pkg	220	15	300	–	0	250	1	–
Wrap Kit Grilled Chicken Caesar	1 pkg	230	14	100	–	0	250	1	–
Wrap Kit Sesame Chicken	1 pkg (6.4 oz)	220	15	0	–	1	100	1	–
Wrap Kit Southwestern Style Chicken	1 pkg	250	15	200	–	9	250	1	–
Wrap Kit Turkey & Bacon Club	1 pkg	250	15	400	–	0	300	1	–
TAKE-OUT									
bacon & egg	1 (6.2 oz)	388	1	830	90	tr	158	3	276
bacon lettuce & tomato w/ mayo	1 (5.8 oz)	344	3	215	74	10	80	2	348
beef barbecue w/ bun	1 (6.7 oz)	417	2	0	94	2	123	5	468
calzone beef & cheese	1 (14 oz)	1476	6	2080	382	0	772	11	683
calzone cheese	1 (15 oz)	1632	5	3200	305	0	1802	9	560
chicken salad	1 (5 oz)	333	2	120	70	1	97	3	210
crab cake w/ bun	1	308	2	260	105	4	174	3	311
croque monsieur	1 (12.4 oz)	765	2	2240	41	9	1089	3	437
egg salad	1 (5.6 oz)	485	1	765	94	0	121	3	157
french dip w/ roll	1 (6.8 oz)	357	1	0	81	0	104	4	347

FOOD	PORTION	CALS	FIBER	VIT A	FOLIC	VIT C	CALCI	IRON	POTAS
fried egg	1 (3.4 oz)	226	1	445	80	0	104	3	117
grilled cheese	1 (2.9 oz)	290	1	645	38	0	235	2	129
gyro	1 (13.7 oz)	593	4	175	164	12	179	6	800
ham & egg	1 (4.4 oz)	272	2	445	82	1	110	3	197
ham w/ cheese w/ lettuce & mayo	1 (5.4 oz)	369	2	102	68	3	260	3	313
peanut butter & jelly	1 (3.3 oz)	327	3	0	78	tr	93	2	222
reuben w/ sauerkraut & cheese	1 (6.4 oz)	463	4	310	63	4	257	3	250
roast beef w/ gravy	1 (7.8 oz)	386	2	0	64	0	91	5	425
sloppy joe pork on bun	1 (6.5 oz)	318	2	10	58	6	93	3	404
tuna melt	1 (5.3 oz)	350	1	315	45	1	165	2	258
tuna salad w/ lettuce	1 (5.9 oz)	289	2	115	68	1	94	3	242
turkey w/ mayo	1 (5 oz)	329	1	54	64	0	100	3	305

SAPODILLA
fresh	1	140	–	102	–	25	36	1	328
fresh cut up	1 cup	199	–	145	–	35	51	2	465

SAPOTES
fresh	1	301	–	923	–	45	88	2	773

SARDINES
CANNED
atlantic in oil w/ bone	2	50	0	54	3	–	92	1	95
atlantic in oil w/ bone	1 can (3.2 oz)	192	0	206	11	–	351	3	365
pacific in tomato sauce w/ bone	1 can (13 oz)	658	0	1351	89	4	887	9	1262
pacific in tomato sauce w/ bone	1	68	0	139	9	tr	91	1	130

Beach Cliff
In Louisiana Hot Sauce	1 can (3.7 oz)	150	0	200	–	0	300	4	–
In Mustard Sauce	1 can (3.7 oz)	150	0	200	–	0	250	5	–
In Olive Oil	1 can (3.7 oz)	200	0	0	–	0	250	2	–
In Tomato Sauce	1 can (3.7 oz)	140	0	200	–	1	250	2	–

FOOD	PORTION	CALS	FIBER	VIT A	FOLIC	VIT C	CALCI	IRON	POTAS
In Water	1 can (3.7 oz)	150	0	200	–	0	250	2	–
Small In Soybean Oil	1 can (3.7 oz)	200	0	200	–	18	100	–	–
Brunswick									
In Louisiana Hot Sauce	1 can (3.7 oz)	150	0	200	–	0	300	4	–
In Mustard Sauce	1 can (3.7 oz)	150	0	200	–	0	250	5	–
In Soybean Oil	1 can (3.7 oz)	110	0	200	–	0	300	2	–
In Spring Water	1 can (3.7 oz)	150	0	200	–	0	250	2	–
In Tomato Sauce	1 can (3.7 oz)	150	0	300	–	1	200	2	220
w/ Hot Green Chilies	1 can (3.7 oz)	180	0	200	–	0	150	3	–
w/ Hot Tabasco Peppers	1 can (3.7 oz)	110	0	100	–	0	250	2	–
Bumble Bee									
In Hot Sauce	¼ cup	90	0	0	–	0	100	1	–
In Mustard	¼ cup	70	1	0	–	0	80	1	–
In Oil	1 can (3.7 oz)	130	0	0	–	0	100	tr	–
In Water	1 can (3.7 oz)	120	0	0	–	0	100	tr	–
Chicken Of The Sea									
In Hot Sauce	1 can (3.75 oz)	130	2	300	–	1	300	1	–
In Mustard Sauce	1 can (3.75 oz)	150	2	0	–	0	300	1	–
In Oil	1 can (3.75 oz)	190	0	0	–	0	200	1	–
In Tomato Sauce	1 can (3.75 oz)	130	2	300	–	2	300	1	–
In Water	1 can (3.75 oz)	100	0	0	–	0	200	1	–
Goya									
In Tomato Sauce	2 pieces (2.2 oz)	50	2	500	–	1	250	1	–

FOOD	PORTION	CALS	FIBER	VIT A	FOLIC	VIT C	CALCI	IRON	POTAS
King Oscar									
In Olive Oil	1 can (3.75 oz)	150	0	450	–	0	220	1	–
Skinless Boneless In Soya Oil	3 pieces (1.9 oz)	120	0	100	–	1	80	1	–
Season									
Brisling In Water	1 can (3.75 oz)	145	0	400	–	0	210	1	–
FRESH									
raw	3.5 oz	135	0	tr	–	–	85	2	–
SAUCE									
JARRED									
fish sauce chinese	1 tbsp	9	0	90	–	0	2	tr	52
fish sauce vietnamese nuoc mam	1 tbsp	6	0	0	9	0	8	tr	52
hoisin	1 tbsp	35	tr	0	4	0	5	tr	19
morroccan tagine	½ cup (4 oz)	70	1	800	–	30	20	1	–
oyster	1 tbsp	8	0	4	2	0	5	tr	9
teriyaki	1 tbsp	15	–	0	4	0	4	tr	41
A Taste Of Thai									
Chili Sauce Garlic Pepper	1 tsp	10	0	100	–	–	–	–	–
Peanut Satay	2 tbsp	80	1	0	–	–	0	–	–
Annie Chun's									
Marinade & Dressing Lemongrass Herb	1 tbsp	25	0	0	–	1	0	0	–
Noodle Sauce & Dressing Sesame Cilantro	1 tbsp	60	0	0	–	0	0	0	–
Shiitake Mushroom	1 tbsp	15	0	0	–	0	0	0	–
Asian Creations									
Marvelous Mango	¼ cup	20	0	750	–	6	0	0	–
Pad Thai Pizzazz	2 oz	110	tr	500	–	6	20	tr	–
Peanut Passion	¼ cup	130	1	500	–	2	20	1	–
Boar's Head									
Ham Glaze Sugar & Spice	2 tbsp	120	0	0	–	0	40	tr	–
Horseradish Sauce Pub Style	1 tsp	15	0	0	0	–	0	0	–

FOOD	PORTION	CALS	FIBER	VIT A	FOLIC	VIT C	CALCI	IRON	POTAS
Bone Suckin'									
Hiccuppin' Hot	1 tsp	10	0	0	–	0	0	0	–
Yaki Stir Fry	1 tbsp	30	0	0	–	0	0	0	–
Carb Options									
Alfredo	¼ cup	110	0	200	–	0	40	0	–
Cheese	¼ cup	90	0	100	–	0	60	0	–
Garden Style	½ cup	80	2	400	–	5	40	1	–
Del Monte									
Seafood Cocktail	¼ cup	100	0	0	–	0	0	0	–
Sloppy Joe Hickory Flavor	¼ cup	60	0	1000	–	1	40	1	–
Sloppy Joe Original	¼ cup	50	0	2250	–	1	20	1	–
Emeril's									
Steak Sauce	1 tbsp	20	–	100	–	1	–	–	–
Fage									
Tzatziki	2 tbsp	30	0	0	–	0	20	0	–
Frank's									
Buffalo Wing Sauce	1 tbsp	5	0	400	–	0	–	–	–
French's									
Worchestershire	1 tsp	0	0	0	–	0	0	0	–
House Of Tsang									
General Tsao	1 tsp	45	0	0	–	0	0	0	–
Hoisin	1 tsp	15	0	0	–	0	0	0	14
Kobe Steak Grill	1 tbsp	50	0	0	–	0	0	0	125
Korean Teriyaki Stir Fry	1 tbsp	35	0	0	–	0	0	0	28
Peanut Sauce Bangkok Padang	1 tbsp	45	0	0	–	0	0	0	41
Spicy Brown Bean	1 tbsp	15	0	0	–	0	0	0	17
Sweet & Sour	1 tbsp	35	0	0	–	0	0	0	20
Sweet Ginger Sesame	1 tbsp	40	0	0	–	0	0	0	47
Thai Peanut	1 tbsp	50	0	0	–	0	0	0	43
Ken's									
Marinade Herb & Garlic	1 tbsp	20	0	0	–	1	0	0	–
Marinade Lemon & Pepper	1 tbsp	10	0	0	–	1	0	0	–
Marinade Teriyaki	1 tbsp	20	0	0	–	0	0	tr	–
Las Palmas									
Enchilada Green	¼ cup	25	0	0	–	4	0	0	–

FOOD	PORTION	CALS	FIBER	VIT A	FOLIC	VIT C	CALCI	IRON	POTAS
Enchilada Mild	¼ cup	20	1	1000	–	0	0	0	–
Red Chili	¼ cup	20	1	500	–	0	0	tr	–
Latino Chef									
Chimichurri Sun Dried Tomato	2 tbsp	120	2	300	–	5	20	1	–
Sofrito	2 tbsp	20	–	300	–	5	–	–	–
Lollipop Tree									
Grilling & Glazing Chipotle	1 tbsp	50	0	100	–	2	0	0	–
Grilling & Glazing Mango Garlic	2 tbsp	60	0	0	–	6	0	0	–
Milo's									
Simmer Sauce Bombay Cabernet	3 oz	35	1	100	–	6	20	1	–
Mrs. Dash									
10 Minute Marinade Mesquite Grille	1 tbsp	25	–	–	–	1	–	–	30
10 Minute Marinade Zesty Garlic Herb	1 tbsp	25	–	–	–	2	–	–	27
Old El Paso									
Enchilada Mild	¼ cup	25	0	100	–	0	0	0	–
Ortega									
Enchilada	¼ cup	15	tr	200	–	–	–	tr	–
Patak's									
Dopiaza	½ cup	90	0	100	–	6	0	tr	–
Jalfrezi Sweet Peppers & Coconut	½ cup	140	1	0	–	4	20	tr	–
Korma Rich Creamy Coconut	½ cup	240	1	0	–	0	0	1	–
Rogan Josh Spicy Tomato & Cardamon	½ cup	90	2	100	–	1	20	tr	–
Tikka Masala Tangy Lemon & Cilantro	½ cup	120	1	0	–	2	0	0	–
Sara Lee									
Horseradish	1 tbsp	20	0	0	–	0	0	0	–
Ty Ling									
Duck	2 tbsp	70	1	–	–	–	–	1	–
Wild Thyme Farms									
Chili Ginger Honey	1 tbsp	30	–	100	–	1	–	–	–

FOOD	PORTION	CALS	FIBER	VIT A	FOLIC	VIT C	CALCI	IRON	POTAS
MIX									
cheese as prep w/ milk	1 cup	307	–	–	–	2	570	tr	554
curry as prep	1 cup	120	–	29	3	1	50	1	99
curry as prep w/ milk	1 cup	270	–	–	–	–	485	–	–
sour cream as prep w/ milk	1 cup	509	–	–	–	–	546	1	733
stroganoff as prep	1 cup	271	–	–	–	–	521	1	672
sweet & sour as prep	1 cup	294	–	–	–	–	41	2	66
teriyaki as prep	1 cup	131	–	–	–	–	112	3	216
white as prep w/ milk	1 cup	241	–	–	–	–	424	tr	443
A Taste Of Thai									
Pad Thai Sauce	2 tbsp	90	1	0	–	–	20	–	–
Peanut Sauce	¼ pkg	45	1	0	–	–	20	–	–
TAKE-OUT									
adobo fresco	2 tbsp	81	1	79	3	2	44	1	67
bearnaise	1 oz	177	tr	–	1	tr	49	tr	63
cucumber yogurt sauce	1½ tbsp	20	0	50	–	4	60	tr	–
enchilada sauce green	¼ cup	46	1	175	0	7	19	tr	134
enchilada sauce red	¼ cup	79	1	390	4	4	16	tr	86
SAUERKRAUT									
canned	½ cup	22	–	21	–	17	36	2	201
B&G									
Sauerkraut	2 tbsp (1 oz)	6	1	0	–	2	0	0	–
Boar's Head									
Sauerkraut	2 tbsp (1 oz)	5	tr	0	–	2	0	0	–
Del Monte									
Bavarian Style	2 tbsp	15	0	0	–	1	0	0	–
Sauerkraut	2 tbsp	0	tr	0	–	1	0	0	–
Eden									
Organic	½ cup	25	3	0	–	12	40	1	160
Hebrew National									
Sauerkraut	2 tbsp	5	1	–	–	2	–	–	–
S&W									
Canned	2 tbsp (1 oz)	5	0	0	–	2	0	0	–
Red Cabbage	2 tbsp (1 oz)	15	0	0	–	1	0	0	–
Silver Floss									
Sauerkraut	½ cup	20	4	0	–	9	0	0	–

FOOD	PORTION	CALS	FIBER	VIT A	FOLIC	VIT C	CALCI	IRON	POTAS
SAUSAGE									
beef & pork	1 link (2.3 oz)	196	0	0	3	0	5	1	187
beef & pork w/ cheddar cheese	1 link (2.7 oz)	228	0	0	2	0	44	1	159
bierschinken	3.5 oz	174	–	–	–	–	15	2	261
bierwurst	3.5 oz	258	0	–	–	–	–	–	–
blutwurst uncooked	3.5 oz	424	0	–	–	–	7	6	38
bockwurst	3.5 oz	276	0	–	–	–	–	–	–
bratwurst pork cooked	1 link (2.5 oz)	226	0	0	4	0	34	1	197
brotwurst pork & beef	1 link (2.5 oz)	226	0	0	4	0	34	1	197
chipolata	3.5 oz	342	0	tr	3	1	16	1	160
chorizo	1 link (2.1 oz)	273	0	0	1	0	5	1	239
fleischwurst	3.5 oz	305	0	–	–	–	14	2	199
free range chicken breakfast	2 links (2.7 oz)	110	0	100	–	0	0	tr	–
gelbwurst uncooked	3.5 oz	363	0	–	–	–	–	–	285
italian pork cooked	1 (2.4 oz)	230	1	21	3	tr	14	1	204
jagdwurst	3.5 oz	211	0	–	–	–	14	3	260
knockwurst pork & beef	1 (2.5 oz)	221	0	0	1	0	8	tr	143
mettwurst uncooked	3.5 oz	483	0	–	–	–	13	2	213
plockwurst uncooked	3.5 oz	312	0	–	–	–	–	–	–
polish kielbasa	2 oz	127	0	0	–	8	–	1	–
pork cooked	2 links (1.7 oz)	163	0	38	1	tr	8	1	141
regensburger uncooked	3.5 oz	354	0	–	–	–	–	–	–
vienna canned	1 can (4 oz)	260	0	0	5	0	11	1	114
vienna canned	1 link (0.5 oz)	37	0	0	1	0	2	tr	16
weisswurst uncooked	3.5 oz	305	0	–	–	–	25	–	122
zungenwurst (tongue)	3.5 oz	285	0	–	–	–	–	–	–
Al Fresco									
Buffalo Style	1 (3 oz)	160	–	500	–	1	20	1	–
Italian Sweet	1 (3 oz)	170	–	100	–	1	20	1	–

FOOD	PORTION	CALS	FIBER	VIT A	FOLIC	VIT C	CALCI	IRON	POTAS
Roasted Garlic	1 (3 oz)	170	–	100	–	1	20	1	–
Sundried Tomato & Basil	1 (3 oz)	180	–	200	–	1	20	1	–
Sweet Apple	1 (3 oz)	160	–	–	–	2	–	1	–
Teriyaki Ginger	1 (3 oz)	180	–	100	–	1	20	1	–
Armour									
Brown'N Serve Lite Original	3	120	0	0	–	0	40	tr	–
Brown'N Serve Turkey	3 links	120	0	0	–	0	40	1	–
Bilinski's									
Chicken Bratworst With Wild Rice	1 (2 oz)	70	0	0	–	1	0	tr	–
Chicken Cajun-Style Andouille	2 oz	80	0	0	–	0	60	1	–
Chicken Italian With Peppers	1 (2 oz)	70	0	100	–	0	60	1	–
Chicken With Apples & Chardonnay	2 oz	70	0	0	–	0	60	1	–
Chicken With Cilantro	2 oz	70	1	300	–	0	–	–	–
Chicken With Jalapenos	2 oz	70	0	100	–	5	–	1	–
Chicken With Pesto	2 oz	90	0	100	–	5	60	1	–
Chicken With Spinach	2 oz	70	1	300	–	0	0	1	–
Chicken With Sun-Dried Tomato	2 oz	70	0	100	–	5	40	1	–
Boar's Head									
Bratwurst	1 (4 oz)	300	0	0	–	0	20	1	–
Hot Smoked	1 (3.2 oz)	250	0	0	–	0	0	1	–
Kielbasa	2 oz	120	0	0	–	0	0	1	–
Knockwurst Beef	1 (4 oz)	310	0	300	–	0	20	1	–
Hebrew National									
Knockwurst Beef	1 (3 oz)	260	0	0	–	0	0	1	–
Jennie-O									
Italian Hot	1 (3.9 oz)	160	–	–	–	–	20	1	–
Turkey Italian Sweet	1 link (3.9 oz)	160	0	0	–	0	20	1	–
Murray's									
Chicken Hot Italian	3 oz	130	–	200	–	0	20	tr	–
Chicken Spinach & Garlic	3 oz	100	–	900	–	5	20	1	–

FOOD	PORTION	CALS	FIBER	VIT A	FOLIC	VIT C	CALCI	IRON	POTAS
Chicken Sun Dried Tomato	3 oz	110	–	100	–	1	20	1	–
Chicken Sweet Italian	3 oz	130	–	0	–	0	20	1	–
Shady Brook									
Turkey Breakfast	1 (2.3 oz)	80	0	–	–	–	–	–	–
Soy Lean									
Pork Breakfast Patty	1 (2 oz)	75	–	0	–	0	20	2	–
Wellshire									
Andouille	1 link (3 oz)	197	0	0	–	0	0	1	–
Andouille Turkey	2 oz	59	0	0	–	0	80	1	–
Chorizo	1 piece (2 oz)	130	0	0	–	0	0	1	–
Chorizo Dried	1 oz	100	0	0	–	0	0	tr	–
Italian Turkey Mild	1 link (2 oz)	70	0	0	–	0	0	1	–
Kielbasa Polska	1 piece (2 oz)	130	0	0	–	0	0	1	–
Kielbasa Turkey	1 piece (2 oz)	59	0	0	–	0	0	1	–
Turkey Maple Breakfast	1 link (2 oz)	70	0	0	–	0	0	1	–

SAUSAGE DISHES
TAKE-OUT

sausage roll	1 (2.3 oz)	311	1	405	–	0	46	1	–

SAUSAGE SUBSTITUTES

meatless	1 patty (1.3 oz)	98	1	0	10	0	24	1	88
meatless	1 link (0.9 oz)	64	1	0	7	0	16	1	58
Boca									
Bratwurst	1 (2.5 oz)	140	1	0	–	0	40	2	–
Breakfast Patties	1 (1.3 oz)	60	2	0	–	0	20	1	–
Breakfast Links	2 (1.6 oz)	70	2	0	–	0	20	1	–
Italian	1 (2.5 oz)	130	1	100	–	0	20	1	–
Lightlife									
Gimme Lean	2 oz	50	2	–	–	–	–	–	–
Smart Brats	1 (2 oz)	120	1	–	–	–	–	–	150
Smart Links Breakfast	2 (2 oz)	100	4	–	–	–	–	–	250

FOOD	PORTION	CALS	FIBER	VIT A	FOLIC	VIT C	CALCI	IRON	POTAS
Smart Links Italian	1 (2 oz)	120	3	–	–	–	–	–	270
Smart Menu Breakfast Patty	1	45	1	–	–	–	–	–	150
Morningstar Farms									
Breakfast Links	2	60	2	0	–	0	0	1	60
Breakfast Patties	1 (1.3 oz)	80	1	0	–	0	0	1	160
Quorn									
Links	2 (1.6 oz)	70	1	0	–	0	30	1	–
Tofurky									
Turkey Beerbrats	1 (3.5 oz)	280	5	0	–	0	40	tr	–
Turkey Breakfast Links	1 (1.6 oz)	130	4	100	–	0	20	1	–
Turkey Italian Sweet	1 (3.5 oz)	280	8	300	–	0	40	3	–
Turkey Kielbasa	1 (3.5 oz)	240	8	0	–	0	40	2	–
Worthington									
Saucettes Breakfast Links	1 (1.3 oz)	90	1	0	–	0	0	1	25
SAVORY									
ground	1 tsp	4	–	72	–	–	30	1	15
SCALLOP									
raw	3 oz	75	–	–	–	–	21	tr	274
TAKE-OUT									
breaded & fried	2 lg	67	–	–	–	–	13	tr	103
SCONE									
Finnegan's									
Irish Raisin	1 (2 oz)	170	1	0	–	0	10	1	–
King Arthur									
Cranberry Orange as prep	1	248	0	81	–	2	116	1	–
English Cream Tea Scone not prep	⅓ cup	180	tr	0	–	0	100	1	–
TAKE-OUT									
apricot	1	232	–	1300	–	–	–	2	–
blueberry	1 (3 oz)	270	2	0	–	0	40	2	–
cheese	1 (3.5 oz)	364	2	850	–	tr	250	2	–
orange poppy	1 (3 oz)	260	2	300	–	0	80	2	–
plain	1 (3.5 oz)	362	2	700	–	tr	180	2	–
raisin	1 (3 oz)	270	2	0	–	0	40	1	–

FOOD	PORTION	CALS	FIBER	VIT A	FOLIC	VIT C	CALCI	IRON	POTAS
SCUP									
fresh baked	3 oz	115	0	–	–	–	44	1	313
SEA CUCUMBER									
dried	1 oz	74	0	37	–	0	87	3	101
fresh	1 oz	20	0	–	–	0	81	4	12
SEA URCHIN									
canned	1 oz	39	0	0	–	0	–	–	–
fresh	1 oz	36	tr	0	–	3	2	tr	51
roe paste	1 tbsp	19	0	24	–	0	6	tr	31
SEAWEED									
agar dried	1 oz	87	–	0	–	0	78	6	321
agar fresh	1 oz	tr	–	0	–	0	15	1	64
hijiki dried	1 tbsp	9	1	16	–	0	70	1	–
irishmoss fresh	1 oz	14	–	–	–	–	21	3	18
kelp fresh	1 oz	12	–	33	51	–	48	1	25
kombu fresh	1 oz	12	–	33	51	–	48	1	25
laver fresh	1 oz	10	–	1483	–	11	20	1	101
nori fresh	1 oz	10	–	1483	–	11	20	1	101
nori sheet dried	1 (8 x 8 in)	5	1	30	–	0	7	1	45
seahair dried	1 tbsp	13	tr	0	–	–	38	–	–
spirulina dried	1 oz	83	–	–	–	13	–	8	388
spirulina fresh	1 oz	7	–	–	–	tr	–	–	36
tangle fresh	1 oz	12	–	33	51	–	48	1	25
wakame fresh	1 oz	13	–	103	–	1	43	1	14
Eden									
Agar Agar Bars	1 bar (7 g)	25	5	–	–	–	–	–	–
Agar Agar Flakes	1 tbsp	0	1	0	–	0	20	tr	10
Arame Wild	½ cup	30	7	500	–	0	100	1	180
Hiziki Wild	½ cup	30	6	0	–	0	100	1	480
Kombu Wild	½ piece (3.3 g)	5	1	0	–	0	20	0	170
Nori Sheets	1 (2.5 g)	10	0	400	–	6	0	0	90
Organic Dulse Flakes	1 tsp	3	0	0	–	0	0	tr	80
SEMOLINA									
dry	1 cup (5.9 oz)	601	7	0	129	0	28	7	311

FOOD	PORTION	CALS	FIBER	VIT A	FOLIC	VIT C	CALCI	IRON	POTAS
SESAME									
seeds	1 tsp	16	–	1	–	–	4	tr	11
sesame butter	1 tbsp	95	1	8	–	0	154	3	93
tahini from roasted & toasted kernels	1 tbsp	89	–	–	–	0	64	1	62
tahini from stone ground kernels	1 tbsp	86	–	–	–	0	63	tr	62
tahini from unroasted kernels	1 tbsp	85	–	–	–	–	20	1	64
MaraNatha									
Raw Tahini	2 tbsp	190	3	0	–	0	20	2	–
Roasted Tahini	2 tbsp	210	2	0	–	0	20	2	–
Peloponnese									
Tahini	1 tbsp	100	1	0	–	0	20	1	–
Sabra									
Tahini Sauce Taratore	1 oz	80	0	0	–	0	20	tr	–
SESBANIA									
flower	1	1	–	0	–	2	1	tr	5
flowers	1 cup	5	–	0	–	15	4	tr	37
flowers cooked	1 cup	23	–	0	–	39	23	1	111
SHAD									
american baked	3 oz	214	0	–	–	–	51	1	418
cooked	1 oz	55	0	185	22	5	7	tr	74
roe baked w/ butter & lemon	1 oz	36	–	–	–	–	4	tr	38
SHARK									
fin dried	1 oz	32	–	0	–	0	48	1	16
raw	3 oz	111	0	198	–	–	29	1	136
TAKE-OUT									
batter-dipped & fried	3 oz	194	–	153	–	–	52	1	132
SHEEPSHEAD FISH									
cooked	1 fillet (6.5 oz)	234	0	–	–	–	70	1	952
cooked	3 oz	107	0	–	–	–	32	1	435
raw	3 oz	92	0	–	–	–	18	tr	344
SHELLFISH SUBSTITUTES									
crab imitation	1 cup (4.4 oz)	144	tr	45	3	0	53	tr	304

FOOD	PORTION	CALS	FIBER	VIT A	FOLIC	VIT C	CALCI	IRON	POTAS
scallop imitation	3 oz	84	–	–	–	–	7	tr	88
shrimp imitation	3 oz	86	–	–	–	–	16	1	76
surimi	3 oz	84	–	–	–	–	7	tr	95
surimi	1 oz	28	–	–	–	–	2	tr	31

Chicken Of The Sea

Imitation Crab	1 pkg (2.5 oz)	40	1	0	–	0	60	0	–

Louis Kemp

Crab Delights	½ cup (3 oz)	80	0	0	–	0	0	0	–
Crab Delights Chunk Style	½ cup (3 oz)	80	0	0	–	0	0	0	–
Crab Delights Easy Shred	½ cup (3 oz)	80	0	0	–	0	450	1	–
Crab Delights Leg Style	½ cup (3 oz)	80	0	0	–	0	0	0	–
Lobster Delights Chunk or Salad Style	½ cup (3 oz)	80	0	0	–	0	0	0	–
Scallop Delights Bay Style	½ cup (3 oz)	80	0	0	–	0	0	tr	–

TAKE-OUT

crab salad	1 cup	395	1	220	19	1	77	1	426

SHELLIE BEANS

canned	½ cup	37	–	278	–	4	36	1	133

SHERBET

orange	1 bar (2.75 fl oz)	91	–	50	3	3	36	tr	63
orange	½ cup (4 fl oz)	132	–	73	4	4	52	tr	92
orange	½ gal	2158	–	1480	111	31	827	2	1585

Blue Bunny

Cool Tubes Orange Sherbet	1 (3 oz)	110	0	–	–	–	–	–	45
Lime	½ cup	110	0	–	–	–	20	–	45
Rainbow	½ cup	110	0	–	–	–	–	–	–
Raspberry	½ cup	110	0	–	–	–	20	–	50

Breyers

Orange	½ cup	120	0	0	–	4	40	0	–
Rainbow	½ cup	120	0	0	–	1	40	0	–

FOOD	PORTION	CALS	FIBER	VIT A	FOLIC	VIT C	CALCI	IRON	POTAS
Hood									
Orange Burst	½ cup	120	0	0	–	0	40	0	–
SHRIMP									
CANNED									
canned	1 can (6 oz)	136	0	100	2	3	67	3	237
chinese shrimp paste	1 tbsp	15	–	0	–	0	125	2	–
Bumble Bee									
Broken Shrimp	¼ cup	40	0	0	–	0	60	tr	–
Medium or Large or Jumbo	¼ cup	40	0	0	–	0	60	tr	–
Small	¼ cup	40	0	0	–	0	60	tr	–
Tiny	¼ cup	40	0	0	–	0	60	tr	–
Chicken Of The Sea									
Tiny Small or Medium	½ can (2 oz)	45	0	0	–	0	40	tr	–
DRIED									
dried	10	15	0	10	0	tr	7	tr	27
FRESH									
broiled	6 med	46	0	130	1	1	19	1	67
steamed	6 med	41	0	95	1	1	20	1	51
FROZEN									
Chicken Of The Sea									
Cooked Large Peeled Deveined Tail On	3 oz	80	0	0	–	0	20	3	–
Large Raw Cleaned Tail Off	4 oz	120	0	0	–	0	60	2	–
Contessa									
Orange Shrimp	11–13 (6 oz)	250	5	0	–	2	60	1	–
Ragin' Cajun	8–10 (4 oz)	170	3	300	–	0	40	3	–
Shrimp Scampi	8–10 (4 oz)	290	2	200	–	0	150	2	–
TAKE-OUT									
breaded & fried	6 med (2.3 oz)	162	tr	41	14	1	43	2	130
cocktail w/ sauce	4 shrimp	87	2	95	9	11	37	1	229
curried	1 cup	295	tr	885	28	3	219	3	427
jambalaya	1 cup	309	1	475	75	13	102	5	413

566   SHRIMP

FOOD	PORTION	CALS	FIBER	VIT A	FOLIC	VIT C	CALCI	IRON	POTAS
scampi	1 cup	310	0	945	3	3	72	3	239
shrimp newburg	1 serv (6.4 oz)	456	tr	1840	37	2	185	2	401
shrimp salad	¾ cup	212	1	170	14	3	66	2	266
shrimp w/ crab stuffing	5	158	tr	250	31	2	66	2	206

SMELT
rainbow cooked	3 oz	106	0	–	–	–	65	1	316
rainbow raw	3 oz	83	0	–	–	–	51	1	247

SMOOTHIES
8th Continent
Refresher Orange Pineapple Banana	8 oz	150	0	500	–	0	200	1	–
Refresher Strawberry Banana	8 oz	150	0	500	–	60	200	1	–

Bolthouse Farms
Green Goodness	8 oz	140	1	6000	–	63	20	3	470
Mango Lemonade	8 oz	120	tr	0	–	9	20	0	35
Passion Fruit Apple Carrot Juice	8 oz	120	2	18250	–	21	20	tr	270
Strawberry Banana Fruit	8 oz	124	tr	5000	–	–	–	1	475

C&W
Berry Blend	½ cup	90	2	100	–	21	150	tr	–
Peach	½ cup	80	1	400	–	5	150	tr	–

E4B
100% Fruit Puree Blueberry Raspberry	4 oz	70	3	0	–	9	20	tr	–
100% Fruit Puree Kiwi	4 oz	70	1	0	–	15	40	tr	–
100% Fruit Puree Mango	4 oz	70	1	400	–	12	20	tr	–
100% Fruit Puree Pear Caramel	4 oz	70	1	0	–	4	40	tr	–
100% Fruit Puree Strawberry Banana	4 oz	70	1	0	–	15	40	tr	–

Hansen's
Apricot Nectar	1 can	170	–	5000	–	60	20	2	250
Cranberry Twist	1 can	180	–	5000	–	60	20	2	–
Energy Island Blast	1 can	170	–	5000	–	60	40	2	230
Guava Strawberry	1 can	170	–	5000	–	60	30	2	130

FOOD	PORTION	CALS	FIBER	VIT A	FOLIC	VIT C	CALCI	IRON	POTAS
Lite Cranberry Raspberry	1 can	50	–	5000	–	60	10	0	130
Mango Pineapple	1 can	170	–	5000	–	60	40	2	130
Peach Berry	1 can	170	–	5000	–	60	30	2	150
Pineapple Coconut	1 can	180	–	5000	–	60	30	2	120
Strawberry Banana	1 can	180	–	5000	–	60	30	2	140
Tropical Passion	1 can	170	–	5000	–	60	30	2	150
Whipped Orange	1 can	180	–	5000	–	60	30	2	180
Horizon Organic									
Tropical Punch	1 bottle (6.2 oz)	120	1	0	–	60	150	0	–
Jammin' Juice									
Mambo Mango	6 oz	92	1	400	–	60	0	1	108
Jammin' Nectars									
C-Beta Carrot	6 oz	96	1	5000	–	60	0	2	193
Ginger Party	6 oz	6	1	–	–	60	–	–	95
Guanabana Limbo	6 oz	78	2	0	–	60	0	0	36
Pure Passion	6 oz	78	1	–	–	60	–	–	7
Razz-Ade	6 oz	89	1	0	–	60	0	2	112
Kidz Dream									
Orange Cream	1 box	120	tr	0	–	6	350	1	240
LightFull									
Satiety Smoothie Cafe Latte	1 (11 oz)	90	5	–	–	–	211	tr	–
Satiety Smoothie Chocolate Fudge	1 (11 oz)	90	6	–	–	–	196	3	–
Satiety Smoothie Peaches & Cream	1 (11 oz)	100	6	498	–	127	217	tr	–
Satiety Smoothie Strawberries & Cream	1 (11 oz)	90	6	–	–	32	202	1	–
Luna									
Berry Pomegranate	1 pkg	140	2	750	200	30	350	0	135
Orange Blossom	1 pkg	130	3	750	200	30	250	0	220
Vanilla Macadamia	1 pkg	150	3	750	200	30	250	0	125
Naked Juice									
Chocolate Karma	8 oz	190	3	500	100	1	20	3	110
Vanilla Chai	8 oz	170	2	500	100	1	300	3	75

FOOD	PORTION	CALS	FIBER	VIT A	FOLIC	VIT C	CALCI	IRON	POTAS
Nutiva									
Organic HempShake Amazon Acai not prep	4 tbsp	100	8	0	–	0	20	5	–
Organic HempShake Chocolate not prep	4 tbsp	80	12	0	–	0	20	3	–
Odwalla									
Blackberry Fruit Shake	8 oz	140	1	100	–	36	20	1	400
Orange Pina	8 oz	140	1	250	–	72	20	tr	–
Sambazon									
Acai Energy Mango Banana	8 oz	190	3	1000	–	72	40	1	–
Acai Soy Energy	8 oz	210	4	1500	–	102	200	3	–
Amazon Cherry	8 oz	156	1	1000	–	900	20	1	–
Mango Uprising	8 oz	190	3	1000	–	72	40	1	–
Protein Warrior Chocolate	8 oz	215	3	550	–	4	50	1	–
Protein Warrior Vanilla	8 oz	215	3	550	–	4	50	1	–
Purple Power	1 bottle (1.05 oz)	155	2	–	–	5	40	1	–
Shaman's Immunity	8 oz	90	1	800	–	1050	10	tr	–
Strawberry Sensation	8 oz	210	2	500	–	5	40	2	–
Supergreens Revolution	8 oz	200	3	1200	–	10	40	2	–
Smooze									
Mango + Coconut	1 box (8.5 oz)	250	0	0	–	60	0	1	–
Passion Fruit + Coconut	1 box (8.5 oz)	225	3	0	–	77	0	1	–
Pineapple + Coconut	1 box (8.5 oz)	200	0	0	–	68	0	1	–
Soy Blendz									
Mango Orange Dream	1 bottle (10 oz)	220	3	11500	–	156	60	2	–
Mixed Berry Medley	1 bottle (10 oz)	210	3	0	–	72	60	2	–
Orange Citrus Splash	1 bottle (10 oz)	220	3	12500	–	150	60	2	0
Strawberry Banana Blast	1 bottle (10 oz)	230	3	0	–	60	40	2	–

FOOD	PORTION	CALS	FIBER	VIT A	FOLIC	VIT C	CALCI	IRON	POTAS
Soy Fusion									
Berry	1 box (8.45 oz)	120	–	1000	40	60	150	1	150
Matcha Green Tea	1 box (8.45 oz)	110	–	2500	100	60	200	1	150
Tropicana									
Fruit Smoothie Mixed Berry	1 bottle (11 oz)	220	2	0	–	120	20	1	630
Fruit Smoothie Tropical Fruit	1 bottle (11 oz)	220	1	0	–	120	20	1	790
WholeSoy & Co.									
Orgainic Soy Strawberry	8 oz	210	0	0	–	1	200	0	–
Organic Soy Peach	8 oz	210	0	0	–	0	200	0	–
Organic Soy Raspberry	8 oz	210	0	0	–	0	200	0	–
Yoplait									
Go-Gurt All Fruit Flavors	1 bottle (5 oz)	120	0	500	–	0	200	–	170
Light All Flavors	1 bottle (8.3 oz)	90	3	750	–	–	200	–	260
Smoothie All Flavors	1 bottle (8.3 oz)	220	3	750	–	–	200	–	280

SNACKS

FOOD	PORTION	CALS	FIBER	VIT A	FOLIC	VIT C	CALCI	IRON	POTAS
cheese puffs	1 oz	157	tr	75	34	0	16	1	47
corn twists cheese	1 oz	157	tr	75	34	0	16	1	47
oriental mix	1 oz	155	–	15	25	tr	22	1	147
pork skins	1 oz	154	0	37	–	tr	8	tr	36
trail mix	1 oz	131	–	5	20	tr	22	1	194
Bowlby's									
Bits Almond	½ cup	100	1	0	–	0	0	1	–
Bits Pecan	½ cup	200	1	0	–	0	0	1	–
Bits Ranch	½ cup	170	0	0	–	0	0	1	–
Bits Salsa	½ cup	170	0	100	–	0	0	1	–
Bits Sour Cream Onion & Dill	½ cup	170	0	0	–	0	0	1	–
Bits'N'Pops	¾ cup	130	1	0	–	1	10	0	–
Mix-Ups Country Mix	½ cup	170	1	0	–	0	0	1	–
Mix-Ups Nuttyest-Of-All	½ cup	160	1	0	–	0	20	1	–
Mix-Ups Trail Mix	½ cup	165	1	0	–	0	0	1	–

FOOD	PORTION	CALS	FIBER	VIT A	FOLIC	VIT C	CALCI	IRON	POTAS
Chester's									
Puffcorn Butter	3 cups	160	tr	100	–	0	0	1	–
Puffcorn Cheese	3 cups	160	0	100	–	0	20	1	–
Chex Mix									
Cheddar	⅔ cup	140	2	–	–	–	–	tr	–
Hot'N Spicy	⅔ cup	130	2	–	–	–	–	–	–
Nacho Fiesta	⅔ cup	120	1	–	–	–	–	–	60
Party Blend Bold	⅔ cup	140	2	–	8	–	–	tr	60
Peanut Lovers	⅔ cup	140	1	–	–	–	–	–	80
Traditional	⅔ cup	130	1	–	8	–	–	tr	–
Garden Of Eatin'									
Organic Baked Cheese Puffs	32 pieces	150	1	0	–	0	20	0	–
Organic Baked Chunchitos	35 pieces	140	1	0	–	0	20	0	–
Good Sense									
Organic Trail Mix Tropical	⅓ cup	160	2	0	–	0	0	1	–
Snack Mix Cajun Corn 'N Sesame	¼ cup	150	2	100	–	0	100	1	–
Trail Mix Dietary Snack Mix	¼ cup	130	2	0	–	0	80	1	–
Gram's Gourmet									
Crunchies Pork Rinds	⅛ pkg (0.5 oz)	70	0	–	–	–	–	–	–
J&J									
Microwave Pork Rinds All Flavors	1 oz	130	0	–	–	–	–	–	–
Kangaroo									
Pita Snackers Crispy Cinnamon	10 pieces (1 oz)	90	1	0	–	1	20	1	–
Pita Snackers Sea Salt	10 pieces (1 oz)	90	1	0	–	1	20	1	–
MaraNatha									
High Energy Mix	¼ cup	120	2	400	–	0	20	tr	–
Organic Harvest Mix	¼ cup	150	2	0	–	0	20	1	–
Organic Nature Mix	¼ cup	150	2	100	–	0	20	1	–
Snack Attack Mix	¼ cup	140	2	0	–	2	20	1	–
Trail Mix Deluxe	¼ cup	150	2	0	–	0	20	1	–
Trail Mix Navajo	¼ cup	140	4	100	–	1	20	1	–

FOOD	PORTION	CALS	FIBER	VIT A	FOLIC	VIT C	CALCI	IRON	POTAS
Trail Mix Olympic w/ Chocolate	¼ cup	140	2	0	–	0	20	1	–
Trail Mix Organic Delight	¼ cup	150	2	0	–	0	20	1	–
Trail Mix Organic Raw	¼ cup	140	2	0	–	0	20	tr	–
Organic Trails									
Trail Mix Summit Blend	¼ cup	150	2	0	–	0	20	1	–
Planters									
Trail Mix Berry Nut & Chocolate	3 tbsp (1 oz)	120	1	0	–	0	20	tr	115
Pumpkorn									
Caramel	⅓ cup	150	2	100	16	0	20	5	–
Chili	⅓ cup	150	2	400	16	0	20	5	–
Curry	⅓ cup	150	2	100	16	0	20	5	–
Maple Vanilla	⅓ cup	150	2	100	16	0	20	5	–
Mesquite	⅓ cup	150	2	100	16	0	20	5	–
Original	⅓ cup	150	2	100	16	0	20	5	–
Sabritones									
Chile & Lime	23 pieces	150	1	300	–	0	20	1	–
Snyder's Of Hanover									
CheddAirs	1 oz	130	tr	0	–	0	20	0	–
MultiGrain Cheese Puffs	1 oz	130	2	0	–	0	0	0	–
SunRise									
Trail Mix Honey Coated	3 tbsp (1 oz)	137	4	0	–	0	30	1	–
Trail Mix w/ Fruit	3 tbsp (1 oz)	130	2	0	–	0	20	1	–
Tumaro's									
Organic Krispy Crunchy Puffs Cheddar	22	120	1	0	–	0	0	0	–
Organic Krispy Crunchy Puffs Natural Corn	22	120	1	0	–	0	0	tr	–
Organic Krispy Crunchy Puffs Ranch & Herb	22	130	tr	0	–	0	0	tr	–
Organic Krispy Crunchy Puffs Tangy BBQ	22	120	tr	100	–	0	0	0	–
SNAIL									
cooked	3 oz	233	–	137	10	–	96	9	590
raw	3 oz	117	–	–	5	–	48	4	295

FOOD	PORTION	CALS	FIBER	VIT A	FOLIC	VIT C	CALCI	IRON	POTAS
TAKE-OUT									
escargot cooked	5	25	0	10	0	0	5	1	95
SNAKE									
fresh	3 oz	78	0	15	–	3	15	3	303
SNAPPER									
cooked	3 oz	109	0	–	–	–	34	tr	444
cooked	1 fillet (6 oz)	217	0	–	–	–	69	tr	887
raw	3 oz	85	0	–	–	–	27	tr	355
SODA									
club	12 oz	0	0	0	0	0	17	–	6
cola	12 oz	151	–	0	0	0	9	tr	4
cream	12 oz	191	–	0	0	0	19	tr	4
diet cola	12 oz	2	–	0	0	0	12	tr	0
diet cola w/ equal	12 oz	2	–	0	0	0	12	tr	0
diet cola w/ saccharin	12 oz	2	–	0	0	0	14	tr	7
ginger ale	12 oz can	124	–	0	0	0	12	tr	5
grape	12 oz	161	–	0	0	0	12	tr	3
lemon lime	12 oz	149	–	0	0	0	9	tr	4
orange	12 oz	177	–	0	0	0	19	tr	9
pepper type	12 oz	151	–	0	0	0	12	tr	2
quinine	12 oz	125	–	0	0	0	5	–	1
root beer	12 oz	152	–	0	0	0	19	tr	3
shirley temple	1 serv	159	0	–	–	–	11	2	23
tonic water	12 oz	125	–	0	0	0	5	–	1
7 Up									
Plus	1 can (12 oz)	10	–	0	–	0	150	0	–
Celsius									
Cola	1 bottle (12 oz)	5	–	–	–	60	50	–	–
Lucozade									
Soda	7 oz	136	0	0	–	0	10	tr	–
Orangina									
Sparkling Citrus	8 oz	90	–	–	–	9	40	tr	–
Santa Cruz									
Organic Cherry	1 can	140	–	–	–	1	–	1	75
Organic Ginger Ale	1 can	150	–	–	–	6	20	–	25
Organic Lemon Lime	1 can	130	–	–	–	4	–	tr	20
							SODA		573

FOOD	PORTION	CALS	FIBER	VIT A	FOLIC	VIT C	CALCI	IRON	POTAS
Organic Orange Mango	1 can	130	–	–	–	12	–	–	45
Organic Root Beer	1 can	150	–	–	–	60	20	–	25
Organic Vanilla Creme	1 can	160	–	–	–	60	–	1	65
Steap									
Green Tea Soda Orange	8 oz	90	–	1500	–	12	–	–	–
Green Tea Soda Root Beer	8 oz	90	–	–	–	36	–	–	–
Organic Green Tea Soda Raspberry	8 oz	90	–	–	–	12	–	–	–
Uno Mas									
All Flavors	1 can (12 oz)	130	0	–	100	–	–	–	–
White Rock									
Organics Raspberry Creme	1 can (12.4 oz)	120	–	–	–	4	–	–	–
Organics Red Peach	1 can (12.4 oz)	120	–	2000	–	1	–	–	–
Yoo-Hoo									
Original	9 oz	150	tr	500	8	6	100	tr	250
SOLE									
cooked	3 oz	99	0	32	–	–	16	tr	292
cooked	1 fillet (4.5 oz)	148	0	48	–	–	23	tr	436
lemon raw	3.5 oz	85	0	–	–	–	–	–	298
TAKE-OUT									
breaded & fried	3.2 oz	211	–	35	51	0	17	2	292
SORGHUM									
sorghum	1 cup (6.7 oz)	651	–	0	–	0	54	8	672
SOUFFLE									
lemon chilled	1 cup	176	–	–	–	–	175	tr	–
raspberry chilled	1 cup	173	–	–	–	–	190	1	–
spinach	1 cup	233	1	3909	99	10	224	2	318
SOUP									
CANNED									
Amy's									
Organic Barley	1 cup	50	2	–	–	–	–	–	–

FOOD	PORTION	CALS	FIBER	VIT A	FOLIC	VIT C	CALCI	IRON	POTAS
Organic Black Bean Vegetable	1 cup	110	5	–	–	–	–	–	–
Organic Cream Of Mushroom	1 cup	120	2	–	–	–	–	–	–
Organic Cream Of Tomato	1 cup	100	4	–	–	–	–	–	–
Organic Lentil	1 cup	130	9	–	–	–	–	–	–
Organic Minestrone	1 cup	90	3	–	–	–	–	–	–
Organic No Chicken Noodle Soup	1 cup	90	2	–	–	–	–	–	–
Organic Vegetable	1 cup	35	1	–	–	–	–	–	–
Boston Market									
Chicken Broth Reduced Sodium	1 cup	15	0	0	–	0	0	1	–
Butterball									
Chicken Broth Reduced Sodium 99% Fat Free	1 cup	10	0	–	–	–	–	–	–
Campbell's									
98% Fat Free Cream of Mushroom	1 cup	70	1	0	–	0	20	0	–
98% Fat Free Cream of Chicken as prep	1 cup	70	1	400	–	0	0	0	–
Cheddar Cheese	1 cup	110	1	750	–	0	40	0	–
Chicken Broth	½ cup	20	0	0	–	0	0	0	–
Chicken Noodle	1 cup	70	tr	500	–	0	0	1	–
Chunky Beef Barley	1 cup	160	2	3500	–	1	20	tr	–
Chunky Beef w/ Country Vegetables	1 cup	150	5	5000	–	1	20	1	–
Chunky Chicken & Dumplings	1 cup	190	3	2500	–	1	20	1	–
Chunky Chicken Corn Chowder	1 cup	230	3	2000	–	0	20	0	–
Chunky Chili Roadhouse Beef & Bean	1 cup	220	7	750	–	1	40	2	–
Chunky Classic Chicken Noodle	1 cup	120	2	2500	–	0	20	1	–
Chunky New England Clam Chowder	1 cup	240	2	0	–	2	20	2	–

FOOD	PORTION	CALS	FIBER	VIT A	FOLIC	VIT C	CALCI	IRON	POTAS
Chunky Old Fashioned Vegetable Beef	1 cup	130	4	5000	–	0	40	1	–
Chunky Sirloin Burger w/ Country Vegetables	1 cup	180	4	3000	–	1	20	1	–
Chunky Vegetable	1 cup	130	4	4000	–	1	40	1	–
Classics Beef Noodle	1 cup	70	1	100	–	0	300	1	–
Classics Minestrone	1 cup	90	3	2000	–	0	20	1	–
Classics Old Fashioned Vegetable	1 cup	90	2	2250	–	0	20	tr	–
Classics Vegetarian Vegetable as prep	1 cup	90	2	2500	–	0	20	1	–
Cream Of Chicken	1 cup	120	2	300	–	0	0	0	–
Cream Of Chicken w/ Herbs	1 cup	90	1	500	–	0	20	tr	–
Double Noodle	1 cup	90	2	1000	–	0	0	1	–
Healthy Request Chicken Noodle as prep	1 cup	60	1	500	–	0	0	tr	–
Healthy Request Chicken Rice as prep	1 cup	60	tr	1250	–	12	0	0	–
Healthy Request Cream Of Chicken as prep	1 cup	80	1	500	–	0	0	0	340
Kitchen Classics Bean With Bacon	1 cup	180	8	500	–	0	60	2	–
Kitchen Classics Chicken Noodle	1 cup	90	2	2500	–	0	20	tr	–
Kitchen Classics Chicken w/ White & Wild Rice	1 cup	100	2	2500	–	0	20	tr	–
Kitchen Classics Lentil	1 cup	120	5	0	–	0	50	3	–
Select Beef w/ Portobello Mushrooms & Rice	1 cup	110	2	500	–	0	20	0	–
Select Blended Red Pepper Black Bean	1 cup	110	4	750	–	4	40	1	–
Select Chicken Rice	1 cup	100	2	3500	–	1	20	0	–
Select Chicken With Egg Noodles	1 cup	90	2	2500	–	0	20	0	–
Select Creamy Potato w/ Roasted Garlic	1 cup	180	2	300	–	0	20	1	–

FOOD	PORTION	CALS	FIBER	VIT A	FOLIC	VIT C	CALCI	IRON	POTAS
Select Fiesta Vegetable	1 cup (8.4 oz)	120	3	2500	–	4	40	1	–
Select Herbed Chicken w/ Roasted Vegetables	1 cup	90	1	1000	–	0	20	tr	–
Select Honey Roasted Chicken w/ Golden Potatoes	1 cup	110	3	1250	–	0	20	tr	–
Select Italian Sausage w/ Pasta & Pepperoni	1 cup	150	2	500	–	0	40	1	–
Select Italian Style Wedding	1 cup	110	2	750	–	0	40	0	–
Select Mexican Chicken Tortilla	1 cup	140	3	300	–	0	40	tr	–
Select Roasted Chicken w/ Rotini & Penne Pasta	1 cup	90	2	1500	–	0	20	tr	–
Select Savory Chicken & Long Grain Rice	1 cup	90	1	0	–	0	20	0	–
Soup At Hand Chicken & Stars	1 pkg	70	2	750	–	0	0	tr	–
Soup At Hand Chicken w/ Mini Noodles	1 pkg (10.75 oz)	80	2	1500	–	0	0	0	–
Soup At Hand Cream of Broccoli	1 pkg (10.75 oz)	160	3	300	–	1	20	1	–
Soup At Hand Creamy Chicken	1 pkg (10.75 oz)	130	4	1500	–	0	0	1	–
Soup At Hand Creamy Tomato	1 pkg	180	4	750	–	24	60	tr	–
Soup At Hand Italian Style Wedding	1 pkg	90	2	2000	–	1	20	tr	–
Soup At Hand Vegetable Medley	1 pkg (10.75 oz)	110	3	8000	–	78	40	1	–
Soup At Hand Velvety Potato	1 pkg (10.75 oz)	160	4	0	–	0	20	tr	–
College Inn									
Beef Broth 99% Fat Free	1 cup	20	0	0	–	0	0	0	–
Beef Broth Fat Free Lower Sodium	1 cup	15	0	0	–	0	0	0	–

FOOD	PORTION	CALS	FIBER	VIT A	FOLIC	VIT C	CALCI	IRON	POTAS
Chicken Broth Light & Fat Free	1 cup	5	0	0	–	0	0	0	–
Gold's									
Borscht Low Calorie	1 cup	20	1	0	–	2	20	tr	–
Borscht Unsalted	1 cup	70	tr	0	–	2	20	tr	–
Hungarian Cabbage	6 oz	70	2	1250	–	24	20	1	–
Schav	1 cup	15	1	1750	–	21	20	1	–
Health Valley									
Organic Split Pea No Salt Added	1 cup	110	8	1250	–	1	20	2	–
Healthy Choice									
Bean & Ham	1 cup	170	6	1000	–	2	80	3	–
Beef & Potato	1 cup	110	2	500	–	2	0	1	–
Chicken & Dumplings	1 cup	130	7	1250	–	1	40	1	–
Chicken & Pasta	1 cup	110	2	1000	–	2	20	1	–
Chicken Corn Chowder	1 cup	140	3	500	–	5	20	1	–
Chicken Fiesta	1 cup	100	3	400	–	4	40	1	–
Chicken w/ Rice	1 cup	90	2	750	–	2	40	0	–
Chicken w/ Roasted Garlic	1 cup	120	2	750	–	2	20	1	–
Chili Beef	1 cup	170	6	500	–	8	60	4	–
Clam Chowder	1 cup	110	4	200	–	2	20	1	–
Country Vegetable	1 cup	110	4	1000	–	2	60	1	–
Creamy Tomato	1 cup	100	2	1000	–	0	20	1	–
Garden Vegetable	1 cup	120	4	1750	–	2	40	2	–
Hearty Chicken	1 cup	120	3	2000	–	0	40	1	–
Italian Bean & Pasta	1 cup	100	3	500	–	2	80	1	–
Old Fashioned Chicken Noodle	1 cup	110	3	0	–	2	20	1	–
Roasted Italian Style Chicken	1 cup	120	4	1000	–	4	60	1	–
Split Pea w/ Ham	1 cup	170	4	1500	–	6	20	1	–
Turkey w/ Rice	1 cup	90	3	750	–	1	40	tr	–
Vegetable Beef	1 cup	130	3	300	–	2	40	1	–
Vegetable Clam Chowder	1 cup	230	3	1250	–	0	40	1	–
Zesty Gumbo	1 cup	100	3	400	–	5	40	1	–
Imagine									
Lobster Bisque	1 cup	130	–	400	–	6	150	tr	–

FOOD	PORTION	CALS	FIBER	VIT A	FOLIC	VIT C	CALCI	IRON	POTAS
Organic Bistro Cuban Black Bean Bisque	1 cup	170	6	100	–	9	40	3	–
Organic Broth Beef	1 cup	20	0	300	–	1	0	tr	–
Organic Broth Free Range Chicken	1 cup	10	0	0	–	0	40	tr	–
Organic Broth Vegetable	8 oz	20	0	0	–	0	20	tr	–
Organic Creamy Butternut Squash	1 cup	90	2	1250	–	0	40	1	–
Organic Creamy Chicken	1 cup	70	1	1250	–	5	20	tr	–
Organic Creamy Sweet Corn	1 cup	120	3	0	–	0	20	1	–
Organic Sweet Potato	1 cup	110	1	13500	–	21	20	1	–
Manischewitz									
Clear Chicken Condensed	½ cup	15	2	0	–	1	0	1	–
Pacific Foods									
Beef Broth	1 cup	20	0	–	–	–	–	–	–
Creamy Butternut Squash	1 cup	90	4	2500	–	5	40	1	–
Creamy Roasted Carrot	1 cup	100	2	10000	–	0	40	–	–
Creamy Roasted Red Pepper & Tomato	1 cup	100	1	500	–	2	10	tr	–
Hearty Beef Barley	1 cup	110	2	100	–	0	40	1	–
Hearty Chicken Noodle	1 cup	80	1	500	–	2	20	2	–
Hearty Chicken Tortilla	1 cup	130	5	500	–	4	10	5	–
Hearty Roasted Red Pepper & Corn Chowder	1 cup	210	3	500	–	9	40	1	–
Organic Creamy Tomato	1 cup	100	1	1000	–	5	10	tr	–
Organic French Onion	1 cup	35	tr	0	–	0	20	–	–
Organic Vegetarian Broth	1 cup	15	tr	–	–	–	20	1	–
Progresso									
50% Less Sodium Chicken Gumbo	1 cup	110	2	750	–	4	20	1	–
50% Less Sodium Chicken Noodle	1 cup	90	1	2250	–	1	20	1	–

FOOD	PORTION	CALS	FIBER	VIT A	FOLIC	VIT C	CALCI	IRON	POTAS
50% Less Sodium Minestrone	1 cup	120	4	750	–	0	40	1	–
99% Fat Free Beef Barley	1 cup	120	4	1000	–	0	20	1	–
Carb Monitor Chicken Vegetable	1 cup	70	1	1250	–	0	20	tr	–
Chicken Rice w/ Vegetable	1 cup	100	1	1000	–	0	20	0	–
Rich & Hearty Beef Pot Roast	1 cup	130	2	1000	–	0	40	1	–
Rich & Hearty Chicken & Homestyle Noodles	1 cup	110	1	1500	–	0	20	1	–
Rich & Hearty Chicken Pot Pie	1 cup	170	2	1000	–	0	20	1	–
Rich & Hearty Sirloin Steak & Vegetables	1 cup	130	2	1250	–	0	20	1	–
Traditional Beef & Vegetable	1 cup	100	2	1000	–	4	40	1	–
Traditional Beef Barley	1 cup	140	2	750	–	0	20	1	–
Traditional Chicken & Herb Dumplings	1 cup	110	1	1250	–	0	20	0	–
Traditional Chicken & Wild Rice	1 cup	100	1	1000	–	0	20	tr	–
Traditional Chicken Noodle	1 cup	100	1	1500	–	0	20	1	–
Traditional Hearty Chicken & Rotini	1 cup	100	1	1000	–	0	20	0	–
Traditional Italian Style Wedding	1 cup	130	1	1500	–	0	40	1	–
Traditional Split Pea w/ Ham	1 cup	140	4	750	–	0	1	1	–
Turkey Noodle	1 cup	90	1	1250	–	0	0	1	–
Vegetable Classics French Onion	1 cup	50	1	100	–	0	20	0	–
Vegetable Classics Green Split Pea w/ Bacon	1 cup	170	5	100	–	0	0	1	–
Vegetable Classics Hearty Tomato	1 cup	110	3	1000	–	5	40	1	–

FOOD	PORTION	CALS	FIBER	VIT A	FOLIC	VIT C	CALCI	IRON	POTAS
Vegetable Classics Lentil	1 cup	150	4	300	–	0	40	3	–
Vegetable Classics Macaroni & Bean	1 cup	160	6	200	–	0	40	2	–
Vegetable Classics Minestrone	1 cup	110	4	1000	–	0	40	1	–
Vegetable Classics Tomato Rotini	1 cup	140	2	1000	–	18	20	1	–
Vegetable Classics Vegetable	1 cup	80	2	1250	–	0	20	1	–
Rienzi									
Chicken & Rice	1 cup	110	2	2000	–	0	20	1	–
Italian Wedding Bell	1 cup	130	tr	750	–	1	20	tr	–
Snow's									
Clam Chowder	1 cup	200	1	200	–	4	40	4	–
Streit's									
Hearty Vegetarian Vegetable	1 cup	90	3	6000	–	0	20	1	–
Mushroom Barley	1 cup	100	3	1000	–	2	20	1	–
Walnut Acres									
Organic Country Corn Chowder	1 cup (8.8 oz)	150	2	300	–	15	80	tr	–
Wolfgang Puck									
Chicken Parmesan w/ Pasta	1 cup	300	1	500	–	0	40	3	–
Hearty Lentil & Vegetable	1 cup	170	6	1000	–	1	40	3	–
FROZEN									
Nature's Entree									
Chowder	1 pkg (12 oz)	230	5	300	–	9	150	3	–
Tortellini Minestrone	1 pkg (12 oz)	360	5	3500	–	9	80	5	–
MIX									
A Taste Of Thai									
Coconut Ginger	2 tsp	15	0	0	–	–	0	–	–
Annie Chun's									
Noodle Bowl Chicken Noodle	1 pkg	260	2	400	–	2	20	tr	–
Noodle Bowl Hot & Sour	1 pkg	280	2	0	–	0	40	1	–

FOOD	PORTION	CALS	FIBER	VIT A	FOLIC	VIT C	CALCI	IRON	POTAS
Noodle Bowl Korean Kimchi	½ pkg	140	1	200	–	0	0	0	–
Noodle Bowl Miso	1 pkg	230	2	500	–	4	40	1	–
Noodle Bowl Thai Tom Yum	½ pkg	150	1	100	–	1	20	0	–
Noodle Bowl Udon	1 pkg	220	1	750	–	4	20	1	–
Azumaya									
Asian Style Thin Noodle	1 cup	120	tr	0	–	0	20	1	–
Asian Style Wide Noodle	1 cup	120	tr	0	–	0	20	1	–
Bean Cuisine									
13 Bean Bouillabaisse	1 cup	220	5	500	–	9	80	6	–
Lots of Lentil	1 cup	230	5	3500	–	18	60	5	–
Mesa Maize	1 cup	160	6	5500	–	5	40	2	–
White Bean Provencal	1 cup	250	11	1000	–	21	150	4	–
Fantastic									
Noodle Bowl Hot & Sour as prep	2 cups	138	1	100	–	5	20	tr	–
Noodle Bowl Miso w/ Tofu as prep	1 cup	100	tr	0	–	0	20	1	–
Noodle Bowl Sesame Miso as prep	2 cups	90	tr	750	–	5	20	1	–
Noodle Bowl Spring Vegetable as prep	2 cups	90	tr	1250	–	12	20	1	–
Noodle Soup Cup Spicy Thai as prep	2 cups	110	1	500	–	5	20	1	–
Noodle Soup Cup Vegetarian Chicken as prep	1 cup	90	1	0	–	0	0	1	–
Soup Cup Italian Tomato as prep	2 cups	130	2	750	–	18	20	1	–
Soup Cup Mandarin Broccoli as prep	2 cups	110	2	200	–	12	20	6	–
Nissin									
Chicken Vegetable as prep	1 pkg	290	2	200	–	0	40	4	–
White Cheddar as prep	1 pkg	290	2	100	–	0	40	3	–

FOOD	PORTION	CALS	FIBER	VIT A	FOLIC	VIT C	CALCI	IRON	POTAS
Nueva Cocina									
Frijoles Negros Con Chipotle Chile	1 cup	140	9	500	–	12	20	2	–
Sopa De Calabaza	1 cup	180	1	200	–	1	20	1	–
Sopa De Frijoles Colorados	1 cup	140	7	400	–	15	40	2	–
Sopa De Frijoles Negros	1 cup	140	9	400	–	12	20	2	–
Sopa De Maiz	1 cup	150	2	100	–	5	40	1	–
Sopa De Tortilla	1 cup	140	2	1250	–	30	40	1	–
Ramen Noodle									
Beef as prep	1 pkg (2.2 oz)	280	3	1662	–	0	31	2	–
Beef Low Fat as prep	1 pkg (2.2 oz)	216	2	1930	–	1	39	3	–
Chicken as prep	1 pkg (2.2 oz)	279	6	897	–	2	27	2	–
Chicken Low Fat as prep	1 pkg (2.2 oz)	216	2	1995	–	1	35	4	–
Oriental Low Fat as prep	1 pkg (2.2 oz)	217	2	2635	–	1	49	3	–
Shrimp as prep	1 pkg (2.2 oz)	294	3	782	–	1	35	2	–
Shrimp Low Fat as prep	1 pkg (2.2 oz)	218	3	2394	–	1	27	3	–
Tomato as prep	1 pkg (2.2 oz)	295	2	932	–	6	37	2	–
Rapunzel									
Cubes Vegetable Bouillon No Salt Added	½ cube	25	0	–	–	–	–	–	–
Cubes Vegetable Bouillon w/ Sea Salt	½ cube	15	0	–	–	–	–	–	–
Cubes Vegetable Bouillon w/ Sea Salt & Herbs	½ cube	15	0	–	–	–	–	–	–
Simply Asia									
Soy Noodle Bowl	1 pkg	70	3	<100	–	0	<20	tr	–
Slim-Fast									
Creamy Broccoli	1 pkg	210	5	1500	120	60	400	3	400

FOOD	PORTION	CALS	FIBER	VIT A	FOLIC	VIT C	CALCI	IRON	POTAS
Creamy Chicken	1 pkg	220	5	1500	120	60	400	3	400
Creamy Potato Cheddar & Chive	1 pkg	220	5	1500	120	60	400	3	400
Thai Kitchen									
Instant Rice Noodle Bangkok Curry	1 pkg	192	0	0	–	0	0	1	–
Rice Noodle Bowl Roasted Garlic	1 bowl	170	0	0	–	0	0	1	–
Rice Noodle Bowl Spring Onion	1 bowl	170	0	0	–	0	0	1	–
Uncle Ben's									
Black Bean & Rice as prep	1 cup	150	7	0	24	0	60	1	–
Broccoli Cheese & Rice as prep	1 cup	110	1	200	24	9	60	tr	–
SHELF-STABLE									
TastyBite									
Tom Yum	½ pkg (5.3 oz)	92	1	0	–	0	20	1	–
TAKE-OUT									
beef stew soup	1 cup (8.8 oz)	221	–	6626	25	14	32	3	527
black bean turtle soup	1 cup	241	10	11	158	0	103	5	801
broccoli cheese	1 cup	165	2	670	53	2	189	tr	425
brunswick stew soup	1 cup (8.5 oz)	232	–	433	21	14	39	2	509
caldo de res beef soup	1 cup	143	2	325	24	11	36	2	674
corn & cheese chowder	¾ cup	215	3	636	12	7	220	1	337
egg drop	1 cup	73	0	205	15	0	22	1	220
gazpacho	1 cup	46	–	–	–	–	28	tr	–
greek lemon	¾ cup	63	2	39	8	4	22	1	45
hot & sour	1 serv (14 oz)	173	1	124	9	1	50	1	197
matzo ball soup	1 cup	118	1	120	19	0	31	1	190
minestrone	1 cup	233	4	390	87	9	45	2	588
miso w/ tofu	1 cup	84	2	1165	58	5	65	2	362
onion soup gratinee	1 serv	492	4	1145	57	11	637	2	528
oxtail	1 cup	68	1	0	10	0	10	tr	81
pasta e fagioll	1 cup (8.8 oz)	194	–	1878	49	12	62	3	522

FOOD	PORTION	CALS	FIBER	VIT A	FOLIC	VIT C	CALCI	IRON	POTAS
ratatouille	1 cup (7.5 oz)	266	–	815	34	41	56	1	485
shrimp bisque	1 cup	263	tr	940	15	2	263	2	436
sopa de albondigas	1 cup	171	1	615	21	12	33	2	431
sopa de feijao portuguese bean & sausage	1 cup	220	6	750	–	9	80	6	–
vietnamese pho beef noodle	1 serv (7.8 oz)	480	1	309	33	50	44	4	334
wonton soup	1 cup	183	1	350	39	3	36	2	321

SOUR CREAM

FOOD	PORTION	CALS	FIBER	VIT A	FOLIC	VIT C	CALCI	IRON	POTAS
sour cream	1 tbsp (0.4 oz)	26	–	95	1	tr	14	tr	17
sour cream	1 cup (8 oz)	493	–	1817	25	2	268	tr	331
Breakstone's									
Sour Cream	2 tbsp (1 oz)	60	0	200	–	0	20	0	–
Cabot									
Light	2 tbsp	35	0	200	–	0	40	0	–
No Fat	2 tbsp	20	0	200	–	0	40	0	–
Sour Cream	2 tbsp	50	0	200	–	0	20	0	–
Crowley									
Sour Cream	2 tbsp	60	0	200	–	0	40	0	–
Daisy									
No Fat	2 tbsp	20	0	200	–	0	40	0	–
Sour Cream	2 tbsp	60	0	200	–	0	20	0	–
Hood									
Fat Free	2 tbsp	20	0	200	–	0	60	0	–
Low Fat	2 tbsp	35	0	200	–	0	60	0	–
Sour Cream	2 tbsp	60	0	200	–	0	40	0	–
Horizon Organic									
Lowfat	2 tbsp	35	0	200	–	0	60	0	–
Sour Cream	2 tbsp	60	0	200	–	0	40	0	–

SOUR CREAM SUBSTITUTES

FOOD	PORTION	CALS	FIBER	VIT A	FOLIC	VIT C	CALCI	IRON	POTAS
nondairy	1 oz	59	–	0	0	0	1	–	46
nondairy	1 cup	479	–	0	0	0	6	–	369

FOOD	PORTION	CALS	FIBER	VIT A	FOLIC	VIT C	CALCI	IRON	POTAS
SOURSOP									
fresh	1	416	–	15	–	129	88	4	1739
fresh cut up	1 cup	150	–	5	–	46	32	1	626
SOY									
lecithin	1 tbsp	104	0	–	–	–	–	–	–
soy milk	1 cup	79	–	77	4	0	10	1	338
soya cheese	1.4 oz	128	0	0	–	0	180	tr	–
Fearn									
Granules	¼ cup	110	8	–	–	–	–	–	–
Powder	¼ cup	100	4	–	–	–	–	–	–
GeniSoy									
Soy Nuts Deep Sea Salted	1 oz	120	5	0	–	0	60	1	–
Soy Nuts Old Hickory Smoked	1 oz	120	5	0	–	0	60	1	–
Soy Nuts Praline	55 pieces (1 oz)	120	2	0	–	0	30	1	–
Soy Nuts Unsalted	1 oz	120	5	0	–	0	60	1	–
Soy Nuts Zesty Barbeque	1 oz	120	5	100	–	0	60	1	–
Good Sense									
Soynuts Honey Roasted	⅓ cup	140	4	0	–	0	40	1	–
Soynuts Roasted & Salted	⅓ cup	140	5	100	–	1	40	1	–
Soynuts Roasted w/o Salt	⅓ cup	140	5	100	–	1	40	1	–
Health Trip									
Soynut Butter Honey Sweet	2 tbsp	170	1	0	–	0	40	1	–
Soynut Butter Original	2 tbsp	180	1	0	–	0	40	1	–
Soynut Butter Unsalted	2 tbsp	180	1	0	–	0	40	1	–
I.M. Healthy									
SoyNut Butter Chocolate	2 tbsp (1.1 oz)	190	4	0	–	0	20	1	–
SoyNut Butter Honey Creamy	2 tbsp (1.1 oz)	170	2	0	–	0	30	1	–
SoyNut Butter Original Creamy	2 tbsp (1.1 oz)	170	1	0	–	0	50	tr	–

FOOD	PORTION	CALS	FIBER	VIT A	FOLIC	VIT C	CALCI	IRON	POTAS
SoyNut Butter Unsweetened Chunky	2 tbsp (1.1 oz)	160	5	0	–	0	60	1	–
SoyNut Butter Unsweetened Creamy	2 tbsp (1.1 oz)	160	5	0	–	0	60	1	–
Revival									
Shake Chocolate Daydream Fructose	1 pkg	240	2	–	–	–	500	3	410
Shake Strawberry Smile Fructose	1 pkg	225	0	–	–	–	500	3	400
Shake Strawberry Smile Splenda	1 pkg	130	0	–	–	–	500	3	400
Shake Strawberry Smile Unsweetened	1 pkg	130	0	–	–	–	500	3	400
Soy Shake Plain	1 pkg	110	0	–	–	–	20	3	20
Soy Shake Vanilla Pleasure	1 pkg	220	0	–	–	–	500	4	230
Soy Shake Vanilla Pleasure Splenda	1 pkg	120	0	–	–	–	500	3	250
Soy Shake Vanilla Pleasure Unsweetened	1 pkg	120	0	–	–	–	500	3	230
Soynuts Chocolate Covered	⅙ cup	70	tr	–	–	–	27	tr	–
Soynuts Hot Jalapeno & Cheddar	⅙ cup	78	2	–	–	–	20	2	–
Soynuts Unsalted	⅙ cup	78	2	–	–	–	29	1	–
Soynuts Yogurt Covered	⅙ cup	720	tr	–	–	–	20	tr	–
Soy Juicy									
All Flavors	8 oz	160	1	500	–	60	200	1	20
Soy Wonder									
Creamy	2 tbsp	170	1	0	–	0	50	tr	–
Crunchy	2 tbsp	170	1	0	–	0	50	tr	–

SOY SAUCE

FOOD	PORTION	CALS	FIBER	VIT A	FOLIC	VIT C	CALCI	IRON	POTAS
shoyu	1 tbsp	9	–	0	3	0	3	tr	32
soy sauce	1 tbsp	7	–	0	2	0	1	tr	27
tamari	1 tbsp	11	–	0	3	0	4	tr	38
Eden									
Organic Shoyu	1 tbsp	15	0	0	–	0	0	0	75

FOOD	PORTION	CALS	FIBER	VIT A	FOLIC	VIT C	CALCI	IRON	POTAS
Organic Shoyu Reduced Sodium	1 tbsp	10	0	0	–	0	0	tr	60
Organic Tamari	1 tbsp	15	0	0	–	0	0	tr	80
House Of Tsang									
Ginger Soy Sauce	1 tbsp	20	0	0	–	0	0	0	49
Less Sodium	1 tbsp	5	0	0	–	0	0	0	19

SOYBEANS

FOOD	PORTION	CALS	FIBER	VIT A	FOLIC	VIT C	CALCI	IRON	POTAS
dried cooked	1 cup	298	–	15	93	3	175	9	886
dry roasted	½ cup	387	–	20	176	4	232	3	1173
green cooked	½ cup	127	4	–	100	–	–	2	485
roasted	½ cup	405	–	172	182	2	119	3	1264
roasted & toasted	1 cup	490	–	216	244	2	149	5	1588
roasted & toasted salted	1 cup	490	–	216	244	2	149	5	1588
sprouts raw	½ cup	43	–	4	60	5	23	1	169
sprouts steamed	½ cup	38	–	5	–	4	28	1	167
sprouts stir fried	1 cup	125	–	17	–	12	82	tr	567
Arrowhead									
Organic not prep	¼ cup	180	10	–	–	–	–	–	–
C&W									
In the Pod	½ cup	110	9	200	–	6	80	3	–
Eden									
Organic Blacksoy	½ cup	120	7	500	24	–	80	3	310
Frieda's									
Edamame	½ cup (2.6 oz)	100	3	500	–	6	40	1	–
Soyafarm									
Edamame Yuba Sticks	7 pieces (2.5 oz)	123	4	–	–	3	50	2	360

SPAGHETTI SAUCE
JARRED

FOOD	PORTION	CALS	FIBER	VIT A	FOLIC	VIT C	CALCI	IRON	POTAS
marinara sauce	1 cup	171	–	2403	–	32	44	2	1061
spaghetti sauce	1 cup	272	–	3055	–	28	70	2	957
Amy's									
Family Marinara	½ cup	50	3	–	–	–	–	–	–
Garlic Mushroom	½ cup	120	3	–	–	–	–	–	–
Puttanesca	½ cup	40	1	–	–	–	–	–	–
Tomato Basil	½ cup	80	3	–	–	–	–	–	–
Wild Mushroom	½ cup	60	2	–	–	–	–	–	–

FOOD	PORTION	CALS	FIBER	VIT A	FOLIC	VIT C	CALCI	IRON	POTAS
Barilla									
Arrabbiata Tomato & Spicy Pepper	½ cup	90	3	200	–	7	60	tr	–
Basilico Tomato & Basil	½ cup	70	3	500	–	9	60	tr	–
Boscaiola Mushrooms & Garlic	½ cup	90	3	400	–	6	60	tr	–
Campagnola Roasted Garlic & Onion	½ cup	60	3	400	–	6	40	tr	–
Restaurant Creations Cheese & Tomatoes	¼ cup	110	1	100	–	2	40	1	–
Restaurant Creations Garlic Herbs & Tomatoes	¼ cup	100	2	0	–	2	20	1	–
Restaurant Creations Pesto & Tomatoes	¼ cup	150	2	200	–	2	40	1	–
Rustica Sweet Peppers & Garlic	½ cup	70	3	750	–	12	60	tr	–
Catelli									
Garden Select Country Mushroom	½ cup	80	3	500	–	12	20	1	–
Garden Select Diced Tomatoes & Basil	½ cup	80	3	500	–	12	40	1	–
Garden Select Fine Herbs	½ cup	80	3	500	–	12	40	1	–
Garden Select Garlic & Onion	½ cup	80	3	500	–	12	40	0	–
Garden Select Parmesan & Romano	½ cup	80	4	500	–	18	60	1	–
Garden Select Zucchini Primavera	½ cup	80	4	500	–	15	40	1	–
Classico									
Italian Sausage	½ cup	90	2	500	–	6	60	2	–
Tomato & Basil	½ cup	60	2	500	–	6	60	1	–
Del Monte									
Chunky Garlic & Herb	½ cup	60	tr	500	–	2	40	1	–
Chunky Italian Herb	½ cup	60	1	500	–	2	40	1	–
Garlic & Onion	½ cup	80	2	1250	–	6	40	1	–
Tomato & Basil	½ cup	70	3	750	–	9	40	1	–
With Four Cheese	½ cup	70	3	750	–	9	40	1	–
With Green Peppers & Mushrooms	½ cup	80	3	1000	–	6	40	1	–

FOOD	PORTION	CALS	FIBER	VIT A	FOLIC	VIT C	CALCI	IRON	POTAS
With Meat	½ cup	60	3	750	–	9	40	1	–
With Mushrooms	½ cup	60	2	750	–	9	40	1	–
Eden									
Organic	½ cup	80	3	2000	–	12	80	1	530
Organic No Salt	½ cup	80	3	2000	–	12	40	1	530
Organic Pizza Pasta Sauce	½ cup	65	5	1000	–	12	40	2	330
Emeril's									
Homestyle Marinara	½ cup	90	3	750	–	0	0	1	–
Roasted Gaaahlic	½ cup	70	2	750	–	0	20	1	–
Sicilian Gravy	½ cup	90	1	750	–	21	40	1	–
Vodka	½ cup	130	2	1000	–	15	40	1	–
Francesco Rinaldi									
Alfredo	¼ cup (2.1 oz)	70	0	100	–	0	80	0	–
Chunky Garden Mushroom & Onion	½ cup (4.4 oz)	80	3	750	–	0	40	2	–
Chunky Garden Mushroom & Peppers	½ cup (4.4 oz)	80	3	750	–	0	40	2	–
Chunky Garden Tomato Garlic & Onion	½ cup	70	tr	1000	–	0	40	1	–
Dolce Sweet & Tasty Tomato	½ cup (4.4 oz)	110	3	1250	–	0	40	1	–
Dulce Super Mushroom	½ cup (4.4 oz)	110	3	1250	–	0	40	1	–
Hearty Diavolo	½ cup (4.4 oz)	70	3	750	–	0	40	1	–
Hearty Mushroom Pepper & Onion	½ cup (4.4 oz)	80	3	750	–	0	40	1	–
Hearty Tomato & Basil	½ cup (4.4 oz)	80	4	750	–	0	60	1	–
Puttanesca	½ cup (4.3 oz)	70	tr	1000	–	0	0	1	–
Three Cheese	½ cup	80	tr	1250	–	0	60	1	–
Tomato Alfredo	¼ cup (2.1 oz)	60	0	750	–	0	40	1	–
Traditional Meat Flavored	½ cup (4.4 oz)	90	3	750	–	0	0	1	–

FOOD	PORTION	CALS	FIBER	VIT A	FOLIC	VIT C	CALCI	IRON	POTAS
Traditional Mushroom	½ cup (4.4 oz)	90	3	750	–	0	0	1	–
Traditional No Salt Added	½ cup (4.4 oz)	70	tr	1250	–	6	40	1	–
Traditional Original	½ cup (4.4 oz)	90	3	750	–	0	0	1	–
Vodka Sauce	¼ cup (2.1 oz)	60	0	500	–	0	0	1	–
Hunt's									
Basil Garlic & Oregano	¼ cup	15	tr	200	–	4	0	tr	180
Cheese & Garlic	½ cup	50	2	400	–	6	40	1	430
Chunky Vegetable	½ cup	50	3	750	–	6	20	2	340
Diced In Tomato Sauce	½ cup	30	1	750	–	12	60	tr	–
Family Favorites Lasagna	¼ cup	30	1	300	–	9	0	tr	180
Four Cheese	½ cup	50	3	500	–	9	40	2	370
Italian Sausage	½ cup	60	3	400	–	12	20	1	–
Light	½ cup	45	3	300	–	9	20	1	400
Meat	½ cup	68	3	400	–	9	20	1	380
No Added Sugar	½ cup	45	3	300	–	12	20	2	380
Roasted Garlic & Onion	½ cup	50	3	400	–	9	20	1	400
Traditional	½ cup	50	2	400	–	9	20	2	–
With Mushrooms	½ cup	45	3	500	–	12	20	3	–
Joey Pots & Pans									
Arrabbiata	½ cup	100	1	1500	–	21	40	1	–
Marinara	½ cup	50	1	750	–	15	40	1	–
Vodka Sauce	½ cup	110	1	1000	–	15	40	1	–
Milo's									
Portobello Shiraz	4 oz	40	2	100	–	9	20	1	–
Muir Glen									
Organic Balsamic Roasted Onion	½ cup (4.4 oz)	50	0	1000	–	9	40	1	–
Organic Cabernet Marinara	½ cup (4.4 oz)	50	0	1000	–	9	40	1	–
Organic Chunky Herb	½ cup (4.4 oz)	50	0	1000	–	9	40	1	–
Organic Garden Vegetable	½ cup (4.4 oz)	50	0	1000	–	9	40	1	–
Organic Garlic & Onion	½ cup (4.4 oz)	55	0	1000	–	9	40	1	–

FOOD	PORTION	CALS	FIBER	VIT A	FOLIC	VIT C	CALCI	IRON	POTAS
Organic Garlic Roasted Garlic	½ cup (4.4 oz)	50	0	1000	–	9	40	1	–
Organic Green Olive	½ cup (4.4 oz)	60	0	1000	–	9	40	1	–
Organic Italian Herb	½ cup (4.4 oz)	55	0	1000	–	9	40	1	–
Organic Mushroom Marinara	½ cup (4.4 oz)	45	0	500	–	6	40	1	–
Organic Portabello Mushroom	½ cup (4.4 oz)	50	0	500	–	6	40	1	–
Organic Sun Dried Tomato	½ cup (4.4 oz)	55	1	1000	–	6	40	1	–
Organic Tomato Basil	½ cup (4.4 oz)	50	0	1000	–	6	40	1	–
Newman's Own									
Bambolina	½ cup	90	tr	1250	–	0	20	1	–
Cabernet Marinara	½ cup	70	2	1000	–	0	60	1	–
Five Cheese	½ cup	80	tr	0	–	0	0	1	–
Italian Sausage & Peppers	½ cup	90	tr	750	–	0	40	1	–
Marinara	½ cup	70	tr	1500	–	0	40	2	–
Marinara w/ Mushrooms	½ cup	70	tr	1250	–	0	40	2	–
Pesto & Tomato Sauce	½ cup	80	tr	1000	–	0	80	1	–
Roasted Garlic & Green Peppers	½ cup	70	4	–	–	–	–	–	–
Sockarooni	½ cup	70	tr	1250	–	0	40	1	–
Tomato & Roasted Garlic	½ cup	70	tr	1000	–	0	40	1	–
Vodka Sauce	½ cup	110	0	–	–	–	–	–	–
Pomi									
Marinara	½ cup	80	3	500	–	18	40	1	–
Prego									
100% Natural Roasted Garlic Parmesan	½ cup	100	3	750	–	1	40	1	–
Organic Mushroom	½ cup	90	4	750	–	5	20	1	–
Ragu									
Chunky Garden Style Tomato Garlic & Onion	½ cup (4.5 oz)	110	2	500	–	5	40	1	–

FOOD	PORTION	CALS	FIBER	VIT A	FOLIC	VIT C	CALCI	IRON	POTAS
Seeds Of Change									
Balsamic Olive & Onion	½ cup	80	2	600	–	2	20	1	–
Garden Vegetable	½ cup	70	2	1000	–	5	10	1	–
Mushroom & Onion	½ cup	70	2	500	–	5	20	1	–
Three Cheese Marinara	½ cup	70	2	1000	–	9	40	1	–
Traditional Herb	½ cup	70	2	1000	–	6	20	1	–
Tuttorosso									
Pasta Sauce Meat	½ cup	90	3	750	–	12	20	1	–
REFRIGERATED									
Buitoni									
Alfredo	¼ cup	140	0	300	–	0	100	0	–
Alfredo Portabello Mushroom	¼ cup	100	0	200	–	0	40	0	–
Alfredo Light	¼ cup	80	0	100	–	0	100	0	–
Marinara	½ cup	80	2	750	–	1	60	tr	–
Marinara Roasted Garlic	½ cup	60	1	500	–	1	60	tr	–
Pesto	¼ cup	330	6	2000	–	2	400	6	–
Pesto w/ Basil	¼ cup	300	2	400	–	0	200	tr	–
Pesto w/ Basil Reduced Fat	¼ cup	230	2	500	–	0	200	tr	–
Pesto w/ Sun Dried Tomatoes	¼ cup	210	2	400	–	0	100	tr	–
Tomato Herb Parmesan	½ cup	120	2	750	–	0	100	1	–
TAKE-OUT									
bolognese	5 oz	195	tr	2260	–	7	36	2	–
SPANISH FOOD									
FROZEN									
Amy's									
Black Bean Vegetable Enchilada	1 (4.75 oz)	130	2	–	–	–	–	–	–
Bowls Santa Fe Enchilada	1 pkg (10 oz)	340	10	–	–	–	–	–	–
Burrito Bean & Cheese	1 (6 oz)	280	6	–	–	–	–	–	–
Burrito Bean & Rice Non-Dairy	1 (6 oz)	270	5	–	–	–	–	–	–
Burrito Black Bean Vegetable	1 (6 oz)	320	4	–	–	–	–	–	–
Burrito Breakfast	1 (6 oz)	210	5	–	–	–	–	–	–

FOOD	PORTION	CALS	FIBER	VIT A	FOLIC	VIT C	CALCI	IRON	POTAS
Cheese Enchilada	1 (4.75 oz)	210	2	–	–	–	–	–	–
Mexican Tamale Pie	1 (8 oz)	150	4	–	–	–	–	–	–
Cedarlane									
Burrito Beans Rice & Cheese	1 (6 oz)	260	7	500	–	15	100	3	–
Contessa									
Fajitas Shrimp	2 (8 oz)	230	5	1000	–	36	100	3	–
Paella w/ Chicken & Seafood	1½ cups	200	2	300	–	5	20	2	–
Seafood Veracruz not prep	1¾ cups	180	6	1000	–	21	60	3	–
El Monterey									
Quesadillas Chicken Breast & Cheese	1 (5 oz)	280	tr	500	–	2	300	2	–
Healthy Choice									
Chicken Enchiladas	1 pkg	360	8	400	–	4	40	1	460
Enchilada Chicken	1 pkg	300	6	200	–	0	100	1	–
Jose Ole									
Burrito Beef & Cheese	1 (5 oz)	300	2	100	–	5	100	3	–
Burrito Chicken Monterey	1 (5 oz)	270	2	200	–	4	80	3	–
Chimichanga Chicken & Cheese	1 (5 oz)	330	2	200	–	1	80	4	–
Chimichanga Shredded Beef	1 (5 oz)	350	2	100	–	5	100	3	–
Mini Burrito Chicken & Cheese	3	200	1	100	–	1	40	2	–
Mini Chimichanga Beef & Cheddar	3	240	1	300	–	2	80	2	–
Mini Quesadilla Grilled Chicken	3	220	1	200	–	0	100	2	–
Mini Tacos Beef & Cheese	4	200	3	300	–	1	100	1	–
Mini Taquitos Beef & Cheese	4	180	2	500	–	4	60	1	–
Soft Taco Beef & Cheese	1 (5 oz)	280	1	200	–	6	100	3	–
Taquitos Beef & Cheese Flour Tortilla	2	220	1	300	–	2	80	2	–

FOOD	PORTION	CALS	FIBER	VIT A	FOLIC	VIT C	CALCI	IRON	POTAS
Taquitos Buffalo Chicken Flour Tortilla	2	200	tr	100	–	4	40	1	–
Taquitos Chicken Flour Tortilla	3	180	2	200	–	0	10	1	–
Taquitos Chicken & Cheese Flour Tortilla	2	220	1	100	–	0	60	2	–
Taquitos Pepperoni Pizza Flour Tortilla	2	240	1	0	–	0	40	1	–
Taquitos Shredded Beef Corn Tortilla	3	180	2	400	–	4	60	1	–
Lean Cuisine									
One Dish Favorites Chicken Enchilada	1 pkg (9 oz)	280	3	200	–	2	150	1	330
Patio									
Beef & Cheese Enchiladas Chili 'N Beans	1 meal (15.5 oz)	670	12	1500	–	0	250	4	–
Beef Enchiladas Chili 'N Beans	1 meal (15.5 oz)	540	12	1500	–	0	250	5	–
Burrito Bean & Cheese	1 (5 oz)	280	5	300	–	0	40	3	–
Burrito Beef & Bean Hot	1 (5 oz)	320	4	200	–	1	20	1	–
Burrito Beef & Bean Medium	1 (5 oz)	300	5	300	–	0	20	2	–
Burrito Beef & Bean Red Chili Pepper Red Hot	1 (5 oz)	320	4	400	–	0	20	1	–
Burrito Chicken	1 (5 oz)	280	2	0	–	0	60	2	–
Enchilada Beef	1 meal (12 oz)	320	9	500	–	4	150	2	–
Enchilada Cheese	1 meal (12 oz)	370	7	500	–	0	150	2	–
Enchilada Chicken	1 meal (12 oz)	400	8	200	–	0	200	2	–
Fiesta	1 meal (12 oz)	350	7	300	–	0	150	2	–
Mexican Style	1 meal (13.25 oz)	470	10	500	–	2	100	3	–

FOOD	PORTION	CALS	FIBER	VIT A	FOLIC	VIT C	CALCI	IRON	POTAS
READY-TO-EAT									
taco shell corn	1 (6.5 in)	98	2	0	28	0	34	1	38
taco shell flour	1 (7 in)	173	1	0	24	0	44	1	46
Ortega									
Tostada Shells	2 (1 oz)	140	1	0	–	0	40	tr	–
SHELF-STABLE									
Fantastic									
Spanish Paella	1 pkg (8 oz)	280	4	1000	–	48	60	3	–
TAKE-OUT									
burrito w/ beans	1 med (5 oz)	295	7	0	106	3	97	3	304
burrito w/ beans & rice	1 (3.5 oz)	221	4	0	76	1	68	2	161
burrito w/ beef	1 sm (3.4 oz)	297	1	0	48	0	74	3	253
burrito w/ beef & beans	1 med (5 oz)	331	6	0	89	3	89	3	364
burrito w/ beef beans & cheese	1 med (5 oz)	379	5	355	78	2	267	3	324
burrito w/ chicken & beans	1 med (5 oz)	295	5	30	84	3	80	3	302
burrito w/ pork & beans	1 med (5 oz)	320	6	5	84	3	82	3	376
chiles rellenos meat & cheese filled	1 (5 oz)	213	2	410	21	32	116	2	345
chimichanga w/ bean cheese lettuce & tomato	1 (4.1 oz)	271	3	285	48	7	150	2	300
chimichanga w/ beef & rice	1 (10 oz)	634	5	260	101	15	118	5	708
chimichanga w/ beef beans lettuce & tomato	1 (4.1 oz)	254	3	90	47	7	53	2	336
chimichanga w/ beef cheese lettuce & tomato	1 (4.1 oz)	337	1	315	35	4	182	2	208

FOOD	PORTION	CALS	FIBER	VIT A	FOLIC	VIT C	CALCI	IRON	POTAS
chimichanga w/ chicken sour cream lettuce & tomato	1 (4 oz)	277	1	350	30	4	74	1	183
enchilada w/ beans	1 (4.1 oz)	179	6	65	68	13	79	2	373
enchilada w/ beans & cheese	1 (4.6 oz)	233	5	315	62	15	199	2	403
enchilada w/ beef	1 (4 oz)	214	3	80	43	13	84	2	401
enchilada w/ beef & beans	1 (4 oz)	195	4	70	57	13	81	2	384
frijoles	1 cup	278	9	375	322	10	88	6	793
frijoles w/ cheese	1 cup	225	–	456	112	2	189	2	605
nachos w/ beans & cheese	1 serv (9.4 oz)	616	13	116	142	8	433	4	608
nachos w/ beef beans cheese & sour cream	1 serv (19 oz)	1620	19	1625	143	14	970	7	1190
pupusa meat filled	1 (3.6 oz)	187	3	45	56	2	66	3	191
quesadilla w/ cheese	1 (5 oz)	498	3	765	57	6	498	3	199
quesadilla w/ meat & cheese	1 (6.5 oz)	605	2	765	61	6	506	4	372
taco de jueye w/ crab meat	1 (4.2 oz)	266	2	280	47	11	160	2	317
taco w/ beans lettuce tomato & salsa	1 (2.8 oz)	117	4	50	49	5	39	1	184
taco w/ chicken lettuce tomato & salsa	1 (2.5 oz)	114	1	75	27	4	32	1	139
taco w/ fish lettuce tomato & salsa	1 (2.7 oz)	101	1	70	32	5	52	1	179
tostada w/ beef lettuce tomato & salsa	1 (2.7 oz)	143	2	60	31	4	40	1	189

SPINACH
CANNED

FOOD	PORTION	CALS	FIBER	VIT A	FOLIC	VIT C	CALCI	IRON	POTAS
drained	1 cup	49	5	20974	210	31	272	5	740
Del Monte									
Whole Leaf	½ cup	30	2	2500	–	15	100	1	–
Popeye									
Spinach	½ cup	45	3	8500	–	15	200	2	220

FOOD	PORTION	CALS	FIBER	VIT A	FOLIC	VIT C	CALCI	IRON	POTAS
S&W									
Spinach	½ cup (4.5 oz)	30	2	3500	–	12	80	3	410
FRESH									
baby raw	2 cups	20	3	1750	–	8	30	2	–
cooked	1 cup	41	4	18866	263	18	245	6	839
malabar cooked	1 cup	10	1	510	50	3	55	1	113
mustard cooked	1 cup	29	4	14760	131	117	284	1	513
new zealand cooked	1 cup	22	–	6520	14	29	86	1	184
raw	1 cup	7	1	2813	58	8	30	1	167
Fresh Express									
Baby Spinach	3 cups	20	2	5500	–	24	80	3	–
Spicy Spinach	3 cups (3 oz)	10	6	4000	100	18	80	5	350
Ready Pac									
Baby	2 cups	20	3	1750	–	8	30	2	–
Microwave Spinach as prep	½ cup	20	tr	3000	–	6	80	0	–
FROZEN									
chopped cooked	1 cup	30	4	11458	115	2	145	2	287
Amy's Organic									
Snacks Spinach Feta	5–6 pieces	170	2	–	–	–	–	–	–
C&W									
Baby Chopped	1 cup	30	1	2500	–	1	80	1	–
Creamed	½ cup	100	4	200	–	9	150	3	–
Fresh Like									
Cut Leaf	3.5 oz	21	1	8194	–	26	108	2	344
Green Giant									
Creamed Low Fat Sauce	½ cup	80	1	4500	–	5	100	tr	–
No Sauce	½ cup	25	1	2500	–	1	60	1	–
Taverna									
Spinach Pie	1 piece (4.8 oz)	190	5	2250	–	6	200	3	–
SHELF-STABLE									
TastyBite									
Kashmir Spinach	½ pkg (5 oz)	170	3	0	–	0	220	1	–
TAKE-OUT									
indian saag	1 serv	28	1	–	–	–	–	–	–

FOOD	PORTION	CALS	FIBER	VIT A	FOLIC	VIT C	CALCI	IRON	POTAS
spanakopita spinach pie	1 serv (3 oz)	148	1	1025	58	6	117	1	215

SPINACH JUICE
| juice | 7 oz | 14 | – | – | – | 58 | 2 | – | 824 |

SPORTS DRINKS
Liv Naturals
| All Flavors | 8 oz | 70 | 0 | – | – | – | – | – | 45 |

SPOT
| baked | 3 oz | 134 | 0 | – | – | – | 15 | tr | 541 |

SPROUTS
kidney bean	½ cup	27	–	2	–	36	16	1	172
lentil sprouts	½ cup	40	–	17	38	6	9	1	122
mung bean	½ cup	16	–	11	32	7	7	tr	77
mung bean canned	½ cup	8	–	14	6	tr	9	tr	17
mung bean cooked	½ cup	13	–	8	–	7	7	tr	63
pea	½ cup	77	–	100	87	6	21	1	229
radish	½ cup	8	–	74	18	6	10	tr	16
Brassica									
Broccoli Sprouts	½ cup (1 oz)	16	1	561	0	20	26	tr	–
TAKE-OUT									
mung bean stir fried	½ cup	31	–	–	–	–	8	1	–

SQUAB
| boneless baked | 1 (4 oz) | 242 | 0 | 155 | 7 | 3 | 19 | 7 | 283 |

SQUASH
CANNED
crookneck sliced	½ cup	14	–	130	11	3	13	1	104
Farmer's Market									
Organic Butternut	½ cup	50	2	2249	–	4	21	tr	–
FRESH									
acorn cooked mashed	½ cup	41	3	315	14	8	32	1	321
acorn cubed baked	½ cup	57	2	437	19	11	45	1	446
butternut baked	½ cup	41	2	7141	20	15	42	1	290
crookneck sliced cooked	½ cup	18	1	259	18	5	24	tr	173
hubbard baked	½ cup	51	3	6156	17	10	17	tr	365

FOOD	PORTION	CALS	FIBER	VIT A	FOLIC	VIT C	CALCI	IRON	POTAS
hubbard cooked mashed	½ cup	35	3	4726	12	8	12	tr	252
scallop sliced cooked	½ cup	14	1	77	19	10	14	tr	126
spaghetti cooked	½ cup	23	2	86	6	3	17	tr	91
Frieda's									
Acorn	¾ cup (3 oz)	35	2	300	–	9	20	1	–
Baby Crookneck	⅔ cup (3 oz)	15	1	300	–	6	0	tr	–
Baby Scallop	⅔ cup (3 oz)	15	1	0	–	15	0	0	–
Eight Ball	2 (4.4 oz)	18	1	200	–	12	20	1	–
Hubbard	¾ cup (3 oz)	35	2	4500	–	9	0	0	–
Mini Pumpkin	¾ cup (3 oz)	20	2	1250	–	9	0	1	–
Spaghetti	¾ cup (3 oz)	30	1	0	–	1	0	0	–
Star Spangled	⅔ cup (3 oz)	20	1	400	–	30	0	0	–
Turban	¾ cup (3 oz)	30	1	3500	–	9	20	tr	–
Glory									
Yellow Sliced	¾ cup	20	1	300	–	6	20	tr	–
Martin Farms									
Butternut Fresh Cut	½ cup	40	1	6500	20	18	40	1	300
FROZEN									
butternut cooked mashed	½ cup	47	3	4007	–	4	23	1	160
crookneck sliced cooked	½ cup	24	–	187	12	7	19	tr	243
C&W									
Butternut	½ cup	45	1	500	–	2	20	tr	–
TAKE-OUT									
fritter	1 (0.8 oz)	81	1	190	13	1	29	1	81
SQUASH SEEDS									
roasted	1 oz	148	–	–	–	–	12	4	229
salted & roasted	1 oz	148	–	–	–	–	12	4	229
seeds dried	1 oz	154	–	108	–	–	12	4	229
seeds whole roasted	1 oz	127	–	–	–	–	16	1	261

FOOD	PORTION	CALS	FIBER	VIT A	FOLIC	VIT C	CALCI	IRON	POTAS
SQUID									
baked	1 cup	192	0	285	8	8	55	1	416
canned in its own ink	1 can (4 oz)	122	0	60	5	4	43	1	260
dried	1 sm (1.5 oz)	147	0	65	8	7	51	1	392
pickled	1 oz	26	0	15	1	1	9	tr	68
steamed	1 cup	147	0	70	6	5	52	1	316
Contessa									
Calamari + Sauce	13 pieces + 2 tbsp sauce	160	1	100	–	0	20	1	–
TAKE-OUT									
arroz con calamares	1 cup	400	1	200	82	42	45	3	326
calamari breaded & fried	1 cup	296	1	130	22	6	87	2	411
SQUIRREL									
roasted	3 oz	147	0	–	–	–	2	6	300
STARFRUIT									
fresh	1	42	–	626	–	27	6	tr	207
Frieda's									
Dried	⅓ cup (1.4 oz)	120	1	1000	–	0	20	1	–
STRAWBERRIES									
CANNED									
in heavy syrup	½ cup	117	–	33	36	40	16	1	109
DRIED									
Frieda's									
Dried	½ cup (1.4 oz)	150	3	0	–	0	20	tr	–
FRESH									
strawberries	1 cup	45	4	41	26	85	21	1	247
strawberries	1 pint	97	–	87	57	182	45	1	530
FROZEN									
sweetened sliced	1 cup	245	–	61	38	106	29	1	249
sweetened sliced	1 pkg (10 oz)	273	–	68	42	118	31	2	277
unsweetened	1 cup	52	–	66	25	61	23	1	220
whole sweetened	1 cup	200	–	70	10	101	29	1	249

FOOD	PORTION	CALS	FIBER	VIT A	FOLIC	VIT C	CALCI	IRON	POTAS
whole sweetened	1 pkg (10 oz)	223	–	78	11	112	32	1	277

C&W
| Ultimate Sliced | ⅔ cup | 50 | 1 | 0 | – | 42 | 20 | 1 | – |

Europe's Best
| Sliced | ¾ cup | 40 | 3 | 0 | – | 78 | 20 | tr | – |

STRAWBERRY JUICE
Adina
| California Kiss Hibiscus Strawberry | 8 oz | 80 | – | – | – | 8 | 20 | tr | – |

Ceres
| Strawberry | 8 oz | 115 | 1 | 0 | – | 60 | 20 | tr | 216 |

Giant Berry Farms
| Just Strawberries | 1 bottle (12 oz) | 140 | 2 | 0 | – | 60 | 40 | 5 | 260 |

STUFFING/DRESSING
Tofurky
| Wild Rice & Mushroom | ½ cup | 110 | 1 | 0 | – | 0 | 20 | 1 | – |

TAKE-OUT
bread	1 cup	352	2	780	66	0	58	2	142
cornbread	½ cup	179	3	340	97	1	26	1	62
oyster	1 cup	304	2	875	50	4	113	5	211
sausage	½ cup	292	1	78	3	2	17	1	96

STURGEON
broiled	3 oz	115	0	744	14	0	14	1	310
roe raw	1 oz	59	–	–	–	5	–	–	–
smoked	1 oz	49	0	265	6	0	5	tr	107

TAKE-OUT
| breaded & fried | 4 oz | 252 | 1 | 955 | 25 | 0 | 41 | 1 | 325 |

SUCKER
| white baked | 3 oz | 101 | 0 | – | – | – | 76 | 1 | 414 |

SUGAR
brown packed	1 cup (7.7 oz)	828	–	0	1	0	167	4	762
brown unpacked	1 cup (5.1 oz)	547	0	0	1	0	123	3	502
brown organic	1 tsp	17	0	–	–	–	–	–	–
cinnamon sugar	1 tsp	16	tr	0	0	0	3	tr	1

FOOD	PORTION	CALS	FIBER	VIT A	FOLIC	VIT C	CALCI	IRON	POTAS
maple	1 piece (1 oz)	99	0	0	0	0	25	tr	77
powdered	1 tbsp (0.3 oz)	31	–	0	0	0	0	0	0
powdered unsifted	1 cup (4.2 oz)	467	–	0	0	0	1	tr	3
raw	1 pkg (5 g)	19	0	0	0	0	4	tr	17
sugarcane stem	3 oz	54	3	–	–	1	2	tr	–
white	1 cup (7 oz)	773	–	0	0	0	2	tr	4
white	1 packet (3 g)	12	0	0	0	0	0	0	0
white	1 tsp (4 g)	15	–	0	0	0	0	0	0

SUGAR SUBSTITUTES
Equal
Sugar Lite	1 tsp	8	0	–	–	–	–	–	–

Fran Gare's
Miracle Sweet	1 tsp	10	0	–	–	–	–	–	–

Keto
Sweet	½ tsp	0	0	–	–	–	–	–	–

Lo Han
Sweet	2 scoops	2	tr	–	–	–	–	–	–

SomerSweet
Sweetener	¼ tsp	0	tr	–	–	–	–	–	–

Splenda
Flavor Blends All Flavors	1 pkg	0	0	–	–	–	–	–	–
No Calorie Granules	1 tsp	0	0	–	–	–	–	–	–
Sweetener	1 pkg	0	0	0	–	0	0	0	–

Steel's
Brown	1 tsp	10	0	–	–	–	–	–	–
Sugar Substitute	1 tsp	10	0	–	–	–	–	–	–

Stevita
Spoonable	⅓ tsp	0	0	–	–	–	–	–	0

Sugar Twin
Spoonable Brown	1 tsp	0	0	–	–	–	–	–	–
Spoonable White	1 tsp	0	0	–	–	–	–	–	–

SweetLeaf
SteviaPlus	1 pkg	0	1	–	–	–	–	–	–

FOOD	PORTION	CALS	FIBER	VIT A	FOLIC	VIT C	CALCI	IRON	POTAS
Whey Low									
Gold	1 tsp	4	0	0	–	0	0	0	–
Granular	1 tsp	4	0	0	–	0	0	0	–
Powder	1 tsp	4	0	0	–	0	0	0	–
SUGAR-APPLE									
fresh	1	146	–	9	–	66	37	1	384
fresh cut up	1 cup	236	–	15	–	91	59	2	619
SUNCHOKE									
fresh raw sliced	½ cup	57	–	15	–	3	10	3	–
Frieda's									
Sunchoke	½ cup (3 oz)	70	1	0	–	4	0	3	–
SUNFISH									
pumpkinseed baked	3 oz	97	0	–	–	–	87	1	381
SUNFLOWER									
seeds dry roasted w/ salt	¼ cup	185	–	85	76	1	39	2	23
seeds dry roasted w/o salt	¼ cup	186	3	3	76	tr	22	1	272
seeds w/ hulls dried	¼ cup	66	1	6	26	tr	13	1	79
David									
Kernals Original	¼ cup	200	2	–	60	–	20	1	–
Seeds BBQ	¼ cup	190	2	–	72	–	20	1	230
Seeds BBQ Sizzlin	¼ cup	190	2	0	–	0	20	1	–
Seeds Jalapeno	¼ cup	190	2	–	–	–	20	1	230
Seeds Nacho Cheese	¼ cup	180	2	–	60	–	20	1	220
Seeds Original	¼ cup	190	2	–	72	–	80	1	230
Seeds Ranch	¼ cup	190	2	–	60	–	40	1	230
Seeds Reduced Sodium	¼ cup	190	2	–	60	–	20	1	230
Frito Lay									
Seeds	3 tbsp	180	2	0	–	0	20	1	–
Good Sense									
Nuts Honey Roasted	¼ cup	190	2	0	–	1	40	1	–
Nuts Raw	¼ cup	170	4	0	–	0	40	2	–
Nuts Roasted & Salted	¼ cup	190	2	–	60	–	40	1	–
Seeds In Shell Roasted & Salted	½ cup	150	13	0	–	0	40	1	260

FOOD	PORTION	CALS	FIBER	VIT A	FOLIC	VIT C	CALCI	IRON	POTAS
Sunflower Nuts Roasted w/o Salt	¼ cup	190	2	–	60	–	40	1	–
MaraNatha									
Tamari Seeds	¼ cup	160	2	0	–	0	20	1	–
SunButter									
Creamy	2 tbsp	200	4	0	–	0	20	1	–
Organic	2 tbsp	220	2	0	–	0	0	1	–
SunGold									
Seeds Roasted Salted	1 oz	172	2	0	–	0	20	1	–

SUSHI
TAKE-OUT

FOOD	PORTION	CALS	FIBER	VIT A	FOLIC	VIT C	CALCI	IRON	POTAS
california roll	1 piece (0.8 oz)	28	–	39	5	1	13	tr	37
fresh salmon rolls	4 pieces	250	3	300	–	9	20	1	–
sashimi	1 serv (6 oz)	198	–	1035	8	4	25	1	668
tuna roll	1 piece (0.7 oz)	23	–	255	1	tr	2	tr	24
vegetable roll	1 piece (1.2 oz)	27	–	371	16	3	20	tr	60
vinegared ginger	⅓ cup (1.6 oz)	48	–	0	5	2	8	tr	189
wasabi	2 tsp (0.3 oz)	5	–	0	0	0	6	tr	28
yellowtail roll	1 piece (0.6 oz)	25	–	57	3	1	12	tr	14

SWAMP CABBAGE

FOOD	PORTION	CALS	FIBER	VIT A	FOLIC	VIT C	CALCI	IRON	POTAS
chopped cooked w/o salt	1 cup	20	2	5096	34	16	53	1	278

SWEET POTATO

FOOD	PORTION	CALS	FIBER	VIT A	FOLIC	VIT C	CALCI	IRON	POTAS
baked w/ skin	1 (3.5 oz)	118	3	24877	26	28	32	1	397
canned in syrup	½ cup	106	–	7014	–	11	16	1	189
canned pieces	1 cup	183	–	15965	33	53	44	2	625
frzn cooked	½ cup	88	–	14441	20	8	31	tr	332
leaves cooked	½ cup	11	–	293	–	1	8	tr	153
mashed	½ cup	172	3	27968	18	28	35	1	301
Farmer's Market									
Organic Puree	½ cup	96	2	15000	–	5	20	1	–

FOOD	PORTION	CALS	FIBER	VIT A	FOLIC	VIT C	CALCI	IRON	POTAS
Glory									
Casserole	½ cup	180	2	16500	–	12	60	tr	–
Cut Fresh	1 serv (5 oz)	140	4	23500	–	18	20	tr	–
Sweet Potatoes	⅔ cup	160	2	9500	–	18	20	1	300
Princella									
In Light Syrup	⅔ cup	160	3	11000	–	5	20	1	–
Royal Prince									
Orange Pineapple	½ cup	160	2	1500	–	1	20	1	–
TAKE-OUT									
candied	3.5 oz	144	–	4399	12	7	27	1	198
SWEETBREAD (PANCREAS)									
beef braised	3 oz	230	0	0	3	17	14	2	209
lamb braised	3 oz	199	0	0	11	17	10	2	247
pork braised	3 oz	186	0	0	4	5	14	2	143
testicals cooked	1 pair (6.8 oz)	241	0	7	39	76	8	2	836
veal braised	3 oz	218	0	0	3	5	15	2	236
SWISS CHARD									
cooked	½ cup	18	–	2762	–	16	51	2	483
raw chopped	½ cup	3	–	594	–	5	9	tr	68
Frieda's									
Bright Lights	1 cup (3 oz)	15	1	3000	–	27	40	1	–
SWORDFISH									
cooked	3 oz	132	0	117	–	1	5	1	314
raw	3 oz	103	0	101	–	1	4	1	245
SYRUP									
corn dark & light	¼ cup	240	0	0	0	0	2	tr	3
date syrup	1 tbsp	63	0	–	–	–	12	1	–
maple	1 tbsp	52	–	–	0	0	13	tr	41
maple	1 cup (11.1 oz)	824	–	–	1	0	211	4	643
raspberry	1 oz	76	–	–	–	8	8	1	45
rose hip	1 oz	9	0	–	–	–	–	–	–
sorghum	1 cup (11.6 oz)	957	–	–	–	–	495	13	3300

FOOD	PORTION	CALS	FIBER	VIT A	FOLIC	VIT C	CALCI	IRON	POTAS
sorghum	1 tbsp (0.7 oz)	61	–	–	–	–	31	1	210
sugar syrup	¼ cup	76	0	0	0	0	1	0	1
Cary's									
Maple	¼ cup	210	–	–	–	–	60	1	–
Eden									
Organic Barley Malt	1 tbsp	60	0	0	–	0	0	0	65
Lundberg									
Organic Sweet Dreams Brown Rice	2 tbsp	110	0	–	–	–	–	–	–
Spectrum									
Balsamic Organic	1 tbsp	35	0	0	–	0	0	0	0

TAMARILLOS
Frieda's

FOOD	PORTION	CALS	FIBER	VIT A	FOLIC	VIT C	CALCI	IRON	POTAS
Gold Or Red	2 (4.2 oz)	40	4	500	–	36	0	0	–

TAMARIND

FOOD	PORTION	CALS	FIBER	VIT A	FOLIC	VIT C	CALCI	IRON	POTAS
dried sweetened pulpitas	½ cup	279	5	5	7	1	74	3	622
dried sweetened pulpitas	1 piece (0.8 oz)	56	1	0	1	tr	15	1	124
fresh	1 (2 g)	5	tr	1	0	tr	1	tr	13
fresh cut up	1 cup	143	3	18	8	2	44	2	377

TAMARIND JUICE

FOOD	PORTION	CALS	FIBER	VIT A	FOLIC	VIT C	CALCI	IRON	POTAS
nectar	1 cup	143	1	0	3	18	25	2	68
Teptip									
Drink	1 can (11.2 oz)	210	0	0	–	0	20	3	–

TANGERINE
CANNED

FOOD	PORTION	CALS	FIBER	VIT A	FOLIC	VIT C	CALCI	IRON	POTAS
in light syrup	1 cup	154	2	2117	13	50	18	1	197
juice pack	1 cup	92	2	2121	12	85	27	1	331

FRESH

FOOD	PORTION	CALS	FIBER	VIT A	FOLIC	VIT C	CALCI	IRON	POTAS
fresh	1 lg (4.2 oz)	64	2	817	19	32	44	tr	199
fresh	1 med (3.1 oz)	47	2	599	14	24	33	tr	146

FOOD	PORTION	CALS	FIBER	VIT A	FOLIC	VIT C	CALCI	IRON	POTAS
fresh	1 sm (2.7 oz)	40	1	518	12	20	28	tr	126
sections	1 cup	103	4	1328	31	52	72	tr	324
Chiquita									
Tangerine	1 med (3.5 oz)	50	2	0	–	30	40	0	–
River Pride									
Sweet	1 (3.8 oz)	50	3	0	–	30	40	0	–
Sunkist									
Fresh	1 (3.8 oz)	50	3	0	–	30	40	0	–

TANGERINE JUICE

FOOD	PORTION	CALS	FIBER	VIT A	FOLIC	VIT C	CALCI	IRON	POTAS
canned sweetened	1 cup	124	1	630	12	55	45	1	443
fresh	1 cup	106	1	625	12	77	44	tr	440
Italian Volcano									
Organic	1 serv (6.75 oz)	94	tr	–	–	64	–	2	–
Naked Juice									
Tangerine Scream	8 oz	110	0	1000	–	78	40	tr	440
Odwalla									
Juice	8 oz	110	0	1000	–	78	40	tr	440

TAPIOCA

FOOD	PORTION	CALS	FIBER	VIT A	FOLIC	VIT C	CALCI	IRON	POTAS
pearl dry	¼ cup (1.3 oz)	136	tr	0	2	0	8	1	4
starch	1 oz	98	–	–	–	0	3	tr	6

TARO

FOOD	PORTION	CALS	FIBER	VIT A	FOLIC	VIT C	CALCI	IRON	POTAS
chips	10 (0.8 oz)	115	–	0	–	1	14	tr	174
leaves cooked	½ cup	18	–	3136	–	26	63	1	341
raw sliced	½ cup	56	–	0	–	2	22	tr	307
shoots sliced cooked	½ cup	10	–	–	–	–	9	tr	240
sliced cooked	½ cup (2.3 oz)	94	–	0	–	3	12	tr	319
tahitian sliced cooked	½ cup	30	–	1200	–	26	101	1	423
Frieda's									
Taro Root	⅔ cup (3 oz)	90	3	0	–	0	40	tr	–

TARPON

FOOD	PORTION	CALS	FIBER	VIT A	FOLIC	VIT C	CALCI	IRON	POTAS
fresh	3 oz	87	0	–	–	–	46	1	306

FOOD	PORTION	CALS	FIBER	VIT A	FOLIC	VIT C	CALCI	IRON	POTAS
TARRAGON									
ground	1 tsp	5	–	67	–	–	18	1	48
TEA/HERBAL TEA									
HERBAL									
chamomile brewed	1 cup	2	0	47	1	0	5	tr	21
Celestial Seasonings									
Dessert Tea English Toffee	1 cup	0	0	–	–	–	–	–	100
Peppermint	1 cup	0	0	–	–	–	–	–	25
Roastaroma Herb	1 cup	0	0	–	–	–	–	–	25
Zinger Lemon	1 cup	0	0	–	–	–	–	–	30
Eden									
Organic Genmaicha Tea	1 tea bag	0	0	0	–	0	0	0	0
Organic Kukicha Tea	1 tea bag	0	0	0	–	0	0	0	0
Silk									
Chai	1 cup	140	0	300	–	0	300	1	–
REGULAR									
brewed tea	6 oz	2	0	0	9	0	0	tr	66
Celestial Seasonings									
Green Antioxidant	1 cup	0	0	1000	–	66	–	–	–
Morning Thunder	1 cup	0	0	–	–	–	–	–	30
TeaHouse Chai Cinnamon Spice as prep	1 serv	110	–	–	–	–	150	–	–
White Tea Antioxidant Plum	1 tea bag	0	0	1000	–	66	–	–	–
Daily Detox									
Original	1 teabag	0	0	–	–	–	–	–	–
Eden									
Organic Bancha Green Tea	1 tea bag	0	0	0	–	0	0	0	0
Organic Hojicha Tea	1 tea bag	0	0	0	–	0	0	0	0
Lipton									
Black Tea as prep	1 teabag	0	0	–	–	–	–	–	25
Black Tea French Vanilla	1 tea bag	0	0	–	–	–	–	–	15
Black Tea Mint	1 tea bag	0	0	–	–	–	–	–	20
Black Tea Orange & Spice	1 tea bag	0	0	–	–	–	–	–	20

FOOD	PORTION	CALS	FIBER	VIT A	FOLIC	VIT C	CALCI	IRON	POTAS
Decaffeinated Black Tea as prep	1 serv	0	0	0	–	0	0	0	20
Earl Grey	1 tea bag	0	0	–	–	–	–	–	20
English Breakfast	1 tea bag	0	0	–	–	–	–	–	25
Green Tea as prep	1 tea bag	0	0	–	–	–	–	–	25
Green Tea Decaffeinated	1 tea bag	0	0	–	–	–	–	–	15
Green Tea Lemon Ginseng	1 tea bag	0	0	–	–	–	–	–	20
Green Tea Mint	1 tea bag	0	0	–	–	–	–	–	15
Low Carb Creations									
Chai as prep	1 cup	25	0	0	–	0	0	tr	–
Oregon									
Chai Latte Cider	½ cup	110	–	0	–	1	0	0	–
Chai Latte Java	½ cup	42	–	0	–	0	0	0	–
Chai Latte Kashmir Green Tea	½ cup	81	–	0	–	0	40	tr	–
Chai Latte Nog	½ cup	90	–	0	–	0	0	0	–
Chai Latte The Original	½ cup	78	–	0	–	0	0	0	–
Pacific Chai									
All Flavors as prep	1 serv	93	0	0	–	0	80	0	–
Tea Tech									
Instant Green Tea All Flavors	1 tube	0	–	–	–	60	–	–	–
XtraGreen Tea Mix All Flavors	1 tube	0	–	–	–	60	–	–	–
Tetley									
British Blend Round Teabags	1 cup	0	0	–	–	–	–	–	31
Decaffeinated Tea Bag as prep	1	0	0	–	–	–	–	–	25
TAKE-OUT									
chai spiced latte decaf	1 cup	130	0	0	–	0	80	0	–
TEMPEH									
tempeh	½ cup	165	–	569	43	0	77	2	305
Lightlife									
Garden Veggie	1 serv (4 oz)	230	10	–	–	–	–	–	340
Organic Flax	1 serv (4 oz)	230	11	–	–	–	–	–	390

FOOD	PORTION	CALS	FIBER	VIT A	FOLIC	VIT C	CALCI	IRON	POTAS
Organic Soy	1 serv (4 oz)	210	10	–	–	–	–	–	240
Organic Three Grain	1 serv (4 oz)	240	8	–	–	–	–	–	290
Organic Wild Rice	1 serv (4 oz)	280	10	–	–	–	–	–	240
Tofurky									
Edamame Veggie	3 oz	145	7	2000	–	0	140	1	–
Five Grain	3 oz	190	6	2500	–	0	80	1	–
Soy	3 oz	160	7	2000	–	0	60	0	–
White Wave									
Five Grain	⅓ block	140	4	0	–	0	20	2	–
Organic Original Soy	⅓ block	150	6	0	–	0	20	2	–
Organic Sea Veggie	⅓ block	120	8	0	–	0	100	3	–
Soy Rice	⅓ block	140	5	0	–	0	20	1	–
THYME									
ground	1 tsp	4	–	53	–	–	26	2	11
TILAPIA									
Beacon Light									
Farm Raised Fillets	3 oz	85	0	0	–	0	110	0	–
TAKE-OUT									
battered & fried	1 filet (4 oz)	206	tr	50	9	2	107	1	302
breaded & fried	1 filet (4 oz)	300	1	120	13	2	138	2	359
broiled	1 filet (3.4 oz)	128	0	185	6	3	90	1	306
TILEFISH									
cooked	½ fillet (5.3 oz)	220	0	–	–	–	39	tr	768
cooked	3 oz	125	0	–	–	–	22	tr	435
raw	3 oz	81	0	–	–	–	22	tr	368
TOFU									
firm	¼ block (3 oz)	118	1	134	24	tr	166	8	192
firm	½ cup	183	2	209	37	tr	258	13	298
fresh fried	1 piece (0.5 oz)	35	tr	0	4	0	48	1	19

FOOD	PORTION	CALS	FIBER	VIT A	FOLIC	VIT C	CALCI	IRON	POTAS
fuyu salted & fermented	1 block (0.3 oz)	13	tr	–	–	–	5	tr	8
koyadofu dried frozen	1 piece (0.5 oz)	82	tr	88	16	tr	62	2	3
okara	½ cup	47	1	0	–	0	49	1	130
regular	¼ block (4 oz)	88	1	99	17	tr	122	6	141
regular	½ cup	94	1	105	19	tr	130	7	150
Azumaya									
Extra Firm	1 serv (2.8 oz)	70	1	0	–	0	150	1	–
Firm	1 serv (2.8 oz)	70	tr	0	–	0	150	1	–
Lite Silken	1 serv (3.2 oz)	40	0	1500	–	0	300	1	–
Lite Extra Firm	1 serv (2.8 oz)	60	1	1500	–	0	300	2	–
Seasoned Oriental Spice	1 serv (3 oz)	90	1	0	–	0	40	1	–
Seasoned Zesty Garlic & Onion	1 serv (3 oz)	90	1	0	–	0	40	1	–
Silken	1 serv (3.2 oz)	40	tr	0	–	0	80	1	160
Eden									
Dried	1 piece (0.4 oz)	50	2	0	–	0	60	tr	5
Nasoya									
Chinese Spice	¼ pkg (3 oz)	90	1	0	–	0	40	1	–
Extra Firm	⅕ pkg (2.8 oz)	80	1	0	–	0	60	1	–
Firm	⅕ pkg (2.8 oz)	70	tr	0	–	0	100	1	–
Garlic & Onion	¼ pkg (3 oz)	90	1	0	–	0	40	1	–
Lite Firm	⅕ pkg (2.8 oz)	40	tr	1500	–	0	300	1	–
Lite Silken	⅕ pkg (3.2 oz)	30	tr	1500	–	0	300	1	–

FOOD	PORTION	CALS	FIBER	VIT A	FOLIC	VIT C	CALCI	IRON	POTAS
Seasoned Ginger Sesame	½ pkg (5.5 oz)	210	2	0	–	0	100	5	–
Seasoned Sweet & Sour	½ pkg (5.5 oz)	190	1	2250	–	0	300	3	–
Seasoned Teriyaki	½ pkg (5.5 oz)	190	2	0	–	0	100	3	–
Seasoned Thai Peanut	½ pkg (5.5 oz)	240	2	0	–	0	100	3	–
Silken	⅕ pkg (3.2 oz)	45	0	0	–	0	60	tr	–
Soft	⅕ pkg (2.8 oz)	60	tr	0	–	0	100	1	–
TofuMate Breakfast Scramble	¼ pkg	15	–	100	–	1	20	tr	–
TofuMate Eggless Salad	¼ pkg	15	–	100	–	0	20	tr	–
TofuMate Mandarin Stirfry	¼ pkg	25	–	0	–	0	60	0	–
TofuMate Mediterranean Herb	¼ pkg	15	–	100	–	4	20	tr	–
TofuMate Szechwan StirFry	¼ pkg	25	–	100	–	1	40	tr	–
TofuMate Texas Taco	¼ pkg	15	0	200	–	0	20	tr	–
Pete's Tofu									
Dessert Peach Mango	1 serv (6 oz)	120	0	–	–	–	40	1	–
Dessert Very Berry	1 serv (6 oz)	120	0	–	–	–	50	1	–
Medium Firm	3 oz	70	0	–	–	–	100	1	–
Soft	3 oz	56	0	–	–	–	20	–	–
Super Firm	3 oz	130	0	–	–	–	100	2	–
Super Firm Italian Herb	3 oz	120	tr	–	–	–	100	2	–
Tofu 2 Go Lemon Pepper	2 pieces + sauce	160	2	–	–	–	300	3	–
Tofu 2 Go Santa Fe	2 pieces + sauce	150	2	–	–	–	300	3	–
Tofu 2 Go Sesame Ginger	2 pieces + sauce	160	2	–	–	–	300	4	–
Tofu 2 Go Thai Tango	2 pieces + sauce	165	2	–	–	–	250	4	–

FOOD	PORTION	CALS	FIBER	VIT A	FOLIC	VIT C	CALCI	IRON	POTAS
Soyafarm									
Baked Tofu	10 pieces (3.5 oz)	147	1	–	–	tr	76	1	300
Nuggets	4 pieces (3.5 oz)	162	1	–	–	3	30	1	110
Tofu & Yuba Patties	1 (3.5 oz)	243	1	–	–	1	44	2	170
White Wave									
Baked Garlic Herb Italian	1 piece	120	1	1250	–	1	40	1	–
Baked Hickory Smoke BBQ	1 piece	75	1	0	–	0	60	1	–
Baked Roma Italian Basil	1 piece	100	2	0	–	0	60	1	–
Baked Teriyaki Oriental	1 piece	120	1	1250	–	1	40	1	–
Baked Thai Style	1 piece	120	1	1250	–	1	40	1	–
Baked Zesty Lemon Pepper	1 piece	120	1	0	–	0	60	1	–
Extra Firm	¼ block	80	1	0	–	0	100	2	–
Organic Extra Firm	⅕ block	90	1	0	–	0	100	2	–
Organic Soft	⅕ block	90	1	0	–	0	100	2	–
Reduced Fat	⅕ block	90	2	0	–	0	40	1	–
TAKE-OUT									
soy sauce marinated & grilled	1 serv (4 oz)	181	1	–	–	–	–	–	–
TOMATILLO									
fresh	1 (1.2 oz)	11	–	39	2	4	2	–	91
fresh chopped	½ cup	21	–	75	4	8	4	–	177
Las Palmas									
Tomatillos Crushed	½ cup	45	2	100	–	12	0	1	–
TOMATO									
CANNED									
paste	½ cup	110	6	3234	–	55	46	4	1221
puree	1 cup	102	6	3402	–	88	37	2	1051
puree w/o salt	1 cup	102	6	3402	–	88	37	2	1051
red whole	½ cup	24	–	725	–	18	32	1	265
sauce	½ cup	37	2	1195	–	16	17	1	452
sauce spanish style	½ cup	40	2	1202	–	11	20	4	576
sauce w/ mushrooms	½ cup	42	–	1165	–	15	16	1	464
sauce w/ onion	½ cup	52	–	1038	–	16	20	1	504

FOOD	PORTION	CALS	FIBER	VIT A	FOLIC	VIT C	CALCI	IRON	POTAS
stewed	½ cup	34	–	710	–	17	47	1	307
w/ green chiles	½ cup	18	–	468	–	8	24	tr	129
wedges in tomato juice	½ cup	34	–	757	–	19	34	1	329
Cento									
Crushed	¼ cup	35	2	400	0	4	0	1	180
Paste	2 tbsp	30	1	500	–	6	0	1	180
Puree	¼ cup	25	1	750	–	9	0	1	–
Contadina									
Crushed w/ Italian Herbs	¼ cup	20	tr	200	–	6	20	tr	–
Italian Paste	2 tbsp	35	1	300	–	6	0	1	–
Italian Paste Roasted Garlic	2 tbsp	35	1	400	–	5	20	1	–
Paste	2 tbsp (1.2 oz)	30	1	500	–	6	0	1	–
Petite Cut Diced	½ cup	25	2	500	–	15	20	tr	–
Puree	¼ cup (2.2 oz)	20	tr	500	–	9	0	tr	–
Stewed	½ cup	35	1	500	–	9	40	1	–
Stewed w/ Celery & Green Peppers	½ cup	35	1	500	–	9	40	1	–
Del Monte									
Chunky Pasta Style	½ cup	45	2	500	–	9	20	tr	–
Diced No Salt Added	½ cup	25	2	500	–	9	20	tr	–
Diced w/ Garlic & Onion	½ cup	40	tr	750	–	9	20	2	–
Diced w/ Green Pepper & Onion	½ cup	40	2	500	–	15	20	tr	–
Diced Zesty Chili Style	½ cup	30	2	500	–	9	20	tr	–
Diced Zesty w/ Mild Green Chilies	½ cup	30	1	750	–	15	20	1	–
Garden Select Petite Diced	½ cup	15	tr	500	–	9	20	tr	–
Organic Diced	½ cup	25	2	500	–	9	20	tr	–
Organic Diced w/ Basil Garlic & Oregano	½ cup	50	tr	750	–	9	80	2	–
Organic Tomato Paste	2 tbsp	30	1	500	–	6	0	1	–
Petite Cut	½ cup	25	2	500	–	9	20	tr	–
Petite Cut Garlic & Olive Oil	½ cup	45	1	750	–	9	20	1	–

FOOD	PORTION	CALS	FIBER	VIT A	FOLIC	VIT C	CALCI	IRON	POTAS
Sauce	¼ cup	20	tr	200	–	5	0	tr	–
Stewed Cajun Recipe	½ cup	35	2	500	–	9	20	tr	–
Stewed Italian Recipe	½ cup	30	2	500	–	9	20	tr	–
Stewed Mexican Recipe	½ cup	35	2	500	–	9	20	tr	–
Stewed No Salt Added	½ cup	35	2	500	–	9	20	tr	–
Stewed Original	½ cup	35	2	500	–	9	20	tr	–
Wedges	½ cup	35	2	500	–	9	20	tr	–
Eden									
Organic Crushed	¼ cup	20	1	750	–	9	20	1	170
Organic Diced	½ cup	30	2	1000	–	18	20	tr	330
Organic Whole Roma	½ cup	30	1	1250	–	21	0	1	260
Hunt's									
Crushed	½ cup	30	2	400	–	12	0	1	400
Diced Original	½ cup	20	tr	300	–	21	40	0	260
Diced w/ Basil Garlic & Oregano	½ cup	25	1	400	–	12	40	tr	530
Diced w/ Green Pepper Celery & Onions	½ cup	45	1	200	–	5	40	1	240
Diced w/ Mild Green Chilies	½ cup	30	2	400	–	9	40	tr	320
Diced w/ Roasted Garlic	½ cup	30	1	300	–	9	40	tr	250
Diced w/ Sweet Onion	½ cup	45	tr	750	–	12	60	1	280
Family Favorites Meatloaf	¼ cup	30	2	200	–	4	0	tr	200
Paste	2 tbsp	25	2	200	–	6	0	tr	–
Paste No Salt Added	2 tbsp	30	2	300	–	4	0	0	–
Paste w/ Basil Garlic & Oregano	2 tbsp	25	2	300	–	5	0	1	–
Petite Diced	½ cup	20	1	300	–	15	40	0	270
Petite Diced w/ Mushrooms	½ cup	40	tr	300	–	9	40	1	–
Puree	½ cup	30	2	400	–	18	60	tr	320
Sauce	¼ cup	15	tr	200	–	5	0	0	–
Sauce Garlic & Herb	½ cup	40	3	300	–	9	20	1	390
Sauce No Salt Added	2 tbsp	30	2	300	–	5	0	0	–
Sauce Roasted Garlic	¼ cup	15	tr	200	–	5	0	0	160
Stewed	½ cup	35	1	300	–	12	60	tr	–
Stewed No Salt Added	½ cup	40	1	300	–	9	40	1	260
Whole No Salt Added	¼ cup	20	1	200	–	6	0	0	150

FOOD	PORTION	CALS	FIBER	VIT A	FOLIC	VIT C	CALCI	IRON	POTAS
Whole No Salt Added	4 oz	20	1	400	–	12	40	0	–
Muir Glen									
Diced Fire Roasted	¼ cup	30	1	500	–	15	20	1	–
Diced w/ Green Chilies	½ cup (4.5 oz)	25	1	500	–	15	0	1	–
Organic Chunky Sauce	¼ cup (2.3 oz)	20	1	500	–	2	0	1	–
Organic Crushed Fire Roasted	¼ cup	20	1	300	–	9	0	tr	–
Organic Diced	½ cup (4.5 oz)	25	1	500	–	15	0	1	–
Organic Diced No Salt Added	½ cup (4.5 oz)	25	1	500	–	15	0	1	–
Organic Diced w/ Basil & Garlic	½ cup (4.5 oz)	25	1	500	–	15	0	1	–
Organic Diced w/ Italian Herbs	½ cup (4.4 oz)	25	1	500	–	15	0	1	–
Organic Ground Peeled	¼ cup (2.3 oz)	10	1	400	–	1	0	tr	–
Organic Paste	2 tbsp (1.2 oz)	30	1	500	–	6	0	1	–
Organic Puree	¼ cup (2.2 oz)	20	1	1000	–	4	0	1	–
Organic Sauce	¼ cup (2.2 oz)	20	1	300	–	2	0	1	–
Organic Sauce No Salt Added	¼ cup (2.2 oz)	20	1	300	–	2	0	1	–
Organic Stewed	½ cup (4.5 oz)	30	tr	200	–	15	40	tr	–
Organic Whole Peeled	½ cup (4.6 oz)	30	1	750	–	15	0	1	–
Whole Peeled w/ Basil	½ cup (4.6 oz)	30	1	750	–	15	0	1	–
Pomi									
Chopped	½ cup	20	3	750	–	15	0	tr	–
Progresso									
Crushed w/ Added Puree	¼ cup (2.1 oz)	20	0	300	–	6	20	1	–
Redpack									
Chunky Style In Puree	½ cup	30	1	500	–	9	0	1	–

FOOD	PORTION	CALS	FIBER	VIT A	FOLIC	VIT C	CALCI	IRON	POTAS
Crushed In Puree	¼ cup	20	1	300	–	6	0	1	–
Diced In Juice	½ cup	25	1	750	–	9	40	1	–
Paste	2 tbsp	0	1	500	–	6	0	1	–
Rienzi									
Paste	2 tbsp	25	1	750	–	15	20	1	–
Ro-Tel									
Diced In Sauce	½ cup	40	tr	1000	–	24	100	1	–
Mexican Festival	½ cup	30	1	400	–	9	20	tr	–
Original	½ cup	20	1	400	–	6	20	tr	–
Tillen Farms									
Sunnyside Tomatoes	3 pieces (1 oz)	40	1	1500	–	0	0	tr	–
Tuttorosso									
Puree	¼ cup	20	1	740	–	5	0	1	–
DRIED									
sun dried	1 piece	5	–	17	1	1	2	–	69
sun dried	1 cup	140	–	472	37	21	60	–	1851
sun dried in oil	1 piece (3 g)	6	–	39	1	3	1	–	47
sun dried in oil	1 cup (4 oz)	235	–	1415	25	112	51	–	1721
Frieda's									
Red Chopped	⅓ cup (1.1 oz)	100	2	1250	–	6	60	1	–
FRESH									
bruschetta	¼ cup	50	tr	800	–	8	0	1	–
cooked	½ cup	32	–	892	16	27	7	1	335
grape tomatoes	20	30	1	750	–	27	0	tr	250
green	1	30	–	789	–	29	16	1	251
red	1 (4.5 oz)	26	2	766	18	24	6	1	273
red chopped	1 cup	35	2	2039	17	32	12	1	372
Chiquita									
Tomato	1 med (5.2 oz)	35	1	1000	–	24	0	tr	–
Earthbound Farm									
Organic Roma	1 med (5.2 oz)	35	1	1000	–	24	20	tr	–
Eurofresh									
Tomatoes On The Vine	1 med (5.2 oz)	35	1	1000	–	24	20	tr	–

FOOD	PORTION	CALS	FIBER	VIT A	FOLIC	VIT C	CALCI	IRON	POTAS
Foxy									
Roma	1 med (5 oz)	35	1	1000	–	24	20	tr	–
Frieda's									
Baby Roma	⅔ cup (3 oz)	120	1	500	–	15	0	tr	–
Tear Drop	⅔ cup (3 oz)	20	1	500	–	15	0	tr	–
TAKE-OUT									
bruschetta on toasted italian bread	1 slice	106	tr	400	–	4	23	1	–
stewed	1 cup	80	–	673	11	18	27	1	249
TOMATO JUICE									
beef broth & tomato	1 can (5.5 oz)	62	tr	215	7	2	18	1	161
clam & tomato	1 can (5.5 oz)	77	–	357	–	7	21	1	149
tomato juice	6 oz	32	–	1012	36	33	16	1	400
tomato juice	½ cup	21	–	678	24	22	10	1	268
Campbell's									
Juice	8 oz	50	2	500	–	60	20	tr	430
Del Monte									
Juice	8 oz	50	1	1750	–	60	40	2	–
Kagome									
Sweet Summer	8 oz	50	1	200	–	30	20	tr	340
Luvli Juices									
Smashing Tomato	1 bottle (10 oz)	125	4	5000	–	60	40	1	870
Spicy Tomato	1 bottle (10 oz)	125	4	5000	–	60	40	1	870
Muir Glen									
Organic	5.5 oz	40	4	200	–	14	20	1	–
TONGUE									
beef simmered	3 oz	241	0	0	6	1	4	2	156
lamb braised	3 oz	234	0	0	3	6	9	2	134
pork braised	3 oz	230	0	0	3	1	16	4	201
veal braised	3 oz	172	0	0	8	5	8	2	138

FOOD	PORTION	CALS	FIBER	VIT A	FOLIC	VIT C	CALCI	IRON	POTAS
TORTILLA									
corn	1 (6 in diam)	56	1	–	4	0	44	tr	39
corn w/o salt	1 (6 in diam)	56	1	–	4	0	44	tr	39
flour w/o salt	1 (8 in diam)	114	1	0	4	0	44	1	46
Alvarado Street Bakery									
Sprouted Wheat Burrito Size	1 (2.2 oz)	170	1	0	–	0	0	1	–
CarbOle									
Low-Carb	1 (2 oz)	100	9	0	–	0	20	5	–
Food For Life									
Sprouted Corn	2 (1.7 oz)	120	4	100	–	0	100	1	–
La Tortilla Factory									
Low Carb Whole Wheat	1 lg	100	15	–	–	–	–	–	–
Low Carb Whole Wheat	1 reg	60	9	–	–	–	–	–	–
Manny's									
Burrito Tortilla	1 (2.1 oz)	180	4	–	–	–	60	2	–
Fajita Tortilla	1 (2 oz)	170	4	–	–	–	40	2	–
Fat Free	1 (1 oz)	65	1	–	–	–	20	1	–
Low Carb	1 (1.7 oz)	140	6	–	–	–	150	1	–
Soft Taco Tortilla	1 (1 oz)	80	tr	–	–	–	20	1	–
Tortilla Wrap Tomato Basil	1 (1.4 oz)	100	2	0	–	0	20	1	–
White Corn Gluten Free	1 (2 oz)	60	tr	–	–	–	20	–	–
Whole Wheat	1 (2 oz)	170	3	–	–	–	40	2	–
Super Bakery									
Organic	1 (2.5 oz)	210	13	0	–	0	50	3	–
Tumaro's									
Low In Carb Garden Vegetable	1 (8 in)	130	10	100	–	0	100	1	–
Low In Carb Green Onion	1 (8 in)	130	11	0	–	0	100	1	–
Low In Carb Multi-grain	1 (8 in)	146	12	0	–	0	150	1	–
Low In Carb Salsa	1 (8 in)	130	12	100	–	0	100	1	–

FOOD	PORTION	CALS	FIBER	VIT A	FOLIC	VIT C	CALCI	IRON	POTAS
TREE FERN									
chopped cooked	½ cup	28	–	142	–	21	6	tr	3
TRIPE									
beef simmered	3 oz	80	0	0	3	0	69	1	36
TAKE-OUT									
mondongo w/ potatoes	1 cup	300	6	615	84	49	123	3	781
TRITICALE									
dry	½ cup (3.4 oz)	323	–	0	70	0	36	2	319
TROUT									
baked	3 oz	162	0	54	13	tr	47	2	393
rainbow cooked	3 oz	129	0	63	–	3	73	2	539
sea trout baked	3 oz	113	0	–	–	–	19	tr	372
TRUFFLES									
fresh	0.5 oz	4	2	–	–	–	12	2	263
TUNA									
CANNED									
light in oil	3 oz	169	0	66	5	–	11	1	176
light in oil	1 can (6 oz)	399	0	134	9	–	23	2	354
light in water	3 oz	99	0	47	3	0	10	1	202
light in water	1 can (5.8 oz)	192	0	92	6	0	19	3	391
white in oil	1 can (6.2 oz)	331	0	–	8	–	8	1	593
white in oil	3 oz	158	0	–	4	–	4	1	283
white in water	3 oz	116	0	–	4	–	–	1	241
white in water	1 can (6 oz)	234	0	–	7	–	–	1	487
Bumble Bee									
Chunk Light In Water	2 oz	60	0	0	–	0	0	tr	–
Chunk Light Touch Of Lemon In Water	¼ cup	60	0	0	–	0	0	tr	–
Chunk Light In Oil	¼ cup	110	0	0	–	0	0	tr	–
Chunk White In Water	¼ cup	60	0	0	–	0	0	0	–
Chunk White In Oil	¼ cup	100	0	0	–	0	0	0	–
Chunk White In Water Very Low Sodium	¼ cup	70	0	0	–	0	0	0	–

FOOD	PORTION	CALS	FIBER	VIT A	FOLIC	VIT C	CALCI	IRON	POTAS
Light In Oil	¼ cup	110	0	0	–	0	0	tr	–
Solid White In Oil	¼ cup	90	0	0	–	0	0	0	–
Solid White In Water	2 oz	70	0	0	–	0	0	0	–
Tonno In Olive Oil	¼ cup	120	0	0	–	0	0	tr	–
Chicken Of The Sea									
Albacore Solid In Water	2 oz	70	0	0	–	0	0	0	–
Chunk Light In Oil	2 oz	110	0	0	–	0	0	tr	–
Chunk Light In Water	¼ cup (2 oz)	60	0	0	–	0	0	tr	–
Chunk White Low Sodium In Spring Water	1 can (3 oz)	80	0	0	–	0	0	tr	–
Chunk White In Spring Water	½ can	60	0	0	–	0	0	0	–
Premium Albacore Pouch	2 oz	60	0	0	–	0	0	0	–
Coral									
Light In Water	¼ cup	60	0	0	–	0	0	tr	–
StarKist									
Chunk Light In Water	¼ cup (2 oz)	60	0	0	–	0	0	tr	–
Solid White Albacore In Water	¼ cup	70	0	0	–	0	0	0	–
Tuna Fillet In Spring Water	¼ cup (2 oz)	60	0	0	–	0	0	0	–
FRESH									
bluefin cooked	3 oz	157	0	2142	–	–	–	1	275
bluefin raw	3 oz	122	0	1856	–	–	–	1	214
skipjack baked	3 oz	112	0	51	–	–	32	1	444
yellowfin baked	3 oz	118	0	58	–	–	17	1	–
MIX									
Chicken Of The Sea									
Salad Kit	1 serv (3.5 oz)	380	1	0	–	0	60	1	–
Tuna Salad Kit Single Mayo & Onion	1 pkg	380	1	0	–	0	60	0	–
SHELF-STABLE									
Bumble Bee									
Steak Entrees Ginger & Soy	1 pkg (4 oz)	170	0	0	–	0	0	1	–

FOOD	PORTION	CALS	FIBER	VIT A	FOLIC	VIT C	CALCI	IRON	POTAS
Steak Entrees Lemon & Cracked Pepper	1 pkg (4 oz)	160	0	0	–	0	0	0	–
Steak Entrees Mesquite Grilled	1 pkg (4 oz)	150	0	0	–	0	0	tr	–

TAKE-OUT

tuna salad	1 cup	383	–	199	15	5	35	2	365

TURBOT

european baked	3 oz	104	0	34	–	–	20	–	259

TURKEY
CANNED

w/ broth	½ can (2.5 oz)	116	0	0	–	1	9	1	–

Valley Fresh

Chunk White	2 oz	80	0	0	–	0	0	0	–

FRESH

back w/ skin roasted	½ back (9 oz)	637	0	0	21	0	87	6	682
breast w/ skin roasted	4 oz	212	0	0	7	0	24	2	323
dark meat w/ skin roasted	3.6 oz	230	0	0	9	0	34	2	285
dark meat w/o skin roasted	1 cup (5 oz)	262	0	0	13	0	45	3	406
dark meat w/o skin roasted	3 oz	170	0	0	9	0	19	2	264
ground cooked	3 oz	188	0	0	5	0	21	2	222
leg w/ skin roasted	2.5 oz	147	0	0	6	0	23	2	199
leg w/ skin roasted	1 (1.2 lbs)	1133	0	0	49	0	176	13	1530
light meat w/ skin roasted	from ½ turkey (2.3 lbs)	2069	0	0	61	0	225	15	2996
light meat w/ skin roasted	4.7 oz	268	0	0	8	0	29	2	388
light meat w/o skin roasted	4 oz	183	0	0	7	0	23	2	356
neck simmered	1 (5.3 oz)	274	0	0	12	0	56	3	226
skin roasted	1 oz	141	0	0	1	0	11	1	51
skin roasted	from ½ turkey (9 oz)	1096	0	0	10	0	87	4	396

FOOD	PORTION	CALS	FIBER	VIT A	FOLIC	VIT C	CALCI	IRON	POTAS
w/ skin roasted	8.4 oz	498	0	0	17	0	63	4	673
w/ skin roasted	½ turkey (4 lbs)	3857	0	0	130	0	488	33	5207
w/ skin neck & giblets roasted	½ turkey (8.8 lbs)	4123	–	4631	409	1	525	40	5473
w/o skin roasted	7.3 oz	354	0	0	16	0	52	4	621
w/o skin roasted	1 cup (5 oz)	238	0	0	10	0	35	2	418
wing w/ skin roasted	1 (6.5 oz)	426	0	0	10	0	44	3	494
Jennie-O									
Ground	4 oz	160	0	100	–	–	40	1	–
Perdue									
Burger Cooked	1 (4 oz)	160	0	–	–	–	60	1	–
Dark Cooked	3 oz	180	0	–	–	–	40	1	–
Drumsticks Cooked	1 (2.2 oz)	110	0	–	–	–	–	1	–
Ground Cooked	3 oz	160	0	–	–	–	–	1	–
Thighs Cooked	1 (3.2 oz)	240	0	100	–	–	–	1	–
White Cooked	3 oz	150	0	–	–	–	0	1	–
Shady Brook									
Tenderloins Turkey Breast Homestyle	4 oz	130	0	0	–	1	20	1	–
FROZEN									
roast boneless seasoned light & dark meat roasted	1 pkg (1.7 lbs)	1213	–	–	–	–	40	13	2332
Jennie-O									
Burger	1 (4 oz)	160	0	100	–	2	60	1	–
READY-TO-EAT									
bologna	1 slice (1 oz)	59	tr	9	3	4	34	1	38
breast	1 slice (0.75 oz)	23	0	0	–	0	1	tr	58
diced light & dark seasoned	1 oz	39	–	–	–	–	0	1	88
prebasted breast w/ skin roasted	1 breast (3.8 lbs)	2175	0	0	–	0	149	11	4281
prebasted breast w/ skin roasted	½ breast (1.9 lbs)	1087	0	0	–	0	75	6	2141
prebasted thigh w/ skin roasted	1 thigh (11 oz)	494	0	0	–	–	25	5	758

FOOD	PORTION	CALS	FIBER	VIT A	FOLIC	VIT C	CALCI	IRON	POTAS
roll light & dark meat	1 oz	42	–	–	–	–	9	tr	77
roll light meat	1 oz	42	–	–	–	–	11	tr	71
salami cooked beef	1 slice (0.9 oz)	67	0	0	1	0	21	1	49
turkey loaf breast meat	1 pkg (6 oz)	187	0	0	–	0	12	1	473
turkey loaf breast meat	2 slices (1.5 oz)	47	0	0	–	0	3	tr	118
turkey salad sandwich spread	¼ cup	104	0	72	3	1	5	tr	95
turkey sticks battered & fried	1 stick (2.3 oz)	178	–	–	–	–	9	1	166
Boar's Head									
Breast 50% Lower Sodium Skin On	2 oz	60	0	0	–	0	0	tr	–
Breast Cracked Pepper Smoked	2 oz	60	0	0	–	0	0	tr	–
Breast Hickory Smoked Black Forest	2 oz	60	0	0	–	0	0	tr	–
Breast Maple Glazed Honey Coat	2 oz	70	0	0	–	0	0	tr	–
Breast Ovengold	2 oz	60	0	0	–	0	0	tr	–
Breast Ovengold Skinless	2 oz	60	0	0	–	0	0	tr	–
Breast Roasted Mesquite Smoked Skinless	2 oz	60	0	0	–	0	0	tr	–
Breast Roasted Salsalito	2 oz	60	0	0	–	0	0	tr	–
Healthy Choice									
Smoked Breast	4 slices (1.8 oz)	60	0	0	–	0	0	0	–
Hebrew National									
98% Fat Free Oven Roasted	5 slices (2 oz)	50	–	–	–	–	0	tr	–
98% Fat Free Smoked Breast	5 slices (2 oz)	60	0	–	–	–	0	tr	–
Oscar Mayer									
Lunchables Turkey Bagels	1 pkg	420	2	300	–	60	250	3	–
Smoked Turkey Breast	2 oz	60	0	–	–	–	–	tr	–

FOOD	PORTION	CALS	FIBER	VIT A	FOLIC	VIT C	CALCI	IRON	POTAS
Turkey Bologna	3 slices (3 oz)	160	–	–	–	–	100	1	–
Turkey Cotto Salami	3 slices (3 oz)	130	–	–	–	–	20	1	–
Perdue									
Breast Sliced Pan Roasted	2 oz	70	0	–	–	–	–	–	–
Sara Lee									
Breast Cracked Pepper	2 oz	50	0	0	–	1	0	tr	–
Breast Honey Roasted	2 slices (1.6 oz)	50	0	0	–	6	0	1	–
Shady Brook									
Turkey Ham Smoked	2 oz	60	0	–	–	–	–	–	–

TURKEY DISHES
FROZEN

FOOD	PORTION	CALS	FIBER	VIT A	FOLIC	VIT C	CALCI	IRON	POTAS
gravy & turkey	1 pkg (5 oz)	95	–	59	–	–	20	1	–
gravy & turkey	1 cup (8.4 oz)	160	–	100	–	–	33	2	–
READY-TO-EAT									
Jennie-O									
Stuffed Breast Cheddar Cheese & Broccoli	1 serv (6 oz)	240	0	200	–	9	150	1	–
Stuffed Turkey Breast Pepper Cheese & Rice	1 piece (6 oz)	250	0	100	–	1	150	1	–
Turkey Breast Roast In Homestyle Gravy	1 serv (5 oz)	110	0	0	–	1	20	tr	–
Mosey's									
Turkey Breast w/ Gravy	1 serv (5 oz)	140	0	0	–	1	20	2	–
TAKE-OUT									
boneless breast w/ cranberry apple stuffing	1 serv (5 oz)	260	1	0	–	1	30	1	–
turkey meatloaf	1 lg slice (5 oz)	243	1	230	29	5	73	2	312

FOOD	PORTION	CALS	FIBER	VIT A	FOLIC	VIT C	CALCI	IRON	POTAS

TURKEY SUBSTITUTES
Lightlife
| Smart Deli Roast Turkey | 4 slices (2 oz) | 80 | 1 | – | – | – | – | – | 160 |

Tofurky
Deli Slices Cranberry	3 slices (1.8 oz)	98	3	0	–	0	20	1	–
Deli Slices Hickory Smoked	3 slices (1.8 oz)	100	3	0	–	0	20	1	–
Deli Slices Italian	3 slices (1.8 oz)	103	4	0	–	0	20	1	–
Deli Slices Original	3 slices (1.8 oz)	103	3	0	–	0	20	1	–
Deli Slices Peppered	3 slices (1.8 oz)	103	3	0	–	0	20	1	–
Deli Slices Philly Steak	3 slices (1.8 oz)	110	3	0	–	0	20	1	–
Roast	1 serv (4 oz)	190	2	0	–	0	150	1	–

Worthington
| Turkee Slices | 3 slices (3.3 oz) | 180 | 0 | 0 | – | 0 | 100 | 4 | 50 |

TURMERIC
| ground | 1 tsp | 8 | – | – | – | 1 | 4 | 1 | 56 |

TURNIPS
canned greens	½ cup	17	–	4196	48	18	138	2	165
cooked mashed	½ cup (4.2 oz)	47	–	674	19	23	58	1	391
cubed cooked	½ cup (3 oz)	33	–	477	13	17	41	tr	277
frzn greens cooked	½ cup	24	2	6540	32	18	125	2	184
greens chopped cooked	½ cup	15	2	3959	85	20	99	1	146
greens raw chopped	½ cup	7	1	2128	54	17	53	tr	83
raw cubed	½ cup (2.4 oz)	25	–	406	14	18	39	tr	236

Allens
| Green Seasoned Southern Style | ½ cup | 30 | 2 | 2250 | – | 4 | 80 | 1 | 240 |

FOOD	PORTION	CALS	FIBER	VIT A	FOLIC	VIT C	CALCI	IRON	POTAS
Glory									
Greens Fresh	2 cups	20	3	6000	–	48	150	1	–
Greens Seasoned canned	½ cup	35	2	4500	–	18	80	1	–
Root Cut Fresh	½ cup	20	1	0	–	15	20	tr	–
Sensibly Seasoned Greens	½ cup	20	2	5500	–	18	100	1	–
TURTLE									
raw	3.5 oz	85	0	–	–	–	107	2	235
TUSK FISH									
raw	3.5 oz	79	0	–	tr	–	17	–	328
VANILLA									
vanilla extract	1 tsp	17	0	–	–	–	–	–	–
VEAL									
breast braised	3 oz	226	0	–	11	–	8	1	231
chop cooked	1 med (6.5 oz)	230	0	0	16	0	20	1	345
chop breaded fried	1 med (6.5 oz)	290	tr	65	34	0	50	2	471
cubed braised	3 oz	160	0	0	14	0	25	1	291
cutlet cooked	3 oz	141	0	0	12	0	5	1	342
ground broiled	3 oz	146	0	0	9	0	14	1	286
leg roasted	3 oz	136	0	0	14	0	5	1	331
loin roasted	3 oz	184	0	0	13	0	16	1	276
patty breaded fried	1 (2.8 oz)	211	tr	6	16	0	31	1	224
shank braised	3 oz	162	0	–	14	–	28	1	259
VEAL DISHES									
TAKE-OUT									
cordon bleu	1 serv (8 oz)	490	1	905	25	4	153	1	497
parmigiana	1 serv (6.4 oz)	362	2	345	31	4	187	2	515
scallopini	1 slice + sauce (3.4 oz)	238	tr	510	12	1	44	1	250
stew	1 serv (8.8 oz)	192	3	605	35	12	40	2	547

FOOD	PORTION	CALS	FIBER	VIT A	FOLIC	VIT C	CALCI	IRON	POTAS
veal marengo	1 serv (8.8 oz)	274	1	565	30	9	23	2	733
veal marsala	1 slice + sauce (3.4 oz)	268	tr	375	12	2	15	1	211
veal paprikash	1 serv (8.6 oz)	280	1	445	27	2	37	2	689
veal picatta	1 piece + sauce (3.5 oz)	154	tr	335	11	tr	8	1	195

VEGETABLE JUICE

FOOD	PORTION	CALS	FIBER	VIT A	FOLIC	VIT C	CALCI	IRON	POTAS
vegetable juice cocktail	6 fl oz	34	–	2130	–	50	20	1	351
vegetable juice cocktail	½ cup	22	–	1416	–	34	13	1	234
Bolthouse Farms									
Vedge Tomato Carrot Celery	8 oz	60	2	7250	–	42	40	1	640
Muir Glen									
Organic	5.5 oz	50	2	6500	–	48	80	1	–
V8									
Lemon Twist	1 bottle (12 oz)	70	3	3000	–	60	40	1	700

VEGETABLES MIXED
CANNED

FOOD	PORTION	CALS	FIBER	VIT A	FOLIC	VIT C	CALCI	IRON	POTAS
mixed vegetables	½ cup	39	–	9551	19	4	22	1	239
peas & carrots	½ cup	48	–	7386	24	8	29	1	128
peas & carrots low sodium	½ cup	48	–	7386	24	8	29	1	128
peas & onions	½ cup	30	–	96	–	2	10	1	57
succotash	½ cup	102	–	187	59	9	15	1	243
Del Monte									
Mixed	½ cup	40	2	2250	–	2	20	1	–
Mixed Vegetables w/ Potatoes	½ cup	45	2	5500	–	6	40	1	–
Peas & Carrots	½ cup	60	2	5000	–	4	20	1	–
Savory Sides Homestyle Vegetable Medley	½ cup	70	2	2000	–	5	40	tr	–
Savory Sides Rio Grande Vegetables	½ cup	70	2	400	–	6	20	1	–

FOOD	PORTION	CALS	FIBER	VIT A	FOLIC	VIT C	CALCI	IRON	POTAS
S&W									
Mixed	½ cup (4.4 oz)	35	2	4500	–	4	20	1	–
Peas & Carrots	½ cup (4.5 oz)	60	2	5000	–	4	20	1	–
Veg-All									
Cajun Mixed	½ cup	50	3	1500	–	1	20	1	–
Original Mixed	½ cup	40	2	6500	–	5	20	1	170
FRESH									
Mann's									
California Stir Fry	1 serv (3 oz)	30	2	7000	32	42	40	1	–
River Ranch									
Broccoli & Carrots	1 cup	25	2	6500	40	48	40	1	–
Broccoli & Cauliflower	1 cup	25	2	1500	60	66	40	1	–
Stir Fry Blend	1 cup	30	2	5000	40	54	40	1	–
Vegetable Medley	1 cup	25	2	8000	40	48	20	tr	–
FROZEN									
mixed vegetables cooked	½ cup	54	2	3892	17	3	22	1	154
peas & carrots cooked	½ cup	38	–	6209	21	7	18	1	127
peas & onions cooked	½ cup	40	–	313	–	6	13	1	–
succotash cooked	½ cup	79	–	196	28	5	13	1	225
Birds Eye									
Broccoli & Cauliflower	1 cup	30	2	0	–	30	20	tr	–
Italian Herb Harvest Vegetables	1¼ cups	90	2	300	–	30	40	1	–
Spring Vegetables In Citrus Sauce	1¼ cups	70	2	1750	–	12	40	1	–
Steamfresh Asian Medley	1 cup	50	2	750	–	15	40	tr	–
Steamfresh Broccoli Cauliflower & Carrots	¾ cup	30	2	750	–	18	20	tr	–
Steamfresh Broccoli Carrots Sugar Snap Peas & Water Chestnuts	¾ cup	35	2	750	–	15	20	tr	–

FOOD	PORTION	CALS	FIBER	VIT A	FOLIC	VIT C	CALCI	IRON	POTAS
Steamfresh Mixed Vegetables	⅔ cup	40	2	1250	–	5	20	tr	–
C&W									
Early Harvest Peas & Baby Carrots	⅔ cup	60	3	1500	–	5	20	1	–
Petite Peas & Pearl Onions	⅔ cup	60	3	300	–	6	20	1	–
Europe's Best									
Zen Garden	¾ cup	60	3	2500	–	18	20	1	–
Fresh Like									
California Blend	3.5 oz	31	1	6797	–	40	38	1	206
Midwestern Blend	3.5 oz	42	1	5388	–	32	33	1	224
Mixed	3.5 oz	69	1	5199	–	10	24	1	212
Oriental Blend	3.5 oz	26	1	1362	–	55	43	1	214
Winter Blend	3.5 oz	26	1	1362	–	55	43	1	214
Green Giant									
Alfredo Vegetables	¾ cup	70	2	1500	–	12	80	tr	–
Cheese Sauce Broccoli Cauliflower Carrots	1 cup (4.1 oz)	60	2	2000	–	18	40	0	–
Seasoned Broccoli & Carrots w/ Garlic & Herbs	½ cup	45	3	2500	–	30	40	tr	–
Lean Cuisine									
Cafe Classics Roasted Potatoes w/ Broccoli & Cheddar Cheese Sauce	1 pkg (10.25 oz)	230	5	400	–	27	250	1	830
McKenzie's									
Gumbo Mixture	1 serv (2.9 oz)	35	2	–	–	–	–	–	–
Okra Tomatoes w/ Onions	1 serv (2.8 oz)	20	2	–	–	–	–	–	–
Melrose Made Gourmet									
Vegetable Souffle Fat Free	1 serv (4 oz)	70	3	3500	–	24	80	1	–
Pictsweet									
Peas & Carrots	⅔ cup	50	3	1250	–	3	20	tr	–

FOOD	PORTION	CALS	FIBER	VIT A	FOLIC	VIT C	CALCI	IRON	POTAS
Roast Works									
Flame Roasted Redskins & Vegetables	1 serv (3 oz)	90	3	200	–	6	100	1	–
SHELF-STABLE									
TastyBite									
Curry Bangkok Red	½ pkg (5.3 oz)	88	1	150	–	0	60	1	–
Curry Patong Yellow	½ pkg (5.3 oz)	118	1	0	–	0	40	1	–
Curry Siam Green	½ pkg (5.3 oz)	63	1	0	–	0	40	1	–
Jaipur Vegetables	½ pkg (5 oz)	220	7	0	–	0	90	1	–
Malabar Mixed	½ pkg (5 oz)	67	1	25	–	8	120	5	–
TAKE-OUT									
buddha's delight	1 serv (16 oz)	174	3	1790	161	64	109	2	668
caponata	¼ cup	28	–	–	–	–	16	–	–
curry	1 serv (7.7 oz)	398	–	7845	–	26	86	2	–
gyoza potstickers vegetable	8 (4.9 oz)	210	5	500	–	0	40	3	–
pakoras	1 (2 oz)	108	3	390	–	3	56	2	–
ratatouille	1 serv (3.5 oz)	96	4	0	36	50	32	1	468
samosa	2 (4 oz)	170	3	500	–	0	20	1	–
succotash	½ cup	111	–	282	–	8	16	1	393
tapenade grilled vegetables	¼ cup	40	tr	800	–	19	0	tr	–
VENISON									
roasted	4 oz	215	0	0	12	0	7	6	353
VINEGAR									
balsamic	1 tbsp	14	–	0	–	0	4	tr	18
cider	1 tbsp	3	0	0	0	0	1	tr	11
white	1 tbsp	3	0	0	0	0	1	0	0
Carapelli									
Balsamic	1 tbsp	15	0	0	–	0	0	0	–

FOOD	PORTION	CALS	FIBER	VIT A	FOLIC	VIT C	CALCI	IRON	POTAS
Red Wine	1 tbsp	5	0	0	–	0	0	0	–
White Wine	1 tbsp	5	0	0	–	0	0	0	–
Eden									
Organic Apple Cider	1 tbsp	0	0	0	–	0	0	0	–
Latino Chef									
Lulo	1 tbsp	35	–	400	–	4	80	–	–
Passion Fruit	1 tbsp	40	tr	–	–	2	–	–	–
Spectrum									
Apple Cider Organic	1 tbsp	7	0	0	–	0	0	0	0
Balsamic Organic	1 tbsp	6	0	0	–	0	0	0	0
Brown Rice Organic	1 tbsp	10	0	0	–	0	0	0	0
White Organic	1 tbsp	2	0	0	–	0	0	0	0

WAFFLES

FROZEN

FOOD	PORTION	CALS	FIBER	VIT A	FOLIC	VIT C	CALCI	IRON	POTAS
buttermilk	1 (4 in sq)	88	1	448	17	0	77	1	43
plain	1 (4 in sq)	88	1	448	17	0	77	1	43
Eggo									
Buttermilk	2	180	1	1000	40	0	100	4	60
Homestyle	2	190	1	1000	40	0	100	4	90
Homestyle Minis	12	250	1	1500	60	0	100	5	130
Nutri-Grain Low Fat Whole Wheat	2	140	3	1000	32	0	100	4	140
Special K	3	190	1	1500	60	0	150	5	190
Waf-Fulls Strawberry	1	150	tr	1000	32	0	100	4	60
EnviroKidz									
Organic Gorilla Banana	2 (2.7 oz)	230	2	0	–	0	20	1	–
Kashi									
Heart To Heart Honey Oat	2 (3 oz)	160	3	1250	400	30	60	2	120
Van's									
Belgian 7 Grain	2	230	7	100	–	0	170	3	–
Belgian Blueberry	2	184	2	0	–	0	200	2	–
Belgian Original	2	172	2	0	–	0	250	2	–
Carb Manager Flax	2	200	6	0	–	0	150	2	–
Carb Manager Homestyle	2	200	6	0	–	0	150	1	–
Gourmet 97% Fat Free	2	230	4	0	–	1	20	1	–
Gourmet Blueberry	2	190	5	50	–	0	130	2	–
Gourmet Buckwheat	2	145	2	0	–	0	250	2	–
Gourmet Flax	2	157	2	0	–	0	200	2	–

FOOD	PORTION	CALS	FIBER	VIT A	FOLIC	VIT C	CALCI	IRON	POTAS
Gourmet Multi Grain	2	260	6	0	–	36	100	2	–
Gourmet Original	2	180	5	50	–	0	130	2	–
Hearty Oat Berry Boost	2	200	4	0	–	0	200	2	–
Hearty Oat Maple Fusion	2	210	4	0	–	0	200	2	–
Hearty Oat Oats 'N Honey	2	200	4	0	–	0	200	2	–
Mini Blueberry	4	110	2	0	–	0	200	2	–
Mini Chocolate Chip	4	119	2	0	–	0	200	2	–
Mini Homestyle	4	116	2	0	–	0	250	2	–
Organic Blueberry	2	240	4	0	–	1	80	1	–
Organic Original	2	190	6	0	–	0	100	2	–
Organic Soy Flax	2	230	6	0	–	1	80	1	–
Wheat Free Blueberry	2	201	5	0	–	0	90	2	–
Wheat Free Cinnamon Apple	2	189	5	0	–	0	90	2	–
Wheat Free Flax	2	230	5	0	–	0	90	2	–
Wheat Free Mini	4	160	tr	0	–	0	150	tr	–
Wheat Free Original	2	189	5	0	–	0	90	2	–
MIX									
plain as prep	1 (7 in diam)	218	1	68	9	tr	93	1	134
READY-TO-EAT									
Kashi									
GoLean Blueberry	2 (3 oz)	170	6	0	–	0	60	1	130
GoLean Original	2 (3 oz)	170	6	0	–	0	60	1	130
Thomas'									
Homestyle	1 (1.6 oz)	140	tr	1000	40	0	300	4	–
TAKE-OUT									
plain	1 (7 in diam)	218	–	140	–	tr	191	2	119
WALNUTS									
black dried chopped	1 cup	759	–	370	–	–	72	4	655
english dried	1 oz	182	1	35	19	1	27	1	142
english dried chopped	1 cup	770	6	148	79	4	113	3	602
halves	14 (1 oz)	190	2	–	24	–	40	1	130
Emerald									
Glazed	¼ cup	140	1	0	–	0	20	tr	65
Good Sense									
Organic Raw Walnuts	¼ cup	210	3	0	–	0	20	1	–

FOOD	PORTION	CALS	FIBER	VIT A	FOLIC	VIT C	CALCI	IRON	POTAS
Sweet Delights									
Walnut Roasters	⅓ pkg (1 oz)	210	2	–		–	–	–	–
WATER									
ice cubes	3	0	0	0	0	0	1	tr	0
tap water	8 oz	0	0	0	0	0	5	tr	0
Absopure									
Natural Spring	8 oz	0	0	–		–	20	–	
Aloe Splash									
All Flavors	8 oz	0	0	–		15	–	–	–
Aquafina									
Essentials Daily C Citrus	8 oz	40	–	–		24	–	–	
Essentials Multi-V Watermelon	8 oz	40	–	–		6	–	–	
Blu Italy									
Sparkling Lemon	8 oz	0	0	–		–	20	–	
Calabria									
Mineral	8 oz	0	0	–		–	0	–	–
Castellina									
Sparkling Spring	8 oz	0	0	–		–	14	–	tr
Dasani									
Purified Water	8 oz	0	0	–		0	0	–	1
w/ Raspberry	8 oz	1	0	–		0	0	–	30
Evamor									
Artesian Water	8 oz	0	0	–		–	–	–	3
Evian									
Spring Water	1 bottle (11.5 oz)	0	0	–		–	20	–	–
Ferrarelle									
Sparkling	8 oz	0	1	–		–	90	–	–
Fiji									
Natural Artesian	1 bottle (16.9 oz)	0	0	–		–	9	–	–
Fruit 2 0									
Natural Berry	8 oz	0	0	–		6	–	–	–
Watermelon Kiwi	8 oz	0	0	–		6	–	–	–
Gerolsteiner									
Sparkling Mineral	8 oz	0	0	–		–	80	–	–
Glaceau Vitamin Water									
Balance Cran Grapefruit	8 oz	50	–	500	–	24	>20	–	–

FOOD	PORTION	CALS	FIBER	VIT A	FOLIC	VIT C	CALCI	IRON	POTAS
Defense	8 oz	50	–	–	–	36	–	–	–
Endurance Peach Mango	8 oz	50	–	500	–	36	–	–	–
Energy Tropical Citrus	8 oz	40	–	1250	–	60	–	–	–
Essential Orange Orange	8 oz	40	–	2500	–	15	20	1	50
Focus Kiwi Strawberry	8 oz	40	–	1250	–	60	–	–	–
Formula 50	8 oz	50	–	–	80	12	–	–	–
Multi-V Lemonade	8 oz	40	–	5000	–	60	20	–	–
Perform Lemon Lime	8 oz	50	–	–	–	24	100	–	100
Power-C Dragonfruit	8 oz	40	–	1250	–	150	–	–	–
Rescue Green Tea	8 oz	40	–	–	–	60	–	–	–
Revive Fruit Punch	8 oz	50	–	500	–	36	–	–	30
Stress-B Lemon Lime	8 oz	40	–	–	–	36	–	–	–
H2Odwalla									
Organic Enhanced Strawberry Kiwi	1 bottle (20 oz)	120	–	–	–	42	–	–	–
Iceland Spring									
Spring Water	1 liter	0	0	–	–	–	5	tr	1
Liquid Salvation									
Ultra Hydrating	1 bottle	0	0	0	–	0	–	0	–
Multi Vitamin Enhanced Water									
All Flavors	8 oz	50	–	750	–	30	–	–	50
No Carb All Flavors	8 oz	0	0	750	–	30	–	–	50
Nui									
All Natural Kid Water	10 oz	90	3	500	–	60	250	–	190
Paradiso									
Slightly Sparkling	8 oz	0	0	–	–	–	10	–	–
Pellegrino									
Mineral Water	8 oz	0	0	–	–	–	40	–	–
Pink2O									
Fortified	1 bottle (20 oz)	0	0	–	252	15	250	–	88
Propel									
Fitness Water All Flavors	1 bottle (23.7 oz)	30	–	–	–	–	300	–	–
Reebok									
Fitness Water Berry	1 bottle (24 oz)	30	0	0	100	0	50	0	70

FOOD	PORTION	CALS	FIBER	VIT A	FOLIC	VIT C	CALCI	IRON	POTAS
Fitness Water Natural	1 bottle (24 oz)	0	0	0	100	0	50	0	70
San Benedetto									
Natural Mineral Water	1 liter	0	0	–	–	–	46	–	1
Sanfaustino									
Mineral	8 oz	0	0	–	–	–	100	–	–
SoBe									
All Flavors	8 oz	50	–	–	–	60	–	–	–
Spa									
Mineral Water Reine	1 bottle (17.5 oz)	0	0	–	–	–	3	–	tr
Special K2O									
Protein Water All Flavors	1 bottle (16.6 oz)	50	–	–	–	–	100	–	–
Speedo Sportswater									
All Flavors	8 oz	10	–	–	100	15	–	–	35
Stacker 2									
Protein Water All Flavors	1 bottle (19.44 oz)	80	0	–	–	–	105	–	90
Sulinka									
Sparkling Mineral	8 oz	0	0	0	–	0	65	0	–
TalkingRain									
Ice All Flavors	8 oz	5	0	0	–	30	0	0	–
Thorpedo									
Ultra Low GI Energy Water	8 oz	45	0	–	80	–	–	–	30
Tipperary									
Mineral Water	1 liter	0	0	–	–	–	37	–	17
Trinity									
Energize	8 oz	50	–	–	–	6	–	–	–
Multi-Essential	8 oz	50	–	1000	–	6	40	–	–
Revive	8 oz	50	–	–	–	6	–	–	–
Strength	8 oz	50	–	–	–	60	–	–	–
Think	8 oz	50	–	1000	–	6	–	–	–
Ty Nant									
Mineral Water	1 liter	0	0	–	–	–	23	tr	1
VitaZest									
All Flavors	8 oz	0	0	250	–	30	20	–	–
Vittel									
Mineral Water	1 bottle	0	0	–	–	–	202	–	1

FOOD	PORTION	CALS	FIBER	VIT A	FOLIC	VIT C	CALCI	IRON	POTAS
Volvic	(18 oz)								
Mineral Water	1 liter	0	0	–	–	–	12	–	6
Voss									
Artesian	8 oz	0	0	–	–	–	1	–	0
W20 For Women									
All Flavors	8 oz	40	0	–	200	30	50	1	–
WaterPlus									
Antioxidants Acai Berry	8 oz	50	–	500	–	–	–	–	–
Electrolytes Fruit Punch	8 oz	50	–	–	–	–	40	–	–
Extra-C Orange Tangerine	8 oz	50	0	–	–	60	–	–	–
Vitamins Dragonfruit Kiwi	8 oz	50	–	500	–	–	–	–	–
Wild Waters									
All Flavors	8 oz	50	–	750	–	60	100	0	40

WATER CHESTNUTS

FOOD	PORTION	CALS	FIBER	VIT A	FOLIC	VIT C	CALCI	IRON	POTAS
chinese sliced canned	½ cup	35	–	3	–	1	3	1	82
fresh sliced	½ cup	66	–	0	–	3	7	tr	362

WATERCRESS

FOOD	PORTION	CALS	FIBER	VIT A	FOLIC	VIT C	CALCI	IRON	POTAS
fresh chopped	½ cup	2	tr	799	–	7	20	tr	56
garden fresh	½ cup	8	–	2325	–	17	20	tr	152
garden fresh cooked	½ cup	16	–	5236	–	16	41	1	240
Frieda's									
Watercress	1 cup	10	2	4000	–	36	100	0	–

WATERMELON

FOOD	PORTION	CALS	FIBER	VIT A	FOLIC	VIT C	CALCI	IRON	POTAS
cut up	1 cup	46	1	876	5	13	11	tr	172
seeds dried	¼ cup	150	–	0	16	0	15	2	175
wedge	1 lg (20 oz)	172	2	800	17	46	40	1	641
wedge	1 med (10 oz)	86	1	400	9	23	20	1	320
wedge	1 sm (2.5 oz)	21	tr	100	2	6	5	tr	80
whole melon	1 (9 lb)	1227	16	5770	123	331	286	10	4581
Dulcinea									
Fresh Mini Seedless	2 cups	88	2	1000	–	15	20	1	–
Frieda's									
Yellow Seedless	½ cup (3 oz)	25	0	300	–	9	0	0	–

FOOD	PORTION	CALS	FIBER	VIT A	FOLIC	VIT C	CALCI	IRON	POTAS
Sundia									
Fresh	2 cups	80	2	1000	–	15	20	1	230
WATERMELON JUICE									
juice	8 oz	71	1	335	7	19	17	1	267
Sundia									
100% Natural	8 oz	110	1	500	–	15	20	tr	360
WHALE									
raw	3.5 oz	134	0	120	–	–	12	4	300
WHEAT									
sprouted	1 cup (3.8 oz)	214	1	0	41	3	30	2	183
starch	3.5 oz	348	–	–	–	0	0	0	16
Bob's Red Mill									
Vital Wheat Gluten	¼ cup	120	0	–	–	–	–	–	–
Hodgson Mill									
Vital Wheat Gluten	4 tsp	40	1	0	–	32	0	0	–
Near East									
Pilaf Mix Wheat as prep	1 cup	220	9	100	–	0	20	1	–
Taboule Salad Mix as prep	⅔ cup	110	5	300	–	9	0	1	–
WHEAT GERM									
plain	¼ cup	108	4	5	99	2	13	3	267
Hodgson Mill									
Untoasted	2 tbsp	55	4	0	40	0	0	1	40
Kretschmer									
Original Toasted	2 tbsp	50	2	–	–	–	–	1	–
Mother's									
Toasted	2 tbsp	50	2	–	80	–	–	1	–
WHEY									
acid dry	1 tbsp	10	0	2	1	0	60	tr	66
sweet dry	1 tbsp	26	0	2	1	tr	60	tr	156
sweet fluid	½ cup	33	0	15	1	tr	58	tr	198
whey cheese	1 oz	126	0	356	–	tr	97	tr	–
Wellements									
Whey Protein Chocolate	1 scoop (1 oz)	120	0	–	–	–	–	–	170
Whey Protein Vanilla	1 scoop (1 oz)	120	0	–	–	–	–	–	170

FOOD	PORTION	CALS	FIBER	VIT A	FOLIC	VIT C	CALCI	IRON	POTAS
WHIPPED TOPPINGS									
cream pressurized	1 tbsp (3 g)	8	–	27	–	0	3	tr	4
cream pressurized	1 cup (2.1 oz)	154	–	548	–	0	61	tr	88
nondairy frzn	1 tbsp	13	–	34	0	0	tr	tr	1
nondairy pressurized	1 tbsp (4 g)	11	–	19	0	0	tr	tr	1
nondairy pressurized	1 cup	184	–	331	0	0	4	tr	13
Cabot									
Whipped Cream	2 tbsp	15	0	0	–	0	0	0	–
Hood									
Light Sugar Free Whipped Cream	2 tbsp	10	0	0	–	0	0	0	–
Whipped Light Cream	2 tbsp	20	0	0	–	0	0	0	–
Reddiwip									
Extra Creamy	2 tbsp	15	0	100	–	–	–	–	–
Soyatoo									
Soy Whip	2 tbsp	10	0	0	–	0	0	0	–
WHITE BEANS									
canned	1 cup	306	–	0	171	0	191	8	1189
dried regular cooked	1 cup	249	–	0	145	0	161	7	1003
dried small cooked	1 cup	253	–	0	245	0	131	5	828
WHITEFISH									
baked	3 oz	146	0	–	–	–	–	tr	345
smoked	3 oz	92	0	162	6	–	15	tr	360
smoked	1 oz	39	0	53	2	–	5	tr	118
WHITING									
cooked	3 oz	98	0	97	13	–	53	tr	369
hake raw	3.5 oz	84	0	–	–	–	41	–	294
raw	3 oz	77	0	84	11	–	41	tr	212
WILD RICE									
cooked	1 cup (5.7 oz)	166	3	0	43	0	5	1	166
Gourmet House									
Cracked not prep	¼ cup	170	2	100	–	0	20	1	120
Hand Harvested not prep	¼ cup	170	2	100	–	0	20	1	120

FOOD	PORTION	CALS	FIBER	VIT A	FOLIC	VIT C	CALCI	IRON	POTAS
Quick Cooking not prep	½ cup	170	2	50	–	0	20	1	120
White & Wild not prep	¼ cup	170	1	0	–	0	20	1	90
Wild & Rice Garden Blend not prep	¼ cup	190	1	1500	–	5	60	1	120
Lundberg									
Organic Quick not prep	¼ cup	150	2	0	–	0	0	tr	–

WINE

FOOD	PORTION	CALS	FIBER	VIT A	FOLIC	VIT C	CALCI	IRON	POTAS
cooking	1 oz	15	0	0	tr	0	3	tr	26
dessert dry	1 glass (4 oz)	179	0	0	0	0	9	tr	109
haiku	1 serv	93	0	–	–	–	3	tr	17
japanese plum	3 oz	139	0	–	–	0	1	tr	–
japanese sake	1 oz	33	0	0	–	0	1	–	1
kir	1 serv	78	0	–	tr	–	8	tr	71
madeira	3.5 oz	169	0	0	–	–	8	1	–
port	3.5 oz	156	0	0	–	0	4	tr	–
red	1 glass (4 oz)	85	0	0	2	0	9	1	132
rose	1 glass (4 oz)	84	0	0	1	0	9	tr	117
sake screwdriver	1 serv	175	tr	372	56	93	24	tr	389
sangria	1 serv	88	tr	23	5	7	7	tr	95
sangria blanco	1 serv	155	3	110	23	27	70	2	267
sweet dessert	1 glass (4 oz)	189	0	0	0	0	9	tr	109
wassail wine	1 serv	142	2	61	17	23	50	2	190
white	1 glass (4 oz)	80	0	0	0	0	11	tr	94
wine cooler	1 serv	218	0	272	8	23	20	1	276
wine spritzer	1 serv	60	0	–	tr	–	9	tr	71

WINGED BEANS

FOOD	PORTION	CALS	FIBER	VIT A	FOLIC	VIT C	CALCI	IRON	POTAS
dried cooked	1 cup	252	–	0	18	0	244	7	481

XANTHAN GUM
Bob's Red Mill

FOOD	PORTION	CALS	FIBER	VIT A	FOLIC	VIT C	CALCI	IRON	POTAS
Xanthan Gum	1 tbsp	8	8	–	–	–	–	–	–

FOOD	PORTION	CALS	FIBER	VIT A	FOLIC	VIT C	CALCI	IRON	POTAS
YAM									
CANNED									
Bruce's									
In Syrup	⅔ cup	150	3	14000	–	18	20	1	–
Glory									
Candied	½ cup	210	1	14000	–	9	40	tr	–
S&W									
Candied	½ cup (4.9 oz)	170	4	2000	–	5	20	1	210
FRESH									
mountain yam hawaii cooked	½ cup	59	–	0	–	0	6	tr	356
yam cubed cooked	½ cup	79	–	0	11	8	9	tr	455
Earthbound Farm									
Organic	1 med (4.6 oz)	130	4	22000	–	18	20	tr	–
Frieda's									
Name	¾ cup	100	3	0	–	15	0	tr	–
YARDLONG BEANS									
sliced cooked w/o salt	1 cup	49	–	488	47	17	46	1	302
YEAST									
baker's compressed	1 cake (0.6 oz)	18	1	0	133	0	3	1	102
baker's dry	1 pkg (7 g)	21	2	0	164	0	4	1	140
baker's dry	1 tbsp	35	3	0	281	0	8	2	240
brewer's dry	1 tbsp	35	3	0	281	0	8	2	240
Hodgson Mill									
Active Dry	1 tsp	30	1	0	–	0	0	tr	–
Fast Rise	1 tsp (9 g)	25	1	0	–	0	0	tr	–
YELLOW BEANS									
fresh cooked w/o salt	1 cup	44	4	101	41	12	58	2	374
fresh raw	1 cup	34	4	119	41	18	41	1	230
Del Monte									
Wax Beans	½ cup	20	2	0	–	4	20	tr	–
S&W									
Wax Beans Cut	½ cup (4.2 oz)	20	2	0	–	4	20	tr	–

FOOD	PORTION	CALS	FIBER	VIT A	FOLIC	VIT C	CALCI	IRON	POTAS
YELLOWTAIL									
baked	4 oz	199	0	110	4	3	31	1	572
YOGURT									
plain low fat	8 oz	143	0	116	25	2	415	tr	531
plain nonfat	8 oz	127	0	16	27	2	452	tr	579
plain whole milk	8 oz	138	0	225	16	1	275	tr	352
tofu yogurt	1 cup	246	1	86	16	7	309	3	123
Axelrod									
Fat Free Lemon	1 pkg (6 oz)	90	0	0	–	0	200	0	–
Fat Free Raspberry	6 oz	90	0	0	–	0	200	0	–
Fat Free Vanilla	1 pkg (6 oz)	90	0	0	–	0	200	0	–
Breyers									
Vanilla 98% Fat Free	½ cup	90	4	200	–	0	80	0	–
Cabot									
Non Fat	8 oz	100	0	1000	–	12	300	0	–
Non Fat Berry Banana	8 oz	130	0	1000	–	12	250	0	–
Non Fat Blueberry	8 oz	130	0	1000	–	12	250	0	–
Non Fat French Vanilla	8 oz	130	0	1000	–	12	250	0	–
Non Fat Lemon	8 oz	130	0	1000	–	12	250	0	–
Non Fat Raspberry	8 oz	130	0	1000	–	12	250	0	–
Non Fat Very Berry	8 oz	130	0	1000	–	12	250	0	–
Colombo									
Fat Free Plain	8 oz	100	0	–	–	–	300	0	440
Fat Free Vanilla	8 oz	160	0	–	–	–	250	–	410
French Vanilla	8 oz	180	0	–	–	–	250	–	370
Fruit On The Bottom Strawberry Banana	8 oz	230	0	0	–	–	200	–	330
Lowfat Plain	8 oz	130	0	–	–	–	300	–	440
Multipack Blended All Flavors	4 oz	110	0	500	–	0	100	0	190
Strawberry	8 oz	190	–	–	–	–	250	–	–
Dannon									
Activia Blueberry	1 pkg (4 oz)	110	0	0	–	0	150	0	210
Activia Mixed Berry	1 pkg (4 oz)	110	0	0	0	0	200	0	220
Activia Peach	1 pkg (4 oz)	110	0	0	–	0	150	0	230
Activia Prune	1 pkg (4 oz)	110	0	100	0	0	150	0	230

FOOD	PORTION	CALS	FIBER	VIT A	FOLIC	VIT C	CALCI	IRON	POTAS
Activia Strawberry	1 pkg (4 oz)	110	0	0	0	0	150	0	220
Activia Vanilla	1 pkg (4 oz)	110	0	0	0	0	150	0	230
All Natural 99% Fat Free Cherry	1 (4 oz)	110	0	0	–	0	150	0	210
Creamy Fruit Blends Raspberry	6 oz	170	tr	–	–	–	150	–	–
La Creme Strawberry	1 pkg (4 oz)	140	–	200	–	–	150	–	240
La Creme Vanilla	1 pkg (4 oz)	140	–	200	–	–	150	–	240
Light 'N Fit Vanilla	6 oz	90	–	300	–	–	150	–	–
Light 'N Fit w/ Fiber Blueberry	4 oz	70	3	400	–	0	100	0	160
Fage									
Sheep & Goat's Milk	1 pkg (7 oz)	190	0	500	–	0	350	0	–
Horizon Organic									
Fat Free Peach	1 pkg (6 oz)	140	1	0	–	2	250	0	–
Fat Free Vanilla	1 cup	180	0	0	–	1	300	0	–
Kids Strawberry	1 pkg (4 oz)	110	1	0	–	1	150	0	–
Lowfat Blended Blueberry	1 pkg (6 oz)	160	2	100	–	1	250	0	–
Tube Lowfat Blueberry	1 (2 oz)	70	0	0	–	0	80	0	–
Whole Milk Plain	1 cup	160	0	300	–	2	350	0	–
LeCarb									
YoCarb Plain	1 pkg (4 oz)	50	–	–	–	–	100	–	–
Redwood Hill Farm									
Goat Milk Apricot Mango	1 cup	180	2	227	–	tr	214	–	–
Goat Milk Cranberry Orange	1 cup	180	2	227	–	tr	214	–	–
Goat Milk Plain	1 cup	130	1	238	–	tr	225	–	–
Goat Milk Strawberry	1 cup	180	2	227	–	tr	214	–	–
Goat Milk Vanilla	1 cup	190	2	230	–	tr	214	–	–

FOOD	PORTION	CALS	FIBER	VIT A	FOLIC	VIT C	CALCI	IRON	POTAS
Silk									
Organic Soy Strawberry	1 pkg (6 oz)	160	1	0	–	3	500	0	–
Soy Apricot Mango	1 pkg	160	1	400	–	2	500	0	–
Soy Banana Strawberry	1 pkg	160	1	0	–	1	500	0	–
Soy Black Cherry	1 pkg	160	1	50	–	0	500	0	–
Soy Blueberry	1 pkg	160	1	0	–	0	500	0	–
Soy Key Lime	1 pkg	170	1	0	–	0	500	0	–
Soy Lemon	1 pkg	160	1	0	–	0	500	0	–
Soy Lemon Kiwi	1 pkg	150	1	0	–	6	500	0	–
Soy Peach	1 pkg	170	1	100	–	0	500	0	–
Soy Plain	8 oz	120	1	50	–	0	700	1	–
Soy Raspberry	1 pkg	160	1	0	–	0	500	0	–
Soy Vanilla	1 pkg (8 oz)	120	1	50	–	0	500	1	–
Spega									
La Natura Low Fat	1 pkg (5.2 oz)	80	0	0	–	0	200	tr	–
Stonyfield Farm									
Kids' Lowfat BaNilla	1 pkg (4 oz)	110	2	0	–	0	200	0	230
Light Black Cherry	1 pkg (6 oz)	100	3	100	–	0	250	0	–
Light Blueberry	1 pkg (4 oz)	100	3	0	–	0	250	0	–
Light Peach	1 pkg (6 oz)	100	3	0	–	0	250	0	–
Light Strawberry	1 pkg (4 oz)	100	3	0	–	0	250	0	–
Nonfat French Vanilla	1 pkg	90	2	0	–	0	200	0	240
Nonfat Strawberry	1 pkg	140	2	0	–	0	300	0	350
O'Soy Chocolate	1 pkg (6 oz)	160	4	100	–	0	100	1	10
O'Soy Peach	1 pkg (4 oz)	100	3	0	–	0	100	1	5
Squeezers Lowfat Strawberry	1 tube (2 oz)	60	tr	0	–	0	100	0	115
Whole Milk French Vanilla	1 pkg (6 oz)	190	3	200	–	0	250	0	330

FOOD	PORTION	CALS	FIBER	VIT A	FOLIC	VIT C	CALCI	IRON	POTAS
Total									
Greek Yogurt 0% Fat	1 pkg (5.3 oz)	80	0	0	–	0	100	0	–
Greek Yogurt 2% Fat	1 pkg (7 oz)	130	0	100	–	0	150	0	–
Greek Yogurt Classic	1 pkg (7 oz)	180	0	750	–	0	150	0	–
Greek Yogurt Light	1 pkg (5.3 oz)	130	0	200	–	0	100	0	–
Honey	1 pkg (3.5 oz)	250	0	500	–	0	100	0	–
Wallaby									
Organic Banana Vanilla	1 pkg (6 oz)	150	0	100	–	0	250	1	–
Organic Lemon	1 pkg (6 oz)	150	0	100	–	2	250	1	–
Organic Maple	1 pkg (6 oz)	150	0	100	–	1	250	1	–
Organic Nonfat Mango Lime	1 pkg (6 oz)	140	0	500	–	5	300	1	–
Organic Nonfat Plain	1 cup	130	0	0	–	0	500	tr	–
Organic Nonfat Vanilla Bean	1 pkg (6 oz)	140	0	0	–	0	250	1	–
Organic Plain	1 cup	150	0	200	–	0	350	tr	–
Organic Raspberry	1 pkg (6 oz)	150	0	100	–	2	250	1	–
Organic Vanilla	1 pkg (6 oz)	150	0	100	–	0	250	1	–
WholeSoy & Co.									
Organic Soy Apricot Mango	1 pkg (6 oz)	160	2	500	–	6	300	4	–
Organic Soy Lemon	1 pkg (6 oz)	160	2	0	–	1	300	1	–
Organic Soy Plain	1 pkg (6 oz)	150	2	0	–	0	300	1	–
Organic Soy Raspberry	1 pkg (6 oz)	170	2	0	–	0	300	1	–
Organic Soy Vanilla	1 pkg (6 oz)	150	2	0	–	0	300	1	–

FOOD	PORTION	CALS	FIBER	VIT A	FOLIC	VIT C	CALCI	IRON	POTAS
Yoplait									
Go-Gurt All Fruit Flavors	1 pkg (2.25 oz)	80	0	0	–	0	100	0	110
Grande 99% Fat Free All Flavors	1 cup	250	0	1000	–	0	250	0	390
Grande Fat Free Plain	1 cup	90	0	0	–	0	400	0	550
Kids Banana Vanilla	1 pkg (4 oz)	100	1	500	–	0	200	0	220
Kids Strawberry Vanilla	1 pkg (4 oz)	100	1	500	–	0	200	0	220
Light All Fruit Flavors	1 pkg (6 oz)	180	0	750	–	0	200	0	250
Light All Indulgent Flavors	1 pkg (6 oz)	110	0	–	–	–	–	–	270
Light Thick & Creamy All Fruit Flavors	1 pkg (6 oz)	100	–	750	–	–	200	–	260
Original All Fruit Flavors	1 pkg (6 oz)	170	0	750	–	0	200	0	260
Original Coconut Cream	1 pkg (6 oz)	190	0	750	–	0	200	0	260
Original Lemon Burst	1 pkg (6 oz)	180	0	750	–	0	200	0	250
Original Pina Colada	1 pkg (6 oz)	170	0	750	–	0	200	0	250
Trix All Fruit Flavors	1 pkg (4 oz)	120	0	500	–	0	100	0	170

YOGURT DRINKS
Dannon

FOOD	PORTION	CALS	FIBER	VIT A	FOLIC	VIT C	CALCI	IRON	POTAS
DanActive	1 bottle (3.5 oz)	90	–	–	–	–	100	–	–
Frusion Smoothie Peach Passion Fruit	1 bottle (10 oz)	270	0	200	–	1	250	0	430
Frusion Smoothie Tropical Fruit	1 bottle (10 oz)	270	0	200	–	4	250	0	430
Stonyfield Farm									
Kids' Juice Smoothie Orange Strawberry Banana Wave	1 bottle (6 oz)	160	2	100	–	60	200	0	320
Smoothie Light Strawberry	1 bottle (10 oz)	130	3	100	–	0	250	0	240

FOOD	PORTION	CALS	FIBER	VIT A	FOLIC	VIT C	CALCI	IRON	POTAS
Smoothie Lowfat Strawberry	1 bottle (10 oz)	250	4	200	–	0	400	0	510
Yo-Goat									
Blueberry	8 oz	150	–	300	–	2	287	0	–
Yoplait									
Nouriche All Fruit Flavors	1 bottle (11 oz)	260	5	1250	100	15	300	3	440

YOGURT FROZEN

FOOD	PORTION	CALS	FIBER	VIT A	FOLIC	VIT C	CALCI	IRON	POTAS
chocolate soft serve	1 cup	230	3	230	16	tr	212	2	376
vanilla soft serve	1 cup	236	0	305	9	1	206	tr	304
Breyers									
Chocolate	½ cup	150	tr	100	–	0	100	tr	–
Vanilla	½ cup	140	0	100	–	0	100	0	–
Vanilla No Sugar Added	½ cup	100	0	100	–	0	100	0	–
Dannon									
Light 'N Fit w/ Fiber Strawberry	4 oz	70	3	400	–	1	100	0	170
Edy's									
Vanilla Chocolate Swirl	½ cup	90	–	–	–	–	100	–	–
Haagen-Dazs									
Lowfat Dulce De Leche	½ cup	190	0	0	–	0	200	1	–
Nonfat Chocolate	½ cup	140	tr	0	–	0	200	1	–
Nonfat Coffee	½ cup	140	0	0	–	0	200	0	–
Nonfat Strawberry	½ cup	140	0	0	–	6	150	0	–
Nonfat Vanilla	½ cup	140	0	0	–	0	200	0	–
Nonfat Vanilla Fudge	½ cup	160	0	0	–	0	150	0	–
Nonfat Vanilla Raspberry Swirl	½ cup	130	tr	0	–	1	100	0	–
Hood									
Fat Free Old Fashioned Vanilla	½ cup	110	tr	200	–	0	100	0	–
Fat Free Strawberry	½ cup	100	tr	200	–	2	100	0	–
Vanilla Swiss Almond	½ cup	150	tr	0	–	0	80	0	–
Turkey Hill									
Chocolate Chip Cookie Dough	½ cup	140	0	100	–	0	100	0	–
Fat Free Chocolate Cherry Cordial	½ cup	100	0	0	–	0	100	0	–
Fat Free Chocolate Marshmallow	½ cup	130	0	0	–	0	80	0	–

FOOD	PORTION	CALS	FIBER	VIT A	FOLIC	VIT C	CALCI	IRON	POTAS
Fat Free Mint Cookie 'N Cream	½ cup	110	0	0	–	0	100	0	–
Fat Free Neapolitan	½ cup	100	0	0	–	0	100	0	–
Fat Free Vanilla Fudge	½ cup	110	0	0	–	0	100	0	–
Peach Raspberry	½ cup	110	0	100	–	0	100	0	–
Tin Roof Sundae	½ cup	140	0	100	–	0	100	0	–
Vanilla & Chocolate	½ cup	110	0	100	–	0	100	0	–
Vanilla Bean	½ cup	110	0	100	–	0	100	0	–
WholeSoy & Co.									
Organic All Flavors	½ cup	120	1	0	–	2	40	tr	–

ZUCCHINI

FOOD	PORTION	CALS	FIBER	VIT A	FOLIC	VIT C	CALCI	IRON	POTAS
baby raw	1 (0.5 oz)	3	tr	78	3	6	3	tr	73
canned italian style	1 cup	66	–	1224	68	5	39	2	622
fresh	1 sm (4.1 oz)	19	1	236	34	20	18	tr	309
pickled	¼ cup	16	1	30	8	8	7	tr	88
raw sliced	1 cup	19	1	226	33	19	17	tr	296
sliced cooked w/o salt	1 cup	29	3	2011	31	8	23	1	455
C&W									
Yellow & Green	⅔ cup	20	tr	100	–	0	20	0	–
Frieda's									
Baby	⅔ cup (3 oz)	20	0	400	–	30	0	1	–
TAKE-OUT									
breaded & fried	6 slices (3 oz)	141	1	50	19	7	20	1	157
indian pakora	1 serv	46	2	–	–	–	–	–	–
sticks breaded & fried	6 (2 oz)	90	1	55	15	5	14	tr	107

INDEX

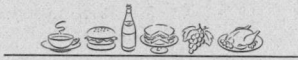

(T) = table